1 8⁵⁵

99BB

PREVENTABLE BRAIN DAMAGE

Brain Vulnerability and
Brain Health

Donald I. Templer, PhD, professor of psychology at California School of Professional Psychology—Fresno, received his doctorate in clinical psychology from the University of Kentucky in 1967. He has contributed to more than 100 publications, most often writing in the areas of neuropsychology, schizophrenia, and death. He has over 1000 citations to his credit, with one of his earlier articles being declared a citation classic by *Current Contents* in 1984. Templer is an author of six assessment instruments. His Death Anxiety Scale has been translated into many languages and used on all six continents. A synthesis of this research is found in the 1986 Lonetto and Templer book *Death Anxiety*. He is a fellow of the American Psychological Association and the American Psychological Society.

Lawrence C. Hartlage, PhD, directs the Augusta Neuropsychology Center in Augusta, GA, and consults to the courts and to rehabilitation hospitals concerning head injuries and their sequelae. He has served as president of the National Academy of Neuropsychology, and of the American Psychological Association division of neuropsychology. His academic appointments have included professor of neurology at the Medical College of Georgia and at Indiana University Medical Center, and Marie Wilson Howell visiting scholar at the University of Arkansas. He has edited the *International Journal of Clinical Neuropsychology*, *Clinical Neuropsychology*, and *Neuropsychology and Special Education*, and served as consulting editor to *Archives of Clinical Neuropsychology*, *International Journal of Psychophysiology*, and the *Journal of Consulting and Clinical Psychology*.

W. Gary Cannon, PhD, received his doctorate in Clinical Psychology from Brigham Young University after completing a neuropsychological rotation at the Veteran's Administration Hospital neuropsychology laboratory in Salt Lake City, Utah. After completing a postdoctoral fellowship with the Devereux Foundation, and teaching at the University of California Santa Barbara, he joined the faculty of the California School of Professional Psychology—Fresno in 1977, where he taught introductory and advanced neuropsychology to clinical psychology graduate students. He became the Provost of CSPP—Fresno in 1982 and continues to be interested in neuropsychological issues.

PREVENTABLE BRAIN DAMAGE

Brain Vulnerability
and
Brain Health

Donald I. Templer
Lawrence C. Hartlage
W. Gary Cannon
Editors

Springer Publishing Company
New York

Springer Publishing Company, Inc.
536 Broadway
New York, NY 10012-3955

92 93 94 95 96 / 5 4 3 2 1

Library of Congress Cataloging-in-Publication Data

Preventable brain damage / [edited by] Donald I. Templer, Lawrence C.
  Hartlage, W. Gary Cannon.
     p.   cm.
  Includes bibliographical references and index.
  ISBN 0-8261-7400-0
  1. Brain damage—Prevention.   I. Templer, Donald I.
II. Hartlage, Lawrence C.   III. Cannon, W. Gary.
  [DNLM: 1. Brain Injuries—etiology.   2. Brain Injuries—prevention
& control.   WL 354 P944]
RC387.5.P74   1991
617.4'8044—dc20
DNLM/DLC
for Library of Congress   91-4816
                                                               CIP

Printed in the United States of America

CONTENTS

Contributors   vii

Introduction   ix

Part I: Impact Damage

1. Brain Injury from Motor Vehicle Accidents   3
   Lawrence C. Hartlage and Gurmal Rattan

2. Contact Sports   15
   Richard H. Drew and Donald I. Templer

3. Noncontact Sports   30
   Donald I. Templer and Richard H. Drew

4. Accidental Injuries of Children   41
   William G. Miller and Frank D. Miller

5. Brain Impairment and Family Violence   58
   Robert Geffner and Alan Rosenbaum

6. Assault   72
   Donald I. Templer

7. Psychosurgery   80
   W. Gary Cannon and Donald I. Templer

8. ECT and Permanent Brain Damage   95
   Donald I. Templer

Part II: Chemical Damage

9. Industrial Toxins   111
   Paula K. Lundberg-Love

10. Agricultural and Domestic Neurotoxic Substances   132
      Raymond Singer

11. Neuropsychology of Alcohol-Induced Brain Damage: 146
      Current Perspectives on Diagnosis, Recovery,
      and Prevention
      Ralph H. B. Benedict and Arthur MacNeil Horton, Jr.

12. Neurological and Neuropsychological Consequences   161
      of Drug Abuse
      Michael W. Lilliquist and Erin D. Bigler

13. Neuropsychological Consequences of Malnutrition   193
      *Rik Carl D'Amato, Mary Mathai Chittooran,
      and Janice D. Whitten*

14. Conclusion: Strategies for Prevention   214
      *Donald I. Templer, Lawrence C. Hartlage,
      and W. Gary Cannon*

Index   225

CONTRIBUTORS

Ralph H. B. Benedict, PhD
Department of Psychiatry
University of Maryland Medical School
Baltimore, Maryland

Erin D. Bigler, PhD
Department of Psychology
Brigham Young University, Provo, Utah

Mary Mathai Chittooran, PhD
Department of Educational Psychology
Mississippi State University
Mississippi State, Mississippi

Rik Carl D'Amato, PhD
Division of Professional Psychology
University of Northern Colorado
Greeley, Colorado

Richard H. Drew, PhD
Private practice
Valley Neuropsychological Services
Sacramento, CA

Robert Geffner, PhD
Family Violence, Research, and Treatment
  Program
Family Violence Department
University of Texas at Tyler
Tyler, Texas

**Arthur MacNeil Horton, Jr., EdD, ABPP
  (CL), ABPN, ABBP (BT)**
National Institute on Drug Abuse
Department of Psychiatry
University of Maryland Medical School
College Park, Maryland

Michael W. Lilliquist, PhD
Department of Psychology
University of Texas at Austin
Austin, Texas

Paula K. Lundberg-Love, PhD
Department of Psychiatry
University of Texas at Tyler
Tyler, Texas

Frank D. Miller, PhD
University of Oklahoma Health Science
  Center
Department of Psychiatry and Behavioral
  Sciences
Children's Hospital of Oklahoma
Oklahoma City, Oklahoma

William G. Miller, PhD
Department of Psychology
Western Maryland College
Westminster, Maryland

Gurmal Rattan, PhD
Indiana University of Pennsylvania
Educational Psychology Department
Indiana, Pennsylvania

Alan Rosenbaum, PhD
University of Massachusetts Medical
  School
Department of Psychiatry
Worcester, Massachusetts

Raymond Singer, PhD
Mt. Sinai School of Medicine
New York, New York

Janice D. Whitten, PhD
Department of Educational Psychology
Mississippi State University
Mississippi State, Mississippi

INTRODUCTION

The 1990s have been designated the "Decade of the Brain." Ninety percent of what we know about the brain has been learned in the last 10 years (Moses, 1989). Brain scanning and other developments have brought us much closer to understanding various types of brain anomalies and their consequences. Literature has ensured on various types of brain injury due to causes as diverse as agriculture, industry, transportation, and sport-related activities and accidents. Interestingly, there has not been a corresponding literature on the prevention of brain injury, although many other aspects of health (e.g., cardiovascular and orthopedic) have witnessed a large public focus in prevention.

The prevention of human brain damage assumes striking importance in the context of recent evidence in seven different but related realms.

1. Many minor blows to the head once regarded as inconsequential now must be viewed as producing consequential long-term and even permanent effects.

2. Many minor blows, such as one observes in boxing, produce cumulative effects.

3. Brain injury makes people highly vulnerable to catastrophic effects produced by a subsequent blow to the head.

4. There is a progression of brain damage that continues long after the trauma, for example, atrophy following a brain injury.

5. There is increasing evidence that a variety of drugs taken during pregnancy produce brain pathology in the fetus and neuropsychological deficits that manifest themselves later in the child's life.

6. Brain damage has an epidemiology.

7. Brain disorder causes "functional" psychiatric disorder.

MINOR HEAD BLOWS

Assault to the brain has traditionally been divided into three types: concussions, contusions, and lacerations. With contusions, bruising occurs and in lacerations the brain tissue tears. Concussions have traditionally been regarded as producing functional rather than structural changes. The "postconcussion syndrome" consists of memory difficulty, concentration difficulty, headache, irritability, anxiety, dizziness, weakness, and depression, months and years after the concussion. This syndrome tended to be regarded as having a heavy psychological component, and in many cases leads to litigation or workmen's compensation. However, accumulating evidence suggests that such assumptions may not be warranted (Rimel, Giodani, Barth, Boll, & Jane, 1981; Rutherford, Merrett, & McDonald, 1979).

Mild brain damage in children may justify even more concern than in adults because of the interference with subsequent neuronal development and concomitant academic proficiency, intellectual development, and interpersonal adjustment (Boll, 1983; Gulbrandsen, 1984; Hartlage, 1990).

Margaret Kennard (1936) reported that cortical lesions in infant monkeys seemed to have a less severe effect on behavior than similar lesions had on adult monkeys' behavior. These findings led to the postulation of the Kennard principle that the earlier that one suffers brain damage, the less severe the behavioral loss. More recent research (Kolb, 1989) suggests that this principle operates only in a very limited way and that behavioral loss is dependent on age or neurodevelopmental phase of the organism at the time of the lesion (there are apparently various developmental windows of vulnerability), type of behavioral assessment employed, the sex of the organism, environmental experiences, size of the brain lesions, and level of endogenous cortical norepinephrine.

Early experimental work with animals has long been consistent with the contention that structural change does take place with concussive blows. The research of Windle and Groat (1945) found that blows of sufficient strength to produce transient loss of the corneal reflex and interruption of respiration in guinea pigs produced disorganization and fragmentation of the Nissl-body pattern and chromatolysis to the point of cytoplasm losing all stainable substance.

The many-faceted vulnerability of the brain may be further illustrated by the case presentation of Fisher (1982) that head impact may not be necessary for brain injury to occur. He described the case of a 67-year-old woman who suffered whiplash associated with amnesia and confusion. He suggested the concussion symptoms resulted from shear strain produced by rotation of the brain within the skull.

CUMULATIVE EFFECTS OF MINOR BRAIN ASSAULTS

For many years, it has been known that electroconvulsive therapy (ECT) can produce permanent brain pathology, and that the resulting impairment is in proportion to the number of ECTs received (Hartelius, 1952; Mosovich &

Katzenebogan, 1948; Meldrum, Horton, & Brierly, 1974; Templer, Ruff, & Armstrong, 1973).

Drew, Templer, Schuyler, Newell, and Cannon (1985) found the number of professional boxing bouts, and the number of professional boxing losses plus draws, to be inversely related to performance on the Halstead-Reitan Neuropsychological Test Battery, the Randt Memory Test, and the Quick Neurological Screening Test. These findings are consistent with the research findings that the number of bouts was positively correlated with electroencephalogram (EEG) abnormality and degree of brain atrophy (Casson, Sham, Campbell, Tablau, & DiDomenico, 1982; Ross, Cole, Thompson, & Kim, 1983). A positive correlation was obtained between duration of solvent abuse and neuropsychological impairment in youngsters (Tsushima & Towne, 1977). Gronwall and Wrightson (1975) found the processing of information of young adults that were studied after a second concussion was significantly inferior to that of first concussed control patients.

SUBSEQUENT BLOWS TO THE HEAD

There is consistent evidence that head trauma can make the person's brain more sensitive to subsequent trauma. Saunders and Harbaugh (1984) reported on a 19-year-old football player who was briefly knocked unconscious during a fist fight 4 days before a football game. A minor blow during the game apparently contributed to his losing consciousness afterward and his dying four days later. Schneider (1966) reported two cases in which football players who had previous concussions died almost immediately after minor second head impacts. Torg, Beer, and Begso (1980) described three cases in which football players who had mononucleosis with encephalitis were devastated by minor head impact.

PROGRESSION OF BRAIN DAMAGE

Atrophy frequently follows brain injury in a process we do not understand well. In Chapter 3, on Contact Sports, our readers will find that cortical atrophy, as demonstrated by computed tomography (CT) scans and pneumoencephalograms, is very common in professional boxers. In a very extensive follow-up study on Finnish war veterans who sustained brain injury, considerable brain atrophy was found. Greater atrophy was apt to be found with a more serious injury (Mantyla, 1981). For 102 veterans, there had been at least two pneumoencephalograms separated by an interval of at least 5 years. Greater progression of atrophy was more likely if there had been an open head injury and if a foreign body remained in the brain. Browder and Hollister (1945) had previously reported on progression of atrophy after an injury. In general, there tends to be displacement of the ventricles toward the site of the injury.

EPIDEMIOLOGY OF BRAIN DAMAGE

There is no doubt about the fact that brain damage has its epidemiology (Frankowski, 1986; Klonox & Thompson, 1969; Field, 1975; Boll & Barth, 1983; Kraus, 1980; Hawthorne, 1978; Annegers & Kurland, 1979; Annegers, Grabou, Hinland, & Laws, 1980; Cooper, Tabado, Houser, Schulman, Feiner, & Factor, 1983). The fact that brain injury is often human-caused is illustrated by its epidemiology, which typically profiles the higher risk person to be a young adult male of below average socioeconomic status. Head injury is more common in blacks and Hispanics than in whites, more common in males than in females, more common from late adolescence to early middle age, and more likely to occur from May through August. Other sorts of brain pathology also have an epidemiology, for example, strokes occurring more frequently in elderly males.

BRAIN DISORDER CAUSING "FUNCTIONAL" PSYCHIATRIC DISORDER

This book focuses primarily on the neuropsychological and neurological effects of preventable brain damage. However, there has been increasing evidence that brain damage and other brain disorders can produce psychiatric disorders that have traditionally been regarded as "functional." In one study, it was found that 63% of patients given a conversion disorder diagnosis were found to have a brain disorder (Whitlock, 1967). There is a report of 78% of temporal lobe epileptics manifesting fugue (Feindel & Penfield, 1954). Pyromaniacs have a high incidence of head injuries and minor neurological abnormalities (Ritvo, Shanok, & Lewis, 1983). Psychopaths demonstrate a disproportionate number of abnormal EEGs and tend to do poorly on neuropsychological tasks that tap frontal lobes functioning (Hare, 1970). Hoenig and Kenna (1979) found that 48% of a group of transsexuals had EEG abnormalities and another 24% had borderline abnormalities, although the authors acknowledged the reasons for such are unclear. A disproportionate number of alcoholics had attentional deficit disorder as children and have children with this disorder. Alcoholics have less alpha rhythm than normal persons; and both alcoholic men and their sons show greater alpha rhythm increase from experimental alcohol consumption than normal control subjects (Pollock, 1983). Anxiety disorder symptoms are prominent in the post-concussion syndrome. Various studies have reported abnormal EEGs ranging from 11% to 65% in obsessive-compulsive patients (Kettl & Marks, 1986).

OBJECTIVE OF PREVENTABLE BRAIN DAMAGE

Most brain injuries result from human error, carelessness, or other action. Comparatively few brain injuries are caused by natural occurrences such as lightning or earthquakes. This book especially focuses on brain damage in which the role of the human factor is large and where the damage could have and should have been prevented. This book examines not only unfortunate occurrences, it offers recommendations for preventive measures.

It is anticipated that the content and presentation of this book will prove appropriate for a wide range of readers that include clinical, counseling, school, and physiological psychologists; neurologists, psychiatrists, and other physicians; educators; athletic directors; and public health officials.

ORGANIZATION OF MATERIAL

Although we do not deny that the brain has notable resilience, we believe that its vulnerability is more striking than its resiliency. The brain is vulnerable to so many things and in so many ways that we must think of it as likened to a chicken that is surrounded by a pack of hungry canines.

We conceptualize the threats to the health of the brain as ranging from clearly external factors such as accidents and assault through less visible impingement such as by environmental neurotoxins and ECT, through ingested substances, through processes originating in the body such as prenatal and nutritional influences, and through processes originating in the brain itself. We ordinarily do not think that internally generated brain conditions such as tumors, strokes, or familial degenerative disorders can be caused by human commission or ommission. However, strokes are more likely to occur in hypertensives who do not take their prescribed medication and do not diet and exercise properly. Research has found that young men who have strokes tend to be abusers of alcohol (Ashley, 1982; Hilbomb & Kaste, 1978, 1981; Taylor & Combes-Orme, 1985). Subsequent chapters will generally proceed from the externally caused to the internally generated brain pathology.

REFERENCES

Annegers, J. F., Garbow, J. D., Kurland, L. T., & Laws, E. R. (1980). The incidence, causes, and secular trends of head trauma in Olmstead County, Minnesota, 1935–1974. *Neurology, 30*, 912–918.

Annegers, J. F., & Kurland, L. T. (1979). The epidemiology of central nervous system trauma. In G. L. Odom (Ed.), *Central nervous system trauma research status report, 1979* (pp. 1–8). Durham, NC: Duke University.

Ashley, M. J. (1982). Alcohol consumption, ischemic heart disease and cerebrovascular disease. *Journal of Studies on Alcohol, 43,* 869-887.

Boll, T. J. (1983). Minor head injury in children—out of sight but not out of mind. *Journal of Clinical Child Psychology, 12,* 74-80.

Boll, T. J., & Barth, J. T. (1983). Mild head injury. *Psychiatric Developments, 3,* 263-275.

Browder, J., & Hollister, N. R. (1945). Air encephalography and ventriculography as diagnostic aids in craniocerebral trauma. *Journal of Nervous and Mental Diseases Proceedings, 24,* 421-436.

Casson, I. R., Sham, R., Campbell, E. A., Tarlau, M., & DiDomenico, A. (1982). Neurological and CT evaluation of knocked-out boxers. *Journal of Neurology, Neurosurgery, and Psychiatry, 45,* 170-174.

Cooper, K. D., Tabaddor, K., Hauser, W. A., Shulman, K., Feiner, C., & Factor, P. R. (1983). The epidemiology of head injury in the Bronx. *Neuroepidemiology, 2,* 70-88.

Drew, R. H., Templer, D. I., Schuyler, B. A., Newell, T. G., & Cannon, W. G. (1986). Neuropsychological deficits in active licensed professional boxers. *Journal of Clinical Psychology, 42,* 520-525.

Feindel, W., & Penfield, W. (1954). Localization of discharge in temporal lobe automatism. *Archives of Neurology and Psychiatry, 72,* 605.

Field, J. H. (1976). *Epidemiology of head injuries in England and Wales: With particular application to rehabilitation.* Department of Health and Social Security. London: Her Majesty's Stationery Office.

Fisher, C. M. (1982). Whiplash amnesia. *Neurology, 32,* 667-668.

Frankowski, R. F. (1986). Descriptive epidemiologic studies of head injury in the United States: 1974-1984. *Advances in Psychosomatic Medicine, 16,* 153-172.

Goldman, H., Gomer, F. E., & Templer, D. I. (1972). Long-term effects of electroconvulsive therapy upon memory and perceptual-motor performance. *Journal of Clinical Psychology, 28,* 32-34.

Gronwall, D., & Wrightson, P. (1981). Memory and information processing capacity after closed head-injury. *Journal of Neurology, Neurosurgery and Psychiatry, 44,* 889-895.

Gulbrandsen, G. B. (1984). Neuropsychological sequelae of light head injuries in older children 6 months after trauma. *Journal of Clinical Neuropsychology, 6,* 257-268.

Hartelius, H. (1952). Cerebral changes following electrically induced convulsions: An experimental study on cats. *Acta Psychiatrica Et Neurologica Scandinavica, 77,* 1-128.

Hartlage, L. C. (1990). *Evaluation of head injury.* Sarasota, Florida: Professional Resource Exchange.

Hare, R. D. (1970). *Psychopathy: Theory and research.* Wiley, New York.

Hawthorne, V. M. (1978). Epidemiology of head injuries. *Scottish Medical Journal, 23,* 1-92.

Hillbom, M., & Kaste, M. (1978). Does ethanol intoxication promote brain infarction in young adults? *Lancet, 2,* 1181-1183.

Hillbom, M., & Kaste, M. (1981). Ethanol intoxication: a risk factor for ischemic brain infarction in adolescents and young adults. *Stroke, 12,* 422-425.

Hoenig, J., & Kenna, J. C. (1979). EEG abnormalities and transsexualism. *British Journal of Psychiatry, 134,* 293-300.

Kennard, M. A. (1936). Age and other factors in motor recovery from precentral lesions in monkeys. *Journal of Neuropsychology, 1,* 477-496.

Kettl, P. A., & Marks-I, M. (1986). Neurological factors in obsessive compulsive disorder: Two case reports and a review of the literature. *British Journal of Psychiatry, 149,* 315-319.

Klonoff, H., & Thompson, G. B. (1969). Epidemiology of head injuries in adults. *Canadian Medical Association Journal, 100,* 235-241.

Kolb, B. (1989). Brain development, plasticity, and behavior. *American Psychologist, 44,* 1203-1212.

Kraus, J. F. (1980). Injury to the head and spinal cord: The epidemiological relevance of the medical literature published 1960 to 1978. *Journal of Neurosurgery, 53,* 53–59.

Meldrum, B. S., Horton, R. W., & Brierley, J. B. (1974). Epileptic brain damage in adolescent baboons following seizures induced by allylglycine. *Brain, 97,* 407–418.

Moses, S. (1989). It's official: 1990's will be 'decade of the brain.' *American Psychological Association Monitor,* October, p. 20.

Mosovich, A., & Katzenelbogan, S. (1948). Electroshock therapy, clinical and electroencephalographic studies. *Journal of Nervous and Mental Disease, 107,* 527–530.

Pollock, V. E. (1983). Relative alpha changes after alcohol among men at risk for alcoholism. *Advances in Biological Psychiatry, 13,* 142–145.

Rimel, R., Giordani, B., Barth, J., Boll, T., & Jane, J. (1981). Disability caused by minor head injury. *Neurosurgery, 9,* 221–227.

Rimel, R. W., Giordani, B., Barth, J. T., Boll, T. J., & Jane, J. A. (1981). Disability caused by minor head injury. *Neurosurgery, 9,* 221–228.

Ritvo, E., Shanok, S. S., & Lewis, D. O. (1983). Firesetting and nonfiresetting delinquents: A comparison of neuropsychiatric, psychoeducational, experiential, and behavioral characteristics. *Child Psychiatry and Human Development, 13,* 259–267.

Ross, R. J., Cole, M., Thompson, J. S., & Kim, K. H. (1983). Boxers—computed tomography, EEG, and neurological evaluation. *Journal of the American Medical Association, 252,* 538–539.

Rutherford, W., Merrett, J., & McDonald, J. (1979). Symptoms at one year following concussion from minor head injury. *Injury, 10,* 225–230.

Saunders, R. L., & Harbaugh, R. E. (1984). The second impact in catastrophic contact-sports head trauma. *Journal of the American Medical Association, 252,* 537–538.

Schneider, R. C. (1966). Serious and fatal neurosurgical football injuries. *Clinical Neurosurgery, 12,* 226–236.

Taylor, J. R., & Combs-Orme, T. (1985). Alcohol and strokes in young adults. *American Journal of Psychiatry, 142,* 116–118.

Templer, D. I., Ruff, C. F., & Armstrong, G. (1973). Cognitive functioning and degree of psychosis in schizophrenics given many electroconvulsive treatments. *British Journal of Psychiatry, 123,* 441–443.

Templer, D. I., & Veleber, D. M. (1982). Can ECT permanently harm the brain? *Clinical Neuropsychology, 4,* 62–66.

Torg, J. S., Beer, L. A., & Begso, J. (1980). Head trauma in football players with infectious mononucleosis. *The Physician and Sports Medicine, 8,* 107–110.

Tsushima, W. T., & Towne, W. S. (1977). Effects of paint sniffing on neuropsychological test performance. *Journal of Abnormal Psychology, 86,* 402–407.

Whitlock, F. A. (1967). The aetiology of histeria. *Acta Psychiatrica Scandinavica, 43,* 144–162.

Windle, W. F., & Groat, R. A. (1945). Disappearance of nerve cells after concussion. *Anatomical Record, 93,* 201–209.

PART I

Impact Damage

CHAPTER 1

BRAIN INJURY
FROM MOTOR VEHICLE ACCIDENTS

Lawrence C. Hartlage and Gurmal Rattan

EPIDEMIOLOGY OF MOTOR VEHICLE ACCIDENTS

Motor vehicle accidents (MVA) represent the single greatest source of brain injury among the general population. Recent statistics compiled by the National Head Injury Foundation (NHIF) indicate that in the United States some 2.7 million people per year, or more than nine thousand individuals per day, may suffer significant brain injury from motor vehicle accidents. This figure of 2.7 million per year actually represents only about 50% of all brain injury from motor vehicle accidents, however, because it does not include "minor" brain injury or brain injury that is ignored due to life-threatening injuries to other organs. In perhaps the most systematic and comprehensive study of head-injury incidence, Caveness' (1979) data suggests a projection of more than 10 million new cases of head injury in the U.S. each year (Hartlage, 1990), with estimates of the percentage of head injury attributable to motor vehicle accidents fairly consistent at or above the 50% level (Annegers, Grabow, Kurland, & Laws, 1980; Gamache & Ducker, 1982; Jagger, Levine, Jane, & Rimel, 1984; Jennett & Teasdale, 1981; Klauber, Barrett-Connor, Marshall, & Bowers, 1981). Thus, current incidence of new head injury cases caused by motor vehicle accidents in the U.S. each year would average somewhere in excess of five million. This translates to an average incidence of one MVA head injury for each person living in the United States, sometime during his life.

Incidence figures compiled from the National Head and Spinal Cord Injury (HSCI) Survey (Kalsbeek, McLauren, Harris, & Miller, 1980) suggest that head injury is much more common than spinal cord injury in motor vehicle accidents, with comparative incidence rates in the range of 35 significant head injuries for each significant spinal cord injury. These incidence figures from surveys of MVAs in the United States cannot, of course, be assumed to apply to other countries. In general, the ratio of 15 MVAs per 100 million kilometers traveled applies to first-world countries, including the United States. By contrast, the Union of South Africa averages a 273/100 million kilometers ratio, with the African nations in the 32/100 million kilometers (Algeria) to 66/100 million kilometers range of Ethiopia (Devilliers, 1984).

The age group most susceptible to head injuries resulting from MVAs consists of individuals between 15 and 24 years of age (Jennett & Teasdale, 1981; Strong, MacMillan, & Jennett, 1978). On the other hand, those sustaining spinal cord injuries as a result of a MVA were in an older age group ranging from 25 to 44 years (Kalsbeek et al., 1980). In both groups, however, males outnumbered females in injuries by a margin of 2 to 1. Similar results were found in other studies previously cited.

The summer months result in the highest rate of head injuries involving MVAs. Kalsbeek et al.'s (1980) data from the HSCI survey found that April represented one peak occurrence while September represented the highest occurrence of head injuries. Not surprisingly, the weekends (i.e., Friday, Saturday, and Sunday) produced the largest number of accidents resulting in head injuries. A study conducted by the University of Virginia for a surrounding 13-county area noted that 25% of the accidents occurred on Saturdays, while Sundays produce an additional 20% (Rimel & Jane, 1983). The peak times for such occurrences were between 3-7 P.M. and resulted in 26% of all reported accidents. In contrast, the lowest occurrence was found between 5-6 A.M. These same researchers also found that 71% of all drivers sustained a head injury and that 59% of the accidents were a result of a single-car collision. Similarly, 58% of the reported accidents occurred on a highway. Overall, the summer months, weekends, and mid-afternoon to early evenings appear to be a critical time during which caution needs to be exercised to avoid a possible mishap.

Motor vehicle accident statistics indicate that male accident victims receive the most severe head injuries that typically involve a longer hospital stay than their female counterparts (Kalsbeek et al., 1980). Once again, the most vulnerable age group was individuals between 15-24 years of age. Long hospital stays were also typical for patients over age 45. In this case, however, other mitigating complications of head injuries such as coma and pneumonia increased the length of hospitalization. Individuals under 15 years of age had the shortest hospital stays, but the cause of their head injuries was usually a fall. Moreover, MVA patients in the 15-24 year age group usually require a hospital stay that is twice as long as those admitted for falls or other causes.

SEQUELAE OF MILD AND MODERATE MVA BRAIN INJURY

Previous mention has been made of "mild" head injury, and some elaboration of this phenomenon is relevant. Specifically, with an incident rate of 10 million new cases annually, and hospitalization of 500,000 cases of head injury per year, it is obvious that approximately 95% of head injuries are sufficiently "mild" that hospital-based treatment is not perceived as necessary (Hartlage, 1990). The sequelae of such injuries are not inconsequential, however (Hartlage, 1984). In a review of two decades of research on intellectual and academic outcome following such injury in children, Goldstein and Levin (1985) concluded that there appeared to be fairly impressive cognitive and academic deficits, with no direct relationship between the severity of the head injury and the ultimate neurocognitive status. Such impairments following head injury in children were not specifically related to age (Klonoff, Crockett, & Clark, 1984). Further, although it has been traditional to use duration of coma as a criterion of severity of head injury, Dubin (1984) found no significant relationship between coma duration and severity of the head injury. Along these same lines, Levin, Benton, and Grossman (1982) found memory deficits among patients whose head injury was so mild that there was no evidence of unconsicousness. Rimel and her associates (Rimel, Giordani, Barth, Boll, & Jane, 1981; Rimel, Giordani, Barth, & Jane, 1982), studying mild versus moderate head injury groups with Halstead-Reitan Neuropsychological Battery measures, found scores indicative of brain injury on 9 of 11 measures with mild head injury versus only 6 of 10 scores indicative of brain injury with moderate head injury. The neurocognitive consequences of mild head injury resulting from motor vehicle accidents are often missed, however, because since IQ tests and similar measures are not sufficiently sensitive to detect the mental processing deficits resultant from such injury (Stuss et al., 1985).

Behaviorally, mild to moderate MVA head injury changes have been noted, and in fact have been recognized as perhaps the most damaging of all such MVA injuries in terms of effects on family life and reintegration into society (Dubin, 1984; Hartlage, 1986; Lewis & Hartlage, 1986; Lezak, 1978; McKinlay, Brooks, Bond, Martinage, & Marshall, 1981). Among behavioral changes reported following MVA head injury have been anxiety, boredom, denial, depersonalization, depression, disinhibition, euphoria, grandiosity, hostility, inhibition, irritability, lability, restlessness, sillinss, suspiciousness, and social withdrawal (Barth et al., 1989; Barth et al., 1983; Boll, 1982; Fordyce, Roueche & Prigatano, 1983; Goethe & Levin, 1984; Grigsby, 1986; Lynch & Mauss, 1981; Oddy, Humphrey, & Luttley, 1978; Sisler, 1978).

A traditional problem in determining the extent to which behavioral problems observed subsequent to an MVA head injury may be attributable to the head injury has involved the lack of information concerning patients' preinjury personality or behavior status. One approach to such information has been pursued by Hartlage and his associates (Hartlage, 1985, 1989; Johnson & Hartlage, 1989; Lewis & Hartlage, 1986). Using an inventory of behaviors suspected of being influenced by head injury with pre- versus postinjury behavioral descriptions provided by parents and teachers of children who had sustained MVA head injury, such injury was found to be associated with significant changes such as becoming more absentminded. agitated, complaining, confused, cross, depressed, disagreeable, distractible, easily upset, forgetful, short-tempered and slow; and less agreeable, calm, cheerful, enthusiastic, good-natured, happy, and pleasant (Hartlage, 1986). In adults, similar changes were found, with significant differences from preinjury on such behaviors as becoming more afraid, agitated, cross, discouraged, down, easily upset, impatient, irritable, tense, tired, and worrisome; and less active, energetic, agreeable, calm, contented, and happy (Speck-Kern & Hartlage, 1986).

Thus research into the neurocognitive and neurobehavioral sequelae of mild to moderate brain injury from motor vehicle accidents suggests that such changes may be expected, and may in fact be demonstrated provided that the appropriate diagnostic and measurement approaches are used.

BIOMECHANICS ASSOCIATED WITH MVA-INDUCED BRAIN INJURY

Brain damage can result from three types of collision injuries. Any or all three types may result from a given accident. In the first type, brain tissue may be destroyed simply by the rapid deceleration of the vehicle without the individual striking any part of the vehicle. The second type involves impact caused by collision of the head with the inside of the vehicle. The third type of collision injury is characterized by the individual being ejected from the vehicle and striking the ground or other outside components of the environment. Recent research into biomechanical criteria for functional brain injury has produced a cortical impact injury model, which, combined with a head-injury criterion previously developed for automotive head injury (Chou & Nyguist, 1974), produced fromulae for calculation of maximum sheer stress and pressure from various types of MVA collisions (Lighthall, Melvin, & Ueno, 1989). Combined with studies of axonal injury related to given directions and velocities (Gennarelli, et al. Thibault, Tomei, Wiser, Graham, & Adams, 1987), it is possible to predict given degrees of axonal shearing. Information about the various types of collisions can be used concomitantly with the biomechanical factors in estimating the severity of the resulting brain injury. The biomechanical sum is a function of the following factors: (1) the impact vectors or angles of the impact to the vehicle during the first collision phase, (2) the kinematics or the amount of resistance the occupants encounter after the first but before the remaining two collisions, (3) the inertial and impact forces imparted to the occupants during the three collision sequence, and (4) the amount, direction, and rate of the negative energy transferred to brain tissue during the accident (Brenner & Enz, 1986). Study of the biomechanical aspects of MVA injuries reveals that, while for slight permanent impairment lower limbs are three times more likely to be involved than the head, for severe and very severe permanent impairment the head is three times more likely to be involved than the lower limbs (Grattan & Hobbs, 1980).

Study of preventable aspects of MVA injuries suggests that information about the human, equipment, and environmental variables also need to be considered in assessing the factors associated with a motor vehicle accident. At the human level, precrash conditions of the driver need to be examined. For example, did the driver disobey any traffic laws such as failing to yield the right of way; did any preexisting psychophysical conditions such as visual acuity or psychomotor coordination hinder driving competence and speed; and did fatigue, drugs, or alcohol impair driving performance. At the equipment level, the primary question is the crashworthiness of the vehicle and its ability to absorb the impact and protect its occupants. Lastly, environmental conditions may mitigate the motor vehicle accident. In this situation, the natural weather conditions (e.g., snow, ice, rain, fog) or human-made conditions (e.g., narrow travel lanes, inadequate shoulder, medians, or traffic signals) that may have facilitated the accident are investigated. By using the combined information noted above, experts in biomechanics can assemble the data to explain the resultant tissue damage to the individual(s) involved in the MVA.

NEUROLOGICAL FEATURES ASSOCIATED WITH MOTOR VEHICLE ACCIDENTS

Head injuries are coded by most countries according to the criteria presented in the International Classification of Diseases (ICD) manual. At present, there are 10 categories that describe the nature of a head injury. Each category uses a three digit "N" code that ranges from "N800 fracture of vault of skull" to "N854 intracranial injury of other and unspecified nature." Motor vehicle accidents are classified under the rubric of "external cause of injury" and are classified using the "BE47" code. Although this classification schema reflects the ninth edition of the ICD, there are limitations to this methodology. As Jennett and Teasdale (1981) point out, some categories are not mutually exclusive, especially with reference to intracranial hematoma. For example, patients can only be classified with this latter disorder if they do not have a skull fracture, yet 75% of hematomas involve skull fractures. Moreover, the variability associated with classifying subjects that present with an identical disorder with different codes such as concussion (N850), unspecified (N854), or unqualified skull fracture (N803) adds to the unreliability of this nosological approach. The above notwithstanding, the ICD does provide structure to enable countries to keep statistics on the incidence of head injuries.

Head injuries suffered from the rapid deceleration of a motor vehicle upon impact typically present with multifocal bilateral lesions without clear indications of lateralization (Levin, Benton, & Grossman, 1982). In a closed head injury, the effects of shearing are also evident. Here, the gray and white matter of the brain separate due to differences in gravity. This effect produces damage to the axons and fibers, and disrupts the vascular flow of blood, nutrients, and waste products. In addition, swelling, atrophy, and degeneration can result and produce significant cognitive deficits as well as emotional disruptions (Hinebaugh, 1986). Additionally, a closed head injury may also result in a rotational acceleration of the brain within the skull and produce a concussion. Based on the HSCI survey, Kalsbeek et al. (1980) found that a higher percentage of concussive head injuries were associated with MVAs in contrast to intracranial hematomas. Given the excessive force imparted on the head or spine, a cerebral concussion may be fatal or result in a loss of daily functioning. Alternatively, in an accident involving a fall, a cerebral hematoma may result and produces swelling or blood clots within the brain. However, the effects of a concussion can also produce hemorrhages, hematomas, and edema that may result in more adverse conditions than the tissue damage caused by the impact (Jennett & Teasdale, 1981).

Injury to the back of the head can result in damage to the temporal lobes and the underside of the frontal lobes. Shearing can occur in both areas and damage to the frontal lobes may lead to broad disruptions in daily living. Because the frontal and prefrontal areas have bidirectional communications with the temporal (processes auditory information), parietal (processes visual-spatial infarction), and occipital (processes visual information) lobes in addition to subcortical links with the limbic system (associated with motivation and arousal), damage to the frontal lobes can be devastating. Disruptions in the following types of behaviors can be evident: (1) loss of initiating behavior due to decreased arousal, orienting response, and slowness; (2) loss of shifting behavior that results in perseveration, disinhibition, and apathy such that the individual cannot shift "gears" and try another alternative or activity; (3) inability to process multiple inputs such that difficulties with planning and processing two or more bits of information simultaneously become apparent; and (4) concrete thinking that results in lack of originality and spontaneity. In addition to the above, emotional disturbances may also be found given the involvement of the limbic structures of the brain. The emotional responses may include flat or diminished affect, depression, apathy, euphoria, inappropriate social behavior, confusion, irritability, explosive outlay of aggression and related behaviors (Hinebaugh, 1986; Lezak, 1983). Overall, the cognitive, emotional, and physical defects resulting from a motor vehicle accident can have devastating consequences on the individual's family, occupation, and general well-being.

No mention thus far has been made of the consequences of very severe brain injury sustained in motor vehicle accidents. Outcome studies indicate that, in very severe brain injury the mortality rate may approach 100%, especially in cases in which patients are both hypotensive and hypoxaemic when they arrive at the neurosurgical unit (Gentleman & Jennett, 1981; Gentleman, Teasdale, & Murray, 1986; Kohi, Mendelow, & Teasdale, 1984). Similar mortality figures have been reported for patients with other complications (Gamache & Ducker, 1982), and poor survival rate was also reported in a large and comprehensive multi-national study by Jennett and colleagues (1977); and the 60% mortality rate reported by Becker (1980) for patients with intracranial hematomas. A prospective study of 200 consecutive patients with severe head injury (Glasgow Coma Scale ≤ 7) who received intracranial pressure monitoring, rapid transport to the neurosurgical center, and cardiopulmonary support, coupled with support from well-trained paramedical and police personnel, showed mortality lowered to 36% (Bowers & Marshall, 1980). This provides the basis for hope that aggressive multifocal attention to severe MVA head injury can improve the survival rate, although it raises some questions concerning the quality of survival that can be achieved (Grossman, 1980).

INTERVENTION AND PREVENTION

Perhaps the single most obvious method of preventing MVA brain injury (and fatalities) is the use of safety belts or airbags (supplemental passive restraint systems) or protective head gear with motorcyclists. Based on the information provided by the National Head Injury Foundation, safety belts are 57% effective in preventing fatal or serious injuries. That is, an individual's chances of survival or avoidance of a serious head injury are more than doubled with the use of safety belts. The automatic belts that are installed on some newer model cars are about 35%–50% effective against fatalities and 40%–50% effective in preventing moderate to severe injuries. The regular use of seat belts, therefore, is estimated to reduce traffic-related head injuries by about 40%. Typically, fewer than 14% of motor vehicle drivers and 58% of motorcycle drivers in collisions were wearing their seat belts or helmets, respectively, even though it is mandatory to wear such equipment in the majority of states. Concomitant with the lack of protective devices, 50% of the patients also reported that they were traveling in excess of the legal 55 MPH speed limit.

A similar picture of fatalities and presumably brain injuries exists in the case of unhelmeted motorcycle drivers. The National Highway Traffic Safety Administration reported that 4,570 fatalities in 1985 and 4,551 in 1986 resulted from motorcycle accidents. The single most important variable determining survival for motorcycle crashes is the use of safety helmets. Yet, fewer than 40% of minors who were fatally injured in motorcycle accidents were wearing helmets, although helmets were mandated by law. It becomes increasingly clear that while there is a causal link between the use of safety equipment and survival in motor vehicle accidents, a large sector of the driving population ignore such statistics. Implementation of a driver safety curriculum within the schools could be a mandatory requirement for future drivers in order to encourage prudence and better judgment when driving. Including driver education curricula to emphasize such safety factors or seat belt use as requirements to obtain and retain driving privileges represent another possibility.

Mandatory seat belt use, while an obvious preventive strategy, is not universally accepted. Wyoming has become the 32nd state to enact a seat-belt-use law for front seat occupants of cars and trucks (AAAM Bulletin, 1989), although the National Highway Transportation Safety Agency (NHTSA) has reiterated its position that safety belts are not needed on large school buses (Federal Register, 1989). Alcohol use contributes to motor vehicle injuries at an incidence estimated at approximately 55 injuries per 100,000 vehicular miles (National Head Injury Foundation, 1984). Some suggested relationship between blood-alcohol concentration and injury severity has been reported (Kraus, Morganstern, Fife, Conroy, & Nourjah, 1989), with the incidence of victims with elevated blood-alcohol concentrations ranging from 30% to 70%. There was overrepresentation of alcohol use in seriously injured patients (Gerberich et al., 1989). Mothers Against Drunk Driving (MADD) has waged a campaign for stricter alcohol legislation and enforcement. Since its organization in 1980, MADD has reported a 17% reduction in fatal crash drivers who were drunk; a 13% decrease in fatal crashes caused by 18–20 year olds as a result of raising the drinking age; and victim compensation and Bill of Rights legislation passage in 45 states (MADD, 1990). Community self-regulation as a voluntary effort has also been reported as reducing alcohol-impaired driving (Worden, Flynn, Merrill, Waller, & Haugh, 1989).

Reduced speed (i.e., 55 MPH speed limit) has been demonstrated to accompany a major decrease in deaths, beginning with the 1974 imposition of the lower speed limits (O'Neill, 1985; Transportation Research Board, 1984). While no statistics concerning specific relationships between given speeds and the incidence of MVA brain injury are available, it is reasonable to conclude that such a relationship exists. Also in the realm of governmental regulation are a number of phenomena with at least suspected potential for reducing MVA and presumably brain injury. For example, deregulation of the airline industry has resulted in increased air passenger miles and decreased auto passenger miles; with air travel injuries/fatalities dramatically lower per mile than auto travel, such deregulation may be expected to have some effect on the incidence of brain injury due to MVA. In an unrelated sphere, governmental requirements for labeling of over the counter (and prescription) medications that can impair driving ability may reasonably be expected to help reduce driving accidents, but no empirical data concerning specific numbers of accidents potentially prevented by such actions are available. Environmental factors, such as the width of highway shoulder berms, have been reported in recent highway safety studies as potentially potent factors in many single vehicle accidents, but no projections concerning cost/benefit ratios for modifications of such factors have yet been developed.

Obviously, the physical characteristics of vehicles, such as "crashworthiness" and improvement of structural protection to occupants are important for prevention of MVA brain and other injury, and manufacturers need to be reminded of driver concern over continued research and modifications by manufacturers.

Finally, to the extent that MVAs resulting in brain injury cannot be prevented or minimized, prompt and knowledgeable intervention can help prevent severe consequences. Given that the first hour of postinjury can be very critical to eventual outcome, better training by the Emergency Medical Technicians (EMT) in maintenance of airways, ventilation, and circulation may add to the survivability of the patient. As suggested by the San Diego prospective study, involving police in training programs emphasizing prompt transport to neurosurgical centers can complement and enhance the effectiveness of EMT efforts.

REFERENCES

Annegers, J. F., Grabow, J. D., Kurland, L. T., & Laws, E. R. (1980). The incidence, causes, and secular trends of head trauma in Olmested County, Minnesota. *Neurology, 30,* 912–919.

Association for the Advancement of Automotive Medicine. (1989). Seat-belt use law passes in Wyoming. *Bulletin, 2*(2), 7.

Barth, J. T., Alves, W. M., Ryan, T. V., Macciocchi, S. N., Rimel, R. W., Jane, J. A., & Nelson, W. E. (1989). Mild head injury in sports: Neuropsychological sequelae and recovery of function. In H. Levin, A. Benton, & H. Eisenberg (Eds.), *Mild head injury* (pp. 257–275). New York: Oxford Press.

Barth, J. T., Macciocchi, S. N., Giordani, B., Rimel, R. W., Jane, J. A., & Boll, T. J. (1983). Neuropsychological sequelae of minor head injury. *Neurosurgery, 13,* 529–533.

Becker, D. P. (1980). Comment. *Neurosurgery, 6*(3), 242.

Boll, T. J. (1982). Behavioral sequelae of head injury. In P. R. Cooper (Ed.), *Head injury* (pp. 363–375). Baltimore: Williams & Wilkins.

Bowers, S. A., & Marshall, L. F. (1980). Outcome in 200 consecutive cases of severe head injury treated in San Diego County: A prospective analysis. *Neurosurgery, 6*(3), 237–242.

Brenner, R., & Enz, B. E. (1986). Classification of information generated in a motor vehicle crash sequence. In A. Sances, D. J. Thomas, C. L. Ewing, S. J. Larson, & F. Unterharnscheidt (Eds.), *Mechanisms of head and spine trauma.* Goshen, NY: Aloray Publisher.

Caveness, W. F. (1977). Incidence of cranio-cerebral trauma in the United States. *Transactions of the American Neurological Association, 102,* 136–138.

Caveness, W. F. (1979). Incidence of craniocerebral trauma in the United States 1976, and trend from 1970–1975. In R. Thompson & J. Green (Eds.), *Advances in neurology* (pp. 1–3). New York: Raven Press.

Chou, C. C., & Nyguist, G. W. (1974). Analytical studies of the head injury criterion. *SAE Technical Paper 740082,* Automotive Engineering Congress.

DeVilliers, J. C. (1984). Head injuries in South Africa. *South African Journal of Surgery, 22*(1), 51–56.

Dubin, W. J. (1984, October). *Prediction of long-term outcome of closed head injury II: Variables which influence the course and extent of recovery.* Paper presented at National Academy of Neuropsychologists, San Diego, CA.

Federal Register. (1989, March 22). FMVS 222, school bus passenger seating and crash protection. *54*(54), 11765.

Fordyce, D. J., Roueche, J. R., & Prigatano, G. P. (1983). Enhanced emotional reactions in chronic head trauma patients. *Journal of Neurology, Neurosurgery and Psychiatry, 46,* 620–624.

Gamache, F. W., & Ducker, T. B. (1982). Alterations in neurological function in head-injured patients experiencing major episodes of sepsis. *Neurosurgery, 10*(4), 468–472.

Gennarelli, T. A., Thibault, G., Tomei, G., Wiser, R., Graham, D., & Adams, J. (1987). *Directional dependence of axonal brain injury due to central and noncentroidal alteration.* Proceedings of 31st Stapp Car Crash Conference, SAE Paper 872197, 49–53.

Gentleman, D., & Jennett, B. (1981). Hazards of inter-hospital transfer of comatose head injured patients. *Lancet, 2,* 853–855.

Gentleman, D., Teasdale, G., & Murray, L. (1986). Cause of severe head injury and risk of complications. *British Medical Journal, 292,* 449.

Gerberich, S., Gerberich, B., Fife, D., Cicero, J., Lilja, G., & Van Berkom, L. (1989). Analyses of the relationship between blood alcohol and nasal breath alcohol concentrations: Implications for assessment of trauma cases. *Trauma, 29,* 338–343.

Goethe, K. E., & Levin, H. S. (1984). Behavioral manifestations during the early and long-term stages of recovery following closed head injury. *Psychiatric Annals, 14,* 540–546.

Goldstein, F. C., & Levin, H. S. (1985). Intellectual and academic outcome following closed head injury in children and adolescents: Research strategies and empirical findings. *Developmental Neuropsychology, 1,* 195–214.

Grattan, E., & Hobbs, J. A. (1980). Permanent disability in road traffic accident casualties. *Transport and Road Research Laboratory Report, 927,* 4.

Grigsby, J. P. (1986). Depersonalization following minor closed head injury. *International Journal of Clinical Neuropsychology, 7,* 65–68.

Grossman, R. G. (1980). Comment. *Neurosurgery, 6*(3), 241–242.

Hartlage, L. C. (1984). Unsuspected consequences of apparently insignificant head injuries. *Auto Torts, 7,* 187–191.

Hartlage, L. C. (1985, October). *Behavioral sequelae of traumatic head injury: Pre-post checklist.* Paper presented at National Academy of Neuropsychologists annual meeting, Philadelphia, PA.

Hartlage, L. C. (1986, April). *Behavioral sequelae of closed head injuries in school-age children.* Paper presented at National Association of School Psychologists, Hollywood, FL.

Hartlage, L. C. (1989). *Behavior change inventory (inventory or pre- versus post-behaviors with brain injury).* Brandon, VT: Clinical Psychology Publishing Company.

Hartlage, L. C. (1990). *Neuropsychological evaluation of head injury.* Sarasota, FL: Practitioner's Resource Exchange.

Hinebaugh, R. L. (1986). Frontal lobe contributions to the psychopathology of closed cranial insults of vehicular origin. *Cognitive Rehabilitation,* 24–27.

Jagger, J., Levine, J. I., Jane, J. A., & Rimel, R. W. (1984). Epidemiologic features of head injury in a predominantly rural population. *Journal of Trauma, 24,* 40–44.

Jennett, B., & Teasdale, G. (1981). *Management of head injuries.* Philadelphia: F. A. Davis.

Jennett, B., Teasdale, G., Galbraith, S., Pickard, J., Grant, H., Braakman, R., Avezaat, C., Maas, A., Minderhout, J., Vecht, C., Heiden, J., Small, R., Caton, W., & Kurze, T. (1977). Severe head injuries in three countries. *Journal of Neurology, Neurosurgery, and Psychiatry, 40,* 291–298.

Johnson, D. J., & Hartlage, L. C. (1989, June). *Specific behavior changes resultant from traumatic head injury.* Paper presented at the first annual meeting, American Psychological Society, Arlington, VA.

Kalsbeek, W. D., McLauren, R. L., Harris, B. S., & Miller, J. D. (1980). The national head and spinal cord injury survey: Major findings. *Journal of Neurosurgery, 53,* S19–S31.

Klauber, M. R., Barrett-Connor, R. E., Marshall, L. F., & Bowers, S. A. (1981). The epidemiology of head injury: A prospective study on an entire community—San Diego County, California. *Journal of Epidemiology, 113,* 353–361.

Klonoff, H., Crockett, D. D., & Clark, C. (1984). Head injuries in children: A model for predicting course of recovery and prognosis. In R. Tarter & G. Goldstein (Eds.), *Advances in clinical neuropsychology* (Vol. 2, pp. 139–157). New York: Plenum.

Kohi, Y. M., Mendelow, A. D., & Teasdale, G. M. (1984). Extracranial insults and outcome in patients with acute head injury—Relationship to the Glasgow Coma Scale. *Injury, 16,* 25–29.

Kraus, J., Morganstern, H., Fife, D., Conroy, C., & Nourjah, P. (1989). Blood alcohol tests, prevalence of involvement and outcomes following brain injury. *American Journal of Public Health, 79,* 294–299.

Levin, H. S., Benton, A. L., & Grossman, R. G. (1982). *Neurobehavioral consequences of closed head injury.* New York: Oxford University Press.

Lewis, P., & Hartlage, L. C. (1986, August). *Objective assessment of behavioral sequelae of head injury.* Paper presented at American Psychological Association, Washington, DC.

Lezak, M. D. (1978). Living with the characterologically altered brain injured patient. *Journal of Clinical Psychiatry, 39,* 592–598.

Lezak, M. D. (1983). *Neuropsychological assessment.* New York: Oxford University Press.

Lighthall, J. W., Melvin, J. W., & Ueno, K. (1989). Toward a biomechanical criterion for functional brain injury. *Research Publication GMR 6680,* General Motors Research Laboratory, Biomedical Science Department, Warren, MI.

Lynch, W. J., & Mauss, N. K. (1981). Brain injury rehabilitation: Standard problem lists. *Archives of Physical Medicine and Rehabilitation, 62,* 223–227.

McKinlay, W. W., Brooks, D. N., Bond, M. B., Martinage, D. P., & Marshall, M. M. (1981). The short-term outcome of severe blunt head injury as reported by relatives of the injured person. *Journal of Neurology, Neurosurgery and Psychiatry, 44,* 527–533.

Mothers Against Drunk Driving. (1990). *Voice of the victim.* Pamphlet.

National Head Injury Foundation. (1984). *Bulletin, 4.*

Oddy, M., Humphrey, M., & Uttley, D. (1978). Subjective impairment and social recovery after closed head injury. *Journal of Neurology, Neurosurgery and Psychiatry, 41,* 611–616.

O'Neil, B. (1985, April). Statement of Insurance Institute for Highway Safety. Chicago, IL. Reported by National Head Injury Foundation, 1985.

Rimel, R. W., Giordani, B., Barth, J. T., Boll, T. J., & Jane, J. A. (1981). Disability caused by minor head injury. *Neurosurgery, 9,* 221–228.

Rimel, R. W., Giordani, B., Barth, J. T., & Jane, J. A. (1982). Moderate head injury: Completing the clinical spectrum of brain trauma. *Neurosurgery, 11,* 344–351.

Rimel, R. W., & Jane, J. A. (1983). Characteristics of the head-injured patient. In M. Tosenthal, E. R. Griffith, M. R. Bond, & J. D. Miller (Eds.), *Rehabilitation of the head injured adult.* Philadelphia: F. A. Davis.

Sisler, G. C. (1978). Psychiatric disorder associated with head injury. *Psychiatric Clinics of North America, 1,* 137–152.

Speck-Kern, E., & Hartlage, L. C. (1986, May). *Behavioral considerations in rehabilitation of head injury.* Paper presented at the Mid-South Conference on Neuropsychology, Memphis, TN.

Strong, I., MacMillan, R., & Jennett, B. (1978). Head injuries in accident and emergency departments at Scottish hospitals. *Injury, 10,* 154–159.

Stuss, D. T., Ely, P., Hugenholtz, H., Richard, M. T., LaRochelle, S., Poirier, C. A., & Boll, I. (1985). Subtle neuropsychological deficits in patients with good recovery after closed head injury. *Neurosurgery, 17*, 41–46.

Transportation Research Board. (1984). 55: A decade of experience. *Special Report 204*, National Research Council, Washington, DC.

Worden, J., Flynn, B., Merrill, D., Waller, J., & Haugh, L. (1989). Preventing alcohol-impaired driving through community self-regulation training. *American Journal of Public Health, 79*, 287–290.

CHAPTER 2

CONTACT SPORTS

Richard H. Drew and Donald I. Templer

Some sports have blows to the head as an expected or even intended "sporting" activity. Included in this category are boxing, wrestling, football, rugby, judo, and karate.

BOXING

A reasonable initial question is whether or not punches to the head have sufficient impact to damage the brain. The research of Atha, Yeadon, Sandover, and Parsons (1985) seems to answer that question in the affirmative. The investigators had Frank Bruno, the top-ranked heavy weight at the time in Britain, deliver punches to a 16-pound cylindrical mass that was considered to be roughly the equivalent of the head and neck of a heavyweight boxer. The mass was padded so as to be roughly the thickness and yield of a human face. The punch traveled about half a meter, attained a velocity of about 9 millimeters per second and had an impact in the neighborhood of half a ton. The authors reasoned that such impact is the equivalent of that provided by a 13-pound wooden mallet swung at 20 miles per hour.

More important that the theoretical issue of punches having sufficient impact is the evidence that brain damage has actually occurred. Research in that area has been going on for many years. Indeed, the literature published concerning the medical aspects of boxing reflects many changes that have taken place in the profession since the punch-drunk syndrome was first identified by Martland (1928). In general, as the medical sequelae to a boxing career became more widely recognized, the rules and medical supervision were adapted to reduce the adverse effects. After this was accomplished, more sensitive measurements were developed and more subtle damage was again detected, which resulted in more rules changes. General changes in the sport that have accompanied the new findings include medical supervision, supervisory governing bodies, elimination of unsupervised "booth" boxing, padded rings and posts, increased glove size, and shorter careers. These changes have undoubtedly been responsible for the reduced incidence of the classic punch-drunk syndrome.

Martland (1928) introduced the term "punch drunk" to the medical profession when he described the symptoms of several aging retired professional boxers. Other terms for the same condition in ring parlance included "cuckoo," "goofy," "cutting paper dolls," "slug nutty," "punchie," "stumble bum," and "slap happy" (Critchley, 1957). The medical profession, in search for more esoteric and less offensive expression, has since coined "traumatic encephalopathy" (Parker, 1934), "demential pugilistica" (Millspaugh, 1937), and "chronic progressive traumatic encephalopathy of boxers" (Critchley, 1957) to indicate the same syndrome. By any name, however, these terms refer to the chronic, progressive consequences of brain tissue damage resulting from the repeated head trauma of boxing.

Neurological examinations of older, retired boxers in the 1920s through the 1960s (Isherwood, Mawdsley, & Ferguson, 1966; Martland, 1928; Mawdsley & Ferguson, 1963; Spillane, 1962) presented a rather stereotyped clinical picture characterized by evidence of damage to one or more of the pyramidal, extrapyramidal or cerebellar systems with associated memory loss, dementia, psychosis, personality change, and in some cases social instability. Symptoms tended to be progressive and developed any time during a boxer's career or as late as many years after retirement from the ring. It is notable that boxers of this period often had several hundred bouts, usually unsupervised by either medical or licensing agencies. Spillane (1962), for example, cited five case studies in which the boxers were reported to have fought 350, 33, 200, 300, and several hundred bouts, and Mawdsley and Ferguson (1963) listed 10 case studies in which professional boxers had from 100 to 600 bouts and one who reported to have fought nearly nightly in boxing booth "blood tanks" for nearly 10 years.

Martland (1928) reported that visible symptoms usually appear first in the extremities with loss of motor control and a general slowing of muscular movements. Progressive cases were next characterized by a peculiar mental attitude including hesitancy in speech, tremors of the hands, and nodding movements of the head, necessitating withdrawal from the ring. Later, in severe cases, there developed a tilting of the head, a marked dragging of one or both legs, a staggering, propulsive gait with facial characteristics of the Parkinsonian syndrome, a backward swaying of the body, tremors, vertigo, and deafness. Finally, marked mental deterioration occasionally set in, necessitating commitment to asylums. Martland cited four such commitments in a list of 23 punch-drunk fighters known to one promoter in 1928. This often quoted classic description of the severe punch-drunk syndrome has been little changed over the years. Older, retired boxers with numerous bouts who fought prior to major changes in the sport (primarily initiated during the 1950s) appear in the literature as recently as 1969 with these severe punch-drunk symptoms (Johnson, 1969b).

Autopsies of these severe cases revealed a pattern of diffuse cortical and subcortical damage consistent with the clinical syndrome. Neubuerger, Sinton, and Denst (1959) reported on two such cases where brain tissue showed severe cortical atrophy and fibral alteration without plaques. Spillane (1962) reported foci of softening in the cerebral and cerebellar cortex in a similar case. Mawdsley and Ferguson (1963) reported on autopsy of a 51-year-old boxer who had had 300 professional bouts. Again, gross diffuse cortical atrophy was the main reported finding, along with a cavum septi pellucidi. The septum pellucidum is a thin, triangular-shaped membrane that separates the lateral ventricles anteriorly, stretching from the corpus callosum down to the anterior commissure of the fornix (Spillane, 1962). A cavum septi pellucidi is not a recognized sequel of acute head injury or of cerebral atrophy. Mawdsley and Ferguson (1963) hypothesized its high incidence in boxers' brains is the result of an abrupt rise in pressure of the ventricular fluid which ruptures the floor or walls of the septum pellucidum, allowing the fluid to communicate with the third or lateral ventricles. Subsequent blows and pressure elevation drive the fluid into the cavum, causing its progressive dilatation and further perforations in its walls, leading eventually to the disappearance of the septum.

Payne (1968), using more refined histological techniques, studied the brains of six retired professional boxers who had experienced long careers. He reported enlarged ventricular systems due to atrophy, miniscars and macroscars in the grey matter and areas of myelin degeneration. He expressed the opinion that these lesions are of sufficient number and amount to account at least in part for the symptoms displayed by ex-boxers.

Corsellis et al. (1973) studied the brains of 15 retired boxers who fought between 1900 and 1940. Over half of these had taken part in over 300 bouts. Fourteen of the 15 (93%) brains had a septum cavum as compared to 3% occurrence in non-boxers. Cerebellar signs included loss of Purkinje cells, atrophy, and well-defined cortical scarring. Degeneration of the substantia nigra was characterized by loss of pigmental neurons and neurofibrillary changes typical of Parkinsonian syndrome. Neurofibrillary tangles (without senile plaques) were spread diffusely through both the brain stem and cerebral cortex, and this combination is reported to be unique to this population. The neurofibrillary tangles, although found in all areas, were more severe in the medial temporal grey matter, including the hippocampal formation. The authors thus concluded that the novel pattern of cerebral damage and degeneration that is concentrated in the septal region, deep in the temporal grey matter and on certain neurons along the cerebellar and nigral pathways account for the combination of clumsiness of speech and movement, memory loss, ataxia, dysarthria, Parkinsonian symptoms, and dementia. This study convincingly ties the diffuse structural alteration due to boxing with the behavioral symptoms associated with the punch-drunk syndrome.

Air encephalographic studies of living retired boxers with extensive careers confirmed evidence of atrophy and cavum septum pellucidum. They were used from the early 1950s until they were replaced by CT scans in the mid-1970s. Spillane (1963), for example, reported that of five retired boxers with extensive careers, air encephalography revealed cerebral atrophy in two, and cavum or perforated septum in three. Mawdsley and Ferguson (1963), in their study of 10 retired professional boxers with similar lengthy careers, found consistent evidence of cerebral and cerebellar atrophy and cavum septi pellucidi using air encephalography. Using the same technique, Isherwood et al. (1966) reported normal encephalogram in three of 16 retired ex-boxers. The other 13 abnormal findings include cavum septi pellucidi in nine cases and evidence of brain atrophy (generalized ventricular enlargement in 11 cases, cerebral cortical atrophy in three cases, cerebellar atrophy in 4 cases. Johnson (1969b) reported similar evidence of brain damage in 13 of 15 ex-professional fighters with extensive careers.

As awareness of the consequence of a long boxing career increased, governing agencies were developed to monitor and control abuses in both amateur and professional bouts.

During this same period, the 1950s and 1960s more research was performed with younger boxers, many still engaged in the sport. The newly developed electroencephalography (EEG) was used in some of these studies. Busse and Silverman (1952) reported the result of EEG examination of 24 active professional boxers obtained as a result of a Colorado law requiring such examination in that state. They reported a significant increase in dysrhythmic patterns in boxers as compared to nonboxers, but were unclear as to what this type of pattern indicated. Larsson et al. (1954) conducted both neurological and EEG examinations of 75 Swedish boxers, 44 of them both before and after matches. The age range of these active amateur fighters was 17–25 years. They found no abnormal neurological findings before matches but temporary amnesia and disorientation in 23 cases (31%) after bouts. EEG findings were abnormal (general flattening or slow irregular waves) in 16% of the cases before and 52% after bouts. They were unable, however, to find any parallel between EEG findings and clinical signs of concussion. Kaplan and Browder (1954) correlated EEG findings of 1,043 professional fighters with age and found it to be not significant with technical knockout (TKO) and knockout (KO). They also found no change in EEG patterns 10 minutes after losing a bout compared to before the bout, nor after a year of professional boxing. Blonstein and Clarke (1954) studied EEG results in 48 amateur boxers and expressed the opinion it was of doubtful value in amateur boxing if rigid medical control is practiced. Blonstein and Clarke (1957) later assessed 29 amateur boxers who had been KOed more than once in 1 year and had suffered from amnesia for 1 month or more (severely concussed) following a bout. They found normal neurological and EEG results in all 29. Nesarajah, Seneviratne, and Watson (1961) compared the EEG records of

50 Ceylonese boxers with 75 control athletes, not boxers. They found 60% of the boxers showed spontaneous discorded activity compared to 8% in the controls. Thomassen, Juul-Jensen, Olivarius, Braemer, and Christensen (1979) compared the EEG findings of 53 amateur champion boxers with a control group of 53 football players who were matched for period of career, age, and occupational level. They found identical neurological and EEG patterns for both the populations. Roberts (1969) assessed the EEG findings of 229 retired professional boxers who were active between 1930 and 1955, 27% of whom had symptoms of boxers' traumatic encephalopathy. He found that abnormal recordings occurred with greater frequency than in the general population. Thus, we see the preliminary EEG studies of boxers showed some abnormalities; however, there seems to be no consistent pattern, and some research suggested the abnormalities to be no more prevalent than in other populations.

By the later 1960s, many researchers felt that major brain damage in boxers was being adequately prevented. In 1966, Blonstein (cited in Harvey & Davis, 1974) reported to the Royal Society of Medicine what "with shorter bouts and modern medical control, the punch-drunk syndrome has not been seen during the last twenty years in active professional boxers" (p. 649). In the same article, Harvey and Davis reported the case of a 25-year-old professional fighter who showed symptoms of traumatic encephalopathy after 16 professional bouts. His symptoms included slurred speech, shuffle gait, stiff legs, slowness on his feet, mood lability, and acute depressive illness with paranoid features necessitating psychiatric hospitalization. Air encephalogram showed mild ventricular dilatation, indications of atrophy and a cavum septum pellucidum.

About this same time, CT scan became available as a more sensitive way to measure structural changes of abnormalities in the brain. Harvey and Davis (1974) used this technique to confirm the ventricular dilatation indicated in the air encephalogram of the previously reported 25-year-old boxer.

This 1974 study by Harvey and Davis is the last reported incidence in the research literature of the classical punch-drunk syndrome with full range of behavioral symptoms. It is noteworthy, however, that this case occurred after most medical precautions were in place, and the fighter was only 25 years old and still fighting, after having completed about 75 amateur bouts and 25 professional bouts. He was reported to have lost only about 10 bouts, took no severe beatings, was never knocked out, and never experienced episodes of amnesia. Studies since that time report much less severe neurological findings. For example, Kaste et al. (1982) reported one case of abnormal neurological findings (apraxia and slight unsteadiness and slight slowness of mental function) in 14 boxers who had been European champions. Casson et al. (1982) reported one case of mild organic syndrome (impaired recent memory and recall, confusion, and dyscalculia) in a study of 10 professional boxers. Ross et al. (1983), after examining 40 ex-boxers, determined standard neurological examination (including detailed history) proved to be a poor tool in assessing brain damage in modern-day boxers, thus again indicating the lack of findings in modern fighters who have experienced more strict medical supervision and fewer bouts.

Nevertheless, many experts on the topic of boxing had contended that by 1980 major neurological impairment in boxers had been an occurrence of the past.

Since 1982, however, a number of research articles have reported continued evidence of brain damage in modern fighters in spite of the lack of gross neurological symptoms. These studies have used a combination of neurological, CT, and EEG evaluations. Using all three methods, Kaste et al. (1982) examined 14 ex-boxers who had been European champions. Six had fought professionally, and 8 were amateurs; only one (an amateur) was still an active boxer. Although only one showed neurological deficits, CT findings revealed brain atrophy in four professionals and one amateur. Two of the professional boxers had EEG abnormalities. Of this group of 14 boxers, five had less than 100 bouts, six between 101 and 150, and three had over 150 total bouts.

Casson et al. (1982) also used detailed neurological examinations as well as EEG and CT scans to examine 10 active professional boxers shortly after being knocked out. They were surprised to find cerebral atrophy in five of the 10 boxers with this finding most common in the boxers with the most bouts.

Ross et al. (1983) examined 40 retired boxers with the same three techniques. They, too, found a significant relationship between the number of bouts fought and CT changes, indicating cerebral atrophy. EEG abnormalities also were significantly correlated with number of bouts, although neurological findings were not.

Sironi and Ravagnati (1983) reported on a study in which they examined 10 young (18–24 years old) Finnish professional boxers, all of whom had normal neurological examinations. Even in these young fighters they found EEG abnormalities in three cases and CT scan signs of atrophy in six. They also reported longitudinal EEG and CT scans on a boxer who had a record of being knocked out. When he had been KOed only two times all findings were normal, but after two more KOs, he showed EEG abnormalities and CT signs of atrophy.

Casson et al. (1984) studied 18 boxers, of whom 13 were ex-professional, two active professional, and three active amateur fighters, using neurological, EEG, CT, and neuropsychological exams. Five of the retired boxers had abnormal neurological findings including disorientation, confusion, and memory loss. Eight had CT findings including cerebral atrophy, and seven of the 13 who had EEG tests showed abnormal findings. The authors found a significant correlation between number of professional bouts and the percentage of impaired or abnormal test results. They concluded that this relationship indicates the cumulative effect of multiple subconcussive blows to the head and that these blows are a likely etiology.

In a study by Jordan and Zimmerman (1990) CTs and magnetic resonance images (MRIs) were compared on 16 active professional, four active amateur, and one retired boxer. Eleven boxers had abnormal CTs and MRIs with seven severely abnormal. Three had abnormal MRIs while the CTs were less definitive. These included subcortical white matter changes, focal contusions, subdural hematoma, and a thalamus cyst. They concluded that the MRI is the imaging study of choice when evaluating central nervous system change in boxers.

It can be seen in recent studies using a combination of techniques, brain damage still occurs in modern-day boxers. These abnormalities appear in CT scans (atrophy), EEG findings (abnormalities), and a few in functional neurological exams (confusion, disorientation, and memory loss). Generally, the deficits were noted in retired boxers and in some cases they tended to correlate with increased number of bouts. With these recent findings there is increasing concern that brain damage may be occurring from early on in a boxer's career when he first experiences subconcussive blows, and that these blows may be resulting in cumulative damage (Casson et al., 1982, 1984; Ross et al., 1983; Sironi & Ravagnati, 1983). With the present techniques this damage cannot be detected until there are gross structural changes such as atrophy of brain tissue, gross electrical abnormalities as measured by EEG or gross behavioral deficits such as disorientation or memory loss. As has been indicated by several authors such as Moore (1980), if a neurologist does find evidence of a deficit, then it is almost always too late. Once damaged, other parts may take over the damaged function, but the damaged part will never repair itself.

Thus, there seems to be no doubt about the fact that boxing can cause brain damage. The only real remaining questions are how common is this brain damage and how does it translate into cognitive and behavioral deficits. To help answer these questions, Drew, Templer, Schuyler, Newell, and Cannon (1985) used neuropsychological tests since, in research on minor head injury outside the area of boxing, brain deficits can often be detected on such instruments before they can be on neurological exams and tests, and on IQ tests. More importantly, they used young, active boxers who only had a mean of 13.7 professional bouts. They administered the most comprehensive neuropsychological test battery to date to 19 young active professional boxers and to 10 control athletes comparable with respect to age, race, and level of education. Fifteen of the 19 boxers and only two of the 10 control athletes were in the impaired range of the Halstead-Reitan Impairment Index. Even though these boxers only had a mean of 13.7 professional bouts there were substantial correlations between number of professional bouts and deficits evidenced from the Quick Neurological Screening Test, the Randt Memory Test, and the Halstead-Reitan Neuropsychological Battery, as displayed in Table 2-1. Although the boxers had a mean of 52.8 amateur bouts, there were no significant correlations between degree of impairment and number of amateur bouts.

Drew et al. (1985, p. 525) concluded: "The findings of the present research suggest that appreciable brain damage and associated neuropsychological deficits in today's active professional boxers may be the rule rather than the exception."

TABLE 2-1 Product-Moment Correlations Between Test Results and Boxing History

	Amateur bouts	Amateur losses plus draws	Professional bouts	Professional losses plus draws
QNST errors	0.31	0.03	0.80****	0.69***
Halstead-Reitan				
Aphasia screening errors	0.00	0.23	0.41	0.51*
Finger tip number writing errors	0.32	0.15	0.60**	0.59**
Trails Test failures	0.34	0.37	0.32	0.49*
Seashore Rhythm failure	0.08	0.06	0.37	0.59**
TPT failures	0.03	0.04	0.45	0.49*
Finger tapping failures	0.44	0.06	0.54*	0.45
Category test failure	0.19	0.29	0.22	0.33
Impairment index	0.22	0.18	0.49*	0.59**
Randt Memory Test				
Acquisition standard score	−0.13	−0.22	−0.58**	−0.47*
Delayed recall standard score	0.02	0.01	−0.51*	−0.47*
Memory index	−0.07	−0.14	−0.62***	−0.52*
Summary scores				
Total errors	0.24	0.19	0.66***	0.68***
Total failures	0.32	0.24	0.61**	0.67***
Total errors plus failures	0.27	0.21	0.68***	0.71****

*$p < 0.05$.
**$p < 0.01$.
***$p < 0.005$.
****$p < 0.001$.

The absence of significant correlations between the number of amateur bouts and neuropsychological test performance in the Drew et al. (1986) study could be interpreted as amateur boxing being safe for the brain. However, subsequent research seems to indicate that brain damage may also occur in amateur boxers. McLatchie, Brooks, Galbraith, Hutchison, Wilson, Melville, and Teasdale (1987) administered a neurological examination, EEG, CT scan, and neuropsychological tests to 20 active British amateur boxers. Seven of the 20 boxers had abnormal neurological examination findings, and abnormality correlated significantly with number of fights. Eight boxers had abnormal EEG's but EEG did not correlate with number of fights. Only one boxer had an abnormal CT scan. The boxers were significantly lower on three neuropsychological tests than a control group of orthopedic outpatients with limb fractures who were also administered the neuropsychological tests. In general, the boxers presented a neurological and neuropsychological profile less favorable than the average person but with appreciable variability. It should be pointed out that these 20 boxers probably had more fights than most American amateur boxers. Two of these British boxers had 200 fights and one had 140. Also, four of the boxers were over the age of 35 with one being 47.

Also relevant to the matter of amateur boxing is the study of Enzenauer and Enzenauer (1989) on boxing injuries in the U.S. Army from 1980 through 1985. During this period 272 (68%) of all 401 boxing injuries requiring hospitalization were head injuries. The head injuries admission diagnoses consisted of intracranial injury (not elsewhere classified), concussion/cerebral contusion, intracranial hemorrhage, skull fracture, fracture of the facial bones, ocular injuries (one necessitating enucleation), and head/neck contusion. There was one death from serious head injury. All of the head injuries listed above were not necessarily injuries to the brain. And, the authors did not provide neurological or neuropsychological test data for all of these head injured soldiers.

They did, however, tie their findings to the growing body of literature indicating permanent brain damage frequently resulting from boxing. They concluded: "When it was deemed that cigarette smoking offered a significant risk to health, cigarettes were no longer included in soldiers' C rations. When physical hazing was determined inappropriate behavior for future officers it was discontinued at the U.S. service academies. Perhaps military boxing, with its definite risks and arguable benefits, will suffer a similar fate" (p. 1466).

In the American Medical News of April 14, 1989, it was revealed that there is growing organizational opposition to boxing. Anti-boxing activists picketed boxing competition sponsored by Notre Dame University and the Tyson-Bruno heavyweight championship fight in Las Vegas. A collation of 242 groups that include the American Medical Association are asking the International Olympic Committee to drop boxing from future Olympic games. These opponents of boxing cite not only the brain damage it causes but the psychological effects upon both child and adult viewers in increasing hostility and willingness to injure other people.

Some states are attempting to protect participants from both acute injuries as well as the more subtle chronic effects of repeated blows to the head from boxing. Most utilize standard neurological examination, and EEG or CT scans. The State of California requires all licensed professional boxers to undergo an annual neurological exam which includes the neuropsychological tests most sensitive to "mental status." Over 1,400 examinations were administered in the 1987–1989 period. Preliminary results indicate that approximately 8% of the participants were showing significant cognitive impairment and were not licensed to box in California.

FOOTBALL AND RUGBY

Bruce, Schut, and Sutton (1982) reported that of the 746,893 injuries from sports in 1975 and 1976 in the United States, 325,957 (44%) were from football. There were 13 football fatalities recorded and only four fatalities in other contact sports. In high school football, about 10% of all injuries are concussions. Football accounts for 40% of all concussion injuries in school sports. Bruce et al. did say that incidence of serious head injuries decreased by about 60% in the last 20 years and this has probably been a function of better equipment.

In a survey regarding 3,064 football players in 103 Minnesota high schools following the 1977 season, 19 percent of the players suffered possible concussions as defined by loss of consciousness or loss of awareness or actual physician diagnoses of concussion. Of the players who suffered loss of consciousness, only 41% were examined by a coach and only 33% were examined by a physician. Sixty-five percent were returned to play the same day. Of the 3,036 football players, 97 experienced loss of unconsciousness, 223 loss of awareness, 464 headaches, 425 dizziness, 162 blurred vision, and 37 double vision that season. Of the players who had concussion symptoms at the time of the injury, 25 reported dizziness, 42 headaches, and 8 blurred vision six months after the injury. Gerberich, Priest, Boen, Straub, and Maxwell (1983) attributed many of the head injuries in their study to the illegal techniques of butt-blocking and face-tackling.

There were a total of 115 head injuries over a period of 8 years in 342 college football players at University of Iowa (Albright, McAuley, Martin, Crowley, & Foster, 1985). One hundred and three of these injuries involved less than 7 days lost time from football, five involved 7-20 days lost time, and seven of these injuries involved over 21 days lost time. In addition, two players were held out of action for a season and two other individuals were permanently restricted from football involvement. One of these permanently restricted players required 2 years to recover full cerebral function after diffuse brain injury. The other developed posttraumatic migraine headaches with aura and transient motor impairment. Players who received a second head injury in college football were apparently more affected by the second injury. The mean time lost was 2.31 days for the first injury and 4.89 days for the second injury. Those players who reported a high school head injury resulting in non-football participation for a day or more were more likley to have lost time for a college head injury, a phenomenon the authors interpreted as sensitization caused by earlier injury. The authors noted that there was a decrease in head injuries from 1977 to 1982. They attributed this to changes in the rules in regard to blocking and tackling, fewer injuries in high school of incoming freshmen that could make them more vulnerable to more serious head injuries, and possibly the fact that University of Iowa football has moved from a ground oriented offense to a more finesse oriented passing offensive.

Although the emphasis of this chapter is more on head injury survivors with deficit than on fatal head injuries, these fatalities do illustrate the severity of head injuries in sports. Gonzales (1951) reported 22 football deaths in New York City from 1918 to 1950. In four of these deaths there was hemorrhage and cerebral compression. Three were deaths from subdural hemorrhage without fracture, and in two of these cases compression symptoms developed shortly after the trauma. In the other case, the characteristics were of a secondary or slow hemorrhage. The player, who was kicked in the head and seemed normal except for intermittent headaches, after 2 weeks began to exhibit the signs of compression with headache, dizziness, vomiting, hemiparesis, and stupor deepening into coma. A large subdural hemorrhage was found at autopsy. The fourth player received a skull fracture and epidermal hemorrhage when he ran into a wall on one side of the field.

Maroon, Steele, and Berlin (1980) recommended that players with a mild concussion, which they described as alteration of consciousness or vision or equilibrium but no loss of consciousness, should be removed from the game for at least several plays. They said that under no circumstances should a mildly concussed player be permitted to resume play until he can move with his usual dexterity and speed, is perfectly oriented, and can answer all questions appropriately. Maroon et al. stated that a player who lost consciousness with complete recovery for five minutes should be removed from the game and should not engage in contact sports for at least several days and should not return if there are headaches or visual disturbances or any neurological abnormality. The authors maintained that players who were rendered unconscious for more than five minutes should be immediately hospitalized and be generally treated like a severely head injured patient. Maroon et al. are generally in agreement with the rule of thumb used by many physicians that three concussions of over five minutes unconsciousness should prohibit a player from playing football again. However, they also maintained that a concussion with structural damage as demonstrated by clinical examination or CT scan should also prohibit return to any contact sport.

Rugby is the sport played in Britain and other Commonwealth countries that is very similar to American football. (Incidentally, when the British say "football" they are usually referring to what Americans call "soccer.") In some respects, rugby is less "rough" than football, but this is offset by the fact that equipment is not worn in rugby. Bruce, Schut, and Sutton (1984) stated that half of all injuries, and almost 100 percent of serious injuries, to children and adolescents are from three collision sports—American football, rugby, and wrestling.

In the study of McKenna, Borman, Findlay, and deBoer (1986), rugby was clearly the sport that produced the most head injuries in New Zealand for all winter sports 1981–1982. Sixty-six percent of all 2,023 head injuries were due to rugby. Also, 45% of all rugby injuries were to the head. Seventeen percent of all rugby injuries were concussions. The authors recommended for sports generally, more widespread adoption of preventative measures by individuals and sporting organizations.

WRESTLING

Regua and Garrick (1981) determined the wrestling injury pattern in four high schools over a 2-year period. The 234 participants sustained 176 injuries for a rate of 75.2 injuries per 100 participants per season. The head injury rate was 2.6 per 100 participants per season. These consisted of 0.4 contusions, 0.4 fractures, 0.9 lacerations, and 0.9 "other." The article does not specify how many of the fractures and "other" injuries were associated with brain injury. Regua and Garrick stated there were no serious brain injuries. However, the authors of the present chapter urge caution in this regard because apparently mild concussions can have substantial residual.

HOCKEY

Pforringer and Smasal (1987) pointed out that hockey is the fastest nontechnical team sport with speeds up to 40 km. They interviewed 88 out of 125 players on six hockey teams in West Germany. The players had a history of 496 injuries, 246 (50%) of which were to the head. Of the 246 head injuries, 111 (45%) cases resulted from being struck with a hockey stick, 27 (11%) from being hit with a fist, and 48 (20%) were the result of a body check. The authors inferred that personal attack is the main reason for head injuries, although only five percent of these injuries included actual fighting. However, the reader should bear in mind that not all of the "head injuries" were necessarily brain injuries. The head injuries consisted of 174 (71%) split injuries, 35 (14%) fractures, 17 (7%) tooth lesions, 17 (7%) concussions, two (1%) eye injuries, and one (0.04%) ear lesion. The Pforringer and Smasal recommendations included more enforcement of the high stick and other rules, a tightly fitted helmet, and avoidance of returning to the game too soon.

Jorgensen and Schmidt-Olsen (1986) administered questionnaires to 210 Danish elite hockey players before the last match of the season. These men received a total of 189 injuries with 53 (14%) being concussions. Such concussions represented the most frequent injury but it received the least medical attention. Only eight percent of concussed players were seen by a physician, although 55 percent were seen by a physiotherapist. (The authors of this chapter have reservations about the adequacy of the training of physiotherapists for attending to a concussion.) Jorgensen and Schmidt-Olsen (1987) recommended stricter enforcement of the rules and making the helmet more shock absorbent.

CONCLUSION

For the most part, our generalizations regarding contact sports are the same as for the non-contact sports. Therefore, the synthesis and recommendations at the end of the non-contact sports chapter also apply to this chapter. However, we believe that the matter of head injuries for the contact sports has more psychological and social implications than the noncontact sports head injuries. This is because the latter may be regarded as accidental injuries, but contact sports injuries tend to less well fit the definition of accidental.

Although the wearing of helmets in sports constitutes a major part of our recommendations at the end of the Non-Contact Sports chapter, we do not at this time recommend helmets or added padding in the gloves for boxers. As the present objective of boxing is to render an opponent unconscious through blows to the head, any attempt to reduce the effectiveness of those blows is going to be controversial. More of a concern is the contention by some that added padding to the hands (gloves) and head (helmet) may actually increase the amount of damage sustained through repeated acceleration/deacceleration of the brain inside the skull. This unresolved argument proposes that the protection results in more blows being sustained with greater force before the hand gives out or the opponent is rendered unconscious. Short of a ban on boxing the most effective method of preventing severe cognitive deficits to boxers may be to limit their careers when early signs of brain impairment can be detected such as is currently being attempted in California. To be successful, such a program will have to be uniformly administered among states.

REFERENCES

Albright, J. P., McAuley, E., Martin, R. K., Crowley, E. T., & Foster, D. T. (1985). Head and neck injuries in college football: An eight-year analysis. *The American Journal of Sports Medicine, 13,* 147-152.

Atha, J., Yeadon, M. R. Sandover, J., & Parsons, K. C. (1985). The damaging punch. *British Medical Journal, 291,* 21-28.

Blonstein, J. L., & Clarke, E. (1954). Medical aspects of amateur boxing. *British Medical Journal, 1,* 1523-1525.

Blonstein, J. L., & Clarke, E. (1957). Further observations on the medical aspects of amateur boxing. *British Medical Journal, 1,* 362-364.

Bruce, D. A., Schut, L., & Sutton, L. N. (1982). Brain and cervical spine injuries occurring during organized sports activities in children and adolescents. *Clinics in Sports Medicine, 1,* 495-514.

Busse, E. W., & Silverman, A. J. (1952). Electroencephalographic changes in professional boxers. *Journal of the American Medical Association, 149,* 1522-1525.

Casson, I. R., Siegel, O., Sham, R., Campbell, E. A., Tarlau, M., & Didomenico, A. (1984). Brain damage in modern boxers. *Journal of the American Medical Association, 251,* 2663-2667.

Casson, I. R., Sham, R., Campbell, E. A., Tarlau, M., & Didomenico, A. (1982). Neurological and CT evaluation of knocked-out boxers. *Journal of Neurology, Neurosurgery, and Psychiatry, 45,* 170-174.

Corsellis, J. A. N., Bruton, C. J., & Freeman-Browne, D. (1973). The aftermath of boxing. *Psychological Medicine, 3,* 270-303.

Critchely, M. (1957). Medical aspects of boxing, particularly from a neurological standpoint. *British Medical Journal, 1*, 357-362.

Drew, R. H., Templer, D. I., Schuyler, B. A., Newell, T. G., & Cannon, W. G. (1986). Neuropsychological deficits in active licensed professional boxers. *Journal of Clinical Psychology, 42*, 520-525.

Enzenauer, R. W., & Enzenauer, R. J. (1989). Boxing-related injuries in the U.S. Army, 1980 through 1985. *Journal of the American Medical Association, 261*, 1463-1466.

Gerberich, S. G., Priest, J. D., Boen, J. R., Straub, C. P., & Maxwell, R. E. (1983). Concussion incidences and severity in secondary school varsity football players. *American Journal of Public Health, 73*, 1370-1375.

Gonzales, T. A. (1951). Fatal injuries in competitive sports. *Journal of the American Medical Association, 146*, 1506-1511.

Harvey, P. K. P., & Davis, J. N. (1974, October). Traumatic encephalopathy in a young boxer. *Lancet, 2*, 995-997.

Isherwood, I., Mawdsley, C., & Ferguson, F. R. (1966). Pneumoencephalographic changes in boxers. *Acta Radiologica: Diagnosis, 5*, 654-661.

Johnson, J. (1969). Organic psychosyndromes due to boxing. *British Journal of Psychiatry, 115*, 45-53.

Johnson, J. (1969). *The EEG in the traumatic encephalopathy of boxers.* Manchester, England: University Department of Psychiatry, Manchester Royal Infirmary.

Jordan, B. D., & Zimmerman, R. D. (1990). Computed tomography and magnetic resonance imaging comparisons in boxers. *Journal of the American Medical Association, 263*, 1670-1674.

Jorgensen, J., & Schmidt-Olsen, S. (1986). The epidemiology of ice hockey injuries. *British Journal of Sports Medicine, 20*, 7-9.

Kaplan, H. A., & Browder, J. (1954). Observations on the clinical and brain wave patterns of professional boxers. *Journal of the American Medical Association, 156*, 1138-1144.

Kaste, M., Kuurne, T., Vilkki, J., Katevuo, K., Santo, K., & Meurala, H. (1982). Is chronic brain damage in boxing a hazard of the past? *Lancet, 2*, 1186-1188.

Lampert, P. W., & Hardman, J. M. (1984). Morphological changes in brains of boxers. *Journal of the American Medical Association, 251*, 1676-1679.

Larsson, L. E., Melin, K. A., Nodstrom-Ohrberg, G., Silfverskiold, B. P., & Ohrberg, K. (1954). Acute head injuries in boxers. *Acta Psychiatrica Et Neurologica Scandinavica Supplementum, 95*, 1-42.

Lundberg, G. D. (1983). Boxing should be banned in civilized countries. *Journal of the American Medical Association, 249*, 250.

Maroon, J. C., Steele, P. B., & Berlin, R. (1980). Football head and neck injuries—an update. *Clinical Neurosurgery, 24*, 414-427.

Martland, H. S. (1928). Punch drunk. *Journal of the American Medical Association, 91*, 1103-1107.

Mawdsley, C., & Ferguson, F. R. (1963). Neurological disease in boxers. *The Lancet, 1*, 795-801.

McKenna, S., Borman, B., Findlay, J., & de Boer, M. (1986). Sports injuries in New Zealand. *New England Medical Journal, 99*, 899-901.

McLatchie, G., Brooks, N., Galbraith, S., Hutchinson, J. S. F., Wilson, L., Melville, I., & Teasdale, E. (1987). Clinical neurological examination, neuropsychology, electroencephalography and computer tomographic head scanning in active amateur boxers. *Journal of Neurology, Neurosurgery and Psychiatry, 50*, 96-99.

Millspaugh, J. A. (1937). Dementia pugilistica. *U.S. Navy Medical Journal, 35*, 297-303.

Moore, M. (1980). The challenge of boxing: Bringing safety into the ring. *The Physician and Sports Medicine, 8*, 101-105.

Moran, L. J., & Mefford, P. B., Jr. (1959). Repetitive psychometric measures. *Psychological Reports, 5*, 269–275.

Nesarajah, M. S., Seneviratne, K. N., & Watson, R. S. (1961). Electroencephalographic changes in Ceylonese boxers. *British Medical Journal, 1*, 866–868.

Neubuerger, K. T., Sinton, D. W., & Denst, J. (1959). Cerebral atrophy associated with boxing. *A.M.A. Archives of Neurology and Psychiatry, 81*, 403–408.

Parker, H. L. (1934). Traumatic encephalopathy ("punch drunk") of professional pugilists. *Journal of Neurology and Psychopathology, 15*, 20–28.

Payne, E. E. (1968). Brains of boxers. *Neurochirurgia, 11*, 173–189.

Pforringer, W., & Smasal, V. (1987). Aspects of traumatology in ice hockey. *Journal of Sports Sciences, 5*, 327–336.

Requa, R., & Garrick, J. G. (1981). Injuries in interscholastic wrestling. *The Physician and Sports Medicine, 9*, 44–51.

Roberts, A. H. (1969). *Brain damage in boxers.* London: Pitman Medical Scientific.

Ross, R. J., Monroe, C., Thompson, J., & Kim, K. H. (1983). Boxers-computed tomography, EEG, and neurological evaluation. *Journal of the American Medical Association, 249*, 211–213.

Sironi, V. A., & Ravagnati, L. (1983). Brain damage in boxers. *The Lancet, 1*, 244.

Spillane, J. D. (1962). Five boxers. *British Medical Journal, 2*, 1205–1210.

Temmes, Y., & Huhmar, E. (1962). Electro-encephalographic changes in boxers. *Acta Psychiatrica Neurologica Scandinavica, 27*, 175–180.

Thomassen, A., Jensen-Juul, P., Olivarius, B. F., Braemer, J., & Christensen, A. L. (1979). Neurological, electroencephalographic and neuropsychological examination of 53 former amateur boxers. *Acta Neurologica Scandinavica, 60*, 352–362.

CHAPTER 3

NONCONTACT SPORTS

Donald I. Templer and Richard H. Drew

The noncontact sports here included are soccer, mountain climbing, equestrian sports, aquatic sports, skiing, golf, and bicycling. This is not to say that all of these sports involve zero body contact. There is certainly some contact in soccer. Also, there is certainly competition in almost all sports. The winners "beat" the losers. More germane to the objectives of this book is the fact that brain damage occurs in these sports.

SOCCER

Soccer is the most widely played team sport in the world. It is rapidly gaining in popularity in the United States. Head injury in soccer can occur from one's head hitting the ground or by being struck by an opponent's head or elbow or boot or hand. Gunther (1974) reported that the more severe head injuries occur during head-on collisions caused by opposing players approaching the ball from opposite directions. However, the deliberate use of the head to propel an object is relatively unique to soccer. It is here parenthetically noted that a good heading in a soccer game draws great applause from the audience. It has been estimated that if a soccer player plays 300 games during his soccer career, he will receive about 2,000 blows to the head from heading (Tyswaer & Slorli, 1981).

It is often claimed that proper heading avoids all ill effects. However, in 10–15-minute demonstrations of proper heading by professionals, five of the 10 developed headaches (Matthews, 1972).

Ashworth (1985) reported three cases of soccer heading produced migraine attacks. Ashworth cited other authors who reported migraines caused by soccer (Matthews, 1972; Morris, 1972) and by a variety of head injuries (Haas, Pineda, & Lourie, 1975; Glesta, Mellinger, & Rooke, 1975; Greenblat, 1973). Typically, in these cases, the migraine onset is at the time of injury followed by a number of attacks over a long period of time. Ashworth stated that the mechanisms of minor head trauma producing migraine attacks are obscure, but he did suggest that some humoral agent is released by the trauma and provokes the attack in susceptible persons. He stated that some professional soccer players have to give up their sport because of migraine attacks.

Abreau (1989) administered the Raven Progressive Matrices, Symbol Digit Modalities Test, and the Paced Auditory Serial Addition Test to 31 collegiate soccer players and to 31 collegiate tennis players who comprised the control group. There were no significant differences between the two groups on these tests. There was, however, within the soccer player group, a significant negative correlation between number of games played and performance of the Paced Auditory Serial Addition Test. Also, a significantly greater number of soccer players than tennis players reported experiencing headaches, blurred vision, dizziness, and passing out after a game. Abreau tied these significant differences to the literature on mild head injury that indicates that such subjective state symptoms without impairment on neuropsychological tests which are less sensitive to very subtle brain damage effects.

Bruce, Schut, and Sutton's (1984) brief review of soccer stated that about five percent of professional soccer players receive a concussion in any given season. They stated that head injuries can occur in soccer from head-to-head contact, falls with the head hitting the ground, and the head being struck by the ball. Bruce et al. (1984) advised that coaches should not encourage children in heading the ball until the children are old enough to be instructed in the correct techniques of heading. (This sounds like good advice, but the present authors are far from certain that there are proper techniques of heading that can guarantee head injuries will not occur.)

In the New Zealand research of McKenna, Borman, Findlay, and de Boer (1986), soccer was the winter sport that contributed the second most head injuries. Thirty-three percent of soccer injuries were to the head.

Nilsson and Roaas (1978) reported on the injuries in the 1975 and 1977 "Norway Cup," an annual international soccer tournament for adolescents. In these two tournaments, 1,547 teams with 25,000 players took part in 2,987 matches. Fifty-four (10%) of the total 522 injuries were to the head and face. Among these were 10 cases of concussion, seven of which required hospitalization. Six of these concussed players were discharged from the hospital after one day and one was discharged after 5 days. The authors noted that there were a disproportionate extent of injuries in the final rounds and they suggested that fatigue could play a factor. They also noted that the girls had a much higher accident rate than the boys. They attributed this to the girls being less experienced in this traditionally male sport and to the fact that, whereas the boys had four age groups, the girls only had two so that some girls had to compete with girls much larger and more mature than themselves.

Pritchett (1981) analyzed 50 serious injuries from soccer covered by the largest insurance company that insures sports injuries in six western states. Six (12%) of these injuries were concussions. However, those concussions, as with the concussions reported by Nilsson and Roaas (1978), probably involved single hard blows to the head rather than deliberate and repeated "heading" of the ball that only recently is receiving attention as likely being injurious to the brain.

Kross, Ohler, and Barolin (1983) performed computerized EEG analyses in ten healthy soccer players after 15 minutes of header training. Eight of the 10 players manifested normal EEG's. However, the EEG of one player had seizure-like abnormality. Another player manifested a focal slowing EEG. The authors suggested that in predisposed persons the microtrauma caused by heading could lead to clinical manifestations.

MOUNTAIN CLIMBING

In mountain climbing, we have the unfortunate situation in which climactic conditions can produce brain dysfunctioning causing poor judgment and resulting injuries to various parts of the body including the head. McLennan and Ungersma (1983) reported that of 215 mountain climbing accidents in the Sierra Nevada mountains over a period of 5 years, 100 (47%) resulted from poor judgment. Of the 215 injuries, 12 (6%) were to the head. The hypoxia bringing about the poor judgment is caused from both the high altitude and the hypothermia. McLennan and Ungersma maintained that most climbers are totally unaware of the dangers of exposure at high altitudes. The authors pointed out that although Arctic explorers spend 3–10% of their day away from shelter, and soldiers spend 10–15% of their time away from shelter in nontactical situations, climbers are exposed to the elements during most of the daylight hours. They recommended that prospective climbers have a physical examination and participate in comprehensive training at least 2 months prior to a climbing trip. They recommended aerobic training to promote tolerance of oxygen deficiencies and isokinetic exercise to promote strength in the leg muscles. McLennan and Ungersma maintained that emergency rescue and treatment in the United States leave much to be desired compared to those in Europe.

Reid, Doyle, Richmond, and Galbraith (1986) reported on the necropsy findings of 42 persons who died in mountaineering accidents in Scotland. In 21 (50%) of these cases, brain injury was a major factor. Seventeen (47%) mountaineers had skull fractures. Twenty-eight (67%) had focal brain damage, 10 with hematomas and 18 with contusions and lacerations. Seventeen (40%) had diffuse brain damage with two cases of diffuse axonal injury, seven of brain swelling, three of hypoxic damage, and five of petechial hemorrhages. Only five (12%) of the mountaineers were wearing crash helmets. The authors offered the conjecture that some of the head injuries could have been prevented if a helmet of satisfactory construction had been worn. However, they said that although a helmet provides protection in glancing blows, it probably does not help in serious falls upon the head.

HORSEBACK RIDING

In the United States, horseback riding (what the British call "horse-riding") is less popular than in Britain and, consequently, associated accidents are less common in the United States. However, Bruce et al. (1984) reported that 66% of these accidents involve children and that 11% of such result in concussion. Their contention that whether or not the rider wears a helmet makes no difference does not support the recommendations of Lindsay, McLatchie, and Jennett (1980) given below. However, the authors of both articles report that horseback riding accidents tend to be more serious than most other sports accidents and are more likely to result in death. Bruce et al. stated that, as with other sports, one-third of injuries occur when no instructor is present. The most frequently occuring injury was that of being dragged by the horse with one foot stuck in the stirrup. Bruce recommended safe quick-release stirrups, more supervision during group riding, and encouraging precaution in children riding ponies.

Lindsay et al. (1980) reported that eight (15%) of 52 brain injuries from sports treated at a hospital in Scotland were from horse-riding. Lindsay et al. recommended that head gear be worn in horse-riding. These authors noted that in an unpublished report of Gleave in Cambridge, 32% of 600 sports brain injuries were from horse-riding. Barber (1973) reported that two-thirds of sports brain injuries to a hospital in England were from horse-riding.

Lloyd's (1987) study was based on 237 patients brought to a British hospital for horse-riding and other equestrian injuries. Such injuries constituted 4.3% of all sports-related injuries. Of these 237 patients, 50 (22%) were admitted to the hospital. Of these 50 patients, 25 (50%) had head injuries. Although most of the head injured persons were admitted after moderate or minor concussions, four head injuries were classified as major. In three of these four cases, the period of post-traumatic amnesia was prolonged beyond four days and in one there was an extradural hematoma that required surgery. Two patients had a skull fracture. In 43 (80%) of the total number of 54 head injuries the cause was a fall, in eight (15%) a kick, and in three (5%) an unknown cause. Lloyd had three safety recommendations. One was that the chin straps of the protective caps be properly used. The second was that the BS4472 cap approved by the British Standard Institute be used. The third was that of adequate supervision of young and inexperienced riders. Muwanga and Dove (1985) reported on 17 cases of horse-riding head injuries brought to a hospital in England. These 17 injuries represented 30% of the 56 sports injuries brought to that hospital in an 18-month period. One of the patients did not have his hat strapped on at the time but he was fortunate insofar as he did not sustain a skull fracture. Of the 16 horse riders with their hat strapped on, six of these had hats that became dislodged and three of them had skull fractures. Of the 10 riders whose hats did not become dislodged, three suffered skull fractures. Although these two proportions did not differ significantly, the authors cautioned about inadequate fixation of the hat. They went on to say that in Britain it is common to see riders with the straps unfastened and that one type of hat has clips on the side to keep the straps up.

AQUATIC SPORTS

Heiser and Kettrcik (1982) pointed out that over 7,000 persons die annually in the United States from drowning. However, 89% of individuals hospitalized for near drowning survive. Heiser and Kettrcik stated that "Permanent and encephalopathic changes are perhaps the most devastating sequelae of the near drowning event" (p. 416). They said that poor neurological outcome tends to be associated with continued need for cardiopulmonary resuscitation on arrival at the hospital, being in a coma, having a pH of less than seven, and requiring mechanical ventilation. The preventive measures of Heiser and Kettrcik are associated with the epidemiology of drowning. Intoxication is often involved in the drowning of adults. In younger adults and adolescents, drownings are often associated with activities reflective of braggadocio, boasting or showing off. The highest incidence of drowning is in the second decade of life. Residential pools are especially dangerous to young children. Half of all who drown in swimming pools are under 10 years of age. Most drownings occur in the summer months. The authors recommended parental and life guard vigilance in addition to the avoidance of areas that are dangerous to the swimmer. Management of the victim, to prevent death and to prevent or lessen brain damage, should focus upon reestablishment of oxygen to the brain.

When one adds together fishermen, fisherwomen, swimmers, divers, scuba divers, deep sea divers, boaters, boat racers, water skiers, and canoeists, we are talking about tens of millions of people in the United States alone that participate in water sports and recreations. Added to these persons at risk of drowning or suffering near-drowning experiences, are the many persons who earn their living on the water such as commercial fishermen, fishing guides, lifeguards, marine scientists, coast guard personnel, and military personnel.

In an article focusing upon spinal cord injury from diving, Albrand and Walker (1975) said all 13 injured divers they studied also received a head injury and 12 of the 13 lost consciousness. The authors recommended that safe-depth requirements should be reevaluated, that public education be carried out, that the fact that some rivers and lakes and reservoirs have shifting depths should be pointed out, and that diving in above ground pools should be prohibited. Albrand and Walker said, "Perhaps the greatest tragedy comes from the diving board in our back yard swimming pools where one can easily overshoot the deep end and project the body into the shallow water" (p. 462).

SKIING

Sherry (1984) reported that of the 1,850 skiing injuries in a recent year in Australia, 17% were to the head/face/neck regions. They did not specify how many of these were brain injuries, but they did say that three percent of all injuries were concussions. Sherry recommended that all skiers wear ski helmets.

GOLF

We hesitated to put a section in this book on golf because we were afraid our fellow Americans would laugh at us. However, in research by Lindsay, McLatchie, and Jennett (1980) 14 (27%) of 52 head injuries through sports seen in a Scottish hospital were from golf. Such a high injury rate from golf probably reflects both the popularity of that sport in Scotland and it being a more dangerous sport than most people realize. Thirteen of the 14 golf injuries were depressed fractures. All but one of the golf injuries were in children under 16 years of age with a mean age of 10. Thirteen of the injuries resulted from being hit by a club and one by a ball. Lindsay et al. said, "The age range of golf club injuries suggests that youngsters should be forewarned of the need to stand well clear when others are wielding golf clubs" (pp. 789–790).

BICYCLING

Only a small fraction of bicycle injuries occur in bicycle racing. However, we are here using sport in a broad sense to include recreation and exercise. It is further acknowledged that in many accidents the bicycle was used in more of a transportation sense than for sport or recreation or exercise. Nevertheless, it was decided to include bicycling because of the very large number of head injuries in the huge number of people who ride bicycles. Head injuries from bicycle riding almost deserves a chapter of its own. It has been estimated that there are now more than 100 million bicycle riders in the United States, and almost half a million accidents a year requiring emergency room visits, and about a thousand fatalities a year (Selbst, Alexander, & Ruddy, 1987; Betz, 1983).

Selbst et al. (1987) determined the epidemiology of the 520 bicycle injuries presenting at The Children's Hospital in Philadelphia from April 1 to October 1 of 1983. Seventy percent of the patients were male. Eighty-four percent of accidents occurred less than five blocks from home. In 36% of the accidents, the patients admitted stunt riding or going too fast. In 36% of the cases, there was a problem with the surface on which they were riding, in 45% of the cases the patient lost control of the bicycle, in 17% the bicycle was hit by a car, and in 10%

a pedestrian was hit by a bicycle. The head or neck was injured in 31% of the cases. The authors did not specify how many of the 31% of cases of head and neck injury involved injury to the brain. However, they did report that 3% of the total cases had a primary diagnosis of concussion. Only three of the 520 children included in the study had head protection equipment on at the time of the accident. The authors recommended that classroom time be devoted to bicycle safety, that posters and reading material on bicycle safety be employed, and that parents and pediatricians should lobby for legislation that mandates helmet use for children riding bicycles.

A study of bicycle injuries in Massachusetts yielded quite similar epidemiological findings as the above study conducted in Philadelphia. Friede, Azzara, Gallagher, and Guyer (1985) also reported that for 573 bicycle injuries 36 (6.3%) involved cerebral injury with 20 concussions, one contusion, and one unspecified injury. They incorporated their findings into a greater context of studies that found head injuries even more salient than in their own study. Forty-nine percent of bicycle injuries brought to a children's hospital in England involved injuries above the necks (Illingsworth, Noble, & Ball, 1981). In a Swedish study head injury was the primary diagnosis in 59% of all injuries requiring hospital admission, and 76% of pediatric bicycle deaths (Thorson, 1974). In a Canadian study, 67% of injured patients had craniocerebral trauma. In an autopsy study in Florida, 81% of deaths had craniocerebral trauma (Guichon & Mules, 1975).

Friede et al. recommended the use of helmets, educational programs, a larger educational role for the pediatrician, greater enforcement of laws, and changes in riding environment. The authors acknowledged that the enforcement of existing bicycle laws has never been popular and that police officers are reluctant to give citations to either children or adults. However, they expressed a favorable opinion about the policy in some states in which violators have to attend a bicycle safety school. They recommended that bicyclists be afforded places of their own to ride that are separated both from pedestrians and from motorized vehicles. They noted that such changes have already been incorporated in the Scandinavian countries with apparently favorable results. They warned of the dangers of alcohol to child and adult bicycle riders and cited a study in Florida in which nine of 31 adult bicycle riders who were fatally injured had elevated blood alcohol concentrations (Fife, Davis, & Tate, 1983).

Wasserman, Waller, Monty, Emery, and Robinson (1988) interviewed 516 bicyclists over the age of 10, with 58% being over the age of 20. Only 19% of the bicyclists owned helmets, and only 8% were wearing helmets at the time of the interview. Riders wearing helmets tended to be more educated, to report car seat belt use, to believe in personal susceptibility to head injury, and to regard head injuries as a serious matter. Twenty-one (4%) of the interviewees struck their head in the past 18 months, and seven of the persons reported sustaining a head injury, with three of these being concussions. Of the 21 bicyclists who reported striking their heads, eight reported wearing helmets and 13 not wearing them.

None of those wearing helmets reported a head injury, but seven of the unhelmeted did. The conclusion of the authors was the very reasonable one that more bicycle riders should wear helmets.

In one study the hospital records in Madison, Wisconsin showed 187 cases of head injury of adult bicycle riders during the fair weather months of 1981–1984 (Belongia, Weiss, Bowman, & Rattanassiri, 1988). Thirty-three percent of the cases consisted of injuries of moderate severity, and 3% of the injuries were severe or life threatening. Thirty-two percent of the patients had evidence of brain injury. Of these patients, 93 percent had a concussion and 7% had an abnormal CT scan. One hundred and four of the respondents were contacted by letters and phone calls, and it was found that most of the serious injuries took place on dry road conditions and in daylight hours and did not involve motor vehicles. Only one of the 104 respondents was wearing a helmet at the time. Our readers can probably guess the recommendation of Belongia et al.—that helmets be worn.

Lind and Wollin (1986) began their article by informing the reader that from 70 to 120 bicyclists are killed in accidents each year and that such represents 10–15% of all traffic fatalities. Twenty to thirty percent of all bicycle accidents in Sweden are related to alcohol consumption, especially among young men bicycling in evening or night hours. For the data that Lind and Wollin analyzed, 61% of the police reported accidents and 39 of nonreported accidents were to the head or face in Sweden. The authors estimated that in 70% of head injuries the injury would have been prevented or lessened if a helmet had been used. Other preventative measures recommended by Lind and Wollin were information campaigns through schools and sports associations and cycling clubs and insurance companies, discouraging children younger than 13 and elderly adults from bicycling in heavy traffic, the strict adherence to traffic regulations, proper road maintenance, and encouraging the sellers of bicycles to stock good-quality bicycles equipped with headlamps and red rear light and reflectors, and good brakes.

There are an increasing number of injuries that parallel the increasing use of bicycle mounted child seats. Sargent, Peck, and Weitzman (1988) reported that of 52 such injuries in California, 22 (42%) were head injuries. Of these 22 head injuries, four were concussion, one internal organ injury, one fracture, one hematoma, two lacerations, and 12 contusions and abrasions. Forty-two percent of the 52 accidents involved the bicycle crashing or tipping over. Twenty-five percent occurred when the child slipped out of the seat.

SYNTHESIS AND RECOMMENDATIONS

What generalizations can be made about which categories of sports are most dangerous to the brain? Contact sports such as boxing, wrestling, football, rugby, hockey, and soccer obviously provide a high risk of brain damage. Sports that have devices for fast locomotion (hockey, skiing, equestrian sports, bicycling, auto racing) contain a high risk. Sports in which there is a danger of falling from a high place, such as diving, mountain climbing, equestrian sports, and skiing, are at a higher risk than those that are played with both feet on level ground. Sports that involve a ball or some type of hard or large projectile such as soccer, baseball, and golf provide higher risk than sports that do not provide such. The sports in which some sort of instrument is wielded such as a golf club or hockey stick or baseball bat have an associated risk of head injury.

The authors believe that the prophylactic recommendations of the various articles concerning various sports are reasonable ones. The following are our recommendations regarding safety precautions over a wide range of sports.

1. Helmets should be worn in most sports, including football, baseball, wrestling, golf, bicycling, horseback riding, skiing, automobile racing, soccer, rugby, mountain climbing, parachute jumping, roller skating, ice skating, judo, and karate. A corollary of our recommendation is that the most protective helmets possible be purchased. However, this is not a simple matter since, as emphasized by Norman (1983) in a review of biomechanical evaluation of sport protective equipment, different investigators have different opinions about the safety of different helmets. Different methods are used in testing the various helmets. These methods differ both in the object, e.g. dummy or cadaver, that receives the blow and the various physical characteristics of the blow. Norman lamented the fact that much of the available safety equipment has not been tested at all and/or the testing results have not been reported in refereed journals. Norman recommended legislation to require manufacturers to document the safety of the instruments they advertise as being safe. He also suggested a tax on each piece of safety equipment sold by companies who cannot document the safety of their equipment, and that such a tax could be used for the testing of equipment.

2. Children and adolescents and beginning participants in a sport should receive good instruction and close supervision. Those doing the instructing and supervision should have a good knowledge of safety procedures and associated hazards.

3. Athletes should be well conditioned for their sport. Fatigue and less than optimal fitness have been mentioned as contributory factors by a number of our authors.

4. Following a head injury, great caution should be exercised before allowing the athlete to resume participation in his or her sport.

5. Participants, parents of participants, and schools and other institutions that sponsor the more dangerous sports, should give serious reflection upon whether or not the benefits balance the associated risks. Such cost analyses should include not only brain injury but injuries to all parts of the body, including the spinal cord. Are a few minutes of glory on a high school football field worth spending the rest of one's life in a wheelchair?

6. Our sixth and last recommendation, which is related to our fifth recommendation, is for a constructive philosophy that makes sports enrich and refresh rather than dominate and dehabilitate our lives. Although the following paragraph from Bruce et al. (1984) pertains primarily to sports played by children and adolescents, we believe it embodies an attitude that is healthy for the mind and healthy for the body, including the health of the brain.

> One further caution is that the teenage athlete is not a pawn to be used by a coach to produce a winning season. Sports activities are designed to produce healthy minds and bodies and when the result of such activity is catastrophic impairment of health, no excuse is acceptable. This leads to a final problem that of forced participation in collision sports. It is clearly unacceptable to allow school aged children to be forced to participate in a sport that has a significant risk of death or severe neurologic damage. No support can or should be given by the medical profession to schools forcing participation of pupils in football, rugby, or wrestling. The role of the pediatrician and the neurologic specialist in the prevention of sports accidents is a significant one. It should be routine at each preschool physical to ask the child about sports injuries, especially concussion or spinal cord or neck injury. Any such injuries may require follow-up with further investigation. In the overall framework of the child's life, organized sports activities are safe and should be encouraged. Stricter concern for the athlete's safety, however, and application of the principles that have been outlined should lead to even greater safety and more enjoyable competition for the school aged athlete. (p. 914)

REFERENCES

Abreau, F. (1989). Psychological assessment of attention and concentration in soccer players [Dissertation]. California School of Professional Psychology–Fresno, CA.

Albrand, O. W., & Walter, J. (1975). Underwater deceleration curves in relation to injuries from diving. *Surgical Neurological, 4*, 461–464.

Ashworth, B. (1985). Migraine, head trauma and sports. *Scottish Medical Journal, 30*, 240–242.

Barber, H. M. (1973). Horse play: a survey of accidents with horse. *British Medical Journal, 3*, 532–534.

Belongia, E., Weiss, H., Bowman, M., & Rattanassiri, P. (1988). Severity and types of head trauma among adult bicycle riders. *Wisconsin Medical Journal, 87*, 11–14.

Betz, C. L. (1983). Bicycle safety: Opportunities for family education. *Pediatric Nurses, 9*, 109–111.

Bruce, D. A., Schut, L., & Sutton, L. N. (1984). Brain and cervical spine injuries occurring during organized sports activities in children and adolescents. *Primary Care, 11*, 175–194.

Fife, D., Davis, L., Tate, L., Wells, J. R., Mohan, D., Williams, A. (1983). Fatal injuries to bicyclists: The experience of Dade County, Florida. *Journal of Trauma, 23*, 745–755.

Friede, A. M., Azzara, C. V., Gallagher, S. S., & Guyer, B. (1985). The epidemiology of injuries to bicycle riders. *Pediatric Clinics of North American, 32*, 141–151.

Glesta, G. G., Mellinger, J. F., & Rooke, E. D. (1975). Familial hemiplegic migraine. *Mayo Clinic Proceedings, 50*, 307-311.

Greenblat, S. H. (1973). Post traumatic transient cerebral blindness. *Journal of American Medical Association, 225*, 1073-1076.

Guichon, D. M., & Mules, J. T. (1975). Bicycle injuries: One-year sample in Calgary. *Journal of Trauma, 15*, 504-506.

Gunther, S. F. (1974). An avoidable soccer injury. *Journal of Sports Medicine, 2*, 167-169.

Hass, D. C., Pineda, G. A., & Lourie, H. (1975). Juvenile head trauma syndromes and their relationship to migraine. *Archives of Neurology, 32*, 727-730.

Heiser, M. S., & Kettrcik, R. G. (1982). Management of the drowning victim. *Clinics in Sports Medicine, 1*, 409-417.

Illingsworth, C. M., Noble, D., Bell, D. et al. (1981). 150 bicycle injuries in children: a comparison with accidents due to other causes. *Injury: The British Journal of Accident Surgery, 13*, 7-9.

Kross, R., Ohler, K., & Barolin, G. S. (1983). Balleinwirkung auf den kopf-eine quantifizie-rende EEG-untersuchung bel fussballern. *Zeitschrift EEG-EMG, 14*, 209-212.

Lind, M. G., & Wollin, S. (1986). Bicycle accidents. *ACTA Chirurgia Scandinavca Supplementum, 531*, 1-47.

Lindsay, K. W., McLatchie, G., & Jennett, B. (1980). Serious head injury in sport. *British Medical Journal, 281*, 789-791.

Lloyd, R. G. (1987). Riding injuries and other equestrian injuries: considerable severity. *British Journal of Sports Medicine, 21*, 22-24.

Matthews, W. B. (1972). Footballer's migraine. *British Medical Journal, 2*, 326-327.

McKenna, S., Borman, B., Findlay, J., & de Boer, M. (1986). Sports injuries in New Zealand. *New England Medical Journal, 99*, 899-901.

Morris, A. M. (1972). Footballer's migraine. *British Medical Journal, 2*, 769-770.

Muwanga, L. C., & Dove, A. F. (1985). Head protection for horse riders: A cause for concern. *Archives of Emergency Medicine, 2*, 85-87.

Nilsson, S., & Roaas, A. (1978). Soccer injuries in adolescents. *The American Journal of Sports Medicine, 6*, 358-361.

Norman, R. W. (1983). Biochemical evaluations of sports protective equipment. In R. L. Tergun (Eds.), *Exercise and sport sciences reviews, vol. 11*, (pp. 232-274). Philadelphia: The Franklin Institute Press.

Pritchett, J. W. (1981). Cost of high school soccer injuries. *The American Journal of Sports Medicine, 9*, 64-66.

Reid, W. A., Doyle, D., Richmond, H. G., & Galbraith, S. L. (1986). Necropsy study of mountaineering accidents in Scotland. *Journal of Clinical Pathology, 39*, 1217-1220.

Sargent, J. D., Peck, M. G., & Weitzman, M. (1988). Bicycle-mounted child seats. *American Journal of Diseases of Children, 142*, 765.

Selbst, S. M., Alexander, D., & Ruddy, R. (1987). Bicycle-related injuries. *American Journal of Diseases of Children, 141*, 140-144.

Sherry, E. (1984). Skiing injuries in Australia. *Medical Journal of Australia, 140*, 530-531.

Thorson, J. (1974). Pedal-cycle accidents. *Scandinavian Journal of Social Medicine, 2*, 121-128.

Tyswaer, A., & Stroli, O. (1981). Association football injuries to the brain: A preliminary report. *British Journal of Sports Medicine, 6*, 267.

Wasserman, R. C., Waller, J. A., Monty, M., Emery, A. B., & Robinson, D. R. (1988). Bicyclists, helmets, and head injuries: A rider-based study of helmet use and effectiveness. *American Journal of Public Health, 78*, 1220-1221.

CHAPTER 4

ACCIDENTAL INJURIES OF CHILDREN

William G. Miller and Frank D. Miller

Injuries among children and adolescents exceed all other diseases as causes of disability and death (Baker, O'Neill, & Karpf, 1984). This fact has been recognized for the past 40 years (Gordon, 1949). Injuries cause approximately 44% of all deaths in children ages 1-4, 51% at ages 5-9, and 58% at ages 10-14 (Waller, Baker, & Szocka, 1989). The National Academy of Sciences has stated: Injury is the principal public health problem in America today; it affects primarily the young and will touch one of every three Americans this year (National Academy of Sciences, 1985).

Despite the frequency of unintentional injuries, there is a relative paucity of national data on medical costs and morbidity. Some rough estimates suggest that over 25% of all emergency department or hospital clinic visits are for the treatment of injuries. For every 1,000 children, there will be approximately 200 emergency department visits each year for injuries (Gallagher, Finison, Guyer, & Goodenough, 1984).

Depending upon the geographical region, the socioeconomic status, and the age group selected for study, some of the leading causes of injury, death, and disability in children are motor vehicle occupancy in an accident, being hit by a vehicle as a pedestrian, bicycle accidents, falls, drowning, house fires, homicides, recreational activities, and competitive sports (Rivara, Calonge, & Thompson, 1989; Waller, Baker, & Szocka, 1989). The largest proportion of injury deaths among adolescents is associated with motor vehicles (Runyan & Gerken, 1989). Adolescents also are disproportionately responsible for the deaths of other nonadolescent drivers, passengers, and pedestrians (Williams, 1985).

This chapter will focus largely on accidents involving motor vehicles, bicyclists, falls, all-terrain vehicles (ATVs), and playground injuries. Child abuse and violence will be discussed in chapter five and sports injuries have been addressed in the preceding two chapters.

INCIDENCE OF HEAD INJURY

Among childhood injuries, head trauma is a major cause of morbidity and mortality. Each year about 100,000 children younger than 15 years of age are admitted to U.S. hospitals and about 90% of these admissions are for mild head injury (Kraus, Fife, & Conroy, 1987). Other studies suggest that 1 million children in the U.S. sustain head injuries each year and that one-sixth of these cases are admitted to hospitals (Eiben et al., 1984).

Age-specific rates for boys increase steadily from about 150 to 200 per 100,000 for those under 5 years of age to greater than 400 per 100,000 for those age 15 years (Klauber, Barrett-Connor, Marshall, & Bowers, 1978). For girls, the rates for those under five years of age ranged from 100 to 170 per 100,000. The rates rose to over 300 per 100,000 for 15-year-old girls (Klauber, Barrett-Conner, Marshall, & Bowers, 1981). Rates for males are consistently about twice as great as for females at all ages, and males tend to have more severe head injury (Annegers, 1983). It has been estimated that the cumulative risk for children through age 15 is 4% for boys and 2.5% for girls (Rivara & Mueller, 1986).

Although the incidence of head injury is generally higher in childhood than at other periods in lifespan, mortality is lower. There are about 10–20 deaths per 100,000 for children under 15 years of age (Rivara & Mueller, 1986). However, some investigators estimate that head injury accounts for approximately 43% of all deaths in children aged five to nine years (Klauber, Marshall, & Toole, 1985).

Injury and death rates may vary also by race and socioeconomic level. The incidence of head injury among nonwhites is nearly 50% higher than among whites (Rivara & Mueller, 1986). Whitman, Coonley-Hoganson, and Desai (1984) compared head injury rates by race in two socioeconomically different areas in Illinois and reported rates for inner city Blacks were slightly higher than those for Blacks living in suburban areas. Rates for suburban Blacks, however, were higher than those for suburban whites. However, Klauber and colleagues (1986) conducted a telephone survey of injuries, including head injuries, and found that education and income of parents were unrelated to the incidence of head injury.

Severity of Injury

The degree of severity of head injury has been lumped into three overlapping categories of mild, moderate, and severe. Kraus and colleagues (1986) classified the severity of head injury according to the Glasgow Coma Scale (GCS) in their San Diego study. Teasdale and Jennett (1974) had developed the GCS to evaluate three components of wakefulness (eye opening, motor response, and verbal response) independently of each other. Coma was defined as the absence of eye opening, inability to obey commands, and failure to utter recognizable words. This definition corresponds to a total GCS score of eight or less (out of a possible

15 points) and is an important watershed because patients with such scores are regarded as having had a "severe" injury (Miller, 1986).

In the San Diego study (Kraus, Fife, Cox, Ramstein, & Conroy, 1986) of 688 children, 606, or 88% had a *mild* brain injury (GCS score 9-15; no intracranial surgery, no abnormal computed tomography (CT) findings, and in hospital less than 48 hours); 46, or 7%, had a *moderate* brain injury (GCS score 9-12; hospitalization longer than 48 hours, intracranial surgery and/or abnormal CT); and 36, or 5% had a *severe* brain injury (GCS score ≤8). The criteria used by Kraus and colleagues for mild injury encompassed a more impaired level of consciousness when compared with other studies (Levin et al., 1988).

Kraus et al. (1986) found that falls were the major cause of injury in children four years and under, whereas recreational activities and motor vehicle accidents accounted for most of the injuries in older children and adolescents. In addition, they found that the incidence of head injury in children reached a peak during the spring and summer months, particularly for bicycle-related injuries. Finally, these authors noted that after the age of 14, there was a significant rise in the percentage of severe injury cases.

Procedures to assess posttraumatic amnesia (PTA) in children have only recently been developed and need refinement pending additional studies of orientation in normal children (Levin, Ewing-Cobbs, & Flethcer, 1989). PTA in adults refers to the time between injury and the recovery of continuous memory. In children, it is somewhat more difficult to establish when full memory for day-to-day events is recovered.

When compared to closed head injury in adults, children differ somewhat with respect to the etiology and the pathophysiology of brain injury (Kraus et al., 1986). Falls are low-velocity injuries and contribute significantly to head injury in young children. Motor vehicle injuries, on the other hand, involve greater acceleration/deceleration forces to the head (Gurdjian, 1971). Intracranial mass lesions are common in older children and adolescents. Investigators have suggested that there are distinctive pathophysiological features of head injury in children, including delayed deterioration in consciousness (Snoek, Minderhoud, & Wilmink, 1984), and more frequent diffuse brain swelling (Bruce, Schut, Bruno, Wood, & Sutton, 1978). Skull fractures are extremely common in infants and small children (Choux, 1986). In addition, assessment of level of consciousness is a more difficult task with infants and young children, and investigators may rely on motor cues rather than "following" verbal commands (Raimondi & Hirschaver, 1984). Vocalizations or cries constitute the ceiling of the verbal portion of the Children's Coma Scale for infants (Raimondi & Hirschaver, 1984).

Kalsbeek et al. (1980) have noted that coma after a head injury secondary to a fall is likely to result in brain compression due to intracranial hematoma. Coma produced by a head injury secondary to a motor vehicle accident is more often due to severe brain damage from acceleration/deceleration forces. Different causal agents produce different complications even when scores on indices such as the GCS are equated (Goldstein & Levin, 1987).

Estimates of severity based on levels of consciousness may vary from six hours to more than seven days of unconsciousness for a *severe* injury (Jennett & Teasdale, 1981). Moderate injury is often defined by exclusion from mild or severe categories. No category such as PROFOUND injury exists for patients who remain unconscious for months. Thus, there is no absolute measure for what constitutes a "severe" injury. Much of the material in this chapter will focus on mild head injuries.

Early Effects of Mild Head Injury

The term "early" refers to findings obtained during initial hospitalization or shortly after discharge. Levin and Eisenberg (1979a) studied children following closed head injury of varying severity, including 14 children 6–12 years of age and 24 adolescents 13–18 years of age. Although these patients had brief or no loss of consciousness and were following commands on admission to the hospital, three children and three adolescents who had computed tomography (CT) had abnormal scans. These preliminary data suggest that cerebral swelling or focal lesions may be present in about one-third of the cases and raise the possibility of performing CTs on all pediatric cases of head injury (Levin, Ewing-Cobbs, & Fletcher, 1989).

Levin and Eisenberg (1979a, b) administered tests to 38 patients to measure the domains of language, visuospatial function, memory, somatosensory function, and motor speed. A neuropsychological deficit was inferred from a score falling two or more standard deviations below the mean for normal children of the same age. For the children age 6–12 years and for the mildly injured adolescents, there were deficits in all areas. Memory deficit was the most frequent neuropsychological residual in severely injured children and adolescents. In the absence of follow-up assessment and the lack of a comparison group, implications of this study for the long-term sequelae of mild head injury are uncertain.

Long-Term Sequelae of Head Injury

In general, the outcome of mild head injury in children has been studied for comparison with severe head injury and has not been the primary focus of inquiry (Rutter, 1982). Rutter et al. (Brown, Chadwick, Shaffer, Rutter, & Troub, 1981; Chadwick, Rutter, Brown, Shaffer, & Troub, 1981; Rutter, Chadwick, Shaffer, & Brown, 1980) found that the mild head injury group had more preexisting school adjustment problems and below average school achievement. Further, boys comprised three-fourths of the mild injury group and were more likely to have had a socially disadvantaged background. Head-injured children, at least in this study in London, are not representative of the pediatric population with respect to psychosocial variables. These studies demonstrate the need to screen for preexisting psychosocial difficulties.

Levin and Benton (1986) reported on scholastic achievement data for children and adolescents who were tested about six months postinjury. The authors excluded children with a preinjury history of a learning disorder or psychiatric problem. Age-percentile reading recognition scores on the Wide-Range Achievement Test (WRAT) were at the average level for both mild-to-moderate and severe head-injured groups. Arithmetic scores, however, fell below reading scores in both groups. The authors attributed this finding to the demands of timed calculation on attention and to information processing speed.

Bawden, Knights, and Winogron (1985), in a study of head injury in children, ages 2.5–17 years, found that the mildly injured children had scores within the average range on the Wechsler Intelligence Scale for Children-Revised (WISC-R), and clearly above the results obtained in severely injured patients. The authors conclude that the mildly injured children recover to within the average range of intelligence. However, there was no control group in this study.

Contrary to the impression of essentially complete recovery after mild head injury, Gulbrandsen (1984), in a study of children ages 9–13 years at injury and tested 4–6 months postinjury, found evidence of neuropsychological deficits with the Reitan-Indiana Neuropsychological Battery. Procedures involving complex sensorimotor integration accounted for most of the impairment.

Levin, High, Ewing-Cobbs, Fletcher, Eisenberg, Miner, and Goldstein (1988) studied three age ranges of pediatric patients with head injuries (6–8, 9–12, and 13–15 years) following resolution of posttraumatic amnesia and one year postinjury using the Selective Reminding Test and the Continuous Recognition Memory Test. The results provided no convincing evidence of persistent memory deficits after mild-to-moderate head injury. However, the severely injured patients manifested deficits.

In a review of the research literature on severe head injury in children, Ewing-Cobbs, Fletcher, and Levin (1985) suggest that cognitive impairment persists despite impressive resolution of focal motor and sensory deficits, and the resumption of daily activities. Persistent intellectual, academic, language, and memory problems are encountered by children after severe head injury. The available data did not permit evaluation of the effect of head injury on cognitive skills at different age periods. However, the authors' considerable combined experience suggests that the type of deficits often vary with age. Preschoolers typically exhibit generalized cognitive impairment, including attentional, motor, intellectual, linguistic, and visuospatial disturbances. In school-age children and adolescents, memory, visuomotor, and attentional difficulties are predominant. Adolescents often exhibit problems with later-developing functions such as planning, social judgment, and use of strategies. Additional research is needed on age-related factors.

Fletcher and Levin (1988) stated that closed head injury in children is associated with major sequelae on performance-based intelligence tests, speeded motoric abilities, memory and attentional skills, and behavioral adjustment.

The latter problem, behavioral adjustment, is frequently mentioned by caretakers and practitioners, but has been the focus of only a few studies. Hartlage (1986) found that head-injured children presented significant changes from preinjury status, including agitation, absent-mindedness, complaining, confusion, forgetfulness, short-temper, and slow-thinking.

Brown, Chadwick, Shaffer, Rutter, and Traub (1981), as noted earlier, found that the mild head-injured children in their study had a higher rate of preinjury behavioral problems than did the severe head injury or the orthopedically injured groups. However, by 2 years postinjury, the rate of behavioral disturbances was three times higher in the severe head injury group than in the other two groups. The study is flawed, however, by the failure to exclude children with antecedent behavioral problems.

In a longitudinal study of 45 children, ages 3-15 years, with mild, moderate, and severe head injuries, Fletcher, Ewing-Cobbs, Miner, Levin, and Eisenberg (1990), concluded that severe head injury is associated with declines in adaptive functioning, but children with mild-to-moderate injuries did not deviate from average levels at any follow-up interval (time of injury, and 6 and 12 months postinjury). This study was based on parent report on two measures of behavioral adjustment, the Child Behavior Checklist and the Vineland Adaptive Behavior Scales. Children with previous head injuries, congenital CNS insults, previous psychological disorder, documented history of abuse or neglect, or evidence of a learning disorder or developmental disability were excluded from the study. The mechanism of injury was consistent with epidemiological studies of pediatric head injury (Annegers, 1983) with a predominance of injuries secondary to falls in the mild group and motor vehicle-related accidents in the severe group. The findings are important because of the absence of evidence linking screened mild head injury cases to behavioral changes beyond three months postinjury and the implication that the effects of head injury on behavioral and cognitive functioning may be somewhat independent.

At Risk for Second Injury

There has been conflicting reports in the literature as to whether children who sustain head injuries are at greater risk for a second injury. Early reports by Partington (1960) and Jamison and Kaye (1974) did not find a greater frequency of previous injury in their samples. However, more recent work by Annegers and colleagues (1980) suggests that the relative risk for a second head injury is age related. Expected incidence rates doubled after a head injury sustained in children under 14 years, tripled through ages 15-24, and was five times the expected rate after age 25. Boys with head trauma have a two-fold risk of subsequent head injury (Annegers, 1983). Increased risk of a second injury is nearly as great in girls. It remains unclear whether the increased risk is a kind of accident proneness, a consequence of the initial injury (slowed reaction times or cognitive changes), the development of behavior patterns, or environmental agents.

PREVENTION

Although medical care for head injuries has improved immensely in the past 20 years, the number of children who sustain serious injury or who die is not likely to decrease solely because of better medical technology. Many persons who die of head injury do so before reaching a hospital center (Rivara & Mueller, 1986). Prevention appears to be of utmost importance.

The most successful injury prevention strategies are passive in nature, that is, agents, vehicles, or environments are changed to protect the population at risk (Robertson, 1983). Airbags, for example, are passive, whereas manual seat belts are active. Active devices requiring some manipulation by the individual are usually less successful. However, passive strategies are not easy to implement. The airbag was highly developed by the late 1960s, but car manufacturers bitterly fought mandated installation of airbags. Overwhelming evidence exists that approximately 10,000 lives could be saved per year if all cars were equipped with airbags (Teret, 1986).

FALLS

Falls are the primary source of head injury in children and account for about 60% of the injuries (Hendrick, Harwood-Nash, & Hudson, 1964). The nature of falls among children less than 15 years of age is age dependent with children under three years old more likely to fall indoors, presumably off furniture or down stairs, whereas older children are more likely to fall while outdoors, for example, falling off bicycles, swings, or other objects (Ivan, Choo, & Ventureyra, 1983). Serious and fatal head injuries from falls are more likely to be due to falls from increased heights (Bergner, Mayer, & Harris, 1971). Most fall-related deaths in children in the United States are due to falls from heights, for example, second-floor apartment windows.

In a study of injuries among 5,300 children in day care centers in Atlanta, Georgia, Sacks et al. (1989) found that the head was the site of 68% of the injuries. Approximately one-third of all injuries resulted from falls on the playground.

Boyce, Sobolewski, Sprunger, and Schaefer (1984) reported that two-thirds of all injuries in the Tucson Unified School District occurred on the playground and that 18% were sustained before or after school hours when there was less supervision available. Climbing equipment injuries are prevalent and often quite serious.

Some Preventive Measures

1. Keep stairs safe by clearing them of toys, laundry, and sundry items. Remove or repair loose carpeting or treads. Install handrails at child levels. Use net gates at stairs (Bosque & Watson, 1988).
2. Install nonskid surfaces in bathtubs.
3. Install locks that limit window opening; install lightweight safety bars or grids in windows (Spiegel & Lindaman, 1977).
4. Utilize energy-absorbing playground surfaces or loose materials such as woodchips or sand (Boyce, Sobolewski, Sprunger, & Schaefer, 1984, Sacks et al., 1989).
5. Install stable, anchored playground swings at safe distances from walls and other obstructions.
6. Instruct recreational/school personnel via workshops in the purchase, installation, maintenance, and supervision of public playgrounds (Fisher, Harris, VanBuren, Quinn, & DeMaio, 1980).

MOTOR VEHICLE OCCUPANT INJURIES

Child restraint systems protect small children, ages 0-4, in motor vehicles from severe injury or death in the event of an accident. Over 600 children aged less than 5 years die each year in the U.S. as passengers in motor vehicle accidents. From age 5 to 29, more that one-fifth of deaths from all causes are caused by motor vehicles (Baker, O'Neill, & Karpf, 1984).

Motor vehicles account for approximately 32% of all head injuries in children. However, in nearly two-thirds of motor vehicle-related pediatric head trauma cases, the child is not an occupant, but a pedestrian (Ivan, Choo, & Ventureyra, 1983). Adolescents are especially at risk for head injuries in motor vehicle accidents.

Between 1977 and 1985, all 50 states passed laws to protect infants and children as occupants of motor vehicles (Teret, Jones, Williams, and Wells, 1986). However, there are serious gaps in the coverage including the exclusion of minivans and pickup trucks, ambiguities in the statutory language about age, restriction of the law to vehicles registered in a particular state, and exempting children held in parents' arms.

Despite the mandatory child passenger safety laws, compliance is much less than 50%. Haaga (1986) reported only a third of children under seven years old were seatbelted on a regular basis, and that usage rates were higher when mothers had more education. However, this study was based on 1981 data and prior to mandated passenger restraints in all 50 states. Williams and Wells (1981) noted that car seat and seat belt use tends to decline as the child ages.

Data suggest that 90% of occupant fatalities to young children under 5 years could be prevented by the use of appropriate restraints, that is, car seats or seat belts (Scherz, 1981). Older children can be protected by the use of air bags (Insurance Institute for Highway Safety, 1981). Lap and shoulder belts can prevent about 50% of the fatalities in children. However, seat belt use nationally is less than 20% (National Highway Traffic Safety Administration, 1986).

Some Preventive Measures

1. Establish uniformity among the laws of the states to reduce ambiguities, facilitate compliance, and enhance protection of children (Teret, Jones, Williams & Wells, 1986).

2. Design the occupant compartment of motor vehicles to maintain its integrity in crashes, to keep occupants inside and protected by energy-absorbing material, and to prevent intrusion by outside objects (Baker, O'Neill, & Karpf, 1984).

3. Installation of automatic seat belts and airbags (driver and passenger) in motor vehicles, including pickup trucks, minivans, and multipurpose vehicles.

4. Continuation of 55 MPH speed limits; demonstrated reduction in death rates among children for 5-year period after mandated 55 MPH limit (Baker, O'Neill, & Karpf. 1984).

5. Provision of hosptal-based or health department clinic-based low cost rental programs of child restraint devices (Coletti, 1983); provide information to new mothers in-hospital and at well-baby clinics.

6. Programs/workshops for parents, physicians, and day care providers to promote continued use of restraint devices for toddlers and older children (Guerin & MacKinnon, 1985).

7. Parent counseling to teach infants and children to accept the restraint system as part of travel (Kanthor, 1976); incentive programs for nursery and elementary school children (Foss, 1989).

8. Placement of child restraint system in center rear seat of vehicle for lowest fatality risk (Evans & Frick, 1988).

9. Purchase of child restraint seats that pass or exceed government compliance tests and were manufactured after 1981; millions of automotive restraint seats are defective according to the Center for Auto Safety. Parents can call a safety hot-line, 1-800-424-9393, to learn if a restraint seat has been recalled and to acquire other information.

10. Make available in clinics, medical/dental offices, daycare centers, shopping malls, and other settings brochures and pamphlets on child safety in motor vehicles (National Highway Traffic Safety Administration, (1981).

11. Legislation to prohibit travel on vehicle exteriors, for example, truck beds (Williams & Goins, 1981).

12. Legislation to increase minimum driving age to 17 or 18; New Jersey's 17-year-old licensing law has been associated with greatly reduced fatal crash involvement (Williams, Karpf, & Zador, 1988); high school driver education is a contributor to earlier licensure and accompanying crash involvement of the 16–17-year-old population (Robertson, 1980).

PEDESTRIAN INJURIES

As noted earlier, in nearly two-thirds of motor vehicle-related pediatric head injury cases, the child is a pedestrian rather than an occupant of a vehicle. Children ages 5 to 9 are at greatest risk because they "dart out" into traffic (*For Kids' Sake*, 1989). Brinson, Wicklund, and Mueller (1988) note that many children are backed over in the home driveway by the family van or light truck driven by a family member. Among all categories of persons injured by motor vehicles, pedestrians have the highest ratio of deaths to injuries (Baker, O'Neill, & Karpf, 1984). Pedestrian collisions are predominately an urban phenomenon.

Some Preventive Measures

1. Separation of pedestrians from traffic by using overpasses/underpasses and/or barriers at sides of roads.

2. Legislation to *not* allow right turns at red lights; right turns on red are a source of pedestrian injuries.

3. Reassess the safety of light trucks and vans as family vehicles in terms of nontraffic pedestrian collisions; possible changes in design and improving visibility (Brinson, Wicklund, & Mueller, 1988)

4. Demand design changes in automobiles; sharp front-corner designs increase risk of death to pedestrians; smooth, sloped hoods and energy absorbing materials in bumpers and windshield rims are the most efficacious designs (Robertson, 1990).

5. Use simulation games and modeling/training at home, in preschool centers, and in elementary school to teach children traffic safety rules (Renaud & Suissa, 1989).

BICYCLE INJURIES

Overall, bicycling injuries account for 1,000 deaths and 500,000 emergency department visits each year in the United States (Wasserman, Waller, Monty, Emery, & Robinson, 1988). Head injuries account for approximately 85% of bicycling deaths (Fife et al., 1983) and about two-thirds of bicycle-related hospital admissions (Guichon & Myles, 1975). Approximately one-third of bicycle-related injuries involve collision with a motor vehicle and brain injuries from these collisions were more severe (Kraus, Fife, & Conroy, 1987). About 90% of all bicyclist deaths involve collision with motor vehicles (Baker, O'Neill, & Karpf, 1984). Two-thirds of all bicyclist deaths occur in the 5–14-year-old age group.

In a study of 3,358 brain injuries in San Diego, California, 7% were bicycle-related, and 86% of these were mild injuries (Kraus, Fife, & Conroy, 1986). These authors found that the annual incidence of bicycle-related brain injury was 13.5 injuries per 100,000 people with the maximum incidence at ages 5–9 for females and at ages 10–14 for males. Among those aged 14 years or less, there were 153 bicycle-related brain injuries, 22% of all brain injuries in this age group.

In a study of 776 persons treated in five hospital emergency rooms for bicycling injuries, 99 patients had brain injuries. Sixty-five percent of these patients were children under the age of 15, and 26% were children under 9 years of age. Sixty-eight percent of the brain injuries classified as "severe" were in riders under the age of 15 (Thompson, Rivara, & Thompson, 1989).

The above study also indicated that bicycle helmets reduce the risk of head injury by 85%. Of the 99 bicyclists with brain injury, only 4% wore helmets. Unfortunately, fewer than 5% of school-aged children wear bicycle helmets (Weiss, 1986).

Some Preventive Measures

1. Legislation at the state or local level to mandate use of safety helmets for bicyclists under 16 years of age. Howard County (Maryland) recently passed such a law. However, the requirement does not apply when the bicyclist is on state, federal, or private roads (*The Sun*, 1990).

2. Peer pressure is an important variable in helmet use; children riding with other children wearing helmets are about 20 times as likely to wear helmets as children riding alone (DiGuiseppi, Rivara, Koepsell, & Polissar, 1989).

3. Purchase safety helmets that meet or surpass American National Standards Institute (ANSI) and the Snell Memorial Foundation standards for impact absorption and strap strength (*Consumer Reports*, 1990).

4. Health professionals should include information about bicycle safety and the importance of helmet use in the health education they provide; bicycle-related deaths in the U.S. exceeds those from accidental poisionings, falls, firearm injuries, and many medical illnesses (Weiss & Duncan, 1986).

5. Provision of bicycle paths for cyclists in effort to reduce motor vehicle-related collisions.

6. A national bicycle helmet campaign sponsored by retailers and the National Head Injury Foundation.

7. Promotion of bicycle safety programs in elementary and middle schools; incentive programs and discounts to purchase and wear bicycle helmets via Parent-Teacher Associations and youth programs.

ALL-TERRAIN VEHICLES INJURIES

All-terrain vehicles (ATVs) are three or four-wheeled motored vehicles that look like riding lawnmowers with handlebars.

Since 1980, over 1,000 persons have been killed and some 340,000 persons injured in ATV mishaps (Christoffel & Christoffel, 1989). About 50% of the fatalities have been children under age 16 and nearly one-fifth were children under age 12.

The American Academy of Pediatrics has termed ATVs a serious hazard to the health and well-being of children (Christoffel & Christoffel, 1989). The Consumer Product Safety Commission (CSPSC) has the authority to restrict the availability of these hazardous products, but after a $2.2 million dollar study of ATV injuries, recommended that the industry stop marketing ATVs to children under age 12. The outrage provoked by this response resulted in the CSPSC asking the U.S. Justice Department to sue the ATV industry. The suit was settled in 1987 when the industry (largely Japanese) agreed to the following: to cease selling three-wheeled ATVs; to recommend adult-sized four wheelers not be used by persons under 16 years of age; to have distributors post warnings and distribute information to buyers; to provide free training to new purchasers, and to conduct a safety advertising campaign (Personal Communication, Trooper Warfield, June, 1990).

The Virginia legislature passed a law effective July, 1989 that included four specific restrictions on ATV riders. The law prohibits children under the age of 16 from riding ATVs larger than a 90 cc engine size, riding double, riding on property without prior written consent from the property owner, and riding without a helmet (*For Kids' Sake*, 1989).

Some Preventive Measures

1. Required enrollment in safety program such as the National 4-H program backed by American Honda Motor Company.
2. Incentive programs, including reduced cost for ATV contingent on completion of a safety workshop.
3. Mandated protective helmet similar to motorcycle helmets.
4. Prohibition of riders other than driver; passengers create instability and do not allow driver to shift positions.
5. Prohibition of riding on pavement or highways.
6. Supervision by parents or responsible adults.

A FINAL NOTE

Sixty years ago, injuries resulting from accidents (unintentional injuries) caused one out of every 10 deaths among children. Today, one out of three childhood deaths is accidental (Bosque & Watson, 1988). Many common childhood diseases have decreased as a result of advanced medical knowledge. Injuries appear to be on the rise. Each year over 250,000 children sustain serious injury from head trauma, and over 4,000 children die from motor vehicle accidents.

Prevention is the best defense against childhood injuries. Haddon (1980) proposed several strategies to prevent the creation of a hazard, including not manufacturing equipment/vehicles that are apt to cause injury, reducing the amount of hazard that is created, separating the hazard from whatever is to be protected by interposing a material barrier, and to modify the relevant basic qualities of the hazard. As noted earlier, the preventive measures most likely to effectively reduce injuries are those that provide built-in, automatic protection, minimizing the amount and frequency of effort required of the persons involved (Baker, O'Neill, & Karpf, 1984).

Health professionals who witness the aftermath of injuries must interact with advocacy groups in designing and promoting *preventive* measures to keep children "safe and sound."

REFERENCES

Annegers, J. F. (1983). The epidemiology of head trauma in children. In K. Shapiro (Ed.), *Pediatric head trauma* (pp. 1-10). Mount Kisco, NY: Futura.

Annegers, J. F., Grabow, J. D., Kurland, L. T., & Laws, E. R. (1980). The incidence, causes, and secular trends of head trauma in Olmsted County, Minnesota, 1935-1974. *Neurology, 30,* 912-919.

Baker, S. P., O'Neill, B., & Karpf, R. S. (1984). *The injury fact book.* Lexington, MA: D. C. Heath & Co.

Bawden, H. N., Knights, R. M., & Winogron, H. W. (1985). Speeded performance following head injury in children. *Journal of Clinical and Experimental Neuropsychology, 7,* 39-54.

Bergner, L., Mayer, S., & Harris, D. (1971). Falls from heights: A childhood epidemic in an urban area. *American Journal of Public Health, 61,* 90.

Bosque, E., & Watson, S. (1988). *Safe & sound.* New York: St. Martin's Press.

Boyce, W. T., Sobolewski, S., Springer, L., & Shaefer, C. (1984). Playground equipment injuries in a large, urban school district. *American Journal of Public Health, 74,* 984-986.

Brinson, R. J., Wicklund, K., & Mueller, B. (1988). Fatal pedestrian injuries to young children: A different pattern of injury. *American Journal of Public Health, 78,* 793-795.

Brown, G., Chadwick, O., Shaffer, D., Rutter, M., & Traub, M. (1981). A prospective study of children with head injuries: III. Psychiatric sequelae. *Psychological Medicine, 11,* 63-78.

Bruce, D. A., Schut, L., Bruno, L. A., Wood, J. H., & Sutton, L. N. (1978). Outcome following severe head injuries in children. *Journal of Neurosurgery, 48,* 679-688.

Chadwick, O., Rutter, M., Brown, G., Shaffer, D., & Traub, M. (1981). A prospective study of children with head injuries: II. Cognitive sequelae. *Psychological Medicine, 11*, 49–61.

Choux, M. (1986). Incidence, diagnosis, and management of skull fractures. In A. J. Raimondi, M. Choux, & C. DiRocco (Eds.), *Head injuries in the newborn and infant* (pp. 163–182). New York: Springer-Verlag.

Christoffel, T., & Christoffel, K. (1989). The Consumer Product Safety Commission's opposition to consumer product safety: Lessons for public health advocates. *American Journal of Public Health, 79*, 336–339.

Coletti, R. B. (1983). Hospital-based rental programs to increase car seat usage. *Pediatrics, 71*, 771–773.

Consumer Reports. (May, 1990). Bike helmets: unused lifesavers. *55*(5), 348–353.

DiGuiseppi, C. G., Rivara, F., Koepsell, T., & Polissar, L. (1989). Bicycle helmet use by children: evaluation of a community-wide helmet campaign. *Journal of The American Medical Association, 262*, 2256–2261.

Eiken, C. F., Anderson, T. P., Lockman, L., Matthews, D. J., Dryja, R., Martin, J., Burrill, C., Gottesman, N., O'Brian, P., & Witte, L. (1984). Functional outcome of closed head injury in children and young adults. *Archives of Physical Medicine Rehabilitation, 65*, 168–170.

Evans, L., & Frick, M. C. (1988). Seating position in cars and fatality risk. *American Journal of Public Health, 78*, 1456–1458.

Ewings-Cobbs, L., Fletcher, J. M., & Levin, H. S. (1985). Neuropsychological sequelae following pediatric head injury. In M. Ylvisaker (Ed.), *Head injury rehabilitation: children and adolescents* (pp. 71–89). San Diego, CA: College-Hill Press.

Fife, D., David, J., Tate, L., Wells, J., Mohan, D., & Williams, A. (1983). Fatal injuries to bicyclists: The experience of Dade County, Florida. *Journal of Trauma, 23*, 745–755.

Fisher, L., Harris, V., VanBuren, J., Quinn, J., & DeMaio, A. (1980). Assessment of a pilot child playground injury prevention project in New York state. *American Journal of Public Health, 70*, 1000–1002.

Fletcher, J. M., Ewing-Cobbs, L., Miner, M. E., Levin, H. S., & Eisenberg, H. M. (1990). Behavioral changes after closed head injury in children. *Journal of Consulting and Clinical Psychology, 58*, 93–98.

Fletcher, J. M., & Levin, H. S. (1988). Neurobehavioral effects of brain injury in children. In D. Routh (Ed.), *Handbook of pediatric psychology* (pp. 258–298). New York: Guilford Press.

For Kid's Sake. (1989). Vol. 7, (3), 1–8. Charlottesville, VA: University of Virginia.

Gallagher, S. S., Finison, K., Guyer, B., & Goodenough, S. (1984). The incidence of injuries among 87,000 Massachusetts children and adolescents: Results of the 1980–81 statewide childhood injury prevention program surveillance system. *American Journal of Public Health, 74*, 1340–1347.

Goldstein, F. C., & Levin, H. S. (1987). Epidemiology of pediatric closed head injury: Incidence, clinical characteristics, and risk factors. *Journal of Learning Disabilities, 20*, 518–525.

Gordon, J. E. (1949). The epidemiology of accidents. *American Journal of Public Health, 39*, 504–595.

Guerin, D., & MacKinnon, D. (1985). An assessment of the California passenger restraint requirement. *American Journal of Public Health, 75*, 142–144.

Guichon, D. M., & Myles, S. T. (1975). Bicycle injuries: A one-year sample in Calgary. *Journal of Trauma, 15*, 504–506.

Gulbrandsen, G. B. (1984). Neuropsychological sequelae of light head injuries in older children 6 months after trauma. *Journal of Clinical Neuropsychology, 6*, 257–268.

Gurdjian, E. S. (1971). Mechanisms of impact injury of the head. In *Head injuries: Proceedings of an international symposium held in Edinburgh and Madrid* (pp. 17-22). Edinburgh, Scotland: Churchill Livingstone.

Haaga, J. (1986). Children's seatbelt usage: Evidence from the National Health Interview Survey. *American Journal of Public Health, 76,* 1425-1427.

Haddon, W., Jr. (1980). The basic strategies for reducing damage from hazards of all kinds. *Hazard Prevention, 16,* 8-12.

Hartlage, L. C. (1986, April). Behavioral sequelae of closed head injuries in school-age children. Paper presented at National Association of School Psychologists, Hollywood, FL.

Hendrick, E. B., Harwood-Nash, D. C., & Hudson, A. R. (1964). Head injuries in children: A survey of 4465 consecutive cases at the Hospital for Sick Children, Toronto, Canada. *Clinical Neurosurgery, 11,* 46-65.

Insurance Institute for Highway Safety. (1981). *Policy options for reducing the motor vehicle crash injury cost burden.* Washington, DC.

Ivan, L. P., Choo, S. H., & Ventureyra, E. C. (1983). Head injuries in childhood: A two-year study. *Canada Medical Association Journal, 128,* 281-284.

Jamison, D. L., & Kaye, H. H. (1974). Accidental head injury in children. *Archives of Disease in Childhood, 49,* 376-381.

Jennett, B., & Teasdale, G. (1981). *Management of head injuries.* Philadelphia: F. A. Davis.

Kalsbeek, W. D., McLaurin, R. L., Harris, B. S., & Miller, J. D. (1980). The national head and spinal cord injury survey: Major findings. *Journal of Neurosurgery, 53*(suppl), 19-31.

Kanthor, H. A. (1976). Car safety for infants: Effectiveness of parental counseling. *Pediatrics, 58,* 320-322.

Klauber, M. R., Barrett-Connor, E., Hofstetter, C. R., & Micik, S. H. (1986). A population-based study of nonfatal childhood injuries. *Preventive Medicine, 15,* 139-149.

Klauber, M. R., Barrett-Connor, E., Marshall, L. F., & Bowers, S. A. (1981). The epidemiology of head injury: A prospective study of an entire community-San Diego County, California, 1978. *American Journal of Epidemiology, 113,* 500-509.

Klauber, M. R., Marshall, L. F., & Toole, B. M. (1985). Cause of decline in head injury mortality rate in San Diego County, California. *Journal of Neurosurgery, 62,* 528-531.

Kraus, J. F., Fife, D., & Conroy, C. (1987a). Incidence, severity, and outcomes of brain injuries involving bicycles. *American Journal of Public Health, 77,* 76-78.

Kraus, J. F., Fife, D., & Conroy, C. (1987b). Pediatric brain injuries: The nature, clinical course, and early outcomes in a defined United States' population. *Pediatrics, 79,* 501-507.

Kraus, J. F., Fife, D., Cox, P., Ramstein, K., & Conroy, C. (1986). Incidence, severity, and external causes of pediatric brain injury. *American Journal of Diseases of Children, 140,* 687-693.

Levin, H. S., & Benton, A. L. (1986). Developmental and acquired dyscalculia in children. In I. Flehmig & L. Stern (Eds.), *Child development and learning behavior* (pp. 317-322). Stuttgart: Gustav Fisher.

Levin, H. S., & Eisenberg, H. M. (1979a). Neuropsychological impairment after closed head injury in children and adolescents. *Journal of Pediatric Psychology, 4,* 389-402.

Levin, H. S., & Eisenberg, H. M. (1979b). Neuropsychological outcome of closed head injury in children and adolescents. *Child's Brain, 5,* 281-292.

Levin, H. S., High, W., Ewing-Cobbs, L., Fletcher, J. M., Eisenberg, H. M., Miner, M. E., & Goldstein, F. (1988). Memory functioning during the first year after closed head injury in children and adolescents. *Neurosurgery, 22,* 1043-1052.

Levin, H. S., Ewing-Cobbs, L., & Fletcher, J. M. (1989) Neurobehavioral outcome of mild head injury in children. In H. S. Levin, H. M. Eisenberg, & A. L. Benton (Eds.), *Mild head injury* (pp. 189-213). New York: Oxford University Press.

Miller, W. G. (1986). The neuropsychology of head injuries. In D. Wedding, A. M. Horton, Jr., & J. S. Webster (Eds.), *The neuropsychology handbook: behavioral and clinical perspectives* (pp. 347-375). New York: Springer.

National Academy of Sciences. (1985). *Injury to America: a continuing public health problem.* Washington, DC: National Academy Press.

National Highway Traffic Safety Administration. (1989). *Child safety in your automobile.* Washington, DC: U.S. Department of Transportation.

National Highway Traffic Safety Administration. (1986). *Traffic safety newsletter.* Washington, DC: Department of Transportation.

Partington, M. W. (1960). The importance of accident-proneness in the aetiology of head injuries in childhood. *Archives of Diseases in Childhood, 35,* 215-223.

Personal communication. (June, 1990). Trooper Buck Warfield, Maryland State Police, Westminster, MD.

Raimondi, A. J., & Hirschauer, J. (1984). Head injury in the infant and toddler: Coma scoring and outcome scale. *Child's Brain, 11,* 12-35.

Renaud, L., & Suissa, S. (1989). Evaluation of the efficacy of simulation games in traffic safety education of kindergarten children. *American Journal of Public Health, 79,* 307-309.

Rivara, F. P., Calonge, N., & Thompson, R. S. (1989). Population-based study of unintentional injury incidence and impact during childhood. *American Journal of Public Health, 79,* 990-994.

Rivara, F. P., & Mueller, B. A. (1986). The epidemiology and prevention of pediatric head injury. *Journal of Head Trauma Rehabilitation, 1,* 7-15.

Robertson, L. S. (1990). Car design and risk of pedestrian deaths. *American Journal of Public Health, 80,* 609-610.

Robertson, L. S. (1983). *Injuries, causes, control strategies and public policy.* Lexington, MA: Lexington Books.

Robertson, L. S. (1980). Crash involvement of teenaged drivers when driver education is eliminated from high school. *American Journal of Public Health, 70,* 599-603.

Runyan, C. W., & Gerken, E. A. (1989). Epidemiology and prevention of adolescent injury: A review and research agenda. *Journal of the American Medical Association, 262,* 2273-2279.

Rutter, M. (1982). Developmental neuropsychiatry: Concepts, issues, and prospects. *Journal of Clinical Neuropsychology, 4,* 91-115.

Rutter, M., Chadwick, O., Shaffer, D., & Brown, G. (1980). A prospective study of children with head injuries: I. Design and methods. *Psychological Medicine, 10,* 633-646.

Sacks, J. J., Smith, J., Kaplan, K., Lambert, D., Sattin, R., & Sikes, R. (1989). The epidemiology of injuries in Atlanta day-care centers. *Journal of the American Medical Association, 262,* 1641-1645.

Scherz, R. G. (1981). Fatal motor vehicle accidents of child passengers from birth through four years of age in Washington state. *Pediatrics, 68,* 572-575.

Snoek, J. W., Minderhoud, J. M., & Wilmink (1984). Delayed deterioration following mild head injury in children. *Brain, 107,* 15-36.

Spiegel, C. N., & Lindaman, F. C. (1977). Children can't fly: A program to prevent childhood morbidity and mortality from window falls. *American Journal of Public Health, 67,* 1143-1147.

Teasdale, G., & Jannett, B. (1974). Assessment of coma and impaired consciousness: A practical scale. *Lancet, 2,* 81-84.

Teret, S. P. (1986). Litigating for the public's health. *American Journal of Public Health, 76,* 1027-1029.

Teret, S. P., Jones, A., Williams, A., & Wells, J. (1986). Child restraint laws: An analysis of gaps in coverage. *American Journal of Public Health, 76,* 31-34.

The Sun. (July 31, 1990). Howard County helmet law amended. Baltimore, MD.

Thompson, R. S., Rivara, F., & Thompson, D. (1989). A case-control study of the effectiveness of bicycle safety helmets. *The New England Journal of Medicine, 320,* 1361-1367.

Waller, J. A. (1985). *Injury control: A guide to the causes and prevention of trauma.* Lexington, MA: Lexington Books.

Waller, A. E., Baker, S. P., & Szocka, A. (1989). Childhood injury deaths: National analysis and geographic variations. *American Journal of Public Health, 79,* 310-315.

Wasserman, R. C., Waller, J., Monty, M., Emery, A., & Robinson, D. (1988). Bicyclists, helmets and head injuries: A rider-based study of helmet use and effectiveness. *American Journal of Public Health, 78,* 1220-1221.

Weiss, B. D. (1986). Bicycle helmet use by children. *Pediatrics, 77,* 677-679.

Whitman, S., Coonley-Hoganson, R., & Desai, B. T. (1984). Comparative head trauma experiences in two socioeconomically different Chicago-area communities: A population study. *American Journal of Epidemiology, 119,* 570-580.

Williams, A. F. (1985). Fatal motor vehicle crashes involving teenagers. *Pediatrician, 12,* 37-40.

Williams, A. F., Karpf, R. S., & Zador, P. (1983). Variations in minimal licensing age and fatal motor vehicle crashes. *American Journal of Public Health, 73,* 1401-1403.

Williams, A. F., & Wells, J. K. (1981). The Tennessee child restraint law in its third year. *American Journal of Public Health, 71,* 163-165.

CHAPTER 5

BRAIN IMPAIRMENT AND FAMILY VIOLENCE

Robert Geffner and Alan Rosenbaum

The purpose of this chapter is to describe the relationship between two problem areas in our society that are often not thought of as being related. These areas are family violence (i.e., child and wife abuse) and brain impairment. Professionals in the health care and social service fields, including physicians, nurses, psychologists/neuropsychologists, and social workers, are responsible for recognizing and treating the trauma associated with both family violence and head injury. However, the connection between these events is not often recognized, and the extent of brain impairment caused by family violence is frequently overlooked. In 1989 the Surgeon General warned physicians that not enough was being done to adequately diagnose family violence so that appropriate referrals could be made.

As a starting point for this chapter, we would like to suggest the possibility that head injury can be caused by domestic aggression. In the course of being abused, a head injury (with subsequent brain impairment) to the victim is not an improbable outcome. Infants are often shaken, dropped, or thrown, and children are bounced off walls or floors or beaten about the head with hands, feet or objects, either intentionally or accidentally, with traumatic consequences to the brain. Battered women are frequently slammed against walls or floors or beaten about the face and head during the abusive incident.

Therefore, this chapter will discuss the incidence rates for such family violence. Its relation to brain impairment, the symptoms and cues that can be used to more accurately diagnose the impairment, the consequences of such impairment, the possible cycle of brain impairment and subsequent family violence (i.e., that brain impairment may be a factor in the aggressiveness of victims who later become batterers), and the need for future research and prevention programs. We will focus on child abuse and brain impairment first, and then discuss wife abuse.

CHILD ABUSE

Numerous reports concerning the incidences and ramifications of child abuse have been written (Gelles, 1978; Kempe & Helfer, 1980). Child abuse for our purposes is defined as the intentional infliction of injury by the parent or other adult family member onto the child. The incidents termed abusive would cause bruises or other injuries to the child's body, and would not include spanking in the buttocks region. Extrapolation from epidemiological studies suggest that nearly 1 million children may be physically abused each year (Starr, 1988), and that these statistics are probably a significant underrepresentation of the incidences of such abuse. Many of the initial reports of child abuse by parents usually involve supposed falls and accidents. Recent research has begun to investigate the likelihood of abusive events involved in emergency room treatment of children's "accidents" or "falls" (Gothard, Runyan, & Hadler, 1985). It appears that many of these "accidents/falls" may actually be the result of child abuse, but the actual incidence rates are difficult to determine due to methodological problems (Reece & Grodin, 1985). Many of these incidences involve trauma to the head.

Brain Injury

Because many child abuse cases involve head injuries, a relevant area would concern epidemiological studies of head trauma and brain injury. It is estimated that head trauma is the cause of almost half of all children's deaths (Rivara & Mueller, 1986), and that about 1 million children sustain head injuries each year from falls, accidents, and abuse (Spivack, 1986; Waaland & Kreutzer, 1988). Unfortunately, it has been difficult to determine the prevalence rates of abuse in these head injuries due to problems in diagnosis. A few small pilot studies have attempted to ascertain these rates, and the results suggest that as many as half of the head injuries in young children (below age 6) may actually be due to abuse (McClelland & Heiple, 1982). One study of children younger than 1 year old indicated that 64% of all head injury cases admitted to their hospital during a 2-year period were due to child abuse (Billmire & Myers, 1985).

Thus, it is very likely that the incidence rates of brain impairment resulting from child abuse is much higher than is often reported or recognized in medicine, psychology, and social services. There appears to be two main types of injuries to children in these cases. One major cause of brain impairment as a consequence of abuse would be injuries resulting from skull fractures and concussions (i.e., closed head injuries). These injuries may be caused by a parent striking children in the head/face region with his fists or other objects, pushing or banging children's heads against another object such as a wall or floor, or by causing children to fall and hit their head. A second major cause of brain impairment has also been recognized: severely shaking the child (Caffey, 1974). One study that reviewed cases over a 20-year period, indicated that 13% of fatal child abuse cases were due to severe shaking (Showers, Apolo, Thomas, & Beavers, 1985). Dykes (1986) reviewed the literature concerning "Whiplash/Shaken Baby Syndrome" and found that these cases are often underdiagnosed by physicians and that the general public is not aware of the dangers of such shaking with respect to brain impairment.

In fact, studies in the child abuse and brain injury fields suggest that there are mistaken views of the consequences of child abuse and brain injury. It appears that the seriousness of the injuries resulting from abuse with respect to brain damage is often overlooked or not even recognized by families, some professionals, and the public (Dykes, 1986; Gouvier, Prestholdt, & Warner, 1988; Waaland & Kreutzer, 1988). However, there have been numerous studies documenting the seriousness of brain impairment as a result of abusive incidents, especially when the abuse occurs repeatedly or the child is under age 6 (Billmire & Myers, 1985; Kriel, Krach, & Panser, 1989; Sinal & Ball, 1987). Recognizing child abuse as well as diagnosing closed head injury have been difficult tasks for the health care professional, and recent studies have attempted to develop such techniques.

Diagnosing Child Abuse and Brain Injury

Recent articles have recommended that health care professionals focus more on the possibility that child abuse may be a possible cause for the injuries of the children they are treating. This appears to be quite important when the particular child or other members of the family also seem to have frequent injuries or "accidents" (Alexander, Crabbe, Sato, Smith, & Bennett, 1990). In addition, greater use of computerized tomography (CT) scans for detecting the possibility of head injury, especially in young children, more thorough intake questionnaires and interviews, and more referrals for neuropsychological evaluations for children age 5 or older are now being recommended in an attempt to better identify brain trauma from child abuse (Boll & Barth, 1983; Gothard et al., 1985; Reece & Grodin, 1985; Sinal & Ball, 1987).

Specific techiques for evaluating head injury in child abuse cases with CT scans, analyses of fractures, and with neurological indicators have been made by Hobbs (1989), Lehman (1989), and McClelland and Heiple (1982). Specific techniques for evaluating the possibility of Shaken Baby Syndrome have also been suggested (Duhaime, Gennarelli, Thibault, & Bruce, 1987; Dykes, 1986). In order to determine the severity of the brain trauma and its functional implications, a comprehensive neuropsychological evaluation, including cognitive, sensory, motor, perceptual, and memory abilities, is recommended when brain impairment is suspected, especially in cases of "mild" head trauma (Bond, 1986; Davidoff, Kessler, Laibstein, & Mark, 1988).

Symptoms and Effects of Brain Impairment

Various types of dysfunctions can occur from child abuse with respect to brain impairment, depending upon the type of injury. Trauma resulting from impact (either being hit in the head or facial region, or falling and having the child's head hit the wall or floor) can produce hematomas, impact seizures, linear or depressed skull fractures, open head wounds, closed head injuries (brain stem and/or concussive), and loss of consciousness (Lehman, 1989). The most difficult to identify are the brain traumas produced by concussions and mild or minor closed head injuries. Substantial research and clinical findings provide evidence for the significant effects and neurobehavioral sequelae of these types of injuries. In fact, these closed head injuries often go undetected and therefore untreated.

It has been suggested in recent years that most head traumas with even brief loss of consciousness in children produce minor closed head injuries with subsequent impairment (Boll & Barth, 1983; Davidoff et al., 1988; Levin, Benton, & Grossman, 1982). The effects of many of these injuries cannot be detected with CT scans, EEGs, or neurological tests. However, the effects are evident with neuropsychological evaluations (Boll & Barth, 1983; Bond, 1986; Hartlage & Telzrow, 1986). The most common symptoms of these closed head injuries and concussions are headache, dizziness, anxiety, reduced concentration, memory deficits, irritability, cognitive and achievement deficits, sleep disturbances, loss of judgment, emotional lability, impulsivity, and other behavioral changes (Eames, 1988; Ewing-Cobbs, Fletcher, & Levin, 1986). These deficits and subsequent behavioral changes have been shown to occur as a result of the brain impairment, and are often still present five years later (Boll & Barth, 1983; Fletcher, Ewing-Cobbs, Miner, Levin, & Eisenberg, 1990).

In the past, these changes were often diagnosed as being emotional reactions to the trauma and merely due to Post Traumatic Stress Disorder (PTSD). In recent years, however, the effects of closed head injuries have been more widely recognized, and it appears that these can occur in conjunction with PTSD (Alves, Colohan, O'Leary, Rimel, & Jane, 1986; Davidoff et al., 1988). These effects have also been documented for child abuse cases, and one recent study indicated that the severity of the impairment was actually worse for children who had head injuries from abuse in comparison to those who had similar injuries but from other causes (Kriel et al., 1989).

Recent reports have suggested that specific remediation techniques, including cognitive rehabilitation, should be initiated as soon as possible following the injury. Many of the studies and clinical reports have shown that the effects of these closed head injuries in children do not disappear. Therefore, it is very important to develop treatment techniques and educational strategies in the rehabilitation plan (Eames, 1988; Ewing-Cobbs et al., 1986; Spivack, 1986). These rehabilitative recommendations have been made for children in general who have experienced closed head injuries. It is probable that modifications would be needed to deal with the emotional aspects of the PTSD due to the abuse as well as the head injury.

Unfortunately, most child abuse victims are never accurately diagnosed, and these mild closed head injuries are usually not recognized nor treated. The subsequent emotional and behavioral changes often reported by family members and school personnel are usually attributed to the family environment rather than due to brain impairment. However, recent research is beginning to investigate the relationship between past abuse, brain impairment, and subsequent aggressiveness.

CYCLE OF ABUSE

It is generally accepted that biological, psychological and sociocultural factors interact in some complex fashion to produce behavior, yet current approaches to understanding the etiology of domestic aggression have all but ignored the possible contributions of biological factors. This is especially surprising given the substantial body of literature supporting a biological substrate for aggressive behavior in both animals and humans. Detre, Kupfer, and Taub (1975), for example, summarized studies involving experimental lesions in animals and clinical reports involving humans, and they concluded that there is convincing evidence of an association between neurological impairment and violent behavior.

If we consider generalized aggression, then the two biological mechanisms that have received the most attention are the effects of head injury and the action of neurotransmitters, especially serotonin. Numerous investigations have established a relationship between reduced serotonergic activity and aggression. Unfortunately, brain levels of serotonin are not directly measured, and indirect measures, such as the level of the serotonin metabolite in the cerebrospinal fluid, are methodologically problemmatic. However, there is substantial evidence that serotonergic activity is reduced in suicide attempters (especially those using violent methods) and subjects showing impulsive aggressive behavior. There is also some evidence that head injury may produce a deficiency of serotonin. Thus, future research will need to focus more on the relationship between neurotransmitter activity and brain impairment.

As stated previously, brain impairment in childhood can produce behavioral changes, including impulsivity and aggressiveness. If the injury resulted from abuse, then it would not be surprising that this impairment could influence the person as an adult; the combination of modeling and the dyscontrol syndrome often seen in the head injured could lead to aggressiveness in relationships (Elliott, 1988). Thus, a batterer or child abuser may be both the past victim and the current offender (Geffner & Rosenbaum, 1990). The suggestion that a head injury may be a cause of domestic aggression may not be easily accepted, though.

The relationship between head injury and aggression does not yet have much empirical support. However, Lewis, Feldman, Jackson, and Bard (1986) reported high percentages of significant head injury among both death row inmates and juvenile murderers (Lewis et al., 1988). They also reported high levels of child abuse (i.e., having been abused as children) among the juvenile murderers. These results are provocative. However, methodological problems (most notably the failure to use interviewers blind to the status of the subjects and the absence of comparison groups) detract from our confidence in the findings. A recent follow-up study of delinquents has led Lewis to propose that a history of child abuse in conjunction with neuropsychological impairment is a better predictor of adult violence (Lewis, Lovely, Yeager, & Femina, 1989).

There are very few studies in the literature examining the relationship between either head injury or other neuropsychological impairment and any form of domestic aggression. Therefore, some of the ideas expressed in this chapter concerning the possible link between being abused as a child and becoming aggressive as an adult are necessarily speculative. Our aim, however, is to stimulate theorizing and research in this poorly understood area. If these speculations are accurate, then being physically abused such that brain impairment occurred would be equivalent to two strikes against the child and would significantly increase their vulnerability.

Critics of this line of reasoning will be quick to point out that head injury would provide a convenient way for batterers to divest themselves of responsibility for their aggressive behavior. We are well aware of the danger here. Shortly after publication of a journal article reporting a relatively high prevalence rate of significant head injury among male batterers (Rosenbaum & Hoge, 1989), Rosenbaum received a letter from an attorney who was defending a batterer. The attorney was "very interested" in these findings as well as any other information about this topic. Attorneys in criminal cases are also interested in "mitigating factors" that may be present in many who commit violent acts directed at others, and this is an area that will probably become increasingly important during the next five years in forensic cases.

The relationship between child abuse, head injury, and brain impairment has now been clinically observed by the senior author of this chapter in about 75% of a small sample of death row inmates neuropsychologically evaluated. Similar results are being reported anecdotally elsewhere in the country, which tends to support the observations of Lewis et al. (1986). The possible role of head injury and child abuse in the production of future aggression will also probably be an unpopular notion. However, if neuropsychological factors are shown to be important in some of these cases, then biological treatments may be useful in reducing this form of aggression. Ignoring this potentially important factor in the etiology of domestic aggression is not wise, and future research needs to explore this possible relationship in more detail.

Wife Abuse, Brain Impairment, and Episodic Dyscontrol

The idea that neuropsychological factors may be relevant to the production of domestic aggression had been suggested over a decade ago. In 1977, Maria Roy prefaced an article, written by Elliott (1977) on the neurology of explosive rage, with the explanation that she was including it in her anthology "because physical disorders of the brain are sometimes responsible for wife battery, though, as yet, there is no data on what proportion of batterers are so affected" (p. 98). Elliott (1977) began that article by asserting that "dyscontrol syndrome" or explosive rage is an important cause of wife and child battery.

The relationship reported by Elliott, however, seems to have been derived more from the similarity between the behaviors identified as dyscontrol syndrome and those behaviors typically displayed by batterers than from any empirical evidence establishing a relationship between the two. According to Elliott, the features of dyscontrol syndrome include "frequent episodes of intense rage which are triggered by trivial irritations and are accompanied by verbal or physical violence. Speech is explosive and marked by unwonted obscenities and profanity. The attack is usually followed by remorse" (p. 104).

Episodic dyscontrol syndrome often develops subsequent to a significant head trauma. Elliott (1982) reported that in 102 of 286 cases of episodic dyscontrol studied, the condition developed following a specific brain insult, including severe head injury. He further reported (Elliott, 1988) that posttraumatic episodic dyscontrol was responsible for incidences of intrafamilial violence in 17% of the cases he evaluated.

Only one study to date has specifically evaluated the prevalence of head injury in perpetrators of domestic aggression. Rosenbaum and Hoge (1989) assessed wife batterers for a history of significant head injury in 31 consecutive referrals to the Men's Educational Workshop, a group program specifically for wife/woman batterers. Nineteen (61%) had histories of severe head injury. Although that study lacked nonabusive comparison groups, we can gain some appreciation of the magnitude by comparing these figures with prevalence estimates for the general population. The annual incidence in the general populaton is about 0.2% (Kraus, 1987), which when multiplied by the average age of the sample (29.7) yields a rough prevalence estimate of about 6%. Thus, the incidence of head injury among wife abusers was substantially higher than that for the population at large. Even taking into account the fact that head injury is most prevalent among young adult males (which would inflate the prevalence in this sample), these appear to exceed conservative estimates of population prevalence. However, even these data do not indicate whether the previous head injuries were due to child abuse, accidents, other traumas, or a combination of threse. This question is still open to debate.

Following up on these findings, Rosenbaum (1990) is currently conducting a larger scale investigation on the prevalence of head injury among partner-abusive males. Data collection is continuing. Preliminary analysis of the data indicated that 52% of the 50 batterers in the sample had a history of significant head injury in contrast to 22% of the 50 nonbatterers (Rosenbaum, 1990). Furthermore, the head injury temporally preceded the aggression in 92% of the cases where there had been a significant head trauma as well as current aggression in the relationship. Although the temporal order does not establish a causal relationship, it is consistent with a causal pattern, especially given that in only one case did the aggression precede the head injury.

In this study, the determination of head injury status was made independently by a physician blind to group membership. This study is the first employing a sample of batterers, appropriate comparison groups (two groups of nonviolent men, one with discordant relationships and one with satisfactory relationships), and assessments of head injury by a physician blind to group membership (as a control for experimenter bias). The research results support the conclusion reported by others that there is a relationship between head injury and aggression. Geffner is in the process of conducting a similar study in a different setting. He is comparing a small sample of batterers to head injured and therapy control group men to determine whether similar results are obtained.

We should also note that in the Lewis et al. (1988) study, 12 (86%) of the 14 juvenile murderers were found to have been abused as children. In the Rosenbaum (1990) study, 30% of the abusers had also been abused as children. We cannot definitively ascertain whether this child abuse caused the head injury. However, if it did, it would support a cyclical process wherein abuse led to head injury which in turn led to abusive behavior as an adult and possibly to head injury in the next generation of victims.

WIFE ABUSE AND BRAIN IMPAIRMENT

We know that woman battering causes physical injury as well as emotional trauma to the victim, and even death in some cases. Victims of marital aggression frequently seek help at hospital emergency rooms or other medical facilities (Stark & Flitcraft, 1988). According to one study, 80% of battered women seek medical help on at least one occasion of battering (Stark & Flitcraft, 1988). Gayford (1975) reported that the majority of battered women frequently visited their physicians. Dickstein (1988) in summarizing several sources, reported that "almost half of all injuries suffered by women in emergency rooms [sic] are due to battering" and that "21% of all women who use emergency rooms are battered women" (p. 612). Although we are not aware of statistics specifically pertaining to head injury among the battered women, the high prevalence of black eyes, facial bruises and missing teeth would attest to the popularity of the head and face as a target.

Indeed, a recent study of battered women attending a hospital emergency department found that the head and face were the most common sites of injury, occurring in 89% of the 117 cases studied (Brismar, Bergman, Larsson, & Strandberg, 1987). However, it does not appear that battering of women in the head region is a recent phenomenon. Dickstein (1988) cites a report by a team of paleontologists from the Medical College of Virginia who found a higher incidence of fractures (30–50%) among women than among men (9–20%) in mummies that were 2,000–3,000 years old. She writes "These fractures, primarily of the skull, were caused by lethal blows as a result of peacetime personal violence" (p. 611).

More recently, Angela Browne presented case histories of several battered women who ultimately killed their abusive husbands (Browne, 1987). These stories exemplify the vulnerability of this population to head trauma, and the likelihood that many battered women have experienced closed head injuries as a result of their abuse:

> He . . . began to hit Molly in the head with his fists. [She] attempted to pull away, but [he] grabbed her by the hair and slammed her head back against the wall with all his force. [She regained consciousness] with [him] throwing water on her. (p. 40)

> In the van [he] knotted one hand in [her] hair and pounded her head against the dashboard. (pp. 56–57)

> Something would just bother him and, like a reflex action, he would begin punching on the right side of her head . . . After the assaults, she would always check to see if she could remember her name, her dog's name, and her street address. (p. 61)

In almost every case described by Browne, there is some instance of head trauma. Summarizing the injuries inflicted on these women, she states: "Injuries to women . . . ranged from bruises, cuts, black eyes, concussions, broken bones, and miscarriages" (p. 69). Permanent injuries included partial loss of hearing or vision. Brismar et al. (1987) reported that the characteristic assault in woman battering is punching in the head, face, and arms. They also reported that 11% of the battered women had suffered a concussion and 11% (not necessarily the same 11%) received their injuries as a result of head-banging against the floor.

Thus, it is likely that this area of family violence also may produce brain impairment, but no research has been conducted to date to evaluate the incidence of such neuropsychological damage as a result of battering of women. It is possible that such damage may explain some of the physical and psychological problems reported by women who have been abused (i.e., battered woman syndrome) over a lengthy time period (Geffner & Pagelow, 1990). Since it is estimated that 20–25% of women in relationships are battered (Stark & Flitcraft, 1988), then the prevalence rates for those who do receive a head injury in this type of situation may be quite large. The recent example reported in the media of

Hedda Nussbaum, who was repeatedly battered so severely that her entire facial appearance was drastically altered, may be illustrative of the likelihood of a closed head injury in these situations.

PREVENTION

The relationship between family violence and brain impairment appears to have merit. It appears that child abuse (both physical battering as well as severe shaking) may be an important factor in many unrecognized head injuries leading to behavioral changes and learning disabilities. There also seems to be a link among this type of abuse, brain impairment and later aggression, delinquent behavior, and adult violence. The connection among child abuse, brain impairment, and adult violence is currently being informally studied for death row inmates and others in prison for violent acts. In clinical and neuropsychological reports of these types of offenders by Geffner and others, the lack of prior recognition of the offenders' history of abuse, head injuries, or other brain impairment is often apparent. Since these traumas were not identified in childhood, no treatment nor remediation occurred.

Therefore, one important component of prevention programs would be to focus more on the identification of children with abuse and possible brain impairment histories. Once properly diagnosed, then treatment and remediation programs may be planned and initiated to help reduce future aggressiveness, psychological disturbances, and antisocial behavior. Educational strategies can then be developed as well to help these children (Eames, 1988; Ewing-Cobbs et al., 1986). Advocacy for these children, taking into account the possibility of brain impairment, has been recommended for quite some time in an effort to educate the public, professionals, and policy makers (Caffey, 1974; Dykes, 1986; Spivack, 1986). This is the first step in the prevention process.

In order to recognize the traumas, it is recommended that physicians, nurses, psychologists, and social workers be trained in the symptoms of both child abuse as well as closed head injuries. This is quite important when evaluating very young children (under age 5) because the research indicates that the effects may be more severe at this stage of development (Billmire & Myers, 1985; Gothard et al., 1985; Kriel et al., 1989). The specific techniques for detecting the possibility of abuse and brain impairment should be a required part of the curriculum at medical and nursing schools to help reduce the effects of repeated abuse. Educating professionals and the public about the long-term consequences of such trauma may increase awareness and therefore reduce the repeated abuse that often occurs in these families.

Unfortunately, prevention of the original trauma is much more difficult to accomplish since such injury/abuse prevention itself is not well developed in this area (Showers et al., 1985; Whitman & McKnight, 1985). Agencies in both the health care and social service fields are continuing to focus on prevention programs, but much more is still needed.

Similarly, the possibility of brain impairment from closed head injuries in wife abuse cases has not been studied nor even recognized. Again it appears to be very important for professionals in a variety of specializations, especially psychology and emergency room treatment, to be adept at identifying victims of this type of abuse. Intake questionnaires have been developed to facilitate this process (e.g., Geffner & Pagelow, 1990), and more emphasis is needed so that continued abuse can be stopped before head injuries and brain impairment do occur.

The only adequate plan for long-term prevention appears to be in the education and legislative arena, so that these traumas can be recognized as epidemics. Funding, diagnostic programs, and treatment/rehabilitation programs can then be provided on a large scale. Perhaps early identification and treatment will lead to reduced aggressiveness in general in our society, which is a major area in need of emphasis. Societal scanctions for aggressiveness may be the only actual possibility of long-term prevention. If the hypotheses presented in this chapter concerning the relationship among abuse, brain impairment, and later violence are supported by research, then a reduction in this type of trauma may impact on violent criminal acts. Rehabilitation programs and/or medication may reduce future violence, which would be preferable to the commission of violent acts and the overcrowded prison conditions.

FUTURE RESEARCH

This chapter has focused on the relationship between family violence and brain impairment. However, much of the information presented has been inferential since there has been minimal research in these areas. Research has documented the relationship between closed head injuries and subsequent brain impairment, but the connection between child abuse and brain impairment has only recently been investigated. Additional research is needed to determine the prevalence rates of head injuries and brain impairment so that the magnitude of this problem can be ascertained. The long-term consequences of such abuse and brain impairment also needs further investigation.

There has been speculation concerning the relationship between child abuse victimization and later violent acts conducted by these victims, but sufficient research is not yet available to confirm a cause and effect link. Similarly, the relationship between brain impairment and the suggested cycle of abuse (i.e., the seemingly high rates of head injury in batterers and violent offenders) is currently being studied by the authors and others to determine whether research data support such hypotheses. The role of neurotransmitters in this process is also in need of investigation. If indeed the results of future research indicates the link among child abuse, brain impairment, and a cycle of violent behavior, then we may be able to add another component in the mounting efforts to reduce such abuse and brain impairment in the long term.

REFERENCES

Alexander, R., Crabbe, L., Sato, Y., Smith, W., & Bennett, T. (1990). Serial abuse in children who are shaken. *American Journal of Diseases of Children, 144*, 58–60.

Alves, W. M., Colohan, A. R. T., O'Leary, T. J., Rimel, R. W., & Jane, J. A. (1986). Understanding posttraumatic symptoms after mild head injury. *Journal of Head Trauma Rehabilitation, 1*, 1–12.

Billmire, M. E., & Myers P. A. (1985). Serious head injury in infants: Accident or abuse? *Pediatrics, 75*, 340–342.

Boll, T. J., & Barth, J. (1983). Mild head injury. *Psychiatric Developments, 1*, 263–275.

Bond, M. R. (1986). Neurobehavioral sequelae of closed head injury. In I. Grant & K. M. Adams (Eds.), *Neuropsychological assessment of neuropsychiatric disorders* (pp. 347–373). New York: Oxford University.

Brismar, B., Bergman, B., Larsson, G., & Strandberg, A. (1987). Battered women: A diagnostic and therapeutic dilemma. *Acta Chirugica Scandinavica, 153*, 1–5.

Browne, A. (1987). *When battered women kill.* New York: MacMillan.

Caffey, J. (1974). The whiplash shaken baby syndrome. *Pediatrics, 54*, 396–403.

Davidoff, D. A., Kessler, H. R., Laibstein, D. F., & Mark, V. H. (1988). Neurobehavioral sequelae of minor head injury: A consideration of post-concussive syndrome versus post-traumatic stress disorder. *Cognitive Rehabilitation, March/April*, 8–13.

Detre, T., Kupfer, D. J., & Taub J. D. (1975). The nosology of violence: III. Biological contributions to family violence. In W. S. Fields & W. H. Sweet (Eds.), *Neural bases of violence and aggression* (pp. 294–316). St. Louis, MO: Green.

Dickstein, L. J. (1988). Spouse abuse and other domestic violence. *Psychiatric Clinics of North America, 11*, 611–628.

Duhaime, A. C., Gennarelli, T. A., Thibault, L. E., & Bruce, D. A. (1987). The shaken baby syndrome; a clinical, pathological, and biomechanical study. *Journal of Neurosurgery, 66*, 409–415.

Dykes, L. J. (1986). The whiplash shaken baby syndrome: what has been learned? *Child Abuse and Neglect, 10*, 211–221.

Eames, P. (1988). Behavior disorders after severe head injury: their nature and causes and strategies for management. *Journal Of Head Trauma Rehabilitation, 3*, 1–6.

Elliott, F. A. (1977). Neurology of explosive rage: The dyscontrol syndrome. In M. Roy (Ed.), *Battered women: A psychosociological study of domestic violence* (pp. 98–109). New York: Guilford Press.

Elliott, F. A. (1982). Clinical approaches to family violence: III. Biological contributions to family violence. *Family Therapy Collections, 3*, 35–58.

Elliott, F. A. (1988). Neurological factors. In V. B. Van Hasselt, R. L. Morrison, A. S. Bellack, & M. Hersen (Eds) *Handbook of family violence* (pp. 359–382). New York: Plenum.

Ewing-Cobbs, L., Fletcher, J. M., & Levin, H. S. (1986); Neurobehavioral sequelae following head injury in children; Educational implications. *Journal of Head Trauma Rehabilitation, 1*, 57–65.

Fletcher, J. M., Ewing-Cobbs, L., Miner, M. E., Levin, H. S., & Eisenberg, H. M. (1990).

Behavioral changes after closed head injury in children. *Journal of Consulting and Clinical Psychology, 58,* 93-98.

Gayford, J. J. (1975). Wife battering; A preliminary survey of 100 cases. *British Medical Journal, 1,* 194-197.

Geffner, R., & Pagelow, M. D. (1990). Victims of spouse abuse. In R. T. Ammerman & M. Hersen (Eds), *Treatment of family violence: A sourcebook* (pp. 182-221). New York: John Wiley & Sons.

Geffner, R., & Rosenbaum, A. (1990). Characteristics and treatment of batterers, *Behavioral Sciences and the Law. 8,* 131-140.

Gelles, R. J. (1978). Violence toward children in the United States. *American Journal of Orthopsychiatry, 48,* 580-592.

Gothard, T. W., Runyan, D. K., & Hadler, J. L. (1985). The diagnosis and evaluation of child maltreatment. *Journal of Emergency Medicine, 3* 181-194.

Gouvier, W. D., Prestholdt, P. H., & Warner, M. S. (1988). A survey of common misconceptions about head injury and recovery. *Archives of Clinical Neuropsychology, 3,* 331-343.

Hartlage, L. C., & Telzrow, C. F. (1986). *Neuropsychological assessment and intervention with children and adolescents.* Sarasota, FL: Professional Resource Exchange.

Hobbs, C. J. (1989). ABC of child abuse: head injuries. British *Medical Journal, 298,* 1169-1170.

Kempe, C. H., & Helfer, R. E. (Eds.). (1980). *Helping the battered child and his family.* 3rd ed. Philadelphia: J. B. Lippincott.

Kraus, J. F. (1987). Epidemiology of head injury. In P. R. Cooper (Ed.), *Head injury* (pp. 1-19). Baltimore, MD: Williams & Wilkins.

Kriel, R. L., Krach, L. E., & Panser, L. A. (1989). Closed head injury: Comparison of children younger and older than 6 years of age. *Pediatric Neurology, 5,* 296-300.

Lehman, L. B. (1989). Neurologic aspects of the abused child syndrome. *Postgraduate Medicine, 85,* 135-137.

Levin, H. S., Benton, A. L., & Grossman, R. G. (1982). *Neurobehavioral consequences of closed head injury.* New York: Oxford University Press.

Lewis, D. O., Lovely, R., Yeager, C., & Femina, D. D. (1989). Toward a theory of the genesis of violence: a follow-up study of delinquents. *Journal of American Academy of Child & Adolescent Psychiatry, 28,* 431-436.

Lewis, D. O., Pincus, J. H., Bard, B., Richardson, E., Prichep, L. S., Feld, M., & Yeager, C. (1988). Neuropsychiatric, psychoeducational, and family characteristics of 14 juveniles condemned to death in the United States. *American Journal of Psychiatry, 145,* 584-589.

Lewis, D. O., Pincus, J. H., Feldman, J., Jackson, L., & Bard, B. (1986). Psychiatric, neurological, and psychoeducational characteristics of 15 death row inmates in the United States. *American Journal of Psychiatry, 143,* 838-845.

McClelland, C. Q., & Heiple, K. G. (1982). Fractures in the first year of life: a diagnostic dilemma? *American Journal of Diseases of Children, 136,* 26-29.

Reece, R. M., & Grodin, M. A. (1985). Recognition of nonaccidental injury. *Pediatric Clinics of North America, 32,* 41-60.

Rivara, R. P., & Mueller, B. A. (1986). The epidemiology and prevention of pediatric head injury. *Journal of Head Trauma Rehabilitation, 1,* 7-15.

Rosenbaum, A. (1990). *Neurological factors in marital aggression.* Preliminary Report, NIMH Grant No. MH44812. Rockville, MD: National Institute of Mental Health.

Rosenbaum, A., & Hoge, S. K. (1989). Head injury and marital aggression. *American Journal of Psychiatry, 146,* 1048-1051.

Showers, J., Apolo, J., Thomas, J., & Beavers, S. (1985). Fatal child abuse: a two-decade review. *Pediatric Emergency Care, 1,* 66-70.

Sinal, S. H., & Ball, M. R. (1987). Head trauma due to child abuse: Serial computerized tomography in diagnosis and management. *Southern Medical Journal, 80*, 1505-1512.

Spivack, M. P. (1986). Advocacy and legislative action for head-injured children and their families. *Journal of Head Trauma rehabilitation, 1*, 41-47.

Stark, E., & Flitcraft, A. (1988). Violence among intimates: An epidemiological review. In V. B. Van Hasselt, R. L. Morrison, A. S. Bellack, & M. Hersen (Eds), *Handbook of family violence* (pp. 293-317). New York: Plenum.

Starr, R. H., Jr. (1988). Physical abuse of children. In V. B. Van Hasselt, R. L. Morrison, A. S. Bellack, & M. Hersen (Eds), *Handbook of family violence* (pp. 119-155). New York: Plenum.

Waaland, P. K., & Kreutzer, J. S. (1988). Family response to childhood traumatic brain injury. *Journal of Head Trauma Rehabilitation, 3*, 51-63.

Whitman, S., & McKnight, J. L. (1985). Ideology and injury prevention. *International Journal of Health Services, 15*, 35-46.

CHAPTER 6

ASSAULT

Donald I. Templer

ASSAULT AND FIGHTING

The fact that serious head injuries can occur in fights and assaults is reflected in the method and instruments used in criminal homicides. In criminal homicides in Philadelphia, 1948–1952, the still widely cited study of Wolfgang (1958) found that 32.5% were a function of beating. Many middle class persons assume that almost all criminal homicides are a function of stabbing and shooting, but these percentages were only 37.5% and 22.9%. A greater percentage of white than black persons take the lives of others through beating, 42.2% and 17.3%, respectively. In 16.1% of these homicides, the hands and/or feet were used as weapons. In 8.9%, a blunt instrument was used. Wolfgang stated, "Many of these beatings appear to have been the results of fighting with no intention on the part of the offender to kill. However, a victim fell from his assailant's blows and fractured his skull on the sidewalk or curb, a condition which, nevertheless, resulted with the assailant being charged with homicide" (p. 86). The present authors note that on television and in the movies (perhaps especially the "Westerns") it is very common for two men to hit each other in the head many times, to be knocked to the ground several times, but to almost always have no more serious injury than a black eye! The present authors believe that children viewing such scenes may grow up with the attitude that fighting is a desirable and manly activity with virtually zero risk of serious injury or death.

A substantial percentage of head injuries in the United States are from assaults. Kraus, Black, Hessol, Ley, Rokaw, Sullivan, Bowers, Knowlton, and Marshall (1984) reported 17.7% for assaults in San Diego county. Cooper, Tabaddor, Hauser, Shulman, Feiner, and Factor (1983) reported 34% for violence in the Bronx. Annergers, Grabow, Kurland, and Laws (1980) reported 4% in Olmstead County, Minnesota from 1935 to 1974. Whitman, Coonly-Hoganson, and Desai (1984) reported 26% for black persons and 10% for white persons in Evanston, Illinois. Whitman et al. (1984) also reported 40% for black persons in Chicago.

The stereotype of Americans being violent receives some support from the fact that the percentage of head injuries from assault tends to be lower in other countries. Klonoff and Thompson (1969) reported 12.54% from assault in Vancouver. Keer, Kay, and Lassman (1971) reported 13% in Newcastle, England. Jamieson (1974) reported 6% in Brisbane, Australia. Rowbotham (1964) reported 3% and Steadman and Graham (1970) reported 7% in England. Barr and Ralston (1964) reported 2% in Scotland.

Socioeconomic status is definitely related to assault risk. In a study of Keer, Kay, and Lassman (1971) the highest two classes (I and II) had 3.8% of head injuries resulting from assaults in marked contrast to 48.1% for the lowest class (V). Gender is another important demographic variable with males having a higher percentage of their head injuries from assaults. Youth is another high-risk variable.

Youthful males, perhaps especially those of below average socioeconomic status, should be told the full story about the effects of fighting and assaults. They should be told that there is nothing manly or macho about poor muscle control, weakness, incoordination, speech difficulty, memory problems, and concentration difficulty. Neither the victor nor the vanquished have anything to be proud of. It is here recommended that persons admired by youth such as professional athletes denounce violence on television and radio just as they denounce substance abuse and dropping out of high school. In general, persons should stay away from "rough" bars, be careful after dark and in high-crime neighborhoods, limit their alcohol consumption, and avoid arguments that could erupt in fighting or assault.

The present author believes that habitual criminals with an extensive history of violence should be monitored even more carefully and not released until they have actually demonstrated substantial behavioral change. For example, such individuals often mellow with old age. This would protect the brains of innocent persons. There are currently no remarkably good methods for the rehabilitation of the chronic criminal. Research regarding impulse and anger control program efficacy should be developed and implemented within our correctional systems. If the research on the efficacy of psychosurgery for violent behavior becomes more impressive than the present literature shows, this also might become a treatment option to consider in selective cases.

TORTURE

Somnier and Genefke (1986) reported on the neuropsychological complaints of 24 Latin-American torture victims who were brought to Denmark. All 24 were males and were described as being in perfect health prior to their torture. In the one case history they provided, "He was battered against the wall until he lost consciousness. This was repeated twice per day for the first three weeks" (p. 326). His torture also included electric shock to various parts of his head and being deprived of food and water. Eighty-three percent of the 24 patients had sleep disturbances, 79% headaches, 79% impaired memory, 75% impaired concentration, 38% vertigo, and 13% tremor. The present author cautions the reader insofar as not all of these symptoms are pathognomonic of brain injury. Nevertheless, a conservative inference is that the sorts of torture described above do not promote brain health. Furthermore, the following illustration reveals sufficient evidence of brutally afflicted damage.

Eitinger (1961) studied 100 persons who survived a German concentration camp during World War II. Fifty of these 100 persons had suffered head injuries with loss of consciousness. "Most of the head injuries were received during interrogations and during work when it was quite usual for prisoners to be knocked down. Only a minority of these injuries were caused by actual accidents, either at work or in traffic" (p. 374). All of the prisoners suffered severe malnutrition. At the time of the Eitinger investigation after the war, 78 persons complained of memory impairment, 53 of headaches, 43 of vertigo, 21 of tremor and other involuntary movements, and 11 of tinnitus.

Eighty-two of these 100 persons were found to have one or more abnormal findings on the neurological exam. Sixty-six persons had cranial nerve involvement, 53 reflex changes, 45 motor function involvement, 19 diminished sensation, and six speech disturbance. Seventy-five of the 100 persons had pneumoencephalographic abnormalities, 29 cerebral spinal fluid abnormalities, and 27 abnormal EEGs. Eitinger attributed these very high rates of pathological findings to mechanical and toxic injuries and to starvation and exhaustion.

WAR

Although the nature of the injuries in war overlap to a substantial extent with civilian head injuries, the former are more likely to be caused by a penetrating foreign body. Sweeney and Smutok (1983) followed up 160 Vietnam War veterans an average of 14 years after penetrating head trauma. One of the notable differences between such penetrating injuries and the closed-head injuries that are more likely to occur in civilian life is that the penetrating injuries are more apt to be associated with less diffuse brain damage that is characterized by early cerebral edema, cerebral atrophy, and hydrocephalus. Twenty-eight percent of the veterans currently had motor impairments, although only two men were not ambulatory. Also, at the time of the follow-up, 50% of the veterans had permanent full-time positions, and 44% were not employed. Nineteen percent were never employed after their injury.

In contrast to the above study that focused upon global functioning, there are two studies that specifically focus upon epilepsy following penetrating head injury during the Vietnam War. Salazar, Jabbari, Vance, Grafman, Amin, and Dillon (1985) found that of 421 veterans who had penetrating wounds 15 years before, 53% had posttraumatic epilepsy, and that half of these continue to have seizures. Meirowsky (1982) reported that 33% of brain-injured Vietnam veterans suffered posttraumatic epilepsy. He grimly pointed out that this percentage is quite similar to that of 32% for World War I, 34% for World War II, and 30% for the Korean War, in spite of apparently relevant medical treatment advances.

Although the present book concerns the living brain damaged rather than the dead, a question of potential theoretical and practical relevance is that of which soldiers live and which die when struck by a penetrating foreign body. The research of Carey, Sacco, and Merhler (1982) described below is directed toward this matter.

During the Vietnam War, the U.S. Army undertook a comprehensive study of wounds incurred by soldiers and marines during combat. By January, 1970, 5,563 cases had been collected and stored. Eighty-three percent of the men had survived their wounds, 2% had died of wounds, and 15% had been killed in action. In 1975, the senior author of that study began a detailed study of fatal and nonfatal combat wounds from this data. One hundred and twenty-nine cases form the basis of his report. Analysis of data obtained from U.S. military personnel who received either a lethal or nonlethal brain or head wound in Vietnam indicate the following:

1. "Bullets caused more fatal brain wounds than did fragments" (p. 355). Eighty-seven percent of all wounds were sustained on offensive operations while only 13% were incurred during defense.

2. "Most bullet wounds were received at close range (mean of 40.9 meters). Most fatal fragment wounds to the brain occurred at very close range, mean of 2.9 meters" (p. 356). The close ranges undoubtedly reflect the jungle warfare of Vietnam where ambushes and unexpected encounters at short ranges were frequent.

3. "Clinically significant intracranial blood clots occurred in only 7% of all fatal brain wounds. Only one man with a nonfatal brain wound had an associated clot" (p. 356). The conclusion here was that fatal brain wounds in combat most often occur as a result of primary brain damage rather than an accumulation of intracranial blood and the effects of intracranial pressure.

4. "Helmets offered no protection against bullets but gave significant protection against fragments. Wearing a helmet appears to have some positive effect" (p. 356).

5. "Men who sustained either fatal or nonfatal brain wounds became immediately militarily noneffective." None of 15 men with nonfatal brain wounds fought after being wounded and only 3/14 (21%) of men receiving head, not brain, wounds were unlikely to continue fighting. Approximately 20% of all "hits" in combat involve the head. Of these, Vietnam data relative to nonfatal head wounds are extrapolated to larger conflicts, then many soldiers may be expected to be militarily noneffective even if they receive a nonfatal head or brain wound" (p. 351).

It is obvious that the prevention of war could prevent associated head injuries. However, such is beyond the scope of this book. It is also apparent that wearing helmets can protect the head. Some helmets presumably are better than others. However, these matters are also beyond the scope of this book. Nevertheless, the author suggests that, if helmets can protect the heads of military personnel, they should be able to protect the heads of police officers and other law enforcement personnel, especially while on high risk assignment. Incidentally, it is quite common for combatants to be hit by fragments in shooting incidents involving police and criminals. Also, perhaps more construction workers should wear helmets.

POLICE BRUTALITY AND VIOLENCE MANAGEMENT

Just as there are good and bad psychologists, there are good and bad police officers. Of the "bad" police officers, only a small minority are all bad, and always violent, sadistic, and antisocial. Some of the bad officers behave badly because of the adverse circumstances they are in at the time. The work of the police officer is not easy work. It is dangerous and stressful. Not all accusations of police brutality are true. There are times when officers are more seriously injured than the suspect in merely attempting to defend himself or herself.

Nevertheless, there can be no doubt that police brutality in the United States occurs. Any person who doubts this should read *Police Riots* by Rodney Stark (1972) that deals with the mass brutality of police such as happened in Chicago at the Democratic Convention in 1968. Anyone familiar with brain fragility is stunned when viewing television news spots showing riot control with brutal night stick blows to unprotected heads.

It is common knowledge that many police officers hit people over the head with their night sticks. In 1967 in Los Angeles, peaceful demonstrators were attacked by the police. Stark wrote, "They beat, herded, and abused a helpless, nonviolent crowd, composed mainly of terrorized, white, middle-class adults who police actions prevented from dispersing. Infants, cripples, pregnant women, the very elderly—none was immune as the crowd was beaten from one cul-de-sac to another while motorcycles and squad cars careened among them" (p. 23). It is not known how many persons were injured. However, of the 178 persons who reported their injuries to the American Civil Liberties Association, forty (22%) reported being hit on the head. On the basis of the growing evidence of brain vulnerability, it seems very unlikely that none of these 40 persons suffered any brain damage or brain dysfunctioning.

An article by Walker (1982) on attitudes of the police toward violence helps us to better understand the violent behavior of police officers. Walker found that police officers had a more favorable attitude toward violence than did psychologists, social workers, college students, doctors, lawyers, and mental patients.

However, this attitude toward violence was less favorable than those of army prisoners, army personnel, college contact sport athletes, high school students, and foremen. The police officers who had more positive attitudes toward violence had more participation in contact sports and were more likely to have received physical punishment from their parents than did officers who had less favorable attitudes. Thus, police officers' attitudes toward violence are neither uniform nor entirely determined by chance. Their attitudes are related to other psychosocial variables, perhaps, especially those pertaining to violence, in a meaningful fashion.

Police officers are in a very dangerous profession. We need not only to concern ourselves with the protection of the brains of nonpolice officers at the hands of the police, but the reverse as well. It has been recommended that the mildly injured officer should be administered a brief neurological screening instrument at the time of debriefing, and that such should be repeated in a serial manner over time (Reed, 1983). The results of such testing should determine when the officer should return to work. Reed maintained that if an officer is demonstrating behavioral abnormalities or performing his work in a substandard fashion following the history of head injury, the immediate supervisor should make a timely referral for further evaluation. I recommend that police officers wear protective head gear when they anticipate being in high-risk situations.

It is my recommendation that the police receive considerable training in how to restrain persons without hitting them on the head. We also recommend that there be close monitoring of physical contact by police departments and by outside authority. This outside authority should include representation of those segments of society that are at higher risk of being assaulted by the police. It is recommended that such issues be considered in the selection and promotion of police officers. It is further recommended that the salary and inducements be sufficient to hire and retain more uniformly high caliber men and women. Most police officers in the Fresno City and County police departments are college graduates. One of the authors (Templer) has observed these officers dealing with highly disturbed individuals in a very professional and compassionate fashion in the emergency room of the county hospital.

FAMILY VIOLENCE

Violence within families is an important category of assault. Child and wife abuse were covered in detail in Chapter 5 and will not be discussed here, but elder abuse will be mentioned. Elder abuse is much more common than most persons realize. Estimates of such abuse in the United States include 500,000 elderly abused every year, 10% of the elderly in a dependent relationship, and between 700,000 and 1,000,000 elderly Americans (Siegel, Plesser, & Jacobs, 1987). Information assembled by the House Select Committee on Aging seems to indicate that in 26% of all injuries there are bruises and welts, and 10% malnutrition, and in 1% there is freezing. It is difficult to estimate how many assaults to the brain this represents. However, the report does indicate that in 1% of the cases there is a known skull fracture.

REFERENCES

Annegers, J. F., Grabow, J. D., Kurland, L. T., & Laws, E. R. (1980). The incidence, causes, and secular trends of head trauma in Olmsted County, Minnesota, 1935-1974. Neurology, 30, 912-928.

Carey, M. E., Sacco, W., & Merkler, J. (1982). An analysis of fatal and non-fatal head wounds incurred during combat in Vietnam by U.S. forces. Acta Chir Scandanavia [Supplemental], 508, 351-356.

Cooper, K., Tabaddor, K., Hauser, W., Shulman, K., Feiner, C., & Factor, P. (1983). The epidemiology of head injury in the Bronx. Neuroepidemiology, 2, 70-88.

Domino, J. V., & Haber, J. D. (1987). Prior physical and sexual abuse in women with chronic headache: Clinical correlates. Headache, 27, 310-314.

Eitinger, L. (1961). Pathology of the concentration camp syndrome: Preliminary report. Archives of General Psychiatry, 5, 371-379.

Fagan, J., & Williams, K. R. (1987). Crime at Home and in the streets: The relationship between family and stranger violence. Violence and Victims, 2, 1-80.

Galles, R. J. (1975). Violence and pregnancy: A note on the extent of the problem and needed services. The Family Coordinator, 24, 81-86.

Hillard, P. J. A. (1985). Physical abuse in pregnancy. Obstetrics and Gynecology, 66, 185-190.

Jamieson, K. G. (1974). Surgical lesions in head injuries: their relative incidence, mortality rates and trends. Australia New Zealand Journal of Surgery, 44, 241-250.

Kerr, T. A., Kay, W. K., & Lassman, L. P. (1971). Characteristics of patients, type of accident, and mortality in a consecutive series of head injuries admitted to a neurosurgical unit. British Journal of Preventative Social Medicine, 25, 179-185.

Kraus, J. F., Black, M. A., Hessol, N., Ley, P., Rokaw, W., Sullivan, C., Bowers, S., Knowlton, S., & Marshall, L. (1984). The incidence of acute brain injury and serious impairment in a defined population. American Journal of Epidemiology, 119, 186-201.

MacLeod, L. (1980). Wife battering in Canada: the vicious circle. Quebec: Canadian Government Publishing Center.

Manlyla, M. (1981). Post-traumatic cerebral atrophy. A study on brain-injured veterans on the Finnish wars of 1939-40 and 1941-45. Annals of Clinical Research, 13, 1-47.

Mierowsky, A. M. (1982). Secondary removal of retained bone fragments in missile wounds of the brain. Journal of Neurosurgery, 57, 617-621.

Morey, M. A., Begleiter, M. L., & Harris, D. J. (1981). Profile of a battered fetus. Lancet, ii, 1294-1298.

Reed, T. B., (1983). Post-concussional syndrome: A disability factor in law enforcement personnel. Psychological Services for Law Enforcement, 17-18, 375-381.

Rowbotham, G. F. (1964). Acute injuries of the head: their diagnosis, treatment, complications, and sequels. 4th ed. Edinburgh: E. & S. Livingstone.

Roy, M. (1977). A current study of 150 cases: battered women. New York: Van Nostrand Reinhold.

Salazar, A. M., Jabbari, B., Vance, S. C., Grafman, J., Amin, D., & Dillon, J. D. (1985).

Epilepsy after penetrating head injury. I. Clinical correlates: A report of the Vietnam Head Injury Study. *Neurology*, *35*, 1406–1414.

Somnier, F. E., & Genefke, I. K. (1986). Psychotherapy for victims of torture. *British Journal of Psychiatry*, *149*, 323–329.

Stark, R. (1972). *Police riots: Collective violence and law enforcement*. Belmont, CA: Focus Books.

Stark, E., Flitcraft, A., & Frazier, W. (1979). Medicine and patriarchal violence: The social construction of a "private" event. *International Journal of Health Services*, *9*, 461–470.

Steadman, J. H., & Graham, J. G. (1970). Head injuries: an analysis and follow-up study. *Proceedings of the Royal Society of Medicine*, *63*, 23–28.

Sweeney, J. K., & Smutok, M. A. (1983). Vietnam head injury study: Preliminary analysis of the functional and anatomical sequelae of penetrating head trauma. *Physical Therapy*, *63*, 2018–2025.

Walker, L. (1979). *The battered woman*. New York: Harper & Row.

Walker, R. O. (1982). Exploratory investigation of police attitudes toward violence. *Journal of Police Science and Administration*, *10*, 93–100.

Whitman, S., Coonly-Hoganson, R., & Desai, B. (1984). Comparative head trauma experiences in two socioeconomically different Chicago-area communities: a population study. *American Journal of Epidemiology*, *119*, 186–201.

Wilcoxen, M. (1981). *Assaulted women: a handbook for health professionals*. Toronto: Support Services for Assaulted Women.

Wolfgang, M. E. (1958). *Patterns in criminal homicide*. Philadelphia: University of Pennsylvania.

CHAPTER 7

PSYCHOSURGERY

W. Gary Cannon and Donald I. Templer

HISTORY OF PSYCHOSURGERY

Psychosurgery was apparently carried out in the stone ages. Archeologists refer to a prehistoric procedure known as "trephining." Trephining, based on the belief of the Incas that mental illness was caused by evil spirits, consisted of making holes in the skull, presumably for the purpose of allowing the evil spirits to exit. The beginning of contemporary psychosurgery, however, is usually traced to Fulton and Jacobsen (1935) who reported that chimpanzees became more tranquil after bilateral frontal context ablation. Moniz and Lima (1937) performed the first lobotomy (frontal lobe incision) upon a human, a 63-year-old Portuguese woman who had been chronically depressed and who reportedly improved considerably after the surgery. Freeman and Watts (1936) performed the first psychosurgery in the United States. Transorbital leukotomy (term used in England, equivalent to lobotomy) was later devised by Freeman (1948). Grantham (1950, 1951) introduced the electrocoagulation of the medial quadrant of the frontal lobes, which he maintained improved the patient's emotional condition without intellectual or personality deterioration. The use of psychosurgery declined in the 1950s due, in large part, to the advent of antipsychotic drugs and the growing controversy of poor results and negative side effects attributed to these surgical procedures of the day.

Flor-Henry (1975) and Bridges and Bartlett (1977) pointed out that since 1950 the psychosurgical techniques have become increasingly refined, sophisticated, and targeted in contrast to the relatively large scale and indiscriminate destruction of the frontal lobes carried out in the earlier era. Areas that have been most often singled out for surgery include the ventromedial segment of the frontal lobe, the anterior cingulum, and the amygdala. Modern stereotaxic procedures have permitted much more discreet lesioning.

EXTENT OF USE

Although the use of psychosurgery declined greatly in the 1950s, it has not been nor is it still an obsolete modality. In 1971 there were 308 psychosurgical procedures in the United States and 22 in Canada. In 1985, it was estimated that less than 100 were carried out in the United States and only five surgical procedures in Canada (McCall, 1989; Donnelly, 1985). Psychosurgery seems to be used more in the United Kingdom than in North America. In fact, in a survey of British psychiatrists, Snaith, Price, and Wright (1984) found that 49% believed that psychosurgery is acceptable and should not be abandoned, 32% asserted that psychosurgery probably still has a place in treatment, 16% thought that psychosurgery should now be abandoned, and only 2% that psychosurgery should never have been countenanced in the first place. Seventy-eight percent of the psychiatrists surveyed said that they either have referred patients for psychosurgery or that they have not referred but may wish to do so.

EFFICACY OF PSYCHOSURGERY

The efficacy of psychosurgery is not central to this chapter. However, a global perspective of the risks of any treatment must take into consideration the benefits derived from that treatment. The literature on the efficacy of psychosurgery provides a rather mixed and unclear picture. In general, the literature based on clinical impression presents a much more favorable picture than the more controlled, research based studies, which incidentally tend to have notable methodological flaws. Consistent with this optimistic view of psychosurgery efficacy is the report of Sachdev, Smith, and Matheson (1988) who found with 11 patients treated for intractable bipolar disorder with the bilateral orbitomedial procedure, that six showed good improvement 3-6 months after surgery, two were slightly improved, and three were largely unchanged. They assert that like Poynton et al. (1988) their findings show greater efficacy with unipolar than with bipolar illness. Some literature reviews conclude that the efficacy of psychosurgery does not have good support (Valenstein, 1977; Templer, 1974; May, 1978; Robin, 1975). Other reviews provide more favorable accounts, but ordinarily do so with caution and qualifications (Blacks, 1982; Tooth & Newton, 1961; Sweet, 1973). The present authors maintain that if psychosurgery were greatly effective for many patients with various disorders the evidence would be stronger than the composite of the literature seems to indicate. On the other hand, there are not many clinicians who believe that psychosurgery should be given to an appreciable percentage of psychiatric patients. The emerging consensus seems to be that psychosurgery is ordinarily indicated in those few patients who are chronically incapacitated, suffering greatly, and fail to respond to all of the more conservative methods of treatment (Bridges & Bartlett, 1988). For example, since affective disorders have 15% risk of death from suicide (Kelly, 1973) psychosurgery may be the most appropriate and safe treatment in some nonresponsive cases.

The current prevalent opinion that schizophrenics profit less from psychosurgery than other patients is consistent with the tabulation of Shevitz (1976) for three different studies (Sykes & Tredgold, 1964; Strom-Olsen & Carlisle, 1971; Golstepe, Young, & Bridges, 1975). Similar findings were reported in the exhaustive study or over 1,000 operations studied by Tooth and Newton (1961). The first study reported 98% of depressive, 20% of obsessional states, 25% of anxiety states, and 13% of schizophrenics improved. Strom-Olsen and Carlisle reported 75%, 20%, 46%, and 5%, respectively. The respective percentages reported by Goktepe et al. were 78%, 18%, 24%, and 4%. Tooth and Newton (1961) collapsed 100 diagnostic descriptions of patients into the 12, which seemed most related to the decision regarding surgery. These 12 were then combined to create five, affective, schizophrenic, organic, neurotic, and paranoid. The last three of which were further combined as a relatively small "other" group to yield three diagnostic categories, schizophrenics (64%), affectives (25%), and others (11%). As has been typical, the schizophrenic group was least improved and the affective the most improved, though details regarding differences due to age, sex, and duration of illness prior to the surgery also contributed to outcome differences. Thus, the overwhelming evidence shows that improvement following psychosurgery seemed most often in depressives and least often with schizophrenic patients.

CONCEPTUAL AND METHODOLOGICAL ISSUES

To ask if psychosurgery is effective and if it has side effects is like asking if psychotropic drugs are effective and if they have side effects. Such a question becomes more meaningful if we ask what drug, in what category of drugs, and at what dosage, is effective for patients of what diagnoses and with what symptoms and history.

Research design for studies assessing the efficacy of psychotropic drugs and psychologically oriented therapy is often a difficult matter but becomes more meaningful when following this "prescriptive" model. Psychosurgery research design is even a more difficult matter. One seldom has the opportunity to randomly assign patients who need and want psychosurgery into treatment and control groups. Furthermore, patients who are ordinarily given psychosurgery (those with affective disorder, schizophrenia, and obsessive-compulsive and other anxiety disorders) have symptoms that wax and wane spontaneously and as a function of treatment, and which can impair some of the same cognitive abilities that are impaired by brain damage. An additional complicating issue is that a large percentage of patients given psychosurgery had a history of ECT. The conclusions which we can draw from reviewing the research to date are limited due to the methodological problems cited above. Also, diagnostic categories for many studies were roughly clumped together as were a wide range of surgical procedures. Due to these limitations we are able to make gross generalization which will not apply in all cases and might require modification, with much improved and more prescriptive approaches to develop. The reader is referred to Joschko's (1986) excellent review for a more thorough discussion of methodological considerations.

DOES BRAIN DAMAGE RESULT FROM PSYCHOSURGERY?

Brain alteration by definition results from psychosurgery just like an appendectomy by definition results in loss of the appendix. Of course, the reduction of white and grey matter when compared to control subjects at autopsy has also been noted (Pakkenberg, 1989). What is of importance clinically and to this review, however, are the *consequences* of this alteration and tissue reduction. The consequences most reported are seizures and other neurological problems, as well as deleterious personality and behavioral changes as assessed by clinical impression. Also reported are the cognitive consequences assessed by clinical impression and by psychological testing. The presentation of the unfavorable consequences of psychosurgery in this chapter is divided into the primitive era of large scale relatively indiscriminate frontal lobe destruction versus the contemporary era of refined stereotaxic surgery. In the earlier era, most of the patients who received psychosurgery were schizophrenics. Contemporary psychosurgery is more often given to obsessive-compulsive, anxious, and depressed patients.

PRIMITIVE ERA OF PSYCHOSURGERY

Rylandes (1948) described the "frontal lobe syndrome" which was associated with early psychosurgery and was comprised of long term sequelae such as disruption of abstract thought and foresight, emotional flattening, euphoria and a loss of initiative. Greenblatt, Arnot, and Popper (1947) reported on 247 leukotomized patients followed up from 6 months to 3½ years postsurgery. Eleven patients died. Two of the 11 deaths were said to have been operative deaths of patients following seizures. In one of these patients, a hemorrhage was found in the operative site of the left hemisphere which ruptured into the left ventricle. The authors reported that 10% of their patients developed seizures. Their description of behavioral side effects were apparently based on clinical impression and did not state how many of their patients developed the stated symptoms—laziness, irritability, untidiness, carelessness, indiscretions of speech, wetting, and weight gain ranging from 5–60 pounds. The Goldstein Block

Designs, Weigl Form Sorting, Color Sorting, and the Shipley test for abstraction were administered to 35 patients before and after surgery. Greenblatt et al. (1947) provided the reader with no test finding information of a quantitative sort but said that most patients exhibited slightly more concrete performance and poorer abstraction.

Friedman, Moore, Ranger, and Russman (1951) reported their 2-year follow-up of 254 leukotomized schizophrenics. They regarded seizures as their most frequent significant complication and they stated that the rate of such with their patients was 12.3%. They incidentally stated that they did not regard this complication as a burdensome one because it can usually be controlled with anticonvulsant drugs. They stated that there were 10 treatment group deaths and that eight of these could be attributed directly to the operation for an incidence of 3.1%. They stated that their operative mortality for over 700 patients was 2.4%.

Wittenborn and Mettler (1951) administered the Wechsler-Bellevue IQ test and the Porteus Maze test to 21 schizophrenics who were leukotomized and to 21 control schizophrenics. The leukotomized patients fell on the Wechsler-Bellevue Verbal scores and the control patients evidenced a gain, and the mean change difference between the groups was significant. The control groups also evidenced more favorable changes on the Performance IQ and Porteus Maze scores but these differences were not significant.

McIntyre, Mayfield, and McIntyre (1954) reported on 30 patients who received the Grantham procedure of prefrontal ventromedial coagulation. However, their description of the side effects and lack of side effects were not described in a precise fashion. They said that the immediate symptoms of disorientation of time and place, confusion, retrograde amnesia, and fecal and urinary incontinence are rarely seen after the Grantham procedure. They also said that the late symptoms associated with the early Freeman and Watts procedure such as loss of sexual inhibitions, bladder and rectal incontinence, and loss of social inhibition are rarely seen with the Grantham procedure. However, they did report loss of sexual and moral inhibition in one patient, persistent inertia in five patients, mild euphoria in five patients, and Korsakoff syndrome in four patients.

Scherer, Winne, and Baker (1955) administered to bilateral prefrontal leukotomized schizophrenic patients the Wechsler Digit Symbol and Digit Span subtests, serial sevens, the Halstead battery, the Bender-Gestalt, the Shipley Hartford, finger dexterity and finger tweezer measures, and other cognitive tasks, for a total of 113 different measures and submeasures. These were administered to both the 28 leukotomized schizophrenics and the 22 schizophrenics who constituted the control group prior to leukotomy, 2 weeks after, 1 year after, and 3 years after. The comparative changes were noted by the number of measures that were higher and lower in both groups. This was primarily presented in tabular form rather than with contemporary statistical techniques. Nevertheless, a visual inspection of their Table 5 shows more similarities than differences between the changes of the two groups, but with a trend for the leukotomized patients to have exhibited more improvement. The authors offered their qualitative impressions that the leukotomized patients tended to be more cooperative but with more childishness, lack of motivation, lack of goal oriented behavior, concrete thinking, and irresponsibility. Scherer, Kett, and Winne (1957) followed up these patients after 5 years and reported that more leukotomized patients had declined over the next 2 years so that at year 5 follow-up there was essentially little difference between the change status of the two groups.

In one of the most comprehensive studies of the period, Tooth and Newton (1981) reviewed 10,365 cases given leukotomy in England and Wales from 1942 to 1954. During that time period, there was a rapid proliferation of operations performed. Initially about 100 operations were performed in a year increasing by approximately 100 per year and leveling off in 1948 at approximately 1,000 per year. Although 36% of men and 44% of women were said to have been at least greatly improved after the procedure, 2% of both sexes were worse, 4% of men, and 3% of women died from factors wholly or partly due to the operation. Moreover, 21% relapsed after the operation, 1.3% developed epilepsy as a result of the operation, though many more experienced transient seizures during the earlier phases of recovery, and 3.1% developed serious adverse personality changes consequent to leukotomy. According to Tooth and Newton (1981), it is these changes, "more than any other factor that accounted for the falling off of the use of leukotomy" (p. 21).

McKenzie and Kaczanowski (1964) provided a 5-year follow-up for 183 predominantly schizophrenic patients who received a prefrontal leukotomy 5 years before. There were no operative deaths. There were nine cases of postoperative epilepsy.

Birley (1964) reviewed 106 cases of patients who received bilateral frontal leukotomy between 1950 and 1957. The patients had primarily depressive and obsessive-compulsive diagnoses. One patient suffered from seizures one year following the surgery. Twenty-six of these patients had unfavorable personality changes. The patients who were regarded as "personality risks" as evidenced by socially undesirable behavior were said to have increased propensities in this regard.

Hirose (1965) followed up 77 patients who received orbitoventromedial undercutting in Japan from 1957 to 1963. There were no operative deaths. There were three cases of seizures, but these seizures were well controlled by anticonvulsant drugs and the patients later became seizure free without drugs. Hirose (1965) stated that the postoperative complications such as confusion, disorientation, amnesia, incontinence, and undesirable personality changes did not occur in his patients. However, he did acknowledge that slight postoperative inertia was observed in some individuals.

Marks, Birley, and Gelden (1966) reported on 22 patients who had a leukotomy for their agoraphobia. Immediately after the surgery one patient had a meningeal reaction, one had headaches, five manifested confusion for several days, one was eneuretic and abnormally interested in his feces for several weeks, and one had a single episode of double incontinence. At the time of follow-up 6 months later, four of the patients exhibited poorer memory or concentration, eight outspokenness or irritability, and six apathy, laziness, or blunting.

Miller (1967) did a follow-up on 116 schizophrenic patients who received prefrontal leukotomy between 1948 and 1952. It was not possible to follow up all 150 patients of this series because of deaths (three from the surgery) and unavailability of the patients. The most common long term negative effects of the surgery were epilepsy (12%) and personality defects (91%). Postoperative complications include hemorrhage (3%) brain abscess (5%) and dementia (5%). The mortality rate was 2%.

Shobe and Bildea (1968) followed up 27 chronically mentally ill patients who received prefrontal leukotomies between 1951 and 1959. One patient developed epilepsy. No other negative effects, either immediately after surgery, or on a long-term basis, were mentioned by the authors.

Post, Rees, and Schurr (1968) evaluated the effects of bimodal leukotomy in 64 patients having primarily neurotic diagnoses. Five persons had died but only one death was said to be a direct result of the leukotomy. One patient developed a subdural hematoma immediately following the surgery. One patient "had attacks very suggestive of petit mal" (p. 1239). Post et al. (1968) maintained that a frontal lobe syndrome occurred in 60% of their cases.

The study by Moser (1969) followed up 147 men who received leukotomies at a Veterans Administration hospital between 1944 and 1955. At the time of the 1966 follow-up, 66 (49%) had recurrent seizures and 33 (15%) were said to have had a severe intellectual loss. Moser stated that 25 (17%) of the men had died, but he did not specify whether or not any of these deaths were a result of the surgery.

Knight (1969) reported on a case apparently treated very successfully by bi-frontal tractotomy. In addition to the substantial lowering of scores on tests assessing psychopathology, changes on four Wechsler-Bellevue verbal subscales and Verbal IQ were also reported. The patient obtained a presurgery scaled score of 13. One and a half months later, the respective scaled scores were 11 and 6 for Digit Span, 10 and 11 for Similarities, 12 and 11 for Vocabulary, and Verbal IQ's of 116 and 107, respectively. Knight quoted the psychologist interpreting the test findings as stating that the falling off of intelligence is more apparent than real because the patient found it difficult to concentrate on the Digit Span subtest. However, the authors of this chapter wish to point out that the Digit Span subtests is one of the Wechsler subtests most sensitive to brain pathology. Furthermore, a few points *gain* in IQ is expected because of the retesting practice effect. On the other hand, it may take much more than a month and a half before the possibly temporary deleterious effects of brain damage are dissipated.

Freeman (1971) reported the follow-up of 415 schizophrenics upon whom he performed frontal leukotomy beginning with his pioneering work in 1936. The bulk of his article consisted of case histories of patients Freeman regarded as greatly helped by the surgery. Freeman stated nothing about side effects except for the fact that there were eight (1.9%) operative deaths. Baker, Young, Gauld, and Fleming (1970) followed up 44 patients with a variety of diagnoses from 1 to 7 years postoperatively. The authors stated that there was almost always a postoperative mild organic brain syndrome, with apathy, silliness, or denial, and some disorientation for 2–3 weeks and occasionally longer. The duration of this organic brain syndrome tended to be longer in older patients. One patient displayed soiling and wetting. One patient had seizures as a result of a staphylo-coccal frontal-lobe abscess. The psychiatric complications were occasional in-crease in appetite with obesity and occasional changes in moral code such as anger, sexuality, or other interpersonal behaviors.

Evans (1971) described two cases of misplaced surgical cuts. The thalamofron-tal radiations had not been severed as intended. Improvement did not occur and both patients eventually committed suicide. Since mistakes are made in all sorts of surgery, the authors of this book do not believe that occasional mistakes alone warrant condemnation of a procedure. However, the possibility of mistakes and unexpected occurrences should be weighed in one's global perspective.

Tan, Marks, and Marset (1971) reported on 24 patients who received bilateral leukotomy for their obsessive-compulsive neurosis. During the first month after surgery, eight patients had transient incontinence of urine, six had headache, of whom three had a meningeal reaction with CSF leucoctybasis, and three had transient confusion. In regard to the "leukotomy effects" at follow-up 6 months after surgery, five patients manifested poor memory or irritability; eight apathy, laziness, or general blunting; one epilepsy; and one a subarachnoid hemorrhage.

Bernstein, Callahan, and Jaranson (1975) followed up 43 patients who re-ceived prefrontal leukotomy between 1948 and 1970. Nine (23%) of the patients had at least one seizure, although only one patient had more than 10 seizures. One patient had a mild but persistent right-sided hemiparesis. Another needed surgery 1 year postoperatively for osteomyelitis of the frontal bone button. Another patient, after a second lobotomy, sustained a hydrocephalus that neces-sitated two shunt procedures. She died 8 months later "after a prolonged vegeta-tive course." Nineteen of the patients developed an organic brain syndrome. Ten patients became obese.

NEWER ERA OF PSYCHOSURGERY

Strom-Olsen and Carlisle (1971) reported follow-up of 210 patients who received bi-frontal stereotaxic tractotomy. Six of their patients who had no history of seizures before surgery had seizures after. In three of the patients, the seizures were attributed to barbiturate withdrawal and the surgery, and all seizures occurred from 1–4 days postsurgery. One patient developed seizures 6 months after surgery and was placed on anticonvulsant medication. One patient had six seizures from 2–6 months postsurgery but had no further seizures after chlorpromazine treatment was stopped. Another patient had a single seizure 18 months postsurgery. Strom-Olsen and Carlisle maintained that, "It may be claimed that at the most one patient had persistent epileptic attacks following tractotomy. In two others the attacks were probably due to prolonged administrations of large dosages of chlorpromazine" (p. 150). Strom-Olsen and Carlisle stated, "Mortality due to operation was nil" (p. 153). However, they did acknowledge that 10 of the patients died between two and 10 months after surgery and they did acknowledge that the surgery "might have contributed to the deaths of some of these patients, all of whom were elderly" (p. 151). The authors apparently reported adverse personality changes as not a major problem, but they did not provide details. Kelly, Richardson, and Mitchell-Heggs (1973) stated that the risk of epilepsy after their stereotaxic limbic leukotomy is "remote." They did not state their definition of remote, but that their patients are routinely placed on anticonvulsants for 6 months postsurgery to mitigate the transient seizures which often follow the procedure. In regard to short-term complications, they did acknowledge that confusion and incontinence may persist for several days.

Goktepe, Young, and Bridges (1975) attempted to follow up 208 patients who had a subcaudate tractotomy 2½ or more years previously. Twenty-five patients had died, 49 were incompletely assessed or could not be interviewed, and 134 were completely assessed and form the main substance of the Goktepe article. Seven of the 134 patients interviewed had one or more postsurgery seizures, but one had a history of one seizure prior to surgery. Four of the seven patients had only one seizure, and three patients had more than one seizure and were placed on anticonvulsive drugs. The incidence of postoperative epilepsy calculated by Goktepe et al. was 2.2%. The authors stated that no socially incapacitating personality effects developed after surgery. However, two patients were reported by their relatives to be eating excessively, two displaying extravagance, two a reduction in social standards, and one a lack of consideration of others.

Curson, Trauer, Bridges, and Gillman (1983) said nothing about unfavorable effects in their study with 34 patients who received stereotaxic tractotomy for depression, anxiety, tension, and obsessive states. However, the patients were administered the Present State Examination, which assesses 48 psychiatric symptoms, a month prior to surgery and a year after surgery. Within the patients judged to have good improvement there was no worsening of any symptom. Within the patients judged to have poor outcome, there were less favorable scores on restlessness, hostile irritability, hypochondriasis, depression, and specific phobias. None of these symptoms are among the more commonly evidenced complications of psychosurgery. There were no mean lowered scores on lost emotions, dulled perception, inefficient thinking, or poor concentration.

Ballantine, Bouckoms, Thomas, and Giriunas (1987) presented follow-up information for 696 patients who received stereotaxic cingulotomy as reported by a series of earlier articles (Ballantine, 1985; Ballantine, Cassidy, Flanagan, &

Marino, 1967; Ballantine, Cassidy, Brodeer, & Giriunas, 1972; Ballantine, Levy, & Giriunas, 1977). It was reported that 0.03% of the patients were rendered hemiplegic and 1% with seizure disorder. There was no surgical mortality. They reported that in an ongoing study "a comparison of preoperative and postoperative scores revealed significant gains in the Wechsler IQ ratings" (p. 358). Poynton, Bridges, and Bartlett (1988) reported on nine patients who received stereotaxic subcaudate surgery. None of these nine patients developed a seizure disorder after the surgery. Furthermore, one patient who had three seizures in the 2 years before the surgery manifested no seizures in the 3 year follow-up period. Poynton et al. said that three patients manifested postsurgery cognitive deficits of mild to moderate degree. They said these deficits were confirmed by psychometric testing but they provided no more specific information about the test findings. Unlike the measures of general intelligence, the measures of neuropsychological deficits revealed some significant declines in ability subsequent to psychosurgical procedure, for example, deficits in abstract thinking ability have been consistently noted (Drewe, 1974; Faillace et al., 1971; Jurco & Andy, 1973; Mirsky & Zack, 1977). On closer look, however, the changes noted may be attributed to other facets of psychiatric treatment, especially electro convulsive shock treatment. Also, deficiencies in attention (Hamlin, 1970) have been reported to result from superior topectomy but *not* from inferior topectomy. Verbal fluency and mnemonic (memory) deficits have also not been consistently related to psychosurgery outcome. Of course, severe memory deficits have long been known to be associated with surgical procedures for the treatment of some types of epilepsy (Saykin, Gur, Sussman, O'Connor, & Gur, 1989). These surgeries lie outside the focus of this chapter. Thus, it is concluded that although earlier psychosurgery results were complicated with notable cognitive changes, more modern treatments have not led reliably to that same result.

SUMMARY OF UNFAVORABLE CONSEQUENCES

It is apparent that the earlier era of psychosurgery had mortality rates and seizure rates that are unacceptable by today's standards. One might be tempted to define this era as bordering on barbaric. However, one must bear in mind that many of these operations were carried out on schizophrenics before the introduction of the antipsychotic drugs. These operations represented desperate attempts to help intractable and unmanageable patients. Undesirable personality changes were very widely reported. However, it is very difficult to estimate their extent because those reported were ordinarily based more on clinical impression than controlled research. There was not much evidence of gross intellectual decline in the typical patient.

It appears that the newer surgical techniques entail a much lower mortality rate and a reduced seizure rate, although seizures are still far from rare. It is difficult to accurately appraise the incidence of personality changes. However, they appear to be less common and less severe than in the earlier operations. There do not appear to be substantial, enduring cognitive deficits.

RECOMMENDATIONS

We neither recommend that psychosurgery be used less than it currently is nor do we recommend that it be used more. What we do recommend is that every patient given psychosurgery should be regarded as a potential research subject both with respect to the side effects of psychosurgery and to its efficacy. We recommend that psychological test findings, historical and clinical material, neurological test and exam findings, symptom and side effect information, and the pertinent neurosurgical facts be recorded, and that as much as possible of this information be recorded presurgery, postsurgery, and at more than one point in the follow-up. A complete neuropsychological assessment prior to surgery and at follow-up is highly recommended. It is also recommended that the treatment team have at least the consultation from a person who is highly knowledgeable about research design and statistics. We view "n of 1" research as scientifically superior to only clinical impression. If the n is large enough, then all psycho-surgery patients in that locality could be used in a study or studies. Since very large numbers of patients are not given psychosurgery, collaboration between investigators at different localities would appear desirable.

We encourage clinicians to continue to be frank with their patients about the possible benefits and possible risks. To guarantee considerable improvement would not be a defensible practice. The risks should neither be overstated nor understated. Psychosurgery should not be given until and unless it is determined that the more standard treatment modalities have been diligently tried and found to be ineffective and when the patient can be assured that the cure is not likely to be worse than the disease.

REFERENCES

Baker, F. F. W., Young, M. P., Gauld, D. M., & Fleming, X. (1970). A new look at bimedial pre-frontal leukotomy. *Canadian Medical Association Journal, 102*, 37–41.

Ball, J., Klett, C. J., & Gresock, C. J. (1959). The Veterans Administration study of prefrontal lobotomy. *Journal of Clinical and Experimental Psychiatry, 20*, 205–217.

Ballantine, H. T., Jr. (1988). Historical overview of psychosurgery and its problematic. *Acta Neurochirugica, Supplementum, 44*, 125–128.

Ballantine, H. T., Jr., Bouckoms, A. J., Thomas, E. K., & Giriunas, I. E. (1987). Treatment of psychiatric illness by stereotactic cingulotomy. *Biological Psychiatry, 22*, 807–819.

Ballantine, H. T., Jr., Cassidy, W. L., Flanagan, N. B., et al. (1967). Sterotaxic anterior cingulotomy for neuropsychiatric illness and intractable pain. *Journal of Neurosurgery*, *26*, 488–495.

Bernstein, I. C., Callahan, W. A., & Jaronson, J. M. (1975). Lobotomy in private practice. *Archives of General Psychiatry*, *32*, 1041–1047.

Black, D. W. (1982). Psychosurgery. *Southern Medical Journal*, *75*, 453–458.

Bouckoms, A. J. (1988). Ethics of Psychosurgery. *Acta Neurochisurgica, Supplementum*, *44*, 173–178.

Bridges, P. K., & Bartlett, J. R. (1977). Psychosurgery: Yesterday and today. *British Journal of Psychiatry*, *131*, 249–260.

Bridges, P. K., & Bartlett, J. R. (1988). Resistant bipolar affective disorder treated by subcaudate tractotomy. *British Journal of Psychiatry*, *152*, 354–358.

Cosyns, P. (1988). Psychosurgery and personality disorders. *Acta Neurochirurgica* [*Supplementum*], *44*, 121–124.

Curson, D. A., Trauer, T., Bridges, P. K., & Gillman, P. K. (1983). Assessment of outcome after psychosurgery using the present state examination. *British Journal of Psychiatry*, *143*, 118–123.

DeMille, R. (1962). Intellectual effects of transorbital versus pre-frontal lobotomy in schizophrenia: A follow-up study. *Journal of Clinical Psychology*, *18*, 61–62.

Donnelly, J. (1985). Psychosurgery. In Kaplan, H. I., Sadock, B. J. (Eds.), *Comprehensive textbook of psychiatry* (pp. 1563–1569). 4th Ed. Baltimore: Williams & Wilkins.

Drewe, E. A. (1974). The effect of type and area of brain lesion on Wisconsin card sorting test performance. *Cortex*, *10*, 159–170.

Evans, P. (1971). Failed leucotomy with misplaced cuts: A clinico-anatomical study of two cases. *British Journal of Psychiatry*, *118*, 165–170.

Faillace, L. A., Allen, R. P., McQueen, J. D., & Northrup, B. (1971). Cognitive deficits from bilateral cingulatomy for intractable pain in man. *Diseases of the Nervous System*, *32*, 171–175.

Flor-Henry, P. (1975). Psychiatric surgery—1935-1973. *Canadian Psychiatric Association Journal*, *20*, 157–167.

Freeman, W. (1948). Transorbital leucotomy. *Lancet*, *ii*, 371–373.

Fulton, J. F., & Jacobsen, C. F. (1935). The functions of the frontal lobes, a comparative study in monkeys, chimpanzees and man. *Advances in Modern Biology*, *4*, 113–123.

Goktepe, E. O., Young, L. B., & Bridges, P. K. (1975). A further review of the results of stereotactic subcaudate tractotomy. 358.

Goldstein, L. H., Canavan, A. G. M., & Polkey, C. E. (1989). Cognitive mapping after unilateral temporal lobectomy. *Neuropsychologia*, *27*, 167–177.

Grantham, E. G. (1950). Frontal lobotomy for relief of intractable pain. *Southern Surgeon*, *16*, 181–190.

Grantham, E. G. (1951). Prefrontal lobotomy for relief of pain. With a report of a new operative technique. *Journal of Neurosurgery*, *8*, 405–410.

Greenblatt, M., Arnot, R. E., Poppen, J. L, & Chapman, W. P. (1947). Report on lobotomy studies at the Boston Psychopathic Hospital. *American Journal of Psychiatry*, *104*, 361–368.

Greenblatt, M., Robertson, E., & Solomon, H. C. (1953). Five year follow-up of one hundred cases of bilateral prefrontal lobotomy. *Journal of American Medical Association*, *151*, 200–202.

Hirose, S. (1965). Orbito-ventromedial undercutting 1957-58: Follow-up cases. *American Journal of Psychiatry*, *121*, 1194.

Jackson, H. (1954). Leucotomy—a recent development. *Journal of Mental Science*, *100*, 62–65.

Joschko, M. (1984). Neuropsychological assessment in neuropsychiatric disorders: clinical methods and emperical findings. In I. Grant and K. M. Adam (Eds.), *Neuropsychological outcome of psychosurgery* (pp. 301–318). New York: Oxford University Press.

Jurko, M. F., & Andy, O. J. (1973). Psychological changes correlated with thalamotomy site. *Journal of Neurology, Neurosurgery, and Psychiatry, 36*, 846–852.

Kelly, D. (1973). Psychosurgery and the limbic system. *Postgraduate Medical Journal, 49*, 825–833.

Knight, G. (1969). Bi-frontal stereotactic tractotomy. *British Journal of Psychiatry, 115*, 257–266.

Laitinen, L. V. (1988). Psychosurgery today. *Acta Neurochirurgica, Supplementum, 44*, 158–162.

Lewin, W. (1961). Observations on selective leukotomy. *Journal of Neurological, Neurosurgery, and Psychiatry, 23*, 37–44.

Logothetis, J. (1968). A long-term evaluation of convulsive seizures following prefrontal lobotomy. *Journal of Nervous and Mental Disease, 146*, 71–79.

Marks, I. M., Birley, J. L. T., & Gelder, M. G. (1966). Modified leukotomy in severe agoraphobia: A controlled serial inquiry. *British Journal of Psychiatry, 112*, 757–769.

May, P. R. A. (1974). Treatment of schizophrenia: III. A survey of the literature on prefrontal leucotomy. *Comprehensive Psychiatry, 15*, 375–387.

McCall, W. V. (1989). Physical treatments in psychiatry: Current and historical use in the Southern United States. *Physical Treatments in Psychiatry, 82*, 345–351.

McKenzie, K. G., & Kaczanowski, G. (1964). Prefrontal leukotomy: A five-year controlled study. *Canadian Medical Association Journal, 91*, 1193–1196.

Median, R. F., Pearson, J. S., & Buchstein, H. F. (1954). The long-term evaluation of prefrontal lobotomy in chronic psychotics. *Journal of Nervous and Mental Disease, 119*, 23–30.

Miller, A. (1967). The lobotomy patient—a decade later: A follow-up study of a research project started in 1948. *Canadian Medical Association Journal, 96*, 1095–1103.

Mindus, P., Bergstrom, K., Levander, S. E., Noren, G., Hindmarsh, T., & Thuomas, K. A. (1987). Magnetic resonance images related to clinical outcome after psychosurgical intervention in severe anxiety disorder. *Journal of Neurology, Neurosurgery, and Psychiatry, 50*, 1288–1293.

Mirsky, A. F., & Orzack, M. H. (1977). Final report on psychosurgery pilot study. In *Psychosurgery, report and recommendations. The national commission for the protection of human subjects of biomedical and behavioral research*: Appendix, Psychosurgery. DHEW publication no. (05) 77-0002. Washington, DC: U.S. Government Printing Office.

Moniz, E. (1937). Prefrontal leukotomy in the treatment of mental disorders. *American Journal of Psychiatry, 93*, 1379–1385.

Moser, H. M. (1969). A ten-year follow-up of lobotomy patients. *Hospital and Community Psychiatry, 20*, 381.

Pakkenberg, B. (1989). What happens in the leucotomised brain? A post-mortem morphological study of brains from schizophrenic patients. *Journal of Neurology, Neurosurgery, and Psychiatry, 52*, 156–161.

Paul, N. L., Fitzgerald, E. N., & Greenblatt, M. (1956). Biomedical lobotomy: Five year evaluation. *Journal of Nervous and Mental Disease, 124*, 49–57.

Paul, N. L., Fitzgerald, E. N., & Greenblatt, M. (1956). The long-term comparative clinical results of three different lobotomy procedures. *American Journal of Psychiatry, 113*, 808–814.

Post, F., Rees, W. L., & Schurr, P. H. (1968). An evaluation of bimedial leucotomy. *British Journal of Psychiatry, 114*, 1223–1246.

Poynton, A., Bridges, P. K., & Bartlett, J. R. (1988). Resistant bipolar affective disorder treated by stereotactic subcaudate tractotomy. *British Journal of Psychiatry, 152,* 354–358.

Robin, A. A. (1958). A controlled study of the effects of leukotomy. *Journal of Neurology, Neurosurgery, and Psychiatry, 21,* 262–269.

Robin, A. A. (1958). A retrospective controlled study of leukotomy in schizophrenia and affective disorders. *Journal of Mental Science, 104,* 1025–1037.

Rosvold, M. E., & Mishkin, M. (1950). Evaluation of the effects of pre-frontal leucotomy on intelligence. *Canadian Journal of Psychiatry, 4,* 122–132.

Rylander, G. (1948). Personality analysis before and after frontal lobotomy. *Associate Research Neuropsychology and Mental Disorders, 27,* 691–705.

Sachdev, P., Smith, J. S., & Matheson, J. (1988). Psychosurgery for bipolar affective disorder. *British Journal of Psychiatry, 153,* 576.

Sano, K., & Mayanagi, Y. (1988). Posteromedial hypothalamotomy in the treatment of violent, aggressive behaviour. *Acta Neurochirurgica, Supplementum, 44,* 145–151.

Saykin, A. J., Gur, R. C., Sussman, N. M., O'Connor, M. J., & Gur, R. E. (1989). Memory deficits before and after temporal lobectomy: Effect of laterality and age of onset. *Brain and Cognition, 9,* 191–200.

Scherer, I. W., Winne, J. F., Clancy, D. D., & Baker, R. W. (1953). Psychological change during the first year following pre-frontal lobotomy. *Psychological Monographs, 67,* 1–24.

Scherer, I. W., Winne, J. F., & Baker, R. W. (1955). Psychological changes over a 3 year period following bilateral pre-frontal lobotomy. *Journal of Consulting Psychology, 19,* 291–298.

Scherer, I. W., Klett, C. J., & Winne, J. F. (1957). Psychological changes over a four year period following bilateral pre-frontal lobotomy. *Journal of Consulting Psychology, 21,* 291–295.

Shevita, S. A. (1976). Psychosurgery: Some current observations. *American Journal of Psychiatry, 133,* 266–270.

Shobe, F. O., & Gildea, M. C. L. (1968). Long-term follow-up of selected lobotomized private patients. *Journal of American Medical Association, 206,* 327–332.

Smith, M. L., & Milner, B. (1988). Estimation of frequency of occurrence of abstract designs after frontal or temporal lobectomy. *Neuropsychologia, 26,* 297–306.

Smith, M. L., & Milner, B. (1989). Right hippocampal impairment in the recall of spatial location: Encoding deficit or rapid forgetting? *Neuropsychologia, 17,* 71–80.

Smith, M. E., & Halgren, E. (1989). Dissociation of recognition memory components following temporal lobe lesions. *Journal of Experimental Psychology, 15,* 50–60.

Snaith, R. P., Price, J. E., & Wright, J. F. (1984). Psychiatrists' attitudes to psychosurgery: Proposals for the organization of a psychosurgical service in Yorkshire. *British Journal of Psychiatry, 144,* 293–297.

Strom-Olsen, R., & Carlisle, S. (1972). Bifrontal stereotaxic tractotomy. A follow-up study. In E. Hitchcock, L., Laitinen, & K. Vaernet (Eds.), *Psychosurgery* (pp. 278–288). Springfield, IL: Charles C. Thomas.

Strom-Olsen, R., & Carlisle, S. (1971). Bi-frontal stereotactic tractotomy: A follow-up of stereotactic subcaudate tractotomy. *British Journal of Psychiatry, 118,* 141–154.

Sykes, M. D., & Tredgold, R. F. (1964). Restricted orbital undercutting: A study of its effects on 350 patients over the ten years 1851–1960. *British Journal of Psychiatry, 110,* 609–640.

Tan, E., Marks, I. M., & Marset, P. (1971). Remedial leucotomy in obsessive-compulsive neurosis: A controlled serial inquiry. *British Journal of Psychiatry, 118,* 155–64.

Templer, D. I. (1974). The efficacy of psychosurgery. *Biological Psychiatry, 9,* 205–209.

Tooth, G. C., & Newton, M. P. (1961). *Leucotomy in England and Wales 1941-1954.* London: Ministry of Health Reports on Public Health and Medical Subjects, no. 104.

Valenstein, E. S. (1974). Brain stimulation and behavior control. *Nebraska Symposium on Motivation, 22,* 251-291.

Waltregny, A. (1988). Regarding the experimental neurophysiological basis of psychosurgery. *Acta Neurochirurgica, Supplement, 44,* 129-137.

Whittenborn, J. R., & Mettler, F. A. (1951). Some psychological changes following psychosurgery. *Journal of Abnormal and Social Psychology, 46,* 548-556.

Whitty, C. W. M., Duffeld, J. E., Tow, P. M., et al. (1952). Anterior cingulectomy in the treatment of mental disease. *Lancet, 1,* 475-481.

CHAPTER 8

ECT AND PERMANENT BRAIN DAMAGE

Donald I. Templer

Electroconvulsive therapy (ECT) is a very controversial treatment. It is a topic for which it is difficult to obtain an objective perspective because emotional undercurrents tend to run strong. It may, in this respect, be comparable to other emotionally laden issues such as ethnic differences in IQ and the bad effects of marijuana. Friedberg (1977), an outspoken critic of ECT, attributed the rise of ECT in the 1930s to the authoritarian political era in Europe in which 275,000 "inmates" in German psychiatric hospitals were starved, beaten, drugged, and gassed to death. On the other hand, Shukla (1981) stated, "Despite abhorrence in some quarters, it is still being practiced as one of the cheapest and safest, and yet one of the most effective, therapeutic techniques in the whole of medical science" (p. 569).

Hoffmann (1986) provided a scholarly discussion of the philosophical differences between those who favor and those who are opposed to ECT. He said that the former have a paternalistic philosophy and those who oppose it have libertarian and Kantian assumptions. He argued, "Paternalism does not pay much attention to patient education or self-esteem and libertarian ethics do not consider patient pain, fear, or dependency." He said that traditionally medicine has operated from a paternalistic point of view and that the attack on ECT can be viewed as arising from the valuing of freedom and autonomy in our society, plus the fact that politically educated persons have little tolerance for obligatory government rule. However, it is here noted by the present author that a study indicated that the psychiatrists and other mental health professionals who were more favorably disposed toward ECT were more experienced and knew more correct facts about ECT (Janicak, Mark, Trimakas, & Gibbons, 1985).

The use of ECT in the United States is decreasing. In fact, there was a 46% decrease from 1975 to 1980. However, even in 1980 there were 33,384 psychiatric patients given ECT (Thompson & Blain, 1987). In California, legislation in 1975 severely restricted the use of ECT. Nevertheless, from 1977 to 1983, 18,627 patients received a total of 99,425 ECT treatments in California, with little year-to-year variation (Kramer, 1985). ECT is far from becoming an obsolete treatment modality. And, because controlled research has demonstrated its efficacy, and because it is especially valued in the recalcitrant cases of depression that do not respond to antidepressant drugs, it is not going to become an obsolete treatment unless and until more effective antidepressant drugs are developed. Janicak, Davis, Gibbons, Ericksen, Chang, and Gallagher (1985) published a meta-analysis that showed ECT to be clearly superior to the tricyclic antidepressants, the monoamine oxidase (MAO) inhibitors, simulated ECT, and placebo for severe depression.

This review covers eight areas relevant to the issue of permanent brain damage caused by ECT. These are (a) subjective report long after ECT, (b) human brain autopsy reports, (c) animal brain studies, (d) the brains of epileptics, (e) spontaneous seizures, (f) psychological test findings in patients with history of many ECT, (g) CT scan findings, and (h) magnetic resonance imaging (MRI) findings.

It is important that the reader be aware of the importance of distinguishing between the modern era of ECT administration with hyperoxygenation, muscle relaxation, and general anaesthesia, and ECT administration before the 1960s, which was less safe for the brain. A number of researchers and authorities have emphasized this distinction (Janicak, Mark, Trimakas, & Gibbons, 1985; Weiner, 1979; d'Elia & Raotma, 1975; Kendell & Pratt, 1983).

It is also important for the reader to bear in mind that unmodified ECT is often administered in third world countries (Weiner, 1984). The brains of poor people in poor countries also deserve protection. Shukla (1981) stated that in India, because of the shortage of anesthesiologists, most psychiatric centers, even in teaching centers, often have to use unmodified ECT that is followed by severe confusion. In India, ECT is used much more often than in the United States and is the mainstay of treatment for schizophrenia.

SUBJECTIVE REPORT

It is common knowledge that most patients complain of memory impairment during and after their course of ECT. There have been at least four studies that have investigated subjective reports of memory deficit long after it is expected that this impairment should have dissipated.

Freeman, Weeks, and Kendell (1980) placed a notice in a local newspaper in the United Kingdom asking for participation of subjects who had ECT at any time in their lives. In addition to the 13 subjects thusly recruited, there were 12 subjects who had been identified as complainers of impairment and referred by local psychiatrists. There were two main sorts of memory complaints. One was forgetfulness of such things as faces, names, phone numbers, and messages. The other was that of holes or gaps in past memories. Furthermore, these subjects' scores on neuropsychological tests were inferior to those of control persons. Needless to say, the generalizability of these findings is very limited because of the subject selection process. Nevertheless, these findings do mesh with other studies concerning the memory complaints of patients who had a past history of ECT.

One hundred and sixty-six patients who had ECT from 1 to 7 years before were interviewed. Although a clear majority of the patients viewed the treatment as beneficial, 30% stated thaty believed the ECT produced lasting memory impairment (Freeman & Kendell, 1980).

Squire and Slater (1983) followed up 31 patients 3 years after ECT. Eighteen (58%) of the respondents said they did not think their memory was as good as for most people their age. Seventeen of these 18 persons attributed their memory difficulty to ECT.

In summary, there is a good accumulation of evidence that many patients complain of memory impairment attributed to their ECT years before. The authors of these studies pointed out that these reports do not provide conclusive evidence that such impairment actually exists. Nevertheless, these reports do legislate against a completely confident bill of health for ECT.

ANIMAL BRAIN STUDIES

Perhaps the most reasonable omnibus generalization is that many animal studies have been carried out, and that some authors have reported permanent damage and some authors have not reported permanent brain damage. In the 15-study review of Hartelius (1952), 13 of the 15 reported pathological findings that were vascular, glial, or neurocytological—or (as was generally the case) in two or three of these domains. However, as Hartelius pointed out, inferences of these studies tended to be conflicting because of different methods used and because of deficient controls. The research that Hartelius himself carried out was unquestionably the outstanding study in the area with respect to methodological sophistication and rigor. Hartelius employed 47 cats, 31 receiving ECT and 16 being control animals. To prevent artifacts associated with the sacrificing of the animals, the cerebrums were removed under anesthesia while the animals were still alive. Brain examinations were conducted blindly with respect to ECT versus control subject. On a number of different vascular, glial, and neuronal variables, the ECT animals were significantly differentiated from the controls. The animals that had 11–16 ECTs had significantly greater pathology than the animals that had received four ECTs. Most of the significant differences were with respect to reversible-type changes. However, some of the significant differences pertained to clearly irreversible changes such as shadow cells and neuronophagia.

The preponderance of human and animal autopsy studies were carried out prior to the modern era of ECT administration that included anesthesia, muscle relaxants, and hyperoxygenation. In fact, animals that were paralyzed and artificially ventilated on oxygen had brain damage of somewhat lesser magnitude than, although similarly patterned as, animals not convulsed without special measures (Meldrum & Brierley, 1973; Meldrum, Vigourocex, & Brierly, 1973).

Needless to say, the generalization from these studies to humans is most difficult because of the great variation in stimulus parameters and other properties of the ECT, the different types of animals, and varying sophistication of design. Nevertheless, there does seem to be one generalization that applies to both animals and humans. It is possible to cause definite permanent brain damage through ECT, and it is possible to administer ECT with minimal or no damage. It is not a matter of whether ECT can produce permanent damage but a matter of in what circumstances it occurs.

HUMAN BRAIN AUTOPSY REPORTS

In the 1940s and 1950s, there were a large number of reports concerning the examination of brains of persons who had died following ECT. Madow (1956) reviewed 38 such cases. In 31 of the 38 cases, there was vascular pathology. However, much of this could have been of a potentially reversible nature. Such reversibility was much less with the 12 patients who had neuronal and/or glial pathology. In one case, the author (Riese, 1948), in addition to giving the neuronal and glial changes, reported numerous slits and rents similar to that seen after execution. Needless to say, patients who died following ECT are not representative of patients receiving ECT. They tended to be in inferior physical health. Madow concluded, on the basis of these 38 cases and five of his own, "If the individual being treated is well physically, most of the neuropathological changes are reversible. If, on the other hand, the patient has cardiac, vascular, or renal disease, the cerebral changes, chiefly vascular, may be permanent" (p. 347).

An interesting autopsy case report was presented by Lippmann et al. (1985). An 89-year-old woman with a long history of psychiatric illness died in 1982 after a documented history of 1250 bilateral treatments beginning in the 1920s. There was also some unsubstantiated evidence of her having received 800 additional ECTs. The authors stated that the moderate cerebral atrophy was consistent with her age and did not show old focal ischemic lesions or any evidence of brain injury resulting from the ECT. The author of the present chapter does believe that these clinical observations, even though based on an apparently nonblind determination, do argue in favor of the brain safety of ECT, especially since many of her treatments were administered prior to the modern era (1960 to present) of ECT administration. However, I raise the question of this woman's aging processes masking the ECT effects upon the brain many years earlier. I note that the authors stated that examination of the frontal lobes failed to reveal the sites of the cannula used in her prefrontal lobotomy in 1953.

CT SCANS

Calloway, Dolan, Jacoby, and Levy (1981) found no significant relationships between history of ECT and CT-scan-determined atrophy and ventricle size. However, a positive significant relationship between ECT and frontal lobe atrophy was found. Borderline significance was obtained with parietal atrophy. However, the authors appropriately raised the possibility that frontal lobe atrophy could have been present before ECT and in some way contributed to the patients receiving ECT.

Calloway, Dolan, and Jacoby (1988) found frontal lobe atrophy assessed by CT scans in 15 of 22 elderly depressed patients who had a history of ECT in contrast to four of 15 control patients without a history of ECT.

Weinberger, Torrey, Neophytides, and Wyatt (1979) found that those patients who had received ECT had significantly higher ventricle brain ratios than patients with no history of ECT.

One study found no relationship between CT scan assessed ventricular enlargement and number of life history of ECT in 27 bipolar patients (Pearlson et al. 1984). However, ECT was a minor part of this study and the authors did not specify how many patients received ECT. The details of ECT administration were also not specified. However, since the patients were from 18 and 40 years of age and presumably living in the United States, a reasonable assumption is that they received modern era administration with oxygenation, sedation, and general anaesthesia.

Kendell and Pratt (1983) presented CT findings on 12 patients who had a history of from 14 and 398 and a median of 94 ECT which were predominantly to the nondominant hemisphere. In two cases, CT scans were performed before history of ECT. In five cases, scans were obtained early in the course of treatment after two to six treatments. In all 12 patients, examinations were made at the end of therapy, which had lasted from over 1–40 years. Neither blind assessment of CT scans nor ventricle measurement pointed to effects of ECT upon the brain. Any increase in atrophy over the years was described as minimal and either bilateral or equally ipsilateral and contralateral to the treated hemisphere. The authors concluded that the absence of CT changes cannot exclude damage but that it is encouraging that CT showed no evidence of this occurring with prolonged courses of ECT taking place over widely varying period of time.

Kolbeinson, Arnoldson, Petruson, and Skulason (1986) found that 22 patients with a history of ECT did not differ in CT scan findings from control patients without a history of ECT. Neither atrophy scores nor ventricle brain ratios differentiated the two groups.

One patient was given a CT scan the day before and 3 hours after multiple ECT that consisted of 10 ECT in a period of 45 minutes (Menken, Safer, Goldfarb, & Varga, 1979). The patient was very confused, disoriented with respect to time and place, and amnestic for events before the day of ECT. Nevertheless, no CT changes were observed. The findings would appear to point to the safeness of the ECT. However, the present author is willing to entertain an alternative explanation. If the CT did not reflect the massive acute brain syndrome with gross disorientation, then it may not be capable of detecting minor changes in patients months or years after the ECT. Perhaps the CT scan is not the most optimal tool for ruling out brain changes resulting from ECT.

A reasonable generalization may be that CT scans have failed to provide a definitive perspective with respect to the matter of permanent brain damage.

MAGNETIC RESONANCE IMAGING

Coffey and colleagues (1988) reported on magnetic resonance imaging before and after ECT administered to nine depressed patients. Blind raters' assessments showed no significant differences between pre- and postECT in cortical atrophy and global comparison. There were also no significant changes in ventricle brain ratios. Furthermore, patients with preexisting brain disease showed no worsening. However, the authors did state: "Still these observations need to be confirmed in a larger number of subjects with techniques that will quantitate even subtle brain changes which might otherwise not be detected by qualitative clinical assessments. Further studies should also include patients with histories of previous ECT (to evaluate any potential cumulative effects) and should involve long-term follow-up studies including both subjective and objective measures of memory function" (p. 706).

A case report of a multiple sclerosis patient with magnetic resonance imaging before and after ECT is reassuring. There was no evidence of changes in white matter lesions visualized on spin-echo images (Coffee, Weiner, McCall, & Heinz, 1987).

In summary, the two studies using magnetic resonance imaging did not provide evidence of permanent brain damage resulting from ECT. However, more studies are needed.

PSYCHOLOGICAL TESTING WITH PAST HISTORY OF MANY ECTS

Goldman, Gomer, and Templer (1972) administered the Bender-Gestalt and the Benton Visual Retention Test to schizophrenics in a VA hospital. Twenty had a past history of from 50 to 219 ECTs, and 20 had no history of ECT. The ECT patients did significantly worse on both instruments. Furthermore, within the ECT groups there were significant inverse correlations between performance on these tests and number of ECTs received. However, the authors acknowledge that

ECT-caused brain damage could not be conclusively inferred because of the possibility that the ECT patients were more psychiatrically disturbed and for this reason received the treatment. (Schizophrenics tend to do poorly on tests of organicity.) In a subsequent study aimed at ruling out this possibility, Templer, Ruff, and Armstrong (1973) administered the Bender-Gestalt, the Benton, and the Wechsler Adult Intelligence Scale to 22 state-hospitalized schizophrenics who had a past history of from 40 to 263 ECTs and to 22 control schizophrenics. The ECT patients were significantly inferior on all three tests. However, the ECT patients were found to be more psychotic. Nevertheless, with degree of psychosis controlled for, the performance of the ECT patients was still significantly inferior on the Bender-Gestalt, although not significantly so on the other two tests.

Thus, the research using psychological tests with patients with history of many ECTs does suggest permanent impairment. However, one should bear in mind that retrospective studies do not permit the same confidence as do prospective studies. Also, the ECT in these studies was administered before the modern era of ECT.

BRAINS OF EPILEPTICS

It would seem that if an epileptic grand mal seizure produces permanent brain changes, then an electrically induced convulsion should also do so. In fact, inspecting the evidence with respect to epileptics may provide us with a conservative perspective in regard to ECT because the latter could produce damage from the externally applied electrical current as well as from the seizure. Experimental research with animals has shown that electric shocks (not to the head) produce more deleterious effects in the central nervous system than any other locality or system of the body. More pertinent are the studies of Small (1974) and of Laurell (1979) that found less memory impairment after inhalant-induced convulsions than ECT. Also, Levy, Serota, and Grinker (1942) reported less EEG abnormality and intellectual impairment with pharmacologically in-duced convulsions. Further argument provided by Friedberg (1977) is the case (Larsen & Vraa-Jensen, 1953) of a man who had been given four ECTs, but did not convulse. When he died 3 days later, a subarachnoid hemorrhage was found in the upper part of the left motor region "at the site where an electrode had been applied" (p. 18).

A number of postmortem reports on epileptics, as reviewed by Meldrum, Horton, and Brierley (1974) have indicated neuronal loss and gliosis, especially in the hippocampus and temporal lobe. However, as Meldrum et al. (1974) pointed out, on the basis of these postmortem reports, one does not know whether the damage was caused by the seizures or whether both were caused by a third factor intrinsic to the epilepsy. To clarify this issue, Meldrum et al. (1974) pharmacologically induced seizures in baboons and found cell changes that corresponded to those in human epileptics.

Gastaut and Gastaut (1976) demonstrated through brain scans that in seven of 20 cases status epilepticus produced brain atrophy. They reasoned, "Since the edema and the atrophy were unilateral and bilateral and related to the localization of the convulsions (unilateral or bilateral chronic seizures), the conclusion can be drawn that the atrophic process depends upon the epileptic process and not on the cause of the status" (p. 18).

A common finding in epileptics and ECT patients is noteworthy. Norman (1964) stated that it is not uncommon to find at autopsy both old and recent lesions in the brains of epileptics. Alpers and Hughes (1942) reported old and recent brain lesions associated with different series of ECT.

SPONTANEOUS SEIZURES

The reports of spontaneous seizures, which appeared in the pre-1960s ECT era, probably do not constitute one of the more definitive domains. However, this section is included to increase breadth of perspective.

It would appear that if seizures that were not previously evidenced appeared after ECT and persisted, permanent brain pathology must be inferred. There have been numerous cases of postECT spontaneous seizures reported in the literature and briefly reviewed by Blumenthal (1955), Pacella and Barrera (1945), and Karliner (1956). It appears that in the majority of cases the seizures do not persist indefinitely, although an exact perspective is difficult to obtain because of anticonvulsant medication employed and the limited follow-up information. Another difficulty is, in all cases, definitively tracing the etiology to the ECT, since spontaneous seizures develop in only a very small proportion of patients given this treatment. Nevertheless, the composite of relevant literature does indicate that, at least in some patients, no evidence of seizure potential existed before treatment and postECT seizures persist for years.

An article that is one of the most systematic and representative in terms of findings is that of Blumenthal (1955) who reported on 12 schizophrenic patients in one hospital who developed postECT convulsions. Six of the patients had previous EEGs with four of them being normal, one clearly abnormal, and one mildly abnormal. The patients averaged 72 ECTs and 12 spontaneous seizures. The time from last treatment to first spontaneous seizure ranged from 12 hours to 11 months, with an average of 2½ months. The total duration of spontaneous seizures in the study period ranged from 1 day to 3½ years, with an average of 1 year. Following the onset of seizures, eight of the 12 patients were found to have a clearly abnormal, and one a mildly abnormal EEG.

Masovich and Katzenelbogen (1948) reported that 20 of their 82 patients had convulsive pattern cerebral dysrhythmia 10 months post-ECT. None had such in their pretreatment EEG. Nine (15%) of the 60 patients who had three to 15 treatments, and 11 (50%) of the 22 patients who had from 16 to 42 treatments

($x^2 = 10.68$; $p < 0.01$, according to our calculations) had this 10-month post-treatment dysrhythmia.

SYNTHESIS

There seems to be little doubt that ECT always produces an acute brain syndrome and that such remits over time. There seems to be little doubt that ECT has, at least in the past, caused permanent brain damage in some patients and has the capacity to continue to do so. There also seems to be little doubt that modern era ECT has greater brain safety than that administered prior to the 1960s. It appears that the overwhelming majority of persons who currently receive ECT in the United States do not suffer from massive cognitive deficits caused by the ECT.

What percentage of persons who receive ECT suffer some permanent impairment? What are, if any, the long-term effects of ECT in the "typical" or "average" ECT patient? Can we tell most of our patients there is absolutely and positively no danger of any permanent brain changes? These are the sort of questions for which we cannot provide confident answers. The present author believes that the difficulties in answering such questions are similar to the questions regarding whether or not alcohol and alcoholism are associated with brain pathology. We do know that a small amount of alcohol produces changes in the brain in all alcoholics and in all normal drinkers. We also know that all or almost all of these effects rather quickly dissipate. We also know that some alcoholics have massive and permanent brain pathology, for example, as seen in Korsakoff's syndrome. We know that a large percentage of newly abstinent alcoholics suffer from neuropsychological deficits. We know that in many of these patients there is improvement in neuropsychological testing over time and in some patients even a retrenchment in cortical atrophy. However, when we attempt to supply the details to answers about the typical or average alcoholic, or even the specification of who are average or typical alcoholics, the situation becomes less clear. This is the difficult situation we face with ECT patients. Some authors argue that ECT is hazardous to the brain and others argue it is safe. I believe they are both right.

The crucial questions at this point in time are those centered around in whom and in what circumstances are the risks higher and lower. We are able to make some generalizations. There is research evidence that type of ECT administration does have an effect upon degree of confusion and amnesia. Higher levels of stimulus intensity, stimulus waveforms that are relatively inefficient in seizure-eliciting properties, and bilateral electrode placement are associated with greater confusion and amnesia (Sackeim, Decena, Prohovnik, Malitz, & Resor, 1983; Cronholm & Ottossom, 1963; Ottossom, 1960; Valentine & Dunne, 1969; Weiner, Rogers, Welch, Davison, Weir, Cahill, & Squire, 1983; Sackeim, Portney, Neeley, Steif, Decema, & Malitz, 1986; Squire & Slater, 1978).

A convergence of evidence indicates the importance of number of ECTs. We have previously referred to the significant inverse correlations between number of ECTs and scores on psychological tests. It is conceivable that this could be a function of the more disturbed patients both receiving more ECTs and doing worse on tests. However, it would be much more difficult to explain away the relationship between number of ECTs received and EEG convulsive pattern dysrhythmia (Mosovich & Katzenelbogen, 1948). No patients had dysrhythmia prior to ECT. Also difficult to explain away is that in Table 1 of Meldrum, Horton and Brierley (1974), the nine baboons who suffered brain damage from experimentally administrated convulsions tended to have recevied more convulsions than the five that did not incur damage. (According to our calculations, $U = 9$, $p < 0.05$.) And, as already stated, Hartelius found greater damage, both reversible and irreversible, in cats that were given 11 to 16 than in those given four ECTs.

Throughout this review the vast individual differences are striking. In the animal and human autopsy studies there is typically a range of findings from no lasting effect to considerable lasting damage with the latter being more of the exception. Most ECT patients do not have spontaneous seizures, but some do. The subjective reports of patients likewise differ from those of no lasting effect to appreciable, although usually not devastating, impairment. The fact that many patients and subjects suffer no demonstrable permanent effects has provided rationale for some authorities to commit the *nonsequitur* that ECT causes no permanent harm.

There is evidence to suggest that preECT physical condition accounts in part for the vast individual differences. Jacobs (1944) determined the cerebrospinal fluid protein and cell content before, during, and after a course of ECT with 21 patients. The one person who developed abnormal protein and cell elevations was a 57-year-old diabetic, hypertensive, arteriosclerotic woman. Jacobs recommended that CSF protein and cell counts be ascertained before and after ECT in patients with significant degree of arteriosclerotic or hypertensive disease. Alpers (1946) reported, "Autopsied cases suggest that brain damage is likely to occur in conditions with pre-existing brain damage, as in cerebral arteriosclerosis" (p. 369). Wilcox (1944) offered the clinical impression that, in older patients, ECT memory changes continue for a longer time than for younger patients. Hartelius (1952) found significantly more reversible and irreversible brain changes following ECT in older cats than younger cats. Mosovich and Katzenelbogen (1948) found that patients with pretreatment EEG abnormalities are more likely to show marked post-ECT cerebral dysrhythmia and to generally show EEGs more adversely affected by treatment.

RECOMMENDATIONS

It is recommended that more research be carried out on the safety and the hazards of ECT. Research on the unmodified ECT given in the developing countries of the world would seem to be especially important. The present author does not have the credentials to make recommendations concerning the brain safety precautions that should be followed. However, I here present the recommendations of Frankel et al. (1978) and those of Weiner (1984).

Weiner (1984) recommended that a careful analysis of risks and benefits be determined; that the possibility of persistent memory defects should be part of the informed consent procedure; that ordinarily unilateral nondominant electrode placement should be used; that EEG monitoring should be carried out; that instruction in sophisticated use of ECT should be in psychiatric residency programs and continuing education opportunities; that inspections of ECT equipment should be made; that the public should be better informed about ECT; and that more research be carried out.

Frankel et al. (1978) recommended that the patients receive a thorough pretreatment medical examination; that there be designated ECT and recovery room areas with availability of equipment, drugs, and personnel in the event of cardiopulmonary or other complications; that ECT be administered with anesthesia and muscle relaxant drugs and ventilatory assistance with a positive pressure bag and 100% oxygen, with EKG, blood pressure and pulse rate monitoring, and with appropriate electrode placement and electrical parameters; that ECT only be used in those conditions for which ECT efficacy has been established; that medical contraindications be considered; that the severity and unremitting nature of the patient's suffering and incapacitation and unresponsiveness to other treatments be taken into account; and that proper informed consent be obtained.

REFERENCES

Alpers, B. J. (1946). The brain changes associated with electrical shock treatment: A critical review. *Lancet, 66*, 363–369.

Blumenthal, I. J. (1955). Spontaneous seizures and related electroencephalographic findings following shock therapy. *Journal of Nervous and Mental Disease, 122*, 581–588.

Calloway, S. P., Dolan, R. J., Jacoby, R. J., & Levy, R. (1981). ECT and cerebral atrophy: A computer tomographic study. *Acta Psychiatrica Scandinavica, 63*, 442–445.

Coffey, C. E., Figiel, G. S., Djang, W. T., Sullivan, D. C., Herfkens, P. V., & Weiner, R. D. (1988). Effects of ECT or brain structure. *American Journal of Psychiatry, 145*, 701–706.

Cronholm, B., & Ottossom, J. O. (1963). Ultrabrief stimulus techniques in ECT. 1. Influence on retrograde amnesia. *Journal of Nervous and Mental Disease, 137*, 117–123.

d'Elia, G., & Frederiksen, S. O. (1980). ACTH4-10 and memory in ECT-treated and untreated patients. I. Effect on consolidation. *Acta Psychiatrica Scandinavica, 62*, 418–428.

d'Elia, G., & Roathma, H. (1975). Is unilateral ECT less effective than bilateral ECT? *British Journal of Psychiatry, 126*, 83–89.

Frankel, F. H., Bidder, T. G., Fink, M., Mandel, M. R., Small, I. F., Wayne, G. J., Squire, L. R., Dutton, E. N., & Gurel, L. (1978). *Electroconvulsive therapy. Report on the task force on electroconvulsive therapy of the American Psychiatric Association.* Washington, DC: American Psychiatric Association.

Freeman, C. P. L., & Kendell, R. E. (1980). Patients' experiences of and attitudes to ECT. *British Journal of Psychiatry, 137,* 8–16.

Freeman, C. P. L., Weeks, D., & Kendell, R. E. (1980). ECT: Patients who complain. *British Journal of Psychiatry, 137,* 17–25.

Friedberg, J. (1977). ECT as a neurologic injury. *Psychiatric Opinion, 14,* 16–19.

Gastaut, H., & Gastaut, J. (1976). Computerized axial tomography in epilepsy. In J. K. Penry (Ed.), *The Eighth International Symposium.* New York: Raven Press.

Goldman, H., Gomer, F. E., & Templer, D. I. (1972). Long-term effects of electroconvulsive therapy upon memory and perceptual-motor performance. *Journal of Clinical Psychology, 28,* 32–34.

Hartelius, H. (1952). Cerebral changes following electrically induced convulsions: An experimental study on cats. *Acta Psychiatrica Et Neuroligica Scandinavica, 77,* 1–128.

Jacobs, J. S. L. (1944). The effect of electric shock therapy upon cerebrospinal fluid pressure, protein and cells. *American Journal of Psychiatry, 101,* 110–112.

Janicak, P. G., Davis, J. M., Gibbons, V. G., Ericksen, S., Chang, S., & Gallagher, P. (1985). Effects of ECT-A meta-analysis. *American Journal of Psychiatry, 142,* 297–302.

Janicak, P. G., Mark, J., Trimakas, K. A., & Gibbons, V. G. (1985). ECT: An assessment of mental health professionals' knowledge and attitudes. *Journal of Clinical Psychiatry, 46,* 262–266.

Karliner, W. (1956). Epileptic states following electroshock therapy. *Journal of Hillside Hospital, 5,* 258–263.

Kendell, B., & Pratt, R. T. C. (1983). *British Journal of Psychiatry, 143,* 99–100.

Kolbeinsson, H., Arnaldsson, O. S., Petursson, H., & Skulason, S. (1986). Computer tomographic scan in ECT patients. *Acta Psychiatrica Scandinavica, 73,* 28–32.

Kramer, B. A. (1985). Use of ECT in California, 1977–1983. *American Journal of Psychiatry, 142,* 1190–1192.

Larsen, E. F., & Vraa-Jensen, G. (1953). Ischaemic changes in the brain following electroshock therapy. *Acta Psychiatrica Et Neuroligica Scandinavica, 28,* 75–80.

Laurell, B. (1970). Flurothyl convulsive therapy. *Acta Psychiatrica Scandinavica, 213,* 5–79.

Levy, N. A., Serota, H. M., & Grinker, R. R. (1942). Disturbance in brain function following convulsive shock therapy. *Archives of Neurology and Psychiatry, 47,* 1000–1029.

Lippmann, S., Manshadi, M., Wehry, M., Byrol, R., Past, W., Keller, W., Schuster, J., Elam, S., Meyer, O., & O'Daniel, R. (1985). 1250 Electroconvulsant treatments without evidence of brain injury. *British Journal of Psychiatry, 147,* 203–204.

Madow, L. (1956). Brain changes in electroshock therapy. *American Journal of Psychiatry, 113,* 337–347.

Meldrum, B. S., & Brierley, J. B. (1973). Prolonged epileptic seizures in primates: Ischaemic cell change and its relation to ictal physiological event. *Archives of Neurology, 28,* 10–17.

Meldrum, B. S., Horton, R. W., & Brierley, J. B. (1974). Epileptic brain damage in adolescent baboons following seizures induced by allylglycine. *Brain, 97,* 407–418.

Meldrum, B. S., Vigouroux, R. A., & Brierley, J. B. (1973). Systemic factors and epileptic brain damage. *Archives of Neurology, 29,* 82–87.

Menken, M., Safer, J., Goldfarb, C., & Varga, E. (1979). Multiple ECT: Morphologic effects. *American Journal of Psychiatry, 136,* 453.

Mosovich, A., & Katzenelbogan, S. (1948). Electroshock therapy, clinical and elctroencephalographic studies. *Journal of Nervous and Mental Disease, 107,* 517–530.

Norman, R. M. (1964). The neuropathology of status epilepticus. *Medicine, Science and the Law, 4,* 46–51.

Ottosson, J. O. (1960). Experimental studies on the mode of action of electroconvulsive therapy. *Acta Psychiatrica et Neuroligica Scandinavica, 35*(suppl 145), 1–141.

Pacella, B. L., & Barrera, S. E. (1945). Spontaneous convulsions following convulsive shock therapy. *American Journal of Psychiatry, 102*, 783–788.

Pearlman, C. A., Sharpless, S. K., & Jarvik, M. E. (1961). Retrograde amnesia produced by anesthetic and convulsant agents. *Journal of Comparative and Physiological Psychology, 54*, 109–112.

Riese, W. (1948). Report of two new cases of sudden death after electric shock treatment with histopathological findings in the central nervous system. *Journal of Neuropathology and Experimental Neurology, 7*, 98.

Sackeim, H. A., Decina, P., Kanzler, M., & Ken, B. (1987). Effects of electrode placement on the efficacy of titrated, low dose ECT. *American Journal of Psychiatry, 144*, 1449–1455.

Sackeim, H. A., Decina, P., Prohovnik, I., Malitz, S., & Resor, S. R. (1983). Anticonvulsant and anti-depressant properties of ECT: A proposed mechanism of action. *Biological Psychiatry, 18*, 310–320.

Shukla, C. D. (1981). Electroconvulsive therapy in a rural teaching general hospital in India. *British Journal of Psychiatry, 139*, 569–571.

Siegel, M. A., Plesser, O. R., & Jacobs, N. R. (1987). *Domestica violena: no longer behind closed doors.* Plano, TX: Information Aids.

Small, J. G. (1974). EEG and neurophysiological studies of convulsive therapies. In M. Fink, S. Kety, J. McGaugh, & T. A. Williams (Eds.), *Psychobiology of Convulsive Therapy, Vol. 63* (pp. 79–86). Washington, DC:

Squire, L. R., & Slater, P. C. (1983). Electroconvulsive therapy and complaints of memory dysfunction: A prospective three-year follow-up study. *British Journal of Psychiatry, 142*, 1–8.

Templer, D. I., Ruff, C. F., & Armstrong, G. (1973). Cognitive functioning and degree of psychosis in schizophrenics given many electroconvulsive treatments. *British Journal of Psychiatry, 123*, 441–443.

Templer, D. I., & Veleber, D. M. (1982). Can ECT permanently harm the brain? *Clinical Neuropsychology, 4*, 62–66.

Thompson, J. W., & Blain, I. D. (1987). Use of ECT in the United States in 1975 and 1980. *American Journal of Psychiatry, 144*, 557–562.

Valentine, M., Keddie, K. M., & Dunne, D. (1968). A comparison of techniques in electroconvulsive therapy. *British Journal of Psychiatry, 114*, 989–996.

Weinberger, D. R., Torrey, E. F., Neophytides, A. N., & Wyatt, R. J. (1979). Lateral cerebral ventricular enlargement in chronic schizophrenia. *Archives of General Psychiatry, 36*, 735–739.

Weiner, R. D. (1979). The psychiatric use of electrically induced seizures. *American Journal of Psychiatry, 136*, 1507–1517.

Weiner, R. D., Rogers, H. J., Welch, C. A., Davidson, J. R. T., Miller, R. D., Weir, D., Cahill, J. F., & Squire, L. R. (1983). ECT stimulus parameters and electrode placement. In B. Lerer, R. D. Weiner, & R. H. Belmaker (Eds.), *ECT: Basic mechanisms.* London: John Libbey.

Weiner, R. D. (1984). Does electroconvulsive therapy cause brain damage? *The Behavioral and Brain Sciences, 7*, 1–54.

Wilcox, P. (1944). The electroshock convulsion syndrome. *American Journal of Psychiatry, 100*, 668–683.

PART II

Chemical Damage

CHAPTER 9

INDUSTRIAL TOXINS

Paula K. Lundberg-Love

Data regarding the impact of environmental toxins on the brain and behavior has appeared only recently in the scientifc literature. Indeed, such reports parallel the emergence of the field of industrial medicine. The fact that scientists have only begun to probe the vulnerability of the brain to environmental toxins is somewhat curious, given that anecdotal accounts of the neurotoxicity of such agents have been chronicled for centuries. For example, toxicity due to the use of lead oxide as a sweetening agent and a preservative for wine, cider, and fruit jucies (Fein, Schwartz, Jacobson, & Jacobson, 1983), has been related to the demise of the Roman empire. In 1535, Anglicus Bartholomaeus described the neurological effects of mercury toxicity (Goldwater, 1972), and as early as 1856 problems attributed to carbon disulfide were described in the medical literature (Wood, 1981).

Nevertheless, the United States has lagged behind European and Scandinavian countries in the basic research, clinical application, and the legislative support of neuropsychological toxicity investigations (Hartmann, 1988). Although Scandinavian countries have recognized the neurotoxic effects of the "organic solvent syndrome" (i.e., memory loss, lowered concentration, loss of initiative), scientists in the United States are still debating its existence (Fisher, 1985). This is unfortunate because Anderson (1982) has estimated that there are at least 20 million United States' workers potentially exposed to the mere 167 substances that the National Institute of Occupational Safety and Health (NIOSH) has deemed to be neurotoxic. Moreover, everyday the population at large is exposed to over 53,000 commercial/industrial chemicals, cosmetics, food additives, pesticides, and prescription drugs, few of which have ever been tested for neurotoxicity (Fisher, 1985). In spite of the fact that the goal of the 1970 Occupational Safety and Health Act (OSHA) was to assure healthful working conditions for all employees (Taft, 1974), and that NIOSH was mandated to conduct research regarding both the motivational and behavioral factors related to occupational safety and health, there are no *requirements* for neuropsychological assessments of industrial toxins (Hartmann, 1988). Nevertheless, public health researchers are beginning to detect and to educate other researchers regarding the importance of neurotoxic syndromes as they relate to the quality of life.

However, there are particular complications inherent in the neuropsychological evaluation of individuals with potential neurotoxic syndromes. Thus, there are caveats that one must keep in mind when interpreting the neuropathological and neuropsychological effects of various industrial toxins (Hartmann, 1988). These include (a) neurophysiological/neurochemical mechanistic unknowns of neurotoxins that compromise the neuropsychologist in optimal test selection, (b) problems with the applicability and generalizability of animal models of neurotoxicity to the neuropsychological deficits observed in human beings, and (c) difficulty assessing the magnitude and chronicity of an individual's exposure to environmental neurotoxins. Thus, when considering anecdotal and research results, the neuropsychologist must consider possible differences between the acute and chronic effects of toxin exposure as well as an individual's level of premorbid functioning. Furthermore, interpretation of neuropsychological test data is complicated by the paucity of relevant test norms for exposure to environmental toxins. Finally, since neuropsychological test results can be the most sensitive indicator of neurotoxic insult, there may be a lack of corroborative medical evidence to support a diagnosis. As a result, differential diagnosis can be problematic.

PREVALENCE/INCIDENCE OF EXPOSURE TO INDUSTRIAL NEUROTOXINS

Given the large numbers of known industrial neurotoxins as well as the myriad industrial substances that are potentially neurotoxic, it is beyond the scope of this chapter to discuss the neuropsychological effects of all these compounds. Hence, the effects of selected members of two major classes of neurotoxic industrial chemicals, metals and organic solvents, will be described. These two types of toxins have been selected because research and clinical data exist, albeit some of it rudimentary, which describe their neuropsychological effects.

The prevalence of neuropsychological sequelae that result from industrial neurotoxin exposure is difficult to assess. Many employees in blue collar, white collar, and professional occupations are at risk for solvent or metal exposure. For example, chemical workers, degreasers, dentists, dental hygienists, dry cleaners, electronics workers, hospital personnel, laboratory workers, painters, plastics workers, printers, rayon workers, steel workers, and transportation personnel are all exposed to metals and/or organic solvents (Hartmann, 1988). Table 9-1 lists estimated numbers of workers exposed to various metallic toxins, and Table 9-2 lists the estimated numbers of workers exposed to organic solvents (Anderson, 1982; Hartmann, 1988). Adding the various categories of individuals at risk in Table 9-1 indicates that approximately 6,928,000 industrial workers are exposed

TABLE 9-1 Numbers of Workers Estimated to be at Risk for Exposure to Neurotoxic Metals

Metallic substance	Individuals at risk
Cadmium	1,400,000
Lead (metallic)	1,394,000
Lead acetate	103,000
Lead carbonate	183,000
Lead napthenate	1,280,000
Lead oxides	1,300,000
Manganese	41,000
Mercury (metallic)	24,000
Mercury (organic)	280,000
Mercuric chloride	51,000
Mercuric nitrate	10,100
Mercury sulfide	8,900
Thallium	853,000

to toxic metals or metallic derivatives, whereas approximately 25,316,000 workers are exposed to toxic solvents. These figures suggest that nearly 13.4% of the United States population is at risk for exposure to only two classes of industrial neurotoxins. When one considers that other potential industrial neurotoxins exist for which data have not yet been collected, it is likely that a conservative estimate of the prevalence of industrial neurotoxic exposure may approach at least 15–20% of the United States population. Clearly, the neuropsychological sequelae of industrial toxin exposure is a significant public health problem.

TABLE 9-2 Numbers of Workers Estimated to be at Risk for Exposure to Neurotoxic Solvents

Solvent	Individuals at risk
Alcohols (industrial)	3,851,000
Aliphatic hydrocarbons	2,776,000
Aromatic hydrocarbons	3,611,000
Carbon disulfide	24,000
Carbon tetrachloride	1,379,000
Dichloromethane	2,175,000
Hexane	764,000
Perchloroethylene	1,596,000
Rubber solvents	600,000
Toluene	4,800,000
Trichloroethylene	3,600,000
Xylene	140,000

CONSEQUENCES OF INDUSTRIAL NEUROTOXIN EXPOSURE

Metals

Arsenic

Although Hamilton and Hardy (1974) have suggested that historically arsenic (As) has been a poison used for criminal purposes, it also has been mentioned as an Assyrian pharmacological agent as early as 1552 BC. Arsenic was used as a curative agent for cancer, fever, herpes, ringworm, eczema, ulcers, and syphillis (Marks & Beatty, 1975). However, its administration often resulted in optic neuritis and encephalopathy (Windebank, McCall, & Dyck, 1984).

NIOSH has estimated that that approximately 1.5 million workers are exposed to inorganic arsenic. Pharmaceutical, agricultural, and iron and steel workers are the primary candidates for arsenic exposure. Bleecker and Bolla-Wilson (1985) have suggested that the central nervous system effects of arsenic resemble those found in thiamine deficiency because arsenic prevents the transformation of thiamine into acetyl-COA and succinyl COA. However, validation for this hypothesis has not been obtained as yet.

Exposure to organic (carbon-containing) arsenic compounds can result in a fluctuating mental state, agitation, and emotional lability (Beckett, Moore, Keogh, & Bleecker, 1986) with progression from drowsiness to confusion and stupor. Organic arsenic intoxication can even result in an organic psychosis resembling paranoid schizophrenia and eventual delirium (Windebank, McCall, & Dyck, 1984).

Lead

The toxicity of lead (Pb) was recognized as early as 200 BC by the physician Nikander of Colophon, who described gastrointestinal effects, nociceptive effects, and swelling/inflammation of the limbs. Currently, the world output of lead exceeds 3.5 million tons per year and is greater than that of any other toxic metal (Hartmann, 1988). Although the practice of adding lead to gasoline has decreased significantly, lead is still a component of paint pigments, ceramic glazes, and batteries. Indeed, more than 800,000 United States workers experience occupational lead exposure, and nearly 20% of these workers have elevated blood lead levels (Schottenfeld & Cullen, 1984). The magnitude of lead exposure is second only to the magnitude of alcohol exposure. As a result there are more data describing the neurological effects of lead than any other neurotoxic metal (Hartmann, 1988).

Lead exposure can occur via inhalation or ingestion. Physiological transportation is effected by the erythrocytes and lead is then deposited in bone and the soft tissue. As a result, the biological half-life of blood lead is relatively short (2–3 weeks) as compared to the biological half-life of bone lead which is estimated to be 10 years (Krigman, Bouldin, & Mushak, 1980). Indeed, 90% of the body burden of lead is contained in bone. Hence, blood lead levels may reflect only a rough approximation of body and brain lead burden. Lilis et al. (1977) have suggested that zinc protoporphyrin (ZPP) level may be a more sensitive index of biologically active lead than blood lead levels, particularly as it relates to the nervous system. ZPP is a substance that accumulates in erythrocytes when lead disrupts the ability of the red blood cell to incorporate iron.

Although the precise mechanisms whereby lead exerts it neuropathologic effects remain unknown, there are several hypotheses. Silbergeld (1982) has suggested that lead may compete with calcium, sodium, and/or magnesium and thus ionically disrupt neural transmission. Or there may be effects on neuronal mitochondria such that the process of phosphorylation is inhibited. Additionally, lead may disrupt processes such as membrane transport, oxidative phosphorylation, and heme synthesis thereby altering neuronal function by depleting precursor supplies, reducing energy sources, or by producing neurotoxic intermediate chemical species.

There are also animal research and human case study data that suggest that lead may be a demyelinating agent (Behse & Carlson, 1978). Also, Nicklowitz (1979) has observed neurofibrillary tangles in lead-exposed animals as well as on autopsy of a 42-year-old survivor of childhood lead encephalopathy. He has suggested that chronic lead exposure may induce an Alzheimer's-like syndrome. Finally, Benson and Price (1985) have reported that lead exposure may result in cerebellar capillary calcification, and it has been found that 84% of 44 patients diagnosed with lead neuropathy at autopsy exhibited cerebellar calcification. Nevertheless, human case study data are sparse in the recent scientific literature. Thus, our knowledge of the neuropathologic mechanisms of lead exposure remains embryonic. Data regarding differential lead toxicity as a function of brain area are lacking, as are data describing the importance of individual differences such as age, gender, diet, and metabolism upon mediation of lead toxicity.

Typically adult lead exposure occurs in the workplace. Lead smelters, individuals involved in battery manufacturing/recycling and auto repair, lead shot manufacturers and painters who use or remove lead-based paint are at greatest risk for toxic lead exposure (Windebank, McCall, & Dyck, 1984). However, lead poisoning also has been documented in Jewish scribes who prepare and use a special lead-containing ink (Cohen et al., 1986).

Describing the neuropsychological effects of lead toxicity is complicated by the fact that there are both organic and inorganic sources of lead in the workplace. Organic lead compounds are those in which lead is covalently bonded to carbon and include leaded gasoline, some solvents, or cleaning fluids. Inorganic lead compounds are those that are ionically bonded to substances other than carbon and include a wide array of chemicals.

Organic lead exposure can result in neuropsychological as well as affective symptoms. The former can include a variety of cognitive deficits such as memory dysfunction and concentration difficulties, whereas the latter can include restlessness, impotence, nightmares, and psychosis with hallucinations. In high concentrations, organic lead exposure can induce delirium, convulsions, and coma (Grandjean, 1983).

Exposure to inorganic lead appears to induce a constellation of neuropathological, cognitive and affective symptoms different from that of exposure to organic lead. Neurotoxicity due to inorganic lead may particularly disrupt the cerebellum and hippocampus and tends to present within the context of a systemic illness with classic symptoms such as abdominal pain, constipation, anemia, neuropathy, and at times, gout (Windebank, McCall, & Dyck, 1984).

The mechanisms of organic lead toxicity are thought to involve interference with neuronal energy and metabolic processes as well as possible direct damage to the hippocampus, amygdala, and pyriform cortex (Grandjean, 1983). Tetraethyl lead, formerly a common additive to gasoline, is metabolized to triethyl lead, which can cross the blood–brain barrier and disrupt central cholinergic and adrenergic neuronal pathways (Bolter, Stanczik, & Long, 1983). However, lead-containing fuels also contain neurotoxic substances such as benzene, xylene, ethylene dichloride, and triorthocresyl so the neuropsychological effects of leaded gasoline may result for triethyl lead and solvent exposure in conjunction with hypoxia, in cases where unconsciousness occurs (Poklis & Burkett, 1977). Typically, unconsciousness is associated with voluntary intoxication. However, two cases of high-dose gasoline exposure via a gasoline storage tank with resultant hypoxia have been described by Bolter, Stanczik, and Long (1983). One subject, who was unconscious for 20 minutes experienced various cerebellar and cortical symptoms including nausea, anxiety, paresthesias, and dysarthria. The results of neuropsychological testing indicated borderline-range intellectual and short-term memory deficits, impaired motor functioning of the right hand, decreased bilateral tactile sensitivity, and impairments of phoneme discrimination, rhythm discrimination, expressive language, abstract reasoning, and sensorimotor functioning. Two-year follow-up examination of the subject revealed headache, numbness and weakness of the right hand, reduced language, verbal memory disabilities, and impaired emotional functioning.

The second subject, who was unconscious for only 2 minutes, exhibited left hemisphere deficits that were apparent three years after the accident. This individual also showed reactive emotional symptomatology that appeared to be linked to the exposure. These symptoms included phobic reaction to gasoline fumes, suspicion, distrust, and withdrawal. The authors speculated that the reduced verbal functioning observed in both subjects was related to a greater relative impairment of left hemisphere functions that, in turn, may reflect greater disruption of cholinergic activity.

Individuals exposed to inorganic lead often fail to report symptoms when blood levels are less than 40 μg/dl. Nevertheless, neurological abnormalities have been detected in the absence of subjective complaint. For example, nerve conduction velocities of median and posterior tibial nerves were significantly correlated with blood lead levels in 39 lead workers with a mean blood lead concentration of 29 μg/dl (Araki & Honma, 1976). Also, significant reductions in visual sensitivity, presumed to reflect optic nerve damage, was found in 35 workers with subclinical blood lead levels (Cavalleri et al., 1982). Such data appear to support Niklowitz's (1979) suggestion that lead can penetrate the brain even at low, subclinical blood lead levels, and that brain tissue is, therefore, exquisitely vulnerable to lead damage.

As in the case of neurological symptomatology, neuropsychological deficits do not necessarily correlate well with blood lead levels or subjective complaint. Neuropsychological effects have been detected at subclinical blood levels of 40–50 μg/dl in the absence of subjective complaints. Hänninen et al. (1979) studied 20 workers whose blood lead levels never exceeded 50 μg/dl, 25 workers whose blood lead levels varied from 50 to 69 μg/dl and compared both groups to a control group. The length of exposure ranged from 2–9 years and subjective complaints were assessed using a Finnish adaptation of the Eysenck Personality Inventory and a questionnaire. The results indicated that workers with low lead exposure reported more postwork fatigue, sleepiness, apathy, and depression as compared to controls. Although higher level lead-exposed workers reported fatigue, restlessness, and apathy, they also described forgetfulness, sensorimotor complaints, and gastrointestinal symptoms (Hänninen, 1979).

Individuals with lead levels exceeding 69 μg/dl tend to report more somatic or emotional symptoms as opposed to cognitive ones. However, it is unclear whether these reports result from the greater saliency of gastrointestinal discomfort and joint pain, or whether attention and abstraction deficits impair the individual's ability to recognize his/her cognitive losses. Nevertheless, the data suggest that neuropsychological assessment is a more sensitive index of lead neurotoxicity than is subjective complaint and can be utilized to detect the effects of low level lead exposure (Hartmann, 1988).

Neuropsychological effects that result from lead exposure include deficits in visuomotor function and visual intelligence (Hänninen et al., 1978), deficits in general intelligence (Grandjean, Arnvig, & Beckmann, 1978) and memory for newly learned material (Feldman, Ricks, & Baker, 1980). Lead-related disruption of information processing appeared to result in decrements in sensory storage memory, Sternberg-type short-term memory scanning, and paired-associate learning (Williamson & Teo, 1986). These data, coupled with lower flicker fusion thresholds, led the authors to interpret their results as being indicative of an arousal deficit and/or a degradation of retinal or visual pathway input. Additionally, deficits in psychomotor speed and dexterity have been documented (Williamson & Teo, 1986), and are thought to result from damage to areas of the motor cortex or reductions in nerve conduction velocity (Hänninen, 1982).

Bleecker et al. (1982) have reported the neuropsychological effects associated with blood lead levels of approximately 30 μg/dl. Workers who had been lead-exposed for a median of 2.5 months (range of 2 weeks to 8 months) exhibited significant deficits on the Block Design and Digit Symbol subtests of the Wechsler Adult Intelligence Scale and marginally significant visual memory impairment on the Wechsler Memory Scale. A reduced rate of learning on the Rey Auditory Verbal Learning Test also was found. Severe lead poisoning can present as a global dementia with generalized memory loss with deficits in attention, concentration and abstract thought processing (Hartmann, 1988).

Lead exposure can result in emotional as well as cognitive changes. Baker et al. (1983) have reported fatigue, confusion, tension, anger, and depression associated with lead exposure. Bleecker et al. (1982) have confirmed these observations in workers with exposure histories of 2 weeks to 8 months. It is important that mental health professionals be aware of the affective sequelae of lead intoxication because a misdiagnosis of affective disorder can delay the appropriate administration of chelation therapy (Schottenfeld & Cullen, 1984).

The precise nature of the central nervous system mechanisms involved in lead-induced emotional alterations remains unknown. However, organic brain dysfunction can produce depression as a result of cortical and/or subcortical neural damage. Schottenfeld and Cullen (1984) have suggested that hypothalamic changes and disruption of catecholamine metabolism may be involved. Affective changes secondary to the recognition of diminished cognitive capacity is also a possibility.

Clearly, research delineating the precise nature of lead associated neuropathy is still needed. However, what is apparent, is that both organic and inorganic forms of lead are potent neurotoxins capable of inducing a wide array of somatic, cognitive, and affective changes. Although neuropsychological testing can detect the effects of lead exposure, and chelation therapy can reduce the body burden of lead, improvements in workplace hygiene and employee education are necessary to prevent lead-induced neural damage.

Manganese

Although manganese (Mn) was once used as a purgative and a treatment for scabies (Marks & Beatty, 1975), in 1837 a Glasgow physician described five workers who had inhaled manganese oxide and subsequently exhibited paraparesis, mask-like facies, drooling, and weak voice in the absence of tremor (Cawte, 1985). Although manganese is not a commonly known neurotoxin, its intoxication can result in significant neurological disturbance (Politis, Schaumberg, & Spencer, 1980). Thousands of workers have developed manganese toxicity with manganese miners, welders and dry cell battery plant employees at high risk for exposure (Grandjean, 1983). Additionally, individuals who work at steel alloy factories and those who use manganese in the production of animal-food additives, antiseptics, ceramics, dyes, fertilizers, glass, germicides, matches, oxidizing solutions, and welding rods may be susceptible to manganese exposure (Katz, 1985).

Symptoms of manganese intoxication can occur in miners over a time period of 6 months to 24 years (Politis, Schaumberg, & Spencer, 1980). Deficits do not necessarily reflect a dose-response relationship. Rather, they appear to be related to a variety of factors including age, nutrition, alcohol ingestion, anemia and genetic predisposition (Cawte, 1985).

Manganese poisoning is associated with three stages of toxicity. The initial symptoms can include sleepiness, poor coordination, ataxia, and speech impairment (Baker, 1983) as well as so-called "manganese mania" consisting of asthenia, anorexia, arousal, insomnia, hallucinations, excitement, aggressive behavior, incoherent talk, judgment, and memory deficits (Rosenstock, Simons, & Meyer, 1971; Politis, Schaumberg, & Spencer, 1980).

Second stage manganese intoxication is characterized by abnormal gait, clumsiness, sleepiness, speech disorder, and mask-like facies. "Manganism" or third stage intoxication consists of Parkinsonian-like symptoms including asthenia, tremor, gait abnormalities, muscular hypertonia, and hypokinesia (Grandjean, 1983) as well as dementia, emotional lability, and frontal lobe dysfunction (Cawte, 1985).

Although the precise mechanisms underlying manganese-induced aggression are not delineated, it has been hypothesized that they may be related to the elevated striatal catecholamines observed in manganese-intoxicated individuals (Chandra, 1983). Cawte (1985) has elaborated this model and suggests that catecholamines are initially displaced in the adrenal medulla which results in CNS "flooding" of catecholamines and the manic-like aspects of the syndrome. Consequent catecholamine depletion is thought to underly the Parkinsonian-like symptoms. Support for this hypothesis lies in the observation that L-dopa can improve many of the neurological symptoms associated with chronic manganism.

Mercury

The recognition of mercury's toxicity bears some similarity to that of lead. Occupational mercury (Hg) poisoning was noted as early as 1700 in miners, gilders, chemists, mirror makers, painters, and those who treated syphilis.

Presently the annual industrial output of mercury in the United States exceeds 11 million pounds, and is used in the manufacture of electrical, pharmaceutical and paint products (Chang, 1980). Although mercury is not readily absorbed from the gastrointestinal tract, its volatility at room temperature renders it easily absorbed via inhalation both indoors and outdoors (Feldman, 1982). Occupations where workers are at risk for exposure to volatile mercury include those involved in the manufacture of barometers or mercury vapor lamps and dental professionals who prepare and utilize dental amalgams (Hartmann, 1988). Indeed, Uzzell, and Oler (1986) have reported that 15-20% of United States dental offices exceed OSHA limits for ambient mercury levels. Additional occupational groups at risk for mercury exposure include: feltmakers, photoengravers, photographers, those involved in the manufacture of electrical switches and batteries, those who use mercuric salts in plating operations, tanners, embalmers and those involved in the production or application of organic mercury compounds such as pesticides, fungicides, disinfectants, or wood preservatives (Hamilton, 1985).

As in the case of lead, the spectrum of neuropathology and neuropsychological deficits vary as a function of whether the source of mercury exposure is organic or inorganic. Methyl mercury, an organic mercury compound, is a significantly more potent neurotoxin than inorganic sources of mercury. A portion of this differential toxicity results from the fact that the gastrointestinal absorption of methyl mercury is nearly complete, while that of inorganic mercury is less than 15% (Hartmann, 1988). Lesions due to methyl mercury poisoning have been found to occur primarily in the calcarine cortex, pre- and postcentral gyrl, superior temporal gyrus and the central area of the cerebellum (Takeuchi, Eto, & Eto, 1979) as well as the basal ganglia (Chaffin & Miller, 1973). Chronic exposure to methyl mercury produces constriction of visual fields, ataxia, dysarthria, partial deafness, tremor, and intellectual impairment (Windebank, McCall, & Dyck, 1984). In a case where a family ate pork derived from animals fed grain treated with a methyl mercury fungicide, several members developed ataxia, agitation, decreased visual acuity, and stupor. Ten years later, the affected parties exhibited blindness, ataxia, retardation, choreoathetosis, myoclonic jerks, and abnormal EEGs (Feldman, 1982).

The neuropathological effects of mercury remain a matter for debate. Feldman (1982) suggests that pathology results from mercury-related enzyme inhibition. Chang (1982) reports that mercury can penetrate and damage the blood–brain barrier. Thus, mercury accumulation may induce structural damage. Although some authors suggest a uniform distribution of mercury in the brain (Hartmann, 1988), Grandjean (1983) postulates that damage may be localized to the occipital cortex and the substantia nigra. The primary observable neurological effect of inorganic mercury exposure is tremor—hand and finger tremor progressing to face and eyelid tremor, and tremor that eventually involves the head and neck (Grandjean, 1983).

Neuropsychological, behavioral, and cognitive deficits are the earliest indicators of chronic mercury intoxication. Tests of visuospatial ability, visual memory, non-verbal abstraction, cognitive efficiency and reaction time appear to be disrupted by mercury toxicity (Angotzi et al., 1982). Hänninen (1982) has found that the Block Design, Digit Symbol and Digit Span subtests of the Wechsler are sensitive measures of mercury toxicity as are the Ravens Progressive Matrices, and tests of visual memory. Reduced eye-hand coordination, decreased finger tapping and foot tapping scores also are obtained (Chaffin & Miller, 1974; Langolf et al., 1978).

The emotional effects of mercury toxicity are varied and can include avoidant behavior, irritability, overly sensitive interpersonal behavior, depression, lassitude, and fatigue (Hänninen, 1982). Six out of nine laboratory technicians exposed to mercury vapor reported irritability while three reported shyness and three were symptom-free (Ross & Sholiton, 1983). Scores on the SCL-90-R differentiated subclinically exposed subjects from controls (Uzzell & Oler, 1986). Hänninen (1982) has reviewed the neuropsychological effects of mercury and concluded that the symptoms fall into three major groups: motor abnormalities (fine motor tremor), intellectual impairment (deterioration of memory, concentration and logical reasoning) and emotional disability.

Tin/Organotin

Inorganic tin (Sn) is used as a plating agent and as a component of metal alloys, solder, and dental amalgam. Organic tin derivatives are utilized in the plastics industry and as a stabilizer for polyvinylchloride. Trisubstituted organic tin derivatives are used as fungicides, miticides, and bactericides (Hartmann, 1988).

Although the toxicity of inorganic tin is very low, due to its poor absorption and rapid tissue turnover organic tin compounds, particularly trimethyl and triethyltin, are neurotoxic. Triethyltin appears to effect neurotoxicity via "massive" myelin edema with consequent increases in intracranial pressure (Reuhl & Cranmer, 1984). Although the mechanism of this edema is not known, it has been observed on autopsy as changes in glial cells (Watanabe, 1980). Additionally, clinical symptoms attributable to elevated intracranial pressure including nausea, vertigo, visual disturbance, papilledema, and convulsions have been reported (Reuhl & Cranmer, 1984).

Although reports of industrial exposure to organotins are uncommon, one study examined 22 workers who were exposed to a trimethyltin chloride spill over a one month period. Ross et al. (1981) found that high-exposure workers reported forgetfulness, fatigue, reduction of libido and motivation, headache and sleep disturbance. Primate exposure to trimethyltin has resulted in hippocampal, amygdala, pyriform cortical, and neuroretinal damage (Reuhl & Cranmer, 1984). It also has been associated with reduced GABA levels in the hippocampus and decreased levels of dopamine in the striatum (Hanin, Krigman, & Mailman, 1984). Neuropsychological deficits associated with trimethyltin chloride have included decrements in verbal memory, finger tapping, fine motor eye-hand coordination, visual-motor integration and learning (Ross et al., 1981).

Data regarding emotional/affective changes due to organotin compounds is somewhat muddied to say the least. Ross et al. (1981) have suggested that workers exposed to trimethyltin chloride exhibited alternating periods of rage and depression lasting several hours to several days. They also said they observed long-term personality deterioration at 9 and 34 months postexposure follow-up. However, the authors indicated that it was impossible to assess what, if any of these symptoms, were related to post-traumatic stress disorder, premorbid factors or coping styles.

This concludes the discussion of the neuropsychological effects of some common neurotoxic metals for which we have data. However, this review is not exhaustive. The reader is encouraged to consult Hartmann (1988) and the scientific literature for data on potentially neurotoxic metals such as aluminum, bismuth, cadmium, gold, nickel, platinum, selenium, silicon, tellurium, thallium, and zinc.

Solvents

The term "organic solvent" is a generic one that is used to describe a group of chemicals that can extract, dissolve or suspend nonwater soluble materials such as fats, lipids, oils, resins, waxes, plastics, polymers, and cellulose derivatives (Arlien-Søberg, 1985). Solvents can be divided into major classes based upon their chemical structure. The names of these classes and representative examples include the following: *aliphatic hydrocarbons* such as pentane, hexane, heptane, octane; *aromatic hydrocarbons* such as benzene, toluene, xylene, styrene; *halogenated* compounds such as carbon tetrachloride, chloroform, methylene chloride, perchloroethylene; *alcohols* such as methanol, ethanol, propanol, butanol; *ethers* such as diethyl ether, dioxane; *glycols* such as ethylene and propyiene glycol; *ketones* such as methyl ethyl ketone, methyl butyl ketone; and *complex* solvents such as varnish, mineral spirits, turpentine, etc. (Hartmann, 1988).

Despite their structural differences, all solvents share some common properties. They tend to be volatile, lipophilic liquids which means that they can traverse various physiological barriers, such as the skin, and cell membranes, including those of the lung, the gastrointestinal tract and nerve tissue, to name a few. They also tend to be soluble in blood. Typically solvents have unobjectionable odors, and are irritating only at high doses. Finally, some solvents are capable of inducing chemical dependence (Curtis & Keller, 1986), which is why voluntary abuse can be a problem.

Many industrial workers are at risk for solvent exposure including those involved in the manufacture of paints, glues, adhesives, dyes, pharmaceuticals, polymers, and synthetic fabrics. Additionally, there are individuals who work directly with solvents including painters, varnishers, and carpet layers (Hartmann, 1988).

Despite a long history of industrial solvent use, current neuropathological and neuropsychological knowledge is not well delineated. Although knowledge of peripheral nervous system solvent toxicity is incomplete, central nervous system effects are even less well-defined (Cherry & Waldron, 1985). As in the case of metal toxicity, a number of individual factors must be taken into consideration when discussing solvent toxicity. These include diurnal metabolic cycles, alcohol use and degree of obesity (Cohr, 1985).

Nevertheless, there are some general neurological and neuropsychological effects of solvent toxicity. All solvents can depress central nervous system activity and thereby induce unconsciousness, coma, or death. Other acute effects can include ataxia, feelings of inebriation and light-headedness (Hartmann, 1988). Neuropsychological deficits reported by solvent-exposed workers via questionnaire and interview include memory impairments, concentration problems, intellectual and problem-solving deficits as well as deficits in speed and initiative. Affective symptoms can include anxiety, fatigue, depression, emotional lability, and irritability. Chronic, prolonged exposure can result in dementia (Mikkelson, 1985).

As in the case of the neuropsychological effects of metals, it is beyond the scope of this chapter to discuss the neuropsychological deficits associated with every industrial solvent for which there are some data. Rather, representative solvents will be discussed. These include carbon disulfide, methyl chloride, styrene, toluene, and trichloroethylene.

Carbon Disulfide

Carbon disulfide CS_2 is a clear liquid with a sweetish, sulfurous odor that was first used to cure natural rubber (Hartmann, 1988). Currently, it is used in soil fumigation, perfume production, as a solvent in the rubber and rayon industries and as a component of lacquers, varnishes, and insecticides (Spyker, Gallanose, & Suratt, 1982). However, the World Health Organization (1979) has indicated that only workers involved in the rayon or cellophane industries are chronically exposed to concentrations of CS_2 that would affect health adversely.

Carbon disulfide appears to be the most neurotoxic of all solvents and one that results in global, nonselective impairment. The primary route of toxic exposure is via inhalation. Doses of 4,800 ppm for a 30-minute period can result in vomiting, narcosis, CNS injury, and death (Spyker, Gallanose, & Suratt, 1982), whereas doses as low as 11 ppm can induce headache. Presently, the United States "safe exposure" limit of 20 ppm has been shown to produce neurological damage (Spyker et al., 1982).

Data concerning CS_2 CNS neuropathology are sketchy. Animals studies have revealed significant damage in the basal ganglia (caudate nucleus, putamen, globus pallidus) and the substantia nigra. Axon degeneration also has been observed (Wood, 1981). Finally, CS_2 appears to cause both cardiovascular and cerebral atherosclerotic changes in workers (Tolonen, 1975). This raises the possibility of neuropathological changes secondary to vasculopathy.

Other mechanisms proposed to account for CS_2 neuropathy include: chelation of essential trace minerals that act as metabolic co-factors, enzyme inhibiton, and disruption of catecholamine, lipid, or vitamin metabolism. (World Health Organization, 1979). However, the precise mechanism whereby CS_2 exerts its toxicity is unknown at this time.

Similarly, the neuropsychological effects of low-level CS_2 exposure are not well-delineated. Although CS_2-exposed subjects reported significantly more symptoms that nonexposed controls on a health inventory, only a neuropsychological eye-hand coordination task differentiated the two groups (Putz-Anderson et al.,

1983). Hänninen et al. (1978) studied a group of workers for an average of 17 years who were exposed to 10-30 ppm of CS_2. They found impairments of motor speed, emotionality, energy level, and psychomotor performance. A study conducted by NIOSH found that reaction time measures, vigilance, visual-motor functions and constructional abilities were correlated with duration of exposure. When Hänninen (1971) examined CS_2 "poisoned" workers, she observed retarded speech, clumsiness, inaccuracy of motor function, diminished intellectual capacity, reduced spontaneous motor activity, and impoverished visualization capacity.

The affective consequences of CS_2 exposure appears to result in stereotyped behavior, neurasthenia, depression, irritability, and insomnia (Wood, 1981). The psychotic and manic-depressive symptoms recorded in the early literature are uncommon now because workplace environments are regulated such that exposure levels are much lower than in the past. Nevertheless, the WHO has concluded that neuropsychological test results are the primary mechanism for determining CNS involvement due to CS_2 exposure.

Methyl Chloride

The most common use of methyl chloride (CS_3Cl) is in the production of methyl silicone compounds and as a fuel additive (Repko, 1981). It is also used as an industrial solvent, an insecticide, propellant, a blowing agent for plastic foams, a refrigerant, and in the production of synthetic rubber, tetramethyl lead, and methyl cellulose (Anger & Johnson, 1985).

The neuropathological effects of methyl chloride consist of profound CNS depression with various degenerative cortical changes including frontal and parietal atrophy, spinal cord damage, edema, and hyperemia. Symptoms of neurotoxicity can remain latent for several hours postexposure. However, patients then report headache, confusion, double vision, somnolence, ataxia, vertigo, tremor, weakness, loss of coordination, euphoria, and chronic personality changes (Repko, 1981).

Repko et al. (1976) performed neuropsychological assessments of 122 workers who manufactured foam products. The mean methyl chloride exposure levels across plants was 34 ppm and mean after-work breath concentration was 13 ppm. The results showed decrements in reaction time, complex parallel processing, and vigilance performance. Exposed workers experienced significant difficulty walking on two different width rails and exhibited performance decrements on the Michigan Eye-Hand Coordination Test.

Styrene

In 1981, the production of styrene ($C_6H_5CHCH_2$) was 6,612 million pounds in the United States. It is estimated that 30,000 to 300,000 workers are exposed to styrene-containing compounds (Hartmann, 1988). Although much of the styrene is used to make plastics, it is also used in the boat-building industry (Baker,

Smith, & Landrigan, 1985), and is a component of floor waxes, polishes, paints, adhesives, putty, metal cleaners, autobody fillers and varnishes. Indeed, even the general population is exposed to styrene via tobacco smoke, automobile exhaust, and polystyrene-wrapped food (Hartmann, 1988).

Exposure to styrene results in a number of effects including nausea, fatigue, giddiness, dizziness, headache, paresthesias, anemia, and memory complaints (Seppäläinen, 1978; Rosen et al., 1978). Since styrene is quite lipophilic, it tends to accumulate in fat tissue and the brain (Savolainen & Pfaffli, 1977). Neuropsychological testing in workers who experienced an average of 5 years exposure to styrene revealed decrements in visuomotor accuracy, psychomotor performance, and vigilance (Härkönen et al., 1978; Lindström, Härkönen, & Kernberg, 1976). A mean exposure at 8.6 years was associated with disrupted performance on a reaction time task, Block Design, Rey's embedded figures, and the Logical Memory and Visual Memory subtests of the Wechsler Memory Scale (Mutti et al., 1984).

Toluene

Toluene ($C_6H_5CH_3$) is an aromatic hydrocarbon that is used as a solvent for paint, varnish, and rubber adhesives, and as a degreaser (Cavanaugh, 1985). Like styrene, toluene has an affinity for brain tissue. Acute exposure to increasing doses of 100–714 ppm in a single test session resulted in decrements in simple and choice reaction time (Gambarale & Hultengren, 1972). Decreased concentration and resultant deficits in perceptual speed occurred at toluene levels of 300 ppm or greater. However, short-term exposures do not mimic chronic workplace exposure because blood toluene levels are cumulative with consistent exposure. Chronic toluene exposure results in general intellectual deficits and increased emotional reactivity. Toluene is also one of the most widely abused solvents and such abuse results in significant brain damage (Hartmann, 1988).

Trichloroethylene

Trichloroethylene (TCE) ($CHClCCL_2$) is used as a degreasing agent, a dry-cleaning solvent, a household cleaner, a component of lubricants and adhesives, and a short-acting dental and obstetric anesthetic (Annau, 1981). Recently, it has become a popular solvent for the electronics industry (Baker & Woodrow, 1984). Hence, nearly 3.5 million workers are exposed to TCE and 100,000 of these are exposed on a full-time basis, 67% under less than adequate safety conditions (NIOSH, 1987).

Much controversy surrounds the precise nature of the neurological effects of TCE. Sensory disturbances and trigeminal anesthesia have been reported (Hartmann, 1988) as have other cranial neuropathies (Firth & Stuckey, 1945; King, 1982). Nevertheless several autopsies on TCE inhalation fatalities revealed no apparent neurological damage. In one subject, however, brain section showed significant brainstem, nerve root and peripheral nerve alterations with extensive myelin degeneration (Annau, 1981). These inconsistencies led Annau to suggest that perhaps dichloroacetylene, a major decomposition product of TCE, is the primary toxicant.

Short-term, low-level experimental exposure to TCE has been associated with deficits in manual dexterity and visuospatial accuracy except these results have not been replicated even when longer exposures to higher concentrations were investigated (Annau, 1981). A 56-year-old male who had been acutely exposed to TCE exhibited reduced general intelligence, concentration difficulties, dyspraxia, dysgraphia, and problems with visual concept formation 2 years postexposure (Steinberg, 1981).

At least two studies of workers chronically exposed to TCE (50 ppm; 110–345 ppm) failed to observe neuropsychological impairment, although sample sizes were small (Maroni et al., 1977; Triebig et al., 1977). However, other researchers have reported several types of psychomotor weakness and impairment of choice reaction time (Konietzko et al., 1975). Examination of 50 workers exposed to TCE for a period of 1 month to 15 years indicated that nine individuals suffered from memory disturbances, cognitive understanding difficulties and affective changes (Lindström, 1982).

Hence, short-term low-level TCE exposure may be devoid of neuropsychological deficits. However, acute exposure to toxic levels may produce trigeminal anesthesia, and the effects of chronic exposure presently are not well-defined. These findings seem somewhat at odds with subjective complaints of headache, dizziness, fatigue, and diplopia (Steinberg, 1981); and tremor, giddiness, lacrimation, alcohol intolerance, anxiety, brachycardia, and insomnia (Spencer & Schaumberg, 1985). Additional research is required to resolve this issue.

FUTURE RESEARCH CONSIDERATIONS

What is most apparent, when reviewing this chapter, is how little we really know regarding the neurotoxicity of industrial toxins. To date, sketchy data exist for ony a paucity of potential neurotoxins. Before practitioners and researchers can make specific recommendations regarding the prevention of industrial toxin-induced brain damage, much research is required. Because it is apparent that the United States lags behind in this endeavor, diligent education of the millions of workers exposed to these chemicals is critical and may be the primary mechanism for prevention of this type of brain insult. Historically, industries have been reluctant to change until its victims are united. However, any additional changes that will mechanically prevent or reduce exposure via inhalation and/or ingestion are preventive measures to reduce brain injury due to industrial toxins. It is also critical that workers understand the importance of *using* the masks and devices that presently exist as opposed to viewing such equipment as cumbersome and unnecessary.

REFERENCES

Anderson, A. (1982). Neurotoxic follies. *Psychology Today, July*, 30-42.

Anger, W. K., & Johnson, B. L. (1985). Chemicals affecting behavior. In J. L. O'Donoghue (Ed.), *Neurotoxicity of industrial and commercial chemicals, volume I* (pp. 52-148). Boca Raton: CRC Press.

Angotzi, G., Camerino, D., Carboncini, F., Cassitto, M. G., Ceccarelli, F., Cioni, R., Paradiso, C., & Sartorelli, E. (1982). Neurobehavioral follow-up study of mercury exposure. In R. Giloli, M. G. Cassitto & V. Foa (Eds), *Neurobehavioral methods in occupational health* (pp. 247-253). New York: Pergamon Press.

Annau, Z. (1981). The neurobehavioral toxicity of trichloroethylene. *Neurobehavioral Toxicology and Teratology, 3*, 417-424.

Araki, S., & Honma, T. (1976). Relationships between lead absorption and peripheral nerve conduction velocities in lead workers. *Scandinavian Journal of Work Environment and Health, 4*, 225.

Arlien-Søberg, P. (1985). Chronic effects of organic solvents on the central nervous system and diagnostic criteria. In Joint WHO/Nordic Council of Ministers Working Group (Eds.), *Chronic effects on organic solvents on the central nervous system and diagnostic criteria* (pp. 197-218). Copenhagen: World Health Organization.

Baker, E. L. (1983). Neurological and behavioral disorders. In B. S. Levys & D. H. Wegman (Eds.), *Occupational health: recognizing and preventing work-related disease* (pp. 317-330). Boston: Little, Brown.

Baker, R., & Woodrow, S. (1984). The clean light image of the electronics industryy: Miracle or mirage? In W. Chavkin (Ed.). *Double exposure: women's health hazards on the job and at home* (pp. 21-36). New York: Monthly Review Press.

Baker, E. L., Smith T. J., & Landrigan, P. J. (1985). The neurotoxicity of industrial solvents: A review of the literature. *American Journal of Industrial Medicine, 8*, 207-217.

Beckett, W. S., Moore, J. L., Keogh, J. P., & Bleecker, M. L. (1986). Acute encephalopathy due to occupational exposure to arsenic. *British Journal of Industrial Medicine, 43*, 66-67.

Behse, F., & Carlson, F. (1978). Histology and ultrastructure of alterations in neuropathy. *Muscle and Nerve, 1*, 368.

Benson, M. D., & Price, J. (1985). Cerebellar calcification and lead. *Journal of Neurology, Neurosurgery and Psychiatry, 48*, 814-818.

Bleecker, M. L. (1984). Clinical neurotoxicology: detection of neurobehavioral and neurological impairments occurring in the workplace and the environment. *Archives of Environmental Health, 39*, 213-218.

Bleecker, M. L., & Bolla-Wilson, K. (1985). Neuropsychological impairment following inorganic arsenic exposure. Unmasking a memory disorder. *Neurobehavioral methods in occupational health. Document 3*, (pp. 173-176). Copenhagen: World Health Organization.

Bolter, J. I., Stanczik, D. F., & Long, C. J. (1983). Neuropsychological consequences at acute, high level, gasoline inhalation. *Clinical Neuropsychology, 5*, 4-7.

Cavalleri, A., Trimarchi, F., Minola, C., & Gallo, G. (1982). Quantitative measurement of visual field in lead exposed workers. In R. Gillioli, M. G. Cassitto, & V. Foa (Eds), *Neurobehavioral methods in occupational health* (pp. 263-269). New York: Pergamon Press.

Cawte, J. (1985). Psychiatric sequelae of manganese exposure in the adult, foetal and neonatal nervous systems. *Australian and New Zealand Journal of Psychiatry, 19*, 211-217.

Chaffin, D. B., & Miller, J. M. (1974). Behavioral and neurological evaluation of workers exposed to inorganic mercury. In C. Xintaras, B. L., Johnson, & I. deGroot (Eds),

Behavioral toxicology: early detection of occupational hazards. Publication No. (NIOSH) 74-126, 213-239. Washington DC: Department of Health ,Education and Welfare.

Chandra, S. V. (1983). Psychiatric illness due to manganese poisoning. *Acta Psychiatrica Scandinavica.* 67, (suppl. 303) 49-54.

Chang, L. W. (1980). Mercury. In P. S. Spencer & H. H. Schaumberg (Eds.) *Experimental and clinical neurotoxicology* (pp. 508-526). Baltimore: Williams & Wilkins.

Cherry, N., & Waldron, H. A. (Eds) (1983). *The neuropsychological effects of solvent exposure.* Havant, Hampshire: Colt Foundation.

Cohen, N., Modai, D., Galik, A., Pik, A., Weissgarten, J., Sigler, E. & Averbukh, Z. (1986). An esoteric occupational hazard for lead poisoning. *Clinical Toxicology,* 24, 59-67.

Cohr, K. H. (1985). Definition and practical limitation of the concept of organic solvents. In Joint WHO/Nordic Council of Ministers Working Group (Eds.), *Chronic effects of organic solvents on the central nervous system and diagnostic criteria. Document 5.* Copenhagen: World Health Organization, Regional Office for Europe.

Curtis, M. F., & Kelier, L. W. (Co-Chairmen). (1986). Exposure issues in the evaluation of solvent effects. *Neurotoxicology,* 7, 5-24.

Fein, G. G., Schwartz, P. M., Jacobson, S. W., & Jacobson, J. L. (1983). Environmental toxins and behavioral development. A new role for psychological research. *American Psychologist,* 1188-1196.

Feidman, R. G. (1982). Central and peripheral nervous system effects of metals: A survey. *Acta Neurologica Scandinavica,* 66, (suppl. 92) 143-166.

Firth, J. B., & Stuckey, R. E. (1945). Decomposition of trilene in closed circuit anesthesia. *Lancet,* 1, 814.

Fisher, K. (December, 1985). Measuring effects of toxic chemicals: A growing role for psychology. *APA Monitor,* 16(12), 13-14.

Gambarale, F., & Hultengren, M. (1972). Toluene exposure: II. Psychophysiological functions. *Work Environment and Health,* 9, 131-139.

Goldwater, L. J. (1972). *Mercury: A history of quicksilver.* Baltimore: York Press.

Grandjean, P. (1983). Behavioral toxicity of heavy metals. In P. Zbinden, V. Cuomo, G. Racagni, & B. Weiss (Eds), *Application of behavioral pharmacology in toxicoloty* (pp. 331-340). New York: Ranen Press.

Grandjean, P., Arnvig, E., & Beckmann, J. (1978). Psychological dysfunctions in lead-exposed workers. *Scandinavian Journal of Work Environment and Health,* 4, 295-303.

Hamilton, A. (1985). Forty years in the poisonous trades. *American Journal of Industrial Medicine,* 7, 3-18.

Hamilton, A., & Hardy, H. L. (1974). *Industrial Toxicology.* Acton, MA: Publishing Sciences Group.

Hanin, I., Krigman, M. R. & Mailman, R. B. (1984). Central neurotransmitter effects of organotin compounds: Trials, tribulations and observations. *NeuroToxicology,* 5, 267-278.

Hänninen, H. (1971). Psychological picture of manifest and latent carbon disulphide poisoning. *British Journal of Industrial Medicine,* 28, 374-381.

Hänninen, H. (1982). Behavioral effects of occupational exposure to mercury and lead. *Acta Neurologica Scandanavica,* 66 (suppl 92), 167-175.

Hänninen, H., Hernberg, S., Mantere, P., Vesanto, R., & Jalkanen, M. (1978). Psychological performance of subjects with low exposure to lead. *Journal of Occupational Medicine,* 20, 683-689.

Hänninen, H., Mantere, P., Hernberg, S., Seppalainen, A. M., & Kock, B. (1979). Subject symptoms to low-level exposure to lead. *NeuroToxicology,* 1, 333-347.

Hänninen, H., Nurminen, M., Tolonen, M., & Martelin, T. (1978). Psychological tests as indicators of excessive exposure to carbon disulfide. *Scandinavian Journal of Psychology,* 19, 163-174.

Härkönen, H., Lindström, K., Seppäläinen, A. M., Sisko, A., & Hernberg, S. (1978). Exposure-response relationship between styrene exposure and central nervous system functions. *Scandinavian Journal of Work Environment and Health*, 4, 53-59.

Hartman, D. (1988). *Neuropsychological toxicology: identification and assessment of human neurotoxic syndromes*. New York: Pergamon Press.

Katz, G. V. (1985). Metals and metalloids other than mercury and lead. In J. L. O'Donoghue (Ed.), *Neurotoxicity of industrial and commerical chemicals, volume 1* (pp. 171-191). Boca Raton: CRC Press.

King, M. (1983). Long term neuropsychological effects of solvent abuse. In N. Cherry & H. A. Waldron (Eds.), *The neuropsychological effects of solvent exposure* (pp. 75-84). Havant, Hampshire: Colt Foundation.

Konietzko, H., Elster, J., Bencsath, A., Drysch, K., & Weichard, H. (1975). Psychomotor responses under standardized trichloroethylene load. *Archives of Toxicology*, 33, 129-139.

Krigman, M. R., Bouldin, T. W., & Mushak, P. (1980). Lead. In P. S. Spencer & H. H. Schaumberg (Eds.), *Experimental and clinical neurotoxicology* (pp. 490-50). Baltimore: Williams & Wilkins.

Langolf, G. D., Chaffin, D. B., Henderson, R., & Whittle, H. P. (1978). Evaluation of workers exposed to elemental mercury using quantitative tests of tremor and neuromuscular functions. *American Industrial Hygiene Association Journal*, 39, 976-984.

Lilis, R. A., Fischbein, A., Diamond, S., Anderson, H. A., Selikoff, I.J., Blumberg, W. E., & Eisinger, J. (1977). Lead effects among secondary lead smelter workers with blood lead levels below 80 μg/100 ml. *Archives of Environmental Health*, 32, 256-266.

Lindström, K. (1982). Behavioral effects of long-term exposure to solvents. *Acta Neurologica Scandinavica*, 66 (suppl 92), 131-141.

Lindström, K., Harkonen, H., & Hernberg, S. (1976). Disturbances in psychological functions of workers occupationally exposed to styrene. *Scandinavian Journal of Work Environment and Health*, 10, 321-323.

Marks, G., & Beatty, W. K. (1975). *The Precious metals of medicine*. New York: Charles Scribner's Sons.

Maroni, M., Bulgheroni, C., Cassitto, M. G., Merluzzi, F., Gilioli, R. & Foa, V. (1977). A clinical, neuropsychological and behavioral study of female workers exposed to 1,1,1-trichloroethane. *Scandinavian Journal of Work Environment and Health*, 3, 16-22.

Mikkelsen, S., Browne, E., Jorgensen, M., & Gyldensted, C. (1985). Association of symptoms of dementia with neuropsychological diagnosis of dementia and cerebral atrophy. In Joint WHO/Nordic Council of Ministers Working Group (Eds.), *Chronic effects of organic solvents on the central nervous system and diagnostic criteria* (pp. 166-184). Copenhagen: World Health Organization.

Mutti, A., Mazzucchi, A., Rustichelli, P., Frigere, G., Arfini, G., & Franchini, J. (1984). Exposure-effect and exposure-response relationships between occupational exposure to styrene and neuropsychological functions. *American Journal of Industrial Medicine*, 5, 275-286.

Nicklowitz, W. J. (1979). Neurotoxicology of lead. In L. Manzo (Ed.), *Advances in neurotoxicology* (pp. 27-34). New York: Pergamon Press.

NIOSH (1987). *Current Intelligence Bulletin 48, Organic Solvent Neurotoxicity*. Publication no. 87-104, Department of Health and Human Services (NIOSH).

Poklis, A., & Burkett, C. D. (1977). Gasoline sniffing: A review. *Clinical Toxicology*, 11, 35-41.

Politis, M. J. Schaumberg, H. H., & Spencer, P. S. (1980). Neurotoxicity of selected chemicals. In P. S. Spencer & H. H. Schaumberg (Eds.), *Experimental and clinical neurotoxicology* (pp. 613-630). Baltimore: Williams & Wilkins.

Putz-Anderson, V., Albright, B. E., Lee, S. T., Johnson, B. L., Chrislip, D. W., Taylor, B. J., Brightwell, W. S., Dickerson, N., Culver, M., Zentmeyer, D., & Smith, P. (1983). A behavioral examination of workers exposed to carbon disulfide. *NeuroToxicology, 4,* 67–78.

Repko, J. D., Corum, C. R., Jones, P. D., & Garcia, L. S. (1978). *The effects of inorganic lead on behavioral and neurologic function.* Publication no. 78–128. Washington, DC: USDHEW (NIOSH).

Repko, J. D., Jones, P. D., Garcia, L. S., Scheider, E. J., Roseman, E., & Corum, C. R. (1976). *Final report of the behavioral and neurological evaluation of workers exposed to solvents: methyl chloride.* DHEW Publications (NIOSH) 77-125, Washington, DC: U.S. Government Printing Office.

Reuhl, K. R.., & Cranmer, J. M. (1984). Developmental neuropathology of organotin compounds. *NeuroToxicology, 5,* 187–204.

Rosen, I., Haeger-Aronsen, B., Rehnstrom, S., & Welinder, H. (1978). Neurophysiological observations after chronic styrene exposure *Scandinavian Journal of Work Environment and Health,* 4 (suppl 2), 184–194.

Rosenstock, H. A., Simons, D. G., & Meyer, J. S. (1971). Chronic manganism. Neurologic and laboratory studies during treatment with levodopa. *Journal of the American Medical Association, 217,* 1354–1358.

Ross, W. D., Emmett, E. A., Steiner, J., & Tureen, R. (1981). Neurotoxic effects of occupational exposure to organotins. *American Journal of Psychiatry, 138,* 1092–1095.

Ross, W. D., & Sholiton, M. C. (1983). Specificity of psychiatric manifestations in relation to neurotoxic chemicals. *Acta Psychiatrica Scandinavian, 67* (suppl 303), 100–104.

Savolainen, H., & Pfaffli, P. (1977). Effects of chronic styrene inhalation on rat brain protein metabolism. *Acta Neuropathologica (Berlin), 40,* 237–241.

Schottenfeld, R. S., & Cullen, M. R. (1984). Organic affective illness associated with lead intoxication. *American Journal of Psychiatry, 41,* 1423–1426.

Seppäläinen, A. M. (1978). Neurotoxicity of styrene in occupational and environmental exposure. *Scandinavian Journal of Work, Environment and Health,* 4 (suppl 2), 181–183.

Silbergeld, E. K. (1982). Neurochemical and ionic mechanisms of lead neurotoxicity. In K. N. Prasad & A. Vernadakis (Eds.), *Mechanisms of actions of neurotoxic substances* (pp. 34–50). New York: Raven Press.

Spencer, P. S., & Schaumberg, H. H. (1985). Organic solvent neurotoxicity. Facts and research needs. *Scandinavian Journal of Work Environment and Health,* suppl 10(1), 53–60.

Spyker, D. A., Gallanose, A. G., & Suratt, P. M. (1982). Health effects of acute carbon disulfide exposure. *Journal of Toxicology-Clinical Toxicology, 19,* 87–93.

Steinberg, W. (1981). Residual neuropsychological effects following exposure to trichloroethylene (TCE): A case study. *Clinical Neuropsychology, 2,* 1–4.

Taft, R., Jr. (1974). Federal commitment to occupational safety and health. In C. Xintarus, B. L. Johnson, & I. deGroot (Eds.), *Behavioral toxicology: early detection of occupational hazards.* Publication no. 74-126. Washington, DC: U.S. Department of Health, Education and Welfare (NIOSH).

Takeuchi, T., Eto, N., & Eto, K. (1979). Neuropathology of childhood cases of methylmercury poisoning (Minamata disease) with prolonged symptoms, with particular reference to the decortication syndrome. *NeuroToxicology, 1,* 1–20.

Tolonen, M. (1975). Vascular effects of carbon disulfide. A review. *Scandinavian Journal of Work Environment and Health, 1,* 63–77.

Triebig, G., Schaller, K. H., Erzigkeit, H. & Valentin, H. (1977). Biochemical investigations and psychological studies of persons chronically exposed to trichloroethylene with regard to non-exposure intervals. *International Archives of Environmental Health, 38,* 149–162.

Uzzell, B., & Oler, J. (1986). Chronic low-level mercury exposure and neuropsychological functioning. *Journal of Clinical and Experimental Neuropsychology, 8,* 581–593.

Watanabe, I. (1980). Organotins (triethyltin). In P. S. Spencer & H. H. Schaumberg (Eds), *Experimental and clinical neurotoxicology* (pp. 545–557). Baltimore: Williams & Wilkins.

Williamson, A. M., & Teo, R. K. C. (1986). Neurobehavioral effects of occupational exposure to lead. *British Journal of Industrial Medicine, 43,* 374–380.

Windebank, A. J., McCall, J. T., & Dyck, P. J. (1984). Metal neuropathy. In P. J. Dyck, P. K. Thomas, E. H. Lambert, R. Bunge (Eds), *Peripheral neuropathy, volume II* (pp. 2133–2161). Philadelphia: W. B. Saunders.

Wood, R. (1981). Neurobehavioral toxicity of carbon disulfide. *Neurobehavioral Toxicology and Teratology, 3,* 397–405.

World Health Organization. (1979). *Carbon disulfide.* Geneva: WHO.

CHAPTER 10

AGRICULTURAL AND DOMESTIC NEUROTOXIC SUBSTANCES

Raymond Singer

Neurotoxicity describes the harmful effects of toxic substances on the nervous system. All parts and aspects of the nervous system are susceptible to neurotoxicity: the peripheral nerves and the brain (central nervous system); the autonomic and voluntary; the sympathetic and parasympathetic; and the sensory organs.

Although few commercial products have been adequately tested for their neurotoxic potential during routine use, many substances are known to be neurotoxic through clinical experience and animal testing. These include agricultural and domestic chemicals, such as pesticides, fumigants, and herbicides.

Two major classes of agricultural pesticides are organophosphate and organochlorine pesticides. Organophosphate pesticides were first designed as nerve gases (Tabun and Sarin) around World War II (Ecobichon & Joy, 1982). After the war, organophosphates were commercially produced as insecticides.

The organochlorine pesticides have the property of persisting in the environment. This persistence was considered beneficial as it reduced the number of times that the poisons needed to be applied. As an expression of the esteem in which organochlorines were once held, the Nobel Prize in Medicine in 1948 was awarded to the inventor of dichlorodiphenyltrichloroethane (DDT) (Ecobichon & Joy, 1982).

Since that time, DDT has been found to have undesirable effects, such as accumulation in animal and human fat due to its lipid solubility. As animals or humans eat other animals contaminated with DDT, the proportion of DDT in body fat increases, a process called "bioaccumulation."

DDT was banned in the U.S. because of health problems among wildlife due to bioaccumulation. Notwithstanding this ban, DDT or its metabolites can be found in the fat of most people. During the period 1970–1975, almost 100% of human tissue samples had detectable amounts of DDT (Schneider, 1979). With appropriate tests, DDT can still be found as residues of the food supply in the U.S., particularly as a contaminant of imported food (NRDC, 1984).

What will be the effect of chronic, low-level neurotoxic chemical exposure on the human nervous system from pesticides? What are the interactive, synergistic or cumulative effects of neurotoxic contaminants of food, air, and water? Because deliberate administration of potentially harmful substances in human experiments may be considered unethical, how can the safety of low-level exposures be proven? Most importantly from the public health perspective, what is the current effect of pesticide residue in food on the mental and emotional function of modern man?

Because a number of questions remain unanswered regarding neurotoxic pesticide safety, we have no assurance that chronic, low-level exposure to neurotoxic substances is not impairing nervous system function in the general population. Evidence mounts that there is no threshold of effect for some neurotoxic substances, such as lead. Add to this uncertainty the effects of many other neurotoxic substances to which we are exposed, and the situation can be seen to pose an important public health concern.

Workers with exposure to neurotoxic substances are at special risk of developing neurotoxicity. They should be carefully monitored for the "early warning signs" of neurotoxicity so that permanent nervous system damage can be averted or minimized.

SYMPTOMS OF NEUROTOXICITY

The symptoms of chronic neurotoxicity are similar for the various substances (Singer, 1990). They include the following:

1. Personality changes
   a. Irritability
   b. Social withdrawal
   c. Amotivation (disturbance of executive function)
2. Mental changes
   a. Problems with memory for recent events
   b. Concentration difficulties
   c. Mental slowness
3. Sleep disturbance
4. Chronic fatigue
5. Headache
6. Sexual dysfunction
7. Numbness in the hands or feet (depends upon the substance)
8. Recognition that there has been a loss of mental function may be present.

Additional symptoms can include the following: motor incoordination, sensory disturbances, and psychosis.

Personality Changes

Irritability can be expressed in many different ways: frequent arguments with friends, family, and neighbors; encounters with police; speeding tickets; or physical fights. Neurotoxicity reduces mental and emotional abilities, resulting in reduced capacity to perceive, remember, ect. These deficits are frustrating and perplexing. The person with neurotoxicity may not be aware that he has been undergoing decrements in mental and emotional function. This unawareness will increase his frustration and resulting irritability.

Social withdrawal occurs as the person with neurotoxicity becomes increasingly frustrated with his functional abilities. He may feel that people are staring at or scrutinizing him. As neurotoxicity develops, there will be gaps in the ability to find words, and in understanding speech.

Amotivation or disturbance of executive function describes the disorganization of behavior that occurs with brain dysfunction and deterioration. Abstract thinking can be impaired, along with less understanding of the relationship between various thoughts, underlying principles, and other cognitive elements. The person appears depressed, with psychomotor slowing and feelings of hopelessness.

Mental Changes

Problems with Memory for Recent Events

This symptom will be expressed as forgetfulness, confusion, absent-mindedness, spells, and a reduced responsiveness to the social and physical environment. Long-term memory may be surprisingly preserved, because neurotoxicity has less effect on this function.

Concentration Difficulties

The affected person will find it hard to keep his mind in focus. His thoughts will drift and seem fuzzy. There will be increased susceptibility to distraction.

Mental Slowness

This symptom can be expressed as dullness, confusion, difficulty in conversing, understanding written material, or following directions.

Chronic Fatigue

Neurotoxicity patients often report that they are constantly tired. They are not able to move about as they had in the past, and have reduced ability to lift, carry, climb stairs, walk distances, or stay awake.

Sleep Disturbance

Sleep patterns are regulated by the secretion of neurohormones that control the degree of wakefulness. These hormones are normally secreted in rhythms corresponding with periods of light and darkness of the day. With diffuse brain dysfunction, such as may occur with pesticide poisoning, the pattern of sleep is disrupted, leading to difficulties in falling asleep or staying asleep. This disturbance creates or contributes to the condition of chronic fatigue seen with neurotoxicity patients.

Headache

These may be diagnosed as migraine, tension, or of mixed origin.

Sexual Dysfunction

Males may have difficulty maintaining an erection. There may also be reduced desire for sexual relations, perhaps secondary to fatigue and irritability. In females, there will be reduced desire for sexual relations.

Numbness in the Hands or Feet

Under conditions of chronic low-level exposure to substances, some neurotoxic agents may damage the peripheral nerves. Because the nerves that serve the feet (and the arms to a lesser extent) have very long axons, the source of nerve vitality tends to be located far from the nerve endings. This results in greater susceptibility to disruption of nerve nutrition and maintenance. When symptoms of peripheral neurotoxicity are present, it tends to affect the feet and legs, and to a lesser extent, the arms and hands. Disruption of the peripheral nervous system may be described by the patient as numbness, tingling, "pin and needles" sensation, or a feeling that the limb "falls asleep."

Recognition of Loss of Mental Function

Unless the damage is severe, an affected person notices that at one time they functioned more effectively, both mentally and interpersonally. They can recall memories of their lives prior to the exposure, due to the retention of long-term memory, and can contrast past intact cognitive and emotional function with current function. For example, family relations often sour after neurotoxicity occurs, yet the person affected can remember when family life was satisfactory. The person may have been an avid reader, yet now cannot read due to visual perception defects or impairment of the ability to concentrate when reading.

This symptom generally does not occur during the early stages of chronic neurotoxicity, as mental impairment may be subtle. The person may have a dim awareness that something is wrong with his mental and emotional capacities, yet be unable to pinpoint the source of his discomfort.

Motor Incoordination

This symptom can be seen as difficulty in walking, manual dexterity, and handling tools, and can progress to motor loss. Neurotoxicity may be diagnosed as multiple sclerosis (MS); "MS-like" disease; amyotrophic lateral sclerosis; opsoclonos-myoclonos; seizures; and other diseases affecting the neuromotor system.

Sensory Disturbances

Blindness, hearing loss, pain, burning sensations, and kinesthetic dysfunction are examples of sensory disturbance that can occur with neurotoxicity. If the peripheral and central nervous system degenerate, the nerves have reduced ability to transmit accurate information to the central nervous system. Any sensory system can be affected, to the point of system failure.

Psychosis

Patients with this condition may be diagnosed as schizophrenic, schizoid, paranoid, and psychotic. They develop hallucinations, impaired ability to communicate, and impaired ability to function in society.

EXPOSURE OF AGRICULTURAL WORKERS TO PESTICIDES

Approximately 1 billion pounds of pesticides are used annually in agriculture in the U.S., costing $5 billion. (Another $2 billion is spend on nonagricultural pesticide products.) Agricultural workers exposed to chemicals include field workers, pesticide applicators, food transporters and storage personnel (OTA, 1990).

An estimated 5 million Americans farm as a primary source of income. Children under the age of 16 are often involved in agriculture. About 3 million workers in the U.S. are migrant and seasonal agricultural workers, and there are an estimated 1 million pesticide handlers that are certified (OTA, 1990).

The estimated prevalence of pesticide poisoning in the U.S. is 300,000 cases, only 1-2% of which are reported (OTA, 1990). However, estimated prevalence rates need to account for the low rate of identification of pesticide neurotoxicity, as few clinicians are trained to diagnose neurotoxicity. Cases of neurotoxicity may (a) not come to the attention of health care workers; (b) be dismissed without a diagnosis; (c) be diagnosed as psychiatric disorders; or (d) be diagnosed as multiple sclerosis or other neurologic disorders.

EXAMPLES OF NEUROTOXIC PESTICIDES

Organophosphate and carbamate pesticides are widely used. Because of their rapid toxicity, they are the most common cause of acute pesticide poisoning. These pesticides affect insects and humans by interfering with the biochemistry of nerve transmission. Acute symptoms can include hyperactivity, breathing difficulties, sweating, tearing, urinary frequency, abnormal heartbeat, anxiety, gastrointestinal disturbance, weakness, dizziness, convulsions, coma, and death. Typical organophosphorus pesticides include Parathion, Thimet, ethyl-P-nitrophenyl phenylphosphonothionate chlorpyrifos, Dursban, dichlovos, and Vapona. Carbamate pesticides include aldicarb, Temik, carbaryl, and Sevin (OTA, 1990).

Organochlorine pesticides are less acutely toxic than organophosphate and carbamate pesticides, but they have a greater potential for chronic toxicity due to their persistence in the environment and in the affected person's body. From 1940 through the 1970s, several organochlorine pesticides were widely used, including DDT, aldrin, mirex, lindane, chlordane and heptachlor. Chlordane, introduced in 1947, was supposed to be banned by EPA in 1974. By 1978, it was banned for most uses except termite control. As of 1990, it may be still not entirely banned (OTA, 1990). Chlordane is highly persistent, and has a half-life of 20 years.

Pyrethroids are a group of insecticides that are highly toxic to insects but less toxic to humans. They will probably be used more frequently due to their lower degree of human toxicity. However, these substances also can be neurotoxic.

Fumigants are gases used to kill insects (including termites) and their eggs, and are the most acutely toxic pesticides used in agriculture. Methyl bromide is a particularly problematic pesticide, as it is colorless, almost odorless, and relatively inexpensive. It has caused death and severe neurotoxic effects in fumigators, applicators and structural pest control workers (exterminators) (OTA, 1990).

Neurotoxic herbicides include 2,4-dichlorophenoxy acetic acid; 2,4,5-trichlorophenoxyasetic acid; and Silvex. Although EPA suspended many of their uses, they continue to be used widely in forest management, and weed control in agricultural and urban settings. These herbicides may be contaminated with dioxins 2,3,7,8-tetrachlorodibenzo-P-dioxin (OTA, 1990).

DOMESTIC EXPOSURE TO PESTICIDES

Neurotoxic pesticides are used to control termites, cockroaches and other household insects. The elderly, adults and children are exposed to these substances in environments including the home, school, public and private offices, restaurants and other public stores, and public parks. Usually, the person being exposed is not aware that an exposure is occurring, nor is there awareness of the potential for neurotoxicity. Additional exposures to pesticides and herbicides can occur during chemical treatment of lawns, golf courses, and playing fields.

Concerning pesticide residues in food, an estimated 17% of the preschool population in the U.S. is exposed to neurotoxic pesticides above levels the Federal government has declared as safe (NRDC, 1989; OTA, 1990). This analysis was based upon raw fruits and vegetables alone, and does not consider other sources of pesticide exposure.

Children are considered to be more at risk of neurotoxicity than adults, because they absorb more pesticides per pound of body weight; their immature development makes them less able to detoxify substances; and their nervous system is developing and may be more vulnerable to permanent disruption (OTA, 1990).

Pesticides banned for use in the U.S. can return to the food supply via produce from other countries with fewer regulations. For example, DDT, which is banned in the U.S., can still be found in our food supply (NRDC, 1984; GAO, 1989a). This phenomena has been termed "banned pesticide rebound."

Third world growers can have difficulty reading the manufacturer's instructions, which may only be available in English, so pesticides may be over-applied. The U.S. Food and Drug Administration is too short-staffed to adequately monitor the pesticide status of imported food (GAO, 1989b).

Pesticides can also contaminate water supplies. Highly persistent pesticides, such as aldicarb, have been found in groundwater supplies (Barrette, 1988).

EFFECTS OF CHRONIC EXPOSURE TO PESTICIDES

Acute exposures, after the acute sickness has run it's course, can leave permanent nervous system damage. The origin of the impairment may be obviously linked in time with the pesticide exposure. However, the effects of chronic exposure to pesticides may be difficult to detect for a number of reasons.

Difficulties for Detection of Neurotoxicity by the Untrained Observer

Mental deterioration from exposure to low-levels of neurotoxic chemicals may not be noticed by the person, because (a) the brain lacks the ability to detect pain resulting from brain cell death or injury, so therefore lacks sensitivity to destruction of brain tissue itself; and (b) mental deterioration often occurs in small increments, so that gradual and subtle change is difficult to notice. Over time, such gradual decrements can cause significant decline in mental function. As the person's mental processes deteriorate, he is less able to use logic, perception, memory and other mental processes to determine the extent or cause of mental deterioration.

Permanency of Neurotoxicity

Injury to neural tissue disrupts function by destroying cells and interrupting nerve fibers. Because dead nerve cells are not replaced, recovery depends upon regrowth of damaged neuronal branches and the reconnection of the surviving cells. In contrast with the peripheral nervous system, there is little fiber regrowth within the CNS, and many of the functional deficits caused by damage to the brain and spinal cord are permanent (Aguayo, 1987).

Lack of Knowledge

To the extent that there is some awareness of neurotoxicity, the generally educated public may be aware of acute effects from pesticides. However, they may not be aware of the subtle effects of neurotoxic chemicals, or the cumulative effects of low-level toxicity. Acute exposures to neurotoxic agents also may have a delayed effect, which further confounds the ability to determine the cause of mental deterioration.

AGRICULTURAL CHEMICALS AND SENILE DEMENTIA

Some scientists have theorized that Alzheimer's disease and other neurological and neuropsychological conditions may be due to exposure to environmental toxins occurring years before the onset of the disease. Determination of the possible relationship between neurotoxic chemical exposure and such neural diseases as senile dementia is hampered by the delayed or cumulative effects of neurotoxicants. We are now aware that some diseases, such as cancer from asbestos exposure, may take 20 years to develop. Without careful study, the causal connection of asbestos and cancer could have been overlooked. Degenerative brain disease could have a long latency period after exposure has occurred.

It seems unlikely that there is a threshold of exposure intensity that must be breached in order for neurotoxicity to occur. A more likely outcome might be the injury of cells at low levels of exposure, and the death of more sensitive nervous tissue at higher exposure levels. Figure 10-1 represents a theoretical exposure level in the sublethal range, where the vast number of cells show no injury, a smaller number show some injury, and a few cells die.

Spencer et al. (1987) have linked an environmental (food) chemical exposure, occurring many years earlier with no apparent effects, with neural disease occurring later, specifically amyotrophic lateral sclerosis—Parkinsonism—dementia. Spencer throught that other environmental chemicals may also act as triggers for neuronal death. Calne et al. (1986) speculated that Alzheimer's disease may be due to environmental damage to the central nervous system. Although damage may remain subclinical for several decades, it may make those affected especially prone to the consequences of age-related neuronal attrition (Lewin, 1987). Arezzo and Schaumburg (1989) also suggested that neurotoxic damage early in life can enhance central nervous system dysfunction that occurs late in life, such as Parkinson's disease.

The relationship between dementia and neurotoxicity was alluded to by Butler (1987), former head of the National Institute of Aging, who stated that a key issue

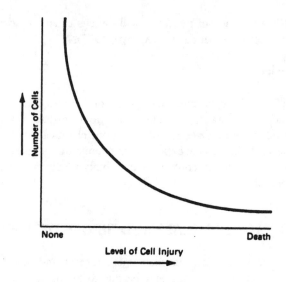

FIGURE 10-1. Sublethal exposure to a neurotoxic substance.

regarding neurotoxicity and aging is the environmentally related effects of neurotoxic chemicals on the CNS, the key pacemaker in old age. Neurotoxic effects are not all-or-nothing effects; with any toxic impact on the central nervous system, symptoms or effects are produced on a continuum.

Chemically induced neurological disorders are often virtually indistinguishable from other causes of disease, suggesting the possibility that environmental chemicals mimic the action of metabolically generated chemical substances circulating in the blood. The decline of neurologic integrity associated with the aging process might be linked with the cumulative effects of endogenous or exogenous poisons (Williams et al., 1987).

The level of pesticide exposure that is necessary to produce dementia is uncertain. However, the total picture may take a long time to become entirely visible. Epidemiologic studies are difficult to accomplish, as neurotoxic exposures are uncontrolled and varied. Control groups are difficult to identify because of the widespread promulgation of neurotoxic substances. Effects can be subtle and below the level of detection with our present measuring instruments.

Some people call for more research to determine a safe exposure level to neurotoxic substances. Other observers believe there is probably a low threshold of effects for many neurotoxic substances and it is time for further control of neurotoxic substances. During the time that these differences of opinion are being worked out, there are a number of important risks to the public health. But some alternatives do exist to reduce the use of neurotoxic substances in agriculture and pest control.

ALTERNATIVES TO NEUROTOXIC PESTICIDES

Integrated pest management (IPM) minimizes the use of pesticides by using less toxic pest control strategies. These include biological controls (natural predators), and improved or more natural agricultural techniques. IPM has also been applied to household and structural pest problems, employing such common sense approaches as habitat modification and the use of relatively benign substances to control pests.

Organic farming does not rely upon synthetic or harmful chemicals to grow food. This approach is designed to produce food without pesticide residue and with less harm to the environment. In 1988, an estimated $1 billion worth of organic produce was marketed. An estimated 84% of Americans would buy organic food if it was available, with 49% willing to pay more for it (organic produce currently costs approximately 10% more than nonorganic produce) (OTA, 1990).

PREVENTION OF OCCUPATIONAL AGRICULTURAL NEUROTOXICITY

Symptom Screening

On logical grounds, symptom screening is probably the single most effective approach to determining the earliest signs of neurotoxicity. Significant alterations in function will probably be reflected in dysfunction that a person could report if asked. Questionnaires can require very little time to administer and score. A limitation of symptom screening is a possible lack of sensitivity to more subtle levels of neurotoxicity.

A questionnaire approach to the monitoring of early disturbances of central nervous system function was explored by Hogstedt et al. (1984). They found testing for symptoms to be valuable in determining the adverse effects of some occupational exposure situations. Other researchers from time to time have published papers on the use of symptom questionnaires in neurotoxicity research.

The *Neurotoxicity Screening Survey* (Singer, 1990) was developed to provide total quantification of both frequency, type and severity of neurotoxicity symptoms. Frequency is determined by a rating scale, ranging from "never" to "most of the time." Type is determined by combining symptoms within functional groups, such as memory, peripheral numbness, and sensory-motor function. Severity is determined by the global score. The test is repeatable. Norms are available comparing normals with diagnosed neurotoxicity cases.

Psychometric Testing

Brief and objective psychometric testing can be used to monitor workers for the early signs of neurotoxicity. Testing could include two to three procedures that could be administered in 20 minutes, such as the Digit Symbol and Block Design tests, and the Embedded Figures test (Valciukas and Singer, 1982). Figure 10-2 shows a sample card of the Embedded Figures test. The subject must identify as many objects possible in 60 seconds.

Other batteries could also be used. Singer (1990) reviews this topic. Singer and Scott (1987) illustrate a typical neuropsychological examination for neurotoxicity.

Peripheral Nerve Testing

The most widely used neurophysiological measure of neurotoxicity is peripheral nerve conduction velocity (NCV) testing. This procedure has been applied to hundreds of studies of neurotoxicity around the world for a number of decades. NCV testing has been found to provide reliable and valid data (Singer et al., 1987, shows an application of NCV).

NCV measures the time it takes for nerve impulses to travel in the arms and legs. The technique is noninvasive, quick, and objective. Electrical activity in the limb is monitored while the nerve is stimulated with an electrical pulse, and the resulting nerve response wave form is stored for measurement. Slowing of response or reduced amplitude of response shows that the nerve function is impaired.

NCV seeks to evaluate the integrity of peripheral nerves by measuring the latency and amplitude of nerve response. Often evaluated nerves include the median motor and median sensory nerves, in the arm and hand, and the sural nerve in the calf. The resulting wave form can be seen in Figure 10-3. The latency of response is reflected by a lack of electrical activity under the sensing electrodes, displayed as a flat line (between the two vertical arrows, Figure 10-3). As the nerve receives the signal, it depolarizes, and its electrical activity is temporarily changed (Figure 10-3, peak amplitude). See Singer (1990) or Kimura (1989) for further details regarding NCV.

The choice of nerves to monitor for neurotoxicity depends upon the following: (a) The sensory nerves seem to be more sensitive than the motor nerves to neurotoxicity, as reflected by slower conduction velocity and reduced amplitude of response; (b) the more distal the nerve segment, the more likely that the nerve will show deterioration; and (c) nerves should be selected that produce a clear, easy to obtain, and reliable reading.

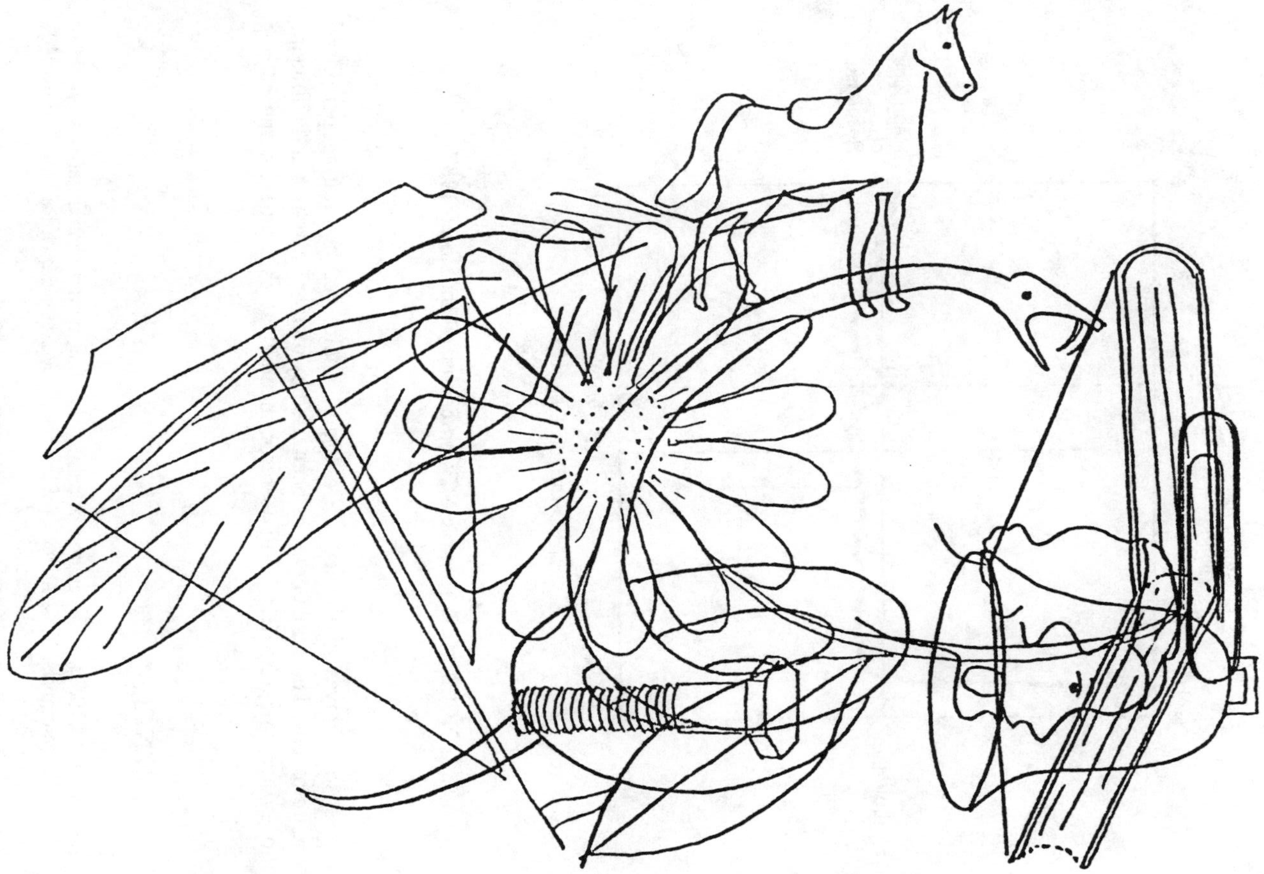

FIGURE 10-2. Sample from the Embedded Figures test (a). (From Valciukas & Singer, 1982).

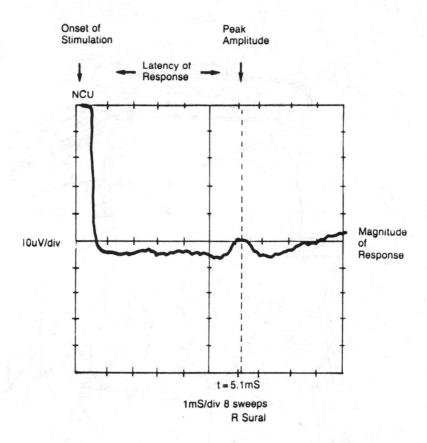

FIGURE 10-3. Sample NCV wave form. (From Singer, 1987).

Sensory nerves of the leg are a logical choice for monitoring peripheral neurotoxicity. The sural nerve has been used by many researchers and clinicians to evaluate neurotoxicity, and is recommended at this time for monitoring programs.

REFERENCES

Aquayo, A. J. (1987). Regeneration of axons from the injured central nervous system of adult mammals. In G. Adelman (Ed.), *Encylopedia of neuroscience* (vol. 2, pp. 1040–1043). Boston: Birkhauser.

Arezzo, J. C., & Schaumburg, H. H. (1989). Screening for neurotoxic disease in humans. *Journal of the American College of Toxicology, 8,* 147–155.

Barrette, B. (1988). The Rhode Island Department of Health (DOH) Private Well Surveillance Program. *Northeast Regional Environmental Public Health Center Newsletter*, 2, 1–2.

Butler, R. (1985). Keynote address. Workshop on Environmental toxicity and the aging process. In S. R. Baker & M. Rogul (Eds.), *Environmental toxicity and the aging process.* Vol. 1. 1st ed. (pp. 11–18). New York: Alan R. Liss.

Calnes, D. B., McGeer, E., Eisen, A., & Spencer, P. (1986). Alzheimer's disease, Parkinson's disease, and motoneurone disease: Abiotropic interaction between ageing and environment? *Lancet*, 2, 1067–1070.

Ecobichon, D., & Joy, R. (1982). *Pesticides and neurological disease.* 1st ed. Boca Raton: CRC Press.

GAO. (1989). *Pesticides: export of unregistered pesticides is not adequately monitored by EPA.* GRD/HRD-89-128. Washington, DC: U.S. General Accounting Office.

GAO. (1989). *Imported foods: opportunities to improve FDA's inspection program.* GAO/HRD-89-128. Washington, DC: U. S. General Accounting Office.

Hogstedt, C., Andersson, K., & Hane, M. (1984). A questionnaire approach to the monitoring Of Early Disturbances In Central Nervous Functions. In A. Aitio, V. Riihimhki, & H. Vaino (Eds.), *Biological monitoring and surveillance of workers* (pp. 275–287). Washington, DC: Hemisphere Publishing.

Kimura, J. (1989). *Electrodiagnosis in diseases of nerve and muscle: principles and practice.* 2nd ed. Philadelphia: F. A. Davis.

Lewin, R. (1987). Environmental hypothesis for brain diseases strengthened by new data. *Science*, 237, Vol. 237 483–484.

NRDC. (1984). *Pesticides in food: what the public needs to know.* San Francisco: National Resources Defense Council.

NRDC. (Ed.). (1989). *Intolerable risk: pesticides in our children's food.* Washington, DC: National Resources Defense Council.

OTA. (1990). *Neurotoxicity. Identifying and Controlling Poisons of the Nervous System.* OTA-BA-436. Washington, DC: Office of Technology Assessment, Congress of the United States.

Schneider, M. J. (1979). *Persistent poisons.* New York: New York Academy of Sciences.

Singer, R. (1990). *Neurotoxicity guidebook.* New York: Van Nostrand Reinhold.

Singer, R., Valciukas, J., & Rosenman, K. D. (1987). Peripheral neurotoxicity in workers exposed to inorganic mercury compounds. *Archives of Environmental Health*, 42, 181–184.

Singer, R., & Scott, N. (1987). Progression of neuropsychological deficits following toluene diisocyanate exposure. *Archives of Neuropsychology*, 2, 135–144.

Spencer, P. S., Nunn, P. B., Hugon, J., Ludolf, C. L., Ross, S. M., Dwijedra, R. I. & Robertson, R. C. (1987). Guam amyotrophic lateral sclerosis—Parkinsonism—dementia linked to a plant excitant neurotoxin. *Science*, 237, 517–522.

Valciukas, J., & Singer, R. (1982). The embedded figures test in epidemiological studies of environmental neurotoxic agents. *Environmental Research*, 28, 183–198.

Williams, J. R., Spencer, P. S., Stahl, S. M., Borzelleca, J. F., Nichols, W., Pfitzer, E., Yunis, E. J., Carchman, R., Opishinski, J. W., & Walford, R. A. (1987). Interactions of aging and environmental agents: The toxicological perspective. In *Environmental toxicity and the aging processes* (pp. 81–135). New York: Alan L. Liss.

CHAPTER 11

NEUROPSYCHOLOGY OF ALCOHOL-INDUCED BRAIN DAMAGE: CURRENT PERSPECTIVES ON DIAGNOSIS, RECOVERY, AND PREVENTION

Ralph H. B. Benedict and Arthur MacNeil Horton, Jr.

Chronic alcohol abuse is now widely recognized as an important medical and social problem that is reaching epidemic proportions. According to the National Institute of Alcohol Abuse and Alcoholism, there are approximately 10.4 million alcoholics in the United States (Williams, Stimson, Parker, Harford, & Noble, 1987) resulting in an economic burden in excess of $100 billion annually (Harwood, Napolitano, Kristiansen, et al., 1984). When viewed in the context of Robins et al.'s, (1984) lifetime prevalence estimate of 13.3%, this alarming cost to American society is not surprising. Moreover, a recent survey of New York high-school students indicates that 67% have had past involvement with illegal or nonmedical substance use (New York State Division of Substance Abuse Services, 1984). The high prevalence rates among teen-agers are of special concern to those professionals interested in the prevention of alcohol-induced brain damage.

The role of neuropsychology in the treatment and prevention of alcohol-induced brain damage appears to be broadening. Indeed, the profound impact of prolonged alcohol abuse on a variety of neuropsychological functions has been firmly established (for review, see Butters & Cermak, 1980; Miller & Saucedo, 1983). Most of these impairments are known to affect the alcohol abuser's ability to recall information, reason effectively, and solve-problems, thereby compromising their capacity to cope with stress and benefit from treatment.

The purpose of this chapter is to introduce the reader to some basic concepts concerning the neuropsychological sequelae of alcohol-induced brain damage,

Dr. Horton's contribution was in his private capacity and was neither endorsed or supported by the federal government.

as well as current perspectives on rehabilitation and prevention. First, we present a brief review of research regarding neuropsychological dysfunction following prolonged alcohol abuse. Second, we provide a discussion of existing evidence for time-dependent recovery of function and the utility of cognitive remediation procedures. Finally, the chapter concludes with a presentation of some current perspectives on the emerging role of neuropsychology in the treatment and prevention of chronic alcohol abuse.

NEUROPSYCHOLOGICAL DYSFUNCTION FOLLOWING ALCOHOL ABUSE

Prolonged alcohol abuse is known to result in significant brain damage, as evidenced by performance deficits on a variety of neuropsychological tests. The degree of brain damage is known to vary according to the amount of alcohol consumed, and the frequency of so-called "bingeing" episodes. Consequently, the severity of cognitive impairment observed in alcoholic subjects has ranged from subtle processing deficits, to severe losses of function such as Korsakoff's amnesia. Whether or not Korsakoff's syndrome is a more severe form of alcohol-induced brain damage, or an etiologically distinct disorder is an issue that has been frequently debated.

Distinguishing Between Korsakoff and NonKorsakoff Alcoholic Brain Damage

In their recent review of the literature, Butters and Granholm (1987) described four cardinal features of Korsakoff's syndrome: (a) anterograde amnesia, (b) retrograde amnesia, (c) visuoperceptive deficits, and (d) problem-solving deficits. Anterograde amnesia refers to a nearly total loss of memory for events occurring after the onset of the disorder. In Korsakoff's patients, recall is often disrupted by interference from previously presented information (i.e., proactive interference). For example, when asked to recall a list of words, Korsakoff's subjects will invariably recall information from previous trials (Butters & Cermak, 1980). Retrograde amnesia is the inability to accurately recall events prior to the onset of the disorder. In Korsakoff's syndrome, this deficit appears to follow what has been described as a temporal gradient. That is, events within a 20-year period of onset are most susceptible to the amnesia. In contrast, childhood memories remain relatively intact (e.g., Albert, Butters, & Levin, 1979). Finally, although trivial in comparison to the aforementioned memory impairments, Korsakoff's patients are also deficient on tasks measuring visuoperceptive, abstract reasoning, and problem-solving skills. Glosser, Butters, and Kaplan (1977), for example, found Korsakoff's subjects to be deficient on the Embedded Figures Test, a visuospatial reasoning task.

Interestingly, similar impairments have also been observed in neurologically intact, chronic alcohol abusers who do not exhibit the pathognomonic signs (e.g., severe anterograde amnesia) of Korsakoff's syndrome. Research has consistently shown this population to be impaired on visuoperceptive and problem-solving tasks such as the Wisconsin Card Sorting, Tactual Performance, and Category Tests (for review, see Ryan & Butters, 1986). There is also evidence for memory dysfunction in nonKorsakoff's, chronic alcohol abusers. Brandt, Butters, Ryan, and Baygog (1983), found detoxified alcoholic subjects to be deficient on the Four Word Short Term Memory Test. On each of 30 trials, their subjects were presented with four words, asked to count backwards by three's for either 15 or 30 seconds, and then asked to recall the four stimulus words. The results indicated that alcoholic subjects were significantly poorer on the task as compared to nonalcoholic controls.

However, because the memory deficits of chronic alcohol abusers are less severe than Korsakoff's amnesia, the prolonged drinker's abstract reasoning, visuoperceptive, and problem-solving deficits comprise the forefront of their cognitive profile. Other qualitative distinctions between Korsakoff's and nonKorsakoff's alcoholics have been demonstrated. For example, unlike Korsakoff's subjects, the chronic alcoholic's episodic recall is characterized by modality-specific deficits, such as poor memory for patterned visual material as opposed to verbal information (Ryan & Butters, 1986). Another distinguishing feature concerns the lack of evidence for the existence of retrograde amnesia in neurologically intact alcoholics. Albert, Butters, and Brandt (1980) examined this issue with the Boston Remote Memory Battery. They found that long-term alcohol abusers performed at a level similar to that of controls on the Famous Faces portion subtest, and were only marginally deficient on the Recall subtest.

The degree of etiologic similarity between Korsakoff's Syndrome and alcoholic brain damage has been frequently debated. Ryback (1971) proposed a continuum of alcohol-induced brain damage with Korsakoff's syndrome at one end, and the normal function of abstinent subjects at the other. Evidence supporting Ryback's hypothesis was derived from studies, such as those mentioned above, investigating visuoperceptive and problem-solving performance. Oscar-Berman (1973), for example, administered a two-choice discrimination task designed to assess hypothesis formation and feedback utilization. The alcoholic group's performance fell between that of the Korsakoff's and normal control groups. Similar results were reported by Becker, Rivoira, Butters, and Ciraulo (1984) on a question and answer problem-solving task. These studies suggest that the pattern of neuropsychological deficits is similar in Korsakoff's and nonKorsakoff's alcoholics.

However, the existence of deficits unique to Korsakoff's syndrome, namely anterograde and retrograde amnesia, do not support the continuity hypothesis. Unlike the memory deficits of neurologically intact alcoholics, these impairments, which may be due to small hemorrhagic lesions in the region of the dorsomedial nucleus of the thalamus (Victor, Adams, & Collins, 1971), appear to have a sudden onset. Both Korsakoff's and nonKorsakoff's patients probably suffer from the effects of cortical atrophy (Butters & Granholm, 1987). Yet the cortical deficits of Korsakoff's syndrome patients appear to be superimposed upon subcortical/limbic neuropathology, a condition that results in severe deficits such as anterograde amnesia.

Features Unique to Alcohol-Induced Brain Damage

It was not long ago that "amnesia" was considered a unitary construct. The reader may recall Cohen and Squire's (1980) description of the "amnesic" as an individual adept at "knowing how," but incapable of "knowing what." Cohen and Squire conceptualized memory as involving either procedural (e.g., motor tasks such as mirror writing) or declarative (e.g., word-list recall) learning, and proposed that amnesics are capable only of the former. After a lengthy review of the research literature, Hirst (1982) concluded that all amnesic subjects manifest the following: (a) rapid forgetting, (b) normal immediate memory, (c) responsiveness to recognition probes, (d) responsiveness to retrieval cues, (e) proactive interference, and (e) preserved skill acquisition. As noted by Hirst, there is a substantial body of literature which supports this definition of a global or "core" amnesia syndrome.

Yet in spite of these commonalties, amnesic patients can be categorized according to certain disease-specific features. For example, Cohen and Squire (1981) observed that Korsakoff's patients, patients receiving electroconvulsive shock therapy, and one patient with medial thalamic damage were all equally impaired in episodic recall, but distinguishable on the basis of their remote memory skills. Moss, Albert, Butters, and Payne (1986) reported that Korsakoff's patients can be distinguished from patients with Alzheimer's and Huntington's disease on the basis of their performance on a recognition memory task. Therefore, in spite of the tendency for Korsakoff's syndrome to meet Hirst's (1982) amnesia criteria, the disorder can be distinguished from other disorders that affect memory performance.

Unlike Korsakoff's patients, neurologically intact alcoholic patients seem to be devoid of pathognomic neuropsychological signs. In general, the pattern of neuropsychological deficits observed in long-term alcoholics is reminiscent of other forms of diffuse brain damage. Therefore, differential diagnosis is best made on the basis of repeated administrations of a neuropsychological test battery in order to rule out the presence of a progressive illness (Ryan & Butters, 1986).

Finally, given that chronic alcohol use causes brain damage, what factors related to drinking behavior are associated with deficits in cognitive function? Research by Eckhardt, Parker, Noble, Fieldman, and Gottschalk (1978) may shed some light on this question. These investigators demonstrated that measures of recent drinking behavior are significantly related to performance on perceptual-motor tasks. Following Eckhardt et al., (1978), Parsons et al. (1987) attempted a more in-depth study by questioning 60 middle-aged alcoholics about their drinking behavior. A linear regression analysis demonstrated that an interaction between "the maximal quantity drunk per occasion" and "the frequency of maximal amount drunk" significantly predicted performance on a series of verbal, memory, and problem-solving neuropsychological tests. Overall, Parson's (1987) data suggest that the neurotoxic effect of frequent high levels of alcohol may be a primary factor in the causation of neuropsychological impairment. That is, individuals who frequently "binge" on excessive amounts of alcohol are at particularly high risk for brain damage.

RECOVERY OF COGNITIVE FUNCTION

Both the extent and the rate of cognitive recovery is remarkably different for Korsakoff's and nonKorsakoff's alcoholic subjects. Concerning the former, Korsakoff's amnesia does not appear to show any recovery over time, regardless of drinking behavior (Butters & Cermak, 1980). Yet a plethora of studies has demonstrated significant cognitive recovery in neurologically intact alcoholics. Goldman (1983), for example, reported improvement in verbal memory abilities within 1 month following detoxification.

Other studies have indicated that the recovery of cognitive function following detoxification is significantly influenced by factors such as subject age and drinking behavior (e.g., Cermak & Ryback, 1976; Goldman, Williams, & Klisz, 1983). Goldman, Klisz, and Williams (1985) studied three groups of alcoholics divided by age (20–29, 30–39, >40). Within 2 weeks following detoxification, the youngest group demonstrated significant recovery of short-term memory. In contrast, the performance of the oldest group remained impaired. The neocortex of older individuals is apparently more vulnerable to alcohol-induced brain damage and less able to compensate for cognitive dysfunction.

Wilkinson and Sanchez-Craig (1981) demonstrated the detrimental effects of drinking during and immediately following the course of treatment. Their data indicated a significant degree of cognitive recovery, as measured by the Digit Symbol Substitution Test, in a group of light-drinking resumers (less than one drink per day) and no improvement in heavy-drinking resumers (greater than 4 drinks per day). In a cross-sectional design, Brandt, Butters, Ryan, and Baygog (1983) compared the performance of three groups of alcoholics: 1–2 months abstinent, 1–3 years abstinent, and 5 years or more abstinent. Significant improvement was found in the 5-year abstinent group on measures of verbal short-term memory and delayed visual-spatial memory.

Yohman, Parsons, and Leber (1985) cleverly isolated the effect of continued drinking on neuropsychological recovery. Thirty-seven alcoholics were compared with controls at 7 weeks and 13 months postdetoxification. The subjects were administered a battery of verbal (e.g., WAIS Comprehension subtest, Shipley

Conceptual Quotient), memory (e.g., paired-associates, digit span), problem-solving (e.g., WAIS Block Design subtest, Wisconsin Card Sorting Test), and perceptual-motor (e.g., Trail Making Test) neuropsychological tests. As expected, the alcoholic group was initially impaired on all four clusters. Although the alcoholic group demonstrated some improvement at 13 weeks, the data analysis indicated that their gains were due to a practice effect. However, dividing the alcoholic group into resumers (having drunk to the point of drunkenness over the past year) and abstainers altered the recovery picture. At 13 months, abstainers were impaired only on perceptual-motor tasks, whereas resumers remained impaired on tests of learning/memory, problem-solving, and perceptual-motor function.

In addition to demonstrating the influence of drinking behavior on cognitive recovery, these studies also suggest that cognitive skills differ in their rate of recovery. Verbal learning functions appear to be among the first skills to recover, often within one month following detoxification. Further support comes from the findings of Goldman (1986) who observed that fixed, verbal abilities such as vocabulary knowledge are seldom impaired after detoxification. In contrast, visuospatial, abstract reasoning, and problem-solving skills, show a slower rate of recovery, and in some individuals may remain impaired. "In general, the more novel, complex, and rapid the information processing the task requires, the longer it takes to recover" (Goldman, 1983, p. 1051).

A full review of this literature is clearly beyond the confines of this chapter (for review, see Goldman, 1986). Nonetheless, this brief review does offer some potential treatment implications. For example, since patients are not adept at processing verbal information during the first few weeks following detoxification, they may not be able to maximally benefit from a lecture based treatment approach. This point may be especially important in the treatment of older and/or frequently resuming patients. We will return to these issues later in a discussion of prevention and treatment issues.

COGNITIVE REHABILITATION

Few neuropsychologists have undertaken the arduous task of evaluating the utility of cognitive rehabilitation interventions with alcoholic subjects. To date, the published reports on this topic have been hindered by a multitude of methodological problems that greatly limit the reliability and generalizability of findings. Certain procedural limitations (e.g., no-treatment control group) have been simply insurmountable in most clinical settings, leading some practitioners to the use of experimental, single-case designs. Woods (1983), for example, presented a multiple-baseline design in which a patient demonstrated improvement in answering a series of personal information and orientation questions over the course of treatment. Although the results of single-case designs cannot be generalized to a patient population, significant findings are often useful in demonstrating the utility of a particular intervention for a particular subject.

Chronic Alcohol Abuse

The existing data suggest that Korsakoff's and nonKorsakoff's alcoholic patients respond differently to cognitive rehabilitation. Beginning with the later, Stringer and Goldman (1984, reported in Goldman, 1987) investigated the effects of cognitive rehabilitation upon the performance of neurologically intact alcoholics, as measured by the Block Design subtest of the Wechsler Adult Intelligence Scale. One group received 80 minutes of a stepwise retraining procedure, including practice on tasks emphasizing discrete components of the cognitive skills necessary to perform the Block Design subtest. The procedure also included training aids to facilitate learning. The control group received unstructured practice with similar training tasks. The data suggested that both interventions had a positive effect on Block Design performance. Unfortunately, statistical analyses were not reported, a problem that seriously limits the validity of the author's conclusions. Goldman and Goldman (1988) employed a quasiexperimental, time-lag design in their investigation of the effects of cognitive retraining. Their results demonstrated improved performance on the Trailmaking Test–Part B, which was significantly greater among the trained group as compared to the untrained controls. However, in view of the lack of a pre-treatment assessment, differences between the groups prior to training may have influenced the results.

Methodological limitations certainly limit definite conclusions regarding the efficacy of cognitive rehabilitation with alcoholics. Nonetheless, the aforementioned reports support the notion that neuropsychological recovery following chronic alcohol abuse may be enhanced with cognitive retraining interventions. Future research should explore this possibility with more rigorous methodology. In addition, efforts at cognitive retraining could be facilitated by including token reinforcement as an adjunct to the rehabilitation process, an idea supported by preliminary findings reported by Dolan and Norton (1977).

Korsakoff's Syndrome

In contrast to nonKorsakoff's alcoholics, Korsakoff's patients have proven to be completely resistant to the effects of cognitive retraining. Nonetheless, Cermak (1980) demonstrated that some subjects can benefit from the use of mnemonic strategies. However, since they were not able to recall and spontaneously use the mnemonic techniques, the subjects did not consistently evidence improved recall. Because the subjects continued to rely on external cues to implement the mnemonic strategies, Cermak's intervention actually functioned as a "compensation" treatment approach. In view of the severity of the dense anterograde amnesia present in Korsakoff's patients, this finding is not surprising.

Acknowledging the resistance of certain types of anterograde amnesia to cognitive retraining, Glisky, Schacter, and Tulving (1986a, 1986b) recently presented a computer based program as a compensatory memory device. Their "vanishing cues" technique was designed to help patients recall domain specific information with the assistance of memory cues. Using this compensation approach, subjects were cued with as many letters of the to-be-remembered target word as needed for recall. The cues were then gradually withdrawn until the target words could be produced with minimal cueing. In the 1986b study, the vanishing cue technique was extended by using interactive computer programs requiring subjects to use target words to operate the computer (i.e., simple computer commands). The amnesic subjects were able to learn how to supply basic computer commands with prompting and examiner-provided retrieval cues.

It should be noted that Glisky et al.'s subjects were not Korsakoff's syndrome patients, but rather victims of severe closed head injury. Yet pretreatment testing did reveal the presence of a dense anterograde amnesia, similar to that commonly observed in Korsakoff's syndrome. Interestingly, one subject, was unable to recall any of his time with the computer (due to a deficit in episodic memory), but retained the information so that he could supply it upon request (i.e., retrieval cues). Future studies investigating the utility of this approach with Korsakoff's patients are recommended.

Conclusion

The lack of evidence supporting the utility of cognitive retraining with Korsakoff's subjects suggests that a compensation approach is appropriate with this population. However, the degree to which the rate of cognitive recovery in neurologically intact alcoholics can be enhanced with cognitive retraining is unknown. Improving the rate of recovery could have a significant impact on the prevention of future drinking binges as well as adaptability to social and vocational stressors. In addition, better cognitive skills would be expected to result in better decision-making during the course of treatment. With this in mind, we now turn to the role of neuropsychology in the treatment and prevention of alcohol-induced brain damage.

ROLE OF NEUROPSYCHOLOGICAL EVALUATION IN TREATMENT

At present, most alcohol treatment programs emphasize education and the acquisition of social problem-solving skills. Yet if patients are neuropsychologically impaired, and therefore deficient in their ability to learn new information, they should not be expected to benefit from such an approach. Therefore, it may be useful to monitor neuropsychologic function throughout the course of treatment, and limit the presentation of new information to patients who are capable of remembering the material.

Although this hypothesis is intuitively appealing, findings obtained from investigations of the predictive validity of neuropsychological evaluation have been inconsistent. Abbott and Gregson (1981) found that neuropsychological test performance is a significant predictor of relapse among alcoholism treatment participants. Similarly, O'Leary, Donovan, Chaney, and Walker (1979) found neuropsychological function to be predictive of completion rate in a rehabilitation program. Yet, negative findings were reported by Donovan, Kiviahan, and Walker (1984). Although neuropsychological function was significantly related to posttreatment employment status, only one of 6 neuropsychological variables (Block design subtest from the WAIS) that comprise the Brain Age Quotient (BAQ) significantly predicted drinking behavior.

Clearly, more research is needed before any definite conclusions can be drawn regarding the predictive validity of neuropsychological variables in the treatment of alcoholism. Future investigators should consider employing measures that are related to adaptive daily living skills and vocational status (Chelune & Moehle, 1986). Future studies should also examine the effects of tailoring treatment programs to accommodate an individual's neuropsychological profile (McCrady & Smith, 1986).

Are alcoholic patients aware of their neuropsychological impairment? Shelton and Parsons (1987) addressed this issue by administering the Patient's Assessment of Own Functioning Inventory (PAOFI), developed by Heaton and Pendleton (1981), to 60 detoxified alcoholics and 60 nonalcoholic controls. The PAOFI provides self-report ratings that are grouped into Memory, Language and Communication, Perceptual-Motor, and Higher Cognitive Functions subscales. Significant between group differences were obtained on all four subscales indicating that alcoholic subjects acknowledge a higher frequency of problems in these areas. Subsequent analyses demonstrated a significant relationship between self-report and extent of alcohol intake over the past 6 months (as measured by the Quantity Frequency Index; Cahalan, Cissin, & Crossly, 1969). In a similar study, Parsons, Tassey, and Schaeffer (reported in Parsons, 1987) employed the Neuropsychological Impairment Scale (NIS) (O'Donnell & Reynolds, 1983) and confirmed the finding that detoxified alcoholics are indeed aware of their cognitive deficits.

If alcoholic patients are capable of becoming more aware of their cognitive deficits, perhaps such information could be used as a motivating force in treatment. That is, patients could receive feedback regarding the extent of brain damage and be counseled accordingly. Because alcohol-induced neuropsychological deficits develop gradually, they may not be readily apparent in the early stages of alcoholism. Bringing these early signs of alcohol abuse to the attention of the alcoholic could enhance awareness of the deleterious effects of alcohol, making educational interventions more successful.

Using neuropsychological data as feedback for the problem drinker and/or alcoholic is not a novel idea. Wilkinson and Sanchez-Craig (1981) described a case study that included such a treatment approach. Their patient was a 53-year-old senior executive who had been consuming 12 to 15 drinks per day prior to treatment. A behavioral modification intervention successfully reduced his intake by 30% at follow-up questioning. The authors then provided feedback regarding the patient's liver (GGTP level) and neuropsychologic function that indicated significant impairment. This intervention prompted the patient to further reduce his alcohol intake; "the client himself noted a reduction in the number of memory lapses (which he previously had experienced) after his drinking was reduced, and he continued to express interest in the results of follow-up testing" (p. 259).

PRIMARY PREVENTION

The most straightforward way to prevent alcohol-induced brain damage is to prevent the use of the substance among children, adolescents, and young adults. Thus far, most primary prevention programs have emphasized either alcohol education, changing social norms and values, enhancing social competence, or a combination of these.

Czechowicz (1987; see also MacDonald, 1984) proposed that chronic substance abuse includes 4 progressive stages. The initial or experimentation phase most often occurs in social settings and is viewed by the user as a safe form of entertainment. In the second stage, the user then begins to seek more regularly the euphoric effects of the substance, leading to habitual use in the third stage. Finally, in the fourth stage, daily use is accompanied by a strong desire to avoid negative feelings associated with sobriety. Assuming that these stages represent a linear progression, it seems logical to promote complete abstinence, thereby avoiding the experimental stage. However, in most settings, experimentation is an enjoyable social norm, making the decision of whether to promote abstinence a difficult one.

Research examining the utility of primary prevention interventions was recently reviewed by Moskowitz (1989). Overall, the available data provide little empirical support for any of these interventions; "although such programs may influence knowledge, beliefs, or attitudes, they generally do not affect behaviors or problems" (p. 79). However, primary prevention efforts might benefit from methods that isolate those individuals "at risk" for developing alcoholism.

There is evidence indicating that some individuals are biologically predisposed to problem-drinking; twin studies, for example, have convincingly demonstrated evidence for a genetic factor in the transmission of alcoholism (e.g., Goodwin et al., 1984). Frances, Tim, and Bucky (1980) found that alcoholics with a family history of alcoholism have an earlier onset of problem drinking, less stable family environment, and poorer academic performance. Children of alcoholics, who are exposed to both genetic and environmental risk factors, are placed at particularly high risk for developing alcoholism. For these individuals, promotion of an alcohol-free lifestyle may be appropriate.

Children at high risk for developing alcoholism may also be more likely to exhibit mental illness and/or learning disability. Tarter, McBride, Buopane, and Schneider (1977) grouped alcoholics into "primary" and "secondary" subtypes using a brief questionnaire. Primary alcoholics included subjects reporting no known precipitating cause for their excessive drinking and at least six of the following eight criteria: (a) increased tolerance, (b) withdrawal symptoms, (c) euphoria after the first drinking experience, (d) euphoria after the first drink following a period of abstinence, (e) no history of social drinking, (f) psychological problems from alcohol before age 40, (g) loss of control over consumption, and (h) excessive drinking prior to age 40. Secondary alcoholics included those subjects not meeting the criteria for primary alcoholism. Tarter et al. (1977) found greater incidence of familial drinking in the primary group. In addition, they reported that primary alcoholics are more likely to report childhood symptoms of hyperkinesis than their secondary counterparts.

More recent data also indicate that neuropsychological differences between primary and secondary alcoholics could contribute to subsequent drinking behavior. After ruling out the effects of current emotional distress, days abstinent, and drinking frequency, DeObaldia and Parsons (1984) found primary alcoholics to exhibit lower educational levels and poorer performance on the Wechsler Memory Scale and the Booklet Category Test. Further, research reported by Tarter, Jacob, and Bremer, (1989), and Whipple, Parker, and Noble (1988) demonstrated impairment in the offspring of alcoholics on neuropsychological tests measuring planning, visuoperceptual, and problem-solving skills. Although inconsistency across studies limits drawing definite conclusions at this time, the available research does suggest the possibility that cognitive characteristics in adolescence may predispose certain individuals to alcoholism. The neuropsychologist could assist in identifying such individuals, who once identified, could receive more individualized preventive and treatment care. Future research should examine the utility of primary prevention interventions that are targeted at these high-risk populations.

CONCLUSION

It would appear quite clear from the foregoing discussion that alcohol use can cause brain damage. It should also be clear that particular characteristics of drinking behavior (e.g., how much per occasion) and individual differences (e.g., age) can influence the degree of brain damage and how quickly cognitive deficits recover, if at all. Also, cognitive rehabilitation efforts with the brain-impaired alcoholic population have shown some interesting results but much more additional research is needed.

Research in the area of treatment and prevention is in its infancy. At present, the role of neuropsychological evaluation in guiding treatment decisions is unclear and additional research will need to be done before any firm conclusions can be drawn. What can be said is that providing direct feedback regarding an alcoholics neuropsychological status is a seductive hypothesis that merits further scrutiny. Similarly, prevention efforts will need to focus on at-risk populations but there is little evidence at present that primary prevention programs can affect the drinking behavior of subjects at-risk for developing alcoholism. The hope and expectation is that this chapter will assist in suggesting potential avenues for future investigation.

REFERENCES

Abbott, M. W., & Gregson, R. A. M. (1981). Cognitive dysfunction in the prediction of relapse in alcoholics. *Journal of Studies on Alcohol, 42*, 230–243.

Albert, M. S., Butters, N., & Brandt, J. (1980). Memory for remote events in alcoholics. *Journal of Studies of Alcohol, 41*, 1071–1081.

Albert, M. S., Butters, N., & Levin, J. (1979). Temporal gradients in the retrograde amnesia of patients with alcoholic Korsakoff's disease. *Archives of Neurology, 36*, 211–216.

Becker, J., Rivoira, P., Butters, N., & Ciraulo, D. (1984). Asking the right questions: Problem solving skills in alcoholics and alcoholics with Korsakoff's syndrome. Paper Presented at the Annual Meeting of the Research Society on Alcoholism, San Antonio, TX.

Brandt, J., Butters, N., Ryan, C., & Baygog, R. (1983). Cognitive loss and recovery in long-term alcohol abusers. *Archives of General Psychiatry, 40*, 435–442.

Butters, N., & Cermak, L. S. (1980). Alcoholic Korsakoff's syndrome: an information processing approach to amnesia. New York: Academic Press.

Butters, N., & Granholm, E. (1987). The continuity hypothesis: Some conclusions and their implications for the etiology and neuropathology of alcoholic Korsakoff's syndrome. In O. A. Parsons, N. Butters, & P. E. Nathan (Eds.), *Neuropsychology of alcoholism: implications for diagnosis and treatment* (pp. 176–206). New York: Guilford Press.

Cahalan, O., Cissin, I., & Crossly, H. (1969). *American drinking practices.* New Brunswick, NJ: Rutgers Center for Alcohol Studies.

Cermak, L. S. (1980). Improving retention in alcoholic Korsakoff's patients. *Journal of Studies on Alcohol, 41*, 159–169.

Cermak, L. S., & Ryback, R. S. (1976). Recovery of verbal short-term memory in alcoholics. *Journal of Studies on Alcohol, 37*, 46–52.

Chelune, G. J., & Moehle, K. A. (1986). Neuropsychological assessment of everyday functioning. In D. Wedding, A. M. Horton, & J. Webster (Eds.), *The neuropsychology handbook* (pp. 489–525). New York: Springer.

Cohen, N. J., & Squire, L. R. (1981). Retrograde amnesia and remote memory impairment. *Neuropsychologia, 1,* 337–356.

Cohen, N. J., & Squire, L. R. (1980). Preserved learning and retention of pattern analyzing skill in amnesia: Dissociation of knowing how and knowing that. *Science, 210,* 207–209.

Czechowicz, D. (1987). Adolescent alcohol and drug abuse and its consequences: An overview. Paper presented at the annual meeting of the American Psychiatric Association, Chicago, Illinois.

Dolan, M. P., & Norton, J. C. (1977). A programmed training technique that uses reinforcement to facilitate acquisition and retention in brain-damaged patients. *Journal of Clinical Psychology, 33,* 496–501.

Donovan, D. M., Kiviahan, D. R., & Walker, R. D. (1984). Clinical limitations of neuropsychological testing in predicting treatment outcome among alcoholics. *Alcoholism: Clinical and Experimental Research, 8,* 470–475.

DeObaldia, R., & Parsons, O. A. (1984). Neuropsychological performance related to primary alcoholism and self-reported symptoms of childhood MBD. *Journal of Studies on Alcohol, 45,* 386–392.

Eckhardt, M. J., Parker, E. S., Noble, E. P., Fieldman, D. J., & Gottschalk, L. A. (1978). Relationship between neuropsychological performance and alcoholic consumption in alcoholics. *Biological Psychiatry, 13,* 551–565.

Glisky, E. L., Schacter, D. L., & Tulving, E. (1986a). Learning and retention of computer-related vocabulary in memory-impaired patients: Method of vanishing cues. *Journal of Clinical and Experimental Neuropsychology, 8,* 292–312.

Glisky, E. L., Schacter, D. L., & Tulving, E. (1986b). Computer learning by memory-impaired patients: Acquisition and retention of complex knowledge. *Neuropsychologia, 24,* 313–328.

Glosser, G., Butters, N., & Kaplan, E. (1977). Visuoperceptual processes in brain-damaged patients on the digit symbol substitution test. *International Journal of Neuroscience, 7,* 59–66.

Goldman, M. (1983). Cognitive impairment in chronic alcoholics: Some cause for optimism. *American Psychologist, 38,* 1045–1054.

Goldman, M. (1986). Neuropsychological recovery in alcoholics: Endogenous and exogenous processes. *Alcoholism: Clinical and Experimental Research, 10,* 136–144.

Goldman, M. S. (1987). The role of time and practice in recovery of function in alcoholics. In O. A. Parsons, N. Butters, & P. E. Nathan (Eds.), *Neuropsychology of Alcoholism: Implications for Diagnosis and Treatment* (pp. 291–321). New York: Guilford Press.

Goldman, R. S., & Goldman, M. S. (1988). Experience-dependent cognitive recovery in alcoholics: A task component strategy. *Journal of Studies on Alcohol, 49,* 142–148.

Goldman, M., Williams, D. L., & Klisz, D. K. (1983). Recoverability of psychological functioning following alcohol abuse: Prolonged visual-spatial dysfunction in older alcoholics. *Journal of Consulting and Clinical Psychology, 51,* 370–378.

Goldman, M., Klisz, D. K., & Williams, D. L. (1985). Experience-dependent recovery of functioning in young alcoholics. *Addictive Behavior, 10,* 169–176.

Harwood, H. J., Napolitano, D. M., Kristiansen, P. L., et al., (1984). *Economic Costs to Society of Alcohol and Drug Abuse and Mental Illness.* Report to the Alcohol, Drug Abuse, and Mental Health Administration, Research Triangle, North Carolina.

Heaton, R. F., & Pendleton, M. D. (1981). Use of neuropsychological tests to predict adult patient's everyday functioning. *Journal of Consulting and Clinical Psychology, 99,* 807–821.

Hirst, W. (1981). The amnestic syndrome: descriptions and explanations. *Psychological Bulletin, 91,* 435–460.

MacDonald, D. I. (1984). Drugs, smoking, and adolescence. *American Journal of Disabled Children, 138*, 117–125.

McCrady, B. S., & Smith, D. E. (1986). Implications of cognitive impairment for the treatment of alcoholism. *Alcoholism: Clinical and Experimental Research, 10*, 145–149.

Miller, W. R., & Saucedo, C. F. (1983). Assessment of neuropsychological impairment and brain damage in problem drinkers. In C. J. Golden, J. A. Moses, J. A. Coffman, W. S. Miller, & F. D. Strider, (Eds.), *Clinical neuropsychology: interface with neurological and psychiatric disorders*, (pp. 141–196). New York: Grune & Stratton.

Moskowitz, J. M. (1989). The primary prevention of alcohol problems: A critical review of the literature. *Journal of Studies on Alcohol, 50*, 54–88.

Moss, M. B., Albert, M. S., Butters, N., & Payne, M. (1986). Differential patterns of memory loss among patients with Alzheimer's disease, Huntington's disease, and alcoholic Korsakoff's syndrome. *Archives of Neurology, 43*, 239–246.

New York State Division of Substance Abuse Services. (1984). *Substance abuse among New York State public and private school students in grades seven through twelve*. Albany, New York.

O'Donnell, W. E., & Reynolds, D. M. (1983). *neuropsychological impairment scale manual*. Annapolis, MD: Annapolis Psychological Service.

O'Leary, M. R., Donovan, D. M., Chaney, E. F., & Walker, R. D. (1979). Cognitive impairment and treatment outcome with alcoholics: Preliminary findings. *Journal of Clinical Psychiatry, 40*, 397–398.

Oscar-Berman, M. (1973). Hypothesis testing and focusing behavior during concept formation by amnesic Korsakoff patients. *Neuropsychologia, 11*, 191–198.

Parsons, O. A. (1987). Neuropsychological consequences of alcohol abuse: Many questions-some answers. In O. A. Parsons, N. Butters, & P. E. Nathan (Eds.), *Neuropsychology of alcoholism: implications for diagnosis and treatment* (pp. 176–206). New York: Guilford Press.

Robins, L. N., Helzer, J. E., Weissman, M. M., Orvaschel, H., Gruenberg, E., Burke, J. D. & Regier, D. A. (1984). Lifetime prevalence of specific psychiatric disorders in three sites. *Archives of General Psychiatry, 41*, 949–958.

Ryan, C. & Butters, N. (1986). The neuropsychology of alcoholism. In D. Wedding, A. M. Horton, & J. Webster (Eds.), *The neuropsychology handbook* (pp. 376–409). New York: Springer.

Ryback, R. (1971). The continuum and specificity of the effects of alcohol on memory: A review. *Quarterly Journal of Studies on Alcohol, 32*, 995–1016.

Shelton, M. D., & Parsons, O. A. (1987). Alcoholic's self-assessment of their neuropsychological function in everyday life. *Journal of Clinical Psychology, 43*, 395–403.

Tarter, R. E., Jacob, T., & Bremer, D. A. (1989). Cognitive status of sons of alcoholic men. *Alcoholism: Clinical and Experimental Research, 13*, 232–235.

Tarter, R. E., McBride, H., Buopane, N., & Schneider, D. U. (1977). Differentiation of alcoholics. *Archives of General Psychiatry, 34*, 761–768.

Victor, M. Adams, R. D., & Collins, G. H. (1971). *The Wernicke-Korsakoff syndrome*. Philadelphia: F. A. Davis.

Whipple, S. C., Parker, E. S., & Noble, E. P. (1988). An atypical neurocognitive profile in alcoholic fathers and their sons. *Journal of Studies on Alcohol, 49*, 240–244.

Wilkinson, D. A. (1987). CT scan and neuropsychological assessments of alcoholism. In O. A. Parsons, N. Butters, & P. E. Nathan (Eds.), *Neuropsychology of alcoholism: implications for diagnosis and treatment* (pp. 176–206). New York: Guilford Press.

Wilkinson, D. A., & Sanchez-Craig, M. (1981). Relevance of brain dysfunction to treatment objectives: Should alcohol-related cognitive deficits influence the way we think about treatment? *Addictive Behaviors, 6*, 253–260.

Williams, G. D., Stinson, F. S., Parker, D. A., Harford, T. C., and Noble, J. (1987). Demographic trends, alcohol abuse and alcoholism 1985-1995. *Alcohol Health and Research World*, *11*, 80-83.

Woods, R. T. (1983). Specificity of learning in reality-orientation sessions: A single-case study. *Behavior Research and Therapy*, *21*, 173-175.

Yohman, J. R., Parsons, O. A., & Leber, W. R. (1985). Lack of recovery in alcoholics' neuropsychological performance one year after treatment. *Alcoholism: Clinical and Experimental Research*, *9*, 114-117.

CHAPTER 12

NEUROLOGICAL AND NEUROPSYCHOLOGICAL CONSEQUENCES OF DRUG ABUSE

Michael W. Lilliquist and Erin D. Bigler

The last few years have witnessed a growth in public concern with the problem of drug abuse in the United States to a level not seen since the drug experimentation days of the 1960s. The political rhetoric has risen to similar heights as evidenced by the much-lauded "war on drugs." Although much has been learned about drug abuse and the drugs themselves since the 1960s, public debate still turns on ideological positions and political opinions.

More directly relevant to the subject of this chapter, drug abuse has often been depicted as being uniformly and unquestionably harmful to the *brain*, producing permanent damage. Although it is beyond the scope of this chapter to discuss the often serious psychological, medical, and sociological problems associated with drug abuse, it is important that the *neurological* and *neuropsychological* consequences of drug abuse be assessed objectively. Review of current knowledge indicates that currently abused drugs constitute a broad spectrum of psychoactive substances that present a wide range of risk factors to brain function. Indiscriminate claims regarding the danger of drug abuse have served only to undermine credibility. By understanding which drugs present a true danger to brain function, we can more convincingly fight abuse of those drugs through informed argument. Just as importantly, the realization that the effects of certain drugs on brain function are potentially reversible provides hope that should guide our rehabilitation efforts with drug users.

The most recent national survey conducted by the National Institute on Drug Abuse concludes that an estimated 72 million Americans have used illicit drugs at some time in their lives, and that some 14 million have done so within the last month (NIDA, 1989). Given numbers such as these, the value of accurate information concerning the long-term risks of drug abuse can hardly be doubted.

This chapter critically reviews the long-term and potentially permanent changes in brain function that may result from drug use/abuse. A distinction is made between the effects of acute intoxication and the enduring results of drug use. Clearly, in as much as abused drugs are psychologically active, they alter brain function. The question is whether brain function remains altered long after the drug has been eliminated from the body, and whether these effects are transient or permanent.

The consequences of drug abuse examined here fall into two broad categories, which we have termed the *neurological* and the *neuropsychological*. By the neurological consequences of drug abuse we mean changes in brain structure and function as measured by physical instruments such as various imaging methods (e.g., computed tomography, or CT), direct physiological measures (e.g., electroencephalography, or EEG), and post mortem neuroanatomical and histopathological methods. The most common gross neurological sign looked for with brain imaging techniques is brain atrophy, as indicated by enlarged cerebral ventricles (fluid-filled cavities within the brain) and enlarged spaces between the convolutions (or *gyri*, singular *gyrus*) of the cerebral cortex. Another neurological complication seen with the abuse of some drugs is cerebrovascular accidents (CVAs), or strokes. In simple terms, CVAs may be due either to hemorrhage within or near the brain, or due to occlusion of a cerebral blood vessel by an *embolus* so that oxygen and nutrients are cut off (*ischemia*) to a part of the brain. In both cases, significant damage to the brain can result, both directly and as a result of further complications.

Neuropsychology concerns itself with brain *function*. Neuropsychological tests examine behaviors that have been empirically associated with the functioning of brain. Typically, these tests evaluate abilities such as verbal and visual reasoning, memory, language function, concentration, concept formation, cognitive flexibility, and perceptual and motor abilities. There are numerous standardized tests that allow the objective assessment of these various functions (Bigler, 1988; Lezak, 1983). A particular deficit in one of these areas may relate to damage or dysfunction in brain regions that subserve that function. Many of the studies that have examined the potental effects of drug abuse on neuropsychological function have relied on the Wechsler Adult Intelligence Scale (WAIS and WAIS-R) and the Halstead-Reitan Neuropsychological Test Battery.

Tests that are considered particularly sensitive to general cerebral dysfunction include the Block Design and Digit Symbol subtests of the WAIS, and the Category Test, Tactual Performance Test, and Trail-Making Test of the Halstead-Reitan battery. The particular sensitivity of these tests occurs because performance on each of them may be affected by damage to any of several areas of the cerebral cortex. The Category Test assesses abstract visual reasoning, which presumably relies upon widely dispersed regions of the cerebral cortex including the frontal lobes and the visual areas of the inferior temporal-occipital cortex. The Trail-Making Test evaluates a subject's concentration and mental flexibility, abilities that also rely upon the functioning of the frontal lobes. The Tactual Performance Test assesses subjects' tactile sensorimotor ability, placing particular burden upon parietal lobe function.

LIMITATIONS OF THE RESEARCH

For obvious ethical reasons, human drug abuse cannot be studied using true experimental designs, characterized by random assignment of subjects and experimenter control over drug dosage and composition.

Even careful human studies must employ quasiexperimental designs, wherein a "control" group is constructed post hoc for comparison with the "experimental" group of drug users. Although these studies are necessarily correlational, causal relationships between drug use and brain damage are often inferred, if not by the authors then by others. Yet only through true experimental designs can causal relationships be empirically demonstrated. In human drug studies, although many variables such as age and educational level can be adequately controlled, the possibility of confounding personality and other premorbid variables remains. In a sense, drug users are self-selected subjects in these studies. It is possible that differences in adaptive ability, perhaps due to premorbid brain dysfunction, may contribute to some individuals' abuse of drugs while demographically similar individuals do not abuse drugs.

A second major limitation of the literature concerning the consequences of drug abuse arises from the method by which the data were gathered. Numerous case studies have been published in which a handful of subjects or even a single drug user is described as developing a particular problem; this is particularly true of the literature concerning the neurological sequelae of drug use. As with quasiexperimental designs, case studies of the occurrence of a neurological disorder in a drug user cannot readily attribute the cause to drug use itself; the relationship is often only circumstantial and correlational. In addition, no comparison group is used, and the base rate for that disorder is often not known or not reported. It is not enough to show that users of a particular drug demonstrate certain neurological problems, but also that these drug users are more likely to experience these problems than similar people who do not use drugs.

An additional problem concerns the reliability of drug use measures. Typically, researchers must rely upon the self-report of drug users themselves. Even in the absence of motives to distort one's history of drug use, self-report measures are notoriously unreliable, and may be particularly unreliable concerning drug use, which often occurs while the person is already intoxicated. Drug users commonly experiment with several drugs, and may have extensive experience with drugs other than the one whose effects are being investigated. Thus, it is not always possible to attribute findings to the abuse of a particular drug. Moreover, heavy use of alcohol is common. While the harmful effects of alcohol abuse are well known (see Horton, this volume), it is not always possible to parcel out its confounding effects, as the effects of alcohol and other drugs of abuse are often presumed to be similar in character.

DIRECT VERSUS INDIRECT RISKS OF DRUG USE

Drug use can contribute to brain dysfunction by many means, only a few of which are directly related to its psychoactive properties. Indirect causes include increased exposure to disease and infection, particularly with intravenous (IV) drug use, and increased likelihood of head trauma from falls and motor vehicle accidents while intoxicated. In this light, AIDS-related dementia is an indirect risk of IV drug use. Intravenous drugs can also serve to provide entry of toxins and contaminants into the blood stream. These contaminants may irritate cerebral blood vessels and contribute to vasculitis (inflammation of the vessel), which can lead to hemorrhage. Drug contaminants may also contribute to the formation of emboli occluding cerebral arteries, leading to infarction (death and subsequent decay) of brain tissue.

Drug use may result in injury to the central nervous system by affecting other systems within the body. For example, the use of cocaine has been associated with heart attacks. In those cases in which the attack does not prove fatal, the temporary loss of blood flow can result in anoxic brain injury. Brain tissue is especially susceptible to such injury because neural tissue contains virtually no stores of nutrients, and is instead wholly dependent upon an uninterrupted supply from the blood stream. Drug use may contribute to metabolic encephalopathy as a consequence of toxic damage to the liver and kidneys.

Drug preparations may also contain substances that are directly toxic to nervous tissue. For example, Wolters et al. (1982) report an epidemic of fatal and near fatal white-matter encephalopathy in heroin abusers due to drug contamination. Lead-induced encephalopathy has been documented in many cases of leaded gasoline sniffing (Valpey, Sumi, Copass, & Goble, 1978; Ross, 1982; Kaelan, Harper, & Vieira, 1986; McGrath, 1986; Rischbieth, Thompson, Hamilton-Bruce, Purdie, & Peters, 1987) in this and several other countries. The appearance of cases of reversible lead poisoning as a result of impure illicit amphetamine use (Allcott, Barnhart, & Mooney, 1987), raises the possibility that after repeated toxic insults from drug impurities the brain may not be able to recover completely. Chronic drug use may produce long-lasting effects in brain function.

MPTP

A particularly striking example of the risks of exposure to neurotoxins in association with drug use is provided by the case of methyl-phenyl-tetrahydo-pyridine (MPTP), a chemical analog of the opiate meperidine (Demerol). A designer drug taken by many users looking for a "new heroin," MPTP has proven to be a powerful and selective neurotoxin that produces permanent and harmful changes in brain tissue. In particular, MPTP permanently destroys neurons which employ dopamine as their neurotransmitter (Kopin, 1988). By damaging the nigrostriatal dopamine system, MPTP produces chronic parkinsonism in both humans (Langston, Ballard, Tetrud, & Irwin, 1983; Wright, Wall, Perry, & Paty, 1984; Ballard, Tetrud, & Langston, 1985) and in experimental monkeys (Crossman, Clarke, Boyce, Robertson, & Sambrook, 1987); Elsworth, Deutch, Redmond, Taylor, Sladek, & Roth, 1989). Parkinsonism is characterized by difficulty with movement, including rigidity, difficulty initiating movements ("freezing"), a shuffling walk, difficulty swallowing, and a general slowing and reduction of movements.

Parkinsonism induced by MPTP can range from mild to severe (Tetrud, Langston, Garbe, & Ruttenber, 1989). In primates, reductions in dopamine activity can be as great as 75% without clear signs of parkinsonism developing (Elsworth et al., 1989), suggesting a surprising robustness of nigrostriatal dopamine function. Damage to dopamine neurons outside the nigrostriatal system, which may contribute to non-movement-related deficits, has also been observed (Gupta, Felton, & Gash, 1984; Crossman et al., 1987). In humans, even in the absence of parkinsonian symptoms, the use of MPTP appears to produce cognitive impairment on neuropsychological tests of executive functions, which require spontaneous generation of novel ideas and the ability to suppress the interfering effects of irrelevant stimuli (Stern, Tetrud, Martin, Kutner, & Langston, 1990). Cognitive deficits in asymptomatic MPTP users may simply reflect the relatively greater vulnerability of higher brain functions compared to the neural systems which govern movement. Given this possibility, it is particularly troublesome that reductions in dopamine activity were found in clinically normal (i.e., no motor symptoms) subjects after a single exposure to MPTP.

POLYDRUG ABUSE

Many people who use illicit drugs have extensive experience with several different kinds of drugs. As discussed above, this has often made it difficult to study the effects of a particular drug. This has led some investigators to chose to investigate the effect of polydrug abuse on brain function.

Compared to normal subjects and to medical patients with no known neurological symptoms, polydrug abusers display neuropsychological deficits in a number of areas, although not consistently on the same tests across studies. Significant deficits have been observed on the Category Test (Judd & Grant, 1975; Adams, Rennick, Schoof, & Keegan, 1975; Grant, Mohs, Miller, & Reitan, 1976), Trail-Making Test part B (Judd & Grant, 1975; Adams et al., 1975), Performance subtests of the WAIS (Adams et al., 1975; Grant et al., 1976), the Tactual Performance Test (Judd & Grant, 1975), and fine-motor control (Adams et al., 1975; Judd & Grant, 1975). However, when adolescent drug abusers were compared to adolescent non-drug-abusers in the same inpatient facility, no differences were found on either the Category or Trail-Making test, regardless of the degree of heavy drug use (Brandt & Doyle, 1983). Similarly, a comparison of prison inmates grouped according to degree of past drug use revealed no intergroup differences (Bruhn & Maage, 1975). The mean score of all groups on the Category Test were within the normal range.

As several authors have pointed out, the comparison of group mean scores can overlook the increased number of abnormal test performances within a group. Studies of polydrug abusers have found that approximately half can be classified as functionally impaired on the basis of neuropsychological testing (Judd & Grant, 1975; Grant, Mohs, Miller, & Reitan, 1976). These neuropsychological deficits do not appear to be due to short-term effects of drug detoxification. In one study, impairment was observed 60 days after the last use of drugs by the subjects (Grant et al., 1976). Subjects classified as impaired 2-3 weeks after admission for drug abuse treatment continued to display neuropsychological deficits 3 months (Grant, Adams, Carlin, Rennick, Judd, & Schoof, 1978) or 5 months later (Grant & Judd, 1976).

In a large collaborative study, investigators subjected the neuropsychological test data from over 150 polydrug abusers to multivariate analysis in order to better characterize the observed deficits (Grant et al., 1978). It is found that neuropsychological deficits correlated significantly with the amount of past use of central nervous system depressants and of opiate drugs. Interestingly, the polydrug abusers studied by Judd and Grant (1975), who displayed particularly large deficits, tended to have had extensive experience with sedatives. It may be that, in the context of multiple drug use, the use of sedatives introduces the greatest risk to brain function. It cannot be ruled out, however, that the observed deficits in polydrug abusers including those especially prone to sedative abuse, are due to some pre-existing factor. Prospective studies are needed to evaluate this possibility.

Neuropsychological deficits observed in polydrug abusers may reflect the additive effects of the individual drugs used, but they may also reflect synergistic interaction between drugs. Minor cerebral damage may result in little or no functional impairment because of the brain's capacity to compensate for deficits in one area by relying upon the intact functioning of other areas. It is possible that, by affecting brain function in different ways, polydrug abuse may circumvent the brain's power to compensate for losses.

CANNABIS

Cannabis, or marijuana, is the most popular illicit drug used in the United States. Recent figures indicate that just over half of all high school seniors have tried marijuana, and 23% of seniors surveyed indicated using marijuana in the last month (NIDA, 1987). Among the general population 65 million Americans have tried marijuana, 11 million smoke marijuana at least once a month, and more than 6 million smoke marijuana on a weekly basis (NIDA, 1989). Other estimates place the figure even higher: 18–20 million Americans may use marijuana on a regular basis (Jones, 1987).

In this country, marijuana has had a mixed reputation. Because cannabis, unlike heroin and other opiates, does not produce clear physiological dependence or carry a risk of lethal overdose, many people have considered marijuana to be a relatively benign, "soft" drug. However, marijuana has also been portrayed as one of the worst "hard" drugs, as it was in the notorious government film "Reefer Madness." In particular, it has been claimed that marijuana is able to provoke chronic psychosis, although the available scientific evidence provides little support for this charge (National Academy of Science, 1982).

The active compound in cannabis is tetrahydrocannabinol (THC). One estimate places the concentration of THC present in marijuana leaf around 1–3% and 3–6% for hashish (Nahas, 1986), although more potent varieties of marijuana have emerged in recent years. Current strains of *sinsemilla* marijuana may contain as high as 6–14% THC (Gold, 1989). Given this increase, early research with cannabis may require reevaluation. When smoked, approximately 18% of the THC is absorbed into the blood stream (Ohlsson, Lindgren, Wahlen, Agurell, Hollister, & Gillespie, 1980). When marijuana is eaten in food on the order of 6% of the THC present is absorbed (Ohlesson et al., 1980). After smoking, the psychological 'high" occurs rapidly and then steadily declines over a four-hour period, mirroring the time course of THC found in circulation. When cannabis is consumed orally, the onset of symptoms is slower, less predictable, and lasts longer, reflecting the less consistent absorption of THC from the gut into circulation. THC is a fat-soluble substance, and so will diffuse into all tissues of the body and remain sequestered there for long periods. The eliminative half-life of THC is approximately one week (Nahas, 1986).

The mechanism by which THC acts has been something of a mystery. THC has properties of both a central nervous stimulant and in higher concentrations acts as a hallucinogen. THC has long been suspected to act on a specific receptor site on particular nerve cells, but until recently evidence has been indirect (Devane, Dysarz, Johnson, Melvin, & Howlett, 1988). THC affects the brain at extremely low concentrations, and even small changes in the THC molecule can alter or elminate its psychoactivity—both properties characteristic of drugs that act on receptor sites. Just recently, researchers announced the identification of a likely receptor molecule for THC and related cannabiniods (Matsuda, Lolait, Brownstein, Young, & Bonner, 1990). The putative receptor appears to bind to cannabinoids in proportion to their known psychoactive potency, and it is found preferentially in those brain regions in which cannabis is presumed to act. THC appears to act by altering metabolic activity within target nerve cells, rather than by affecting neurotransmission between cells directly (Howlett, 1985; Howlett, Johnson, Melvin, & Milne, 1987).

Neurochemical studies of chronic cannabis treatment in experimental animals have failed to demonstrate persistent alterations in neurotransmitter function after detoxification. For example, a 90-day regimen of 20 mg of THC failed to result in changes in transmitter binding for dopamine serotonin, acetylcholine, GABA or opiate transmitter systems (Ali, et al. 1989). These results do not rule out the possibilities that other aspects of transmitter function or that unexamined neurotransmitter and neuromodulatory systems may be affected.

The first published report of neurologic abnormalities associated with cannabis use (Campbell, Evans, Thomson, & Williams, 1971) sparked a lively period of academic debate by reporting the presence of cerebral atrophy in a sample of 10 young cannabis users. However, this study has serious methodological flaws. Nearly half of their drug users were included in the study because they were already known to have cerebral abnormalities. Three of the cannabis users had histories of head trauma, and all showed evidence of psychopathology, both of which are associated independently with cerebral abnormalities. At the same time, the "control" group was intentionally selected from among patients whose neuroradiological exams were known to be normal.

Subsequent studies have failed to support the existence of cerebral atrophy in cannabis users. Using CT scanning technology that was not available to Campbell et al. (1971), Kuehnle, Mendelson, Davis, and New (1977) found no evidence of cerebral atrophy, as determined by ventrical size and separation of cortical gyri, in any of 19 men with long histories of heavy marijuana use. Co, Goodwin, Gado, Mikhail, and Hill (1977) also failed to find signs of atrophy in their sample of 12 heavy cannabis users. It should be noted that these studies used linear measures of brain and ventricle size, usually measured from a single representative CT section through the brain. As studies with other patient populations have shown, volumetric techniques that take into account many more CT sections through the brain are more sensitive to changes in brain morphology.

EEG studies to date have failed to demonstrate consistent abnormalities associated with cannabis use (Rubin & Comitas, 1975; Karacan, Fernadez-Salas, Coggins, Carter, Williams et al., 1976; Stefanis, Dornbush, & Fink, 1977). One study that reported the absence of any differences, however, was methodologically flawed by its selection of cannabis subjects from a pool of high-functioning medical students (Rodin, Domino, & Porzak, 1970).

Neuropsychological investigations of cannabis use have yielded similarly negative results. Currently available data do not provide convincing evidence that cannabis users display more deficits on neuropsychological tests than comparable individuals drawn from the general population (for review, see Wert & Raulin, 1986), although the existence of reports suggesting deficits provides a basis for concern.

The findings of many early studies of the effects of cannabis use are called into question by the existence of methodological flaws. For example, Agarwal, Sethi, and Gupta (1975) examined 40 cannabis users in India using several tests, but employed no control group. The small number of subjects who scored in the impaired range in this study may simply represent the expected number, given a random sample of subjects from the general population. Soueif (1976) examined 850 cannabis users and compared their performances with 839 control subjects. Given such large sample sizes, even very small differences may be *statistically* significant. The author failed to present data indicating the *magnitude* of the differences (reporting only the probabilities) or give arguments that these differences represent clinically meaningful "deficits."

A number of studies employed tests that have received little validation as neuropsychological measures. The primary example is the Bender Visual Motor Gestalt test, which has been shown to be a limited indicator of brain function (Bigler & Ehrfurth, 1980), and yet has been used to indicate "organic" impairment by numerous investigators (e.g., Rodin et al., 1970; Argarwal et al., 1975; Soueif, 1976; Wig & Varma, 1977; Mendhiratta, Wig, & Verma, 1978; Varma, Malhotra, Dang, Das, & Nehra, 1988). Several studies have been conducted in nonEnglish speaking countries. This has often necessitated the use or invention of tests that have received limited prior psychometric validation, and in most cases no validation as a *neuro*psychological measure. Examples include the Time Perception Test, in which the subject is asked to say when he believes two minutes have elapsed (Varma et al., 1988) and the Tool Matching Test, purported to assess accuracy of form perception (Soueif, 1976). While such tests may provide measures of cognitive function, conclusions about brain function per se cannot be based upon their results.

Another issue in the interpretation of study findings arises from the use of tests of memory, attention, concentration, and psychomotor speed—areas in which apparent deficits have been most consistently observed. Such tests are heavily influenced by variables such as anxiety and poor motivation, which may be expected to play a role when users of an illicit drug, who may react suspiciously to people in positions of authority, are brought before a researcher to receive formal testing. Such variables may have played a role in the findings of Soueif (1976) of deficits among Egyptian prison inmates. The existence of concurrent psychopathology and residual intoxication may also affect tests of shortterm memory, attention, concentration, and psychomotor speed. The subjects studied by Varma et al. (1988), for example, were abstinent for as little as 12 hours prior to testing. The observed deficits in perceptual motor speed may have been due to low levels of THC remaining in circulation. Significantly, the same investigators failed to find evidence of deficits on intelligence or memory tests in their sample of cannabis users. Notwithstanding, other investigators using tests weighing heavily on attention and motor speed have failed to observe differences between cannabis users and control subjects (Ray, Prabhu, Mohan, Nath, & Neki, 1978, 1979).

Numerous studies have appeared which report no evidence of cognitive or neuropsychological differences between cannabis users and controls. However, a number of these studies are not without methodological shortcomings themselves. Specifically, several studies with negative findings examined cannabis users drawn from populations of medical or college students, where the rate of cerebral dysfunction should be low by a process of selection (Culver & King, 1974; Grant, Rochford, Fleming, & Stunkard, 1973; Rochford, Grant, & LaVigne, 1977). Notably, those studies that have employed empirically validated neuro-psychological measures and sound methodology have failed to demonstrate deficits among cannabis users (Satz, Fletcher, & Sutker, 1976; Carlin & Trupin, 1977). One study involving members of a religious sect who smoked large amounts of potent (THC greater than 8%) marijuana for an average of seven years not only failed to find evidence of cognitive impairment, but documented superior intellectual performance (Schaeffer, Andrysiak, & Ungerleider, 1981). These superior performances were achieved even though most subjects had not completed college. It may be significant that these subjects led active lives, ate a largely vegetarian diet, and avoided all other psychoactive drugs including alcohol.

Can it be concluded, then, that cannabis use presents little danger to brain function? The inconsistent and largely negative nature of the data suggest that cannabis use may not produce notable permanent impairment in brain function. Methodological shortcomings of many studies invite caution, however, As other authors have cautioned before, it remains to be seen if subtler and more specific deficits have been overlooked and may be demonstrated using improved experi-mental designs and more sophisticated measures.

COCAINE

Cocaine is a nervous system stimulant that acts primarily by preventing the reuptake of catecholamine transmitter molecules, norepinephrine and dopa-mine, from the synaptic cleft. As a result, the normal chemical signals from neurons using these transmitters are prolonged, so that the postsynaptic cell receives greater excitation. These effects are observed both in the peripheral nervous system, where cocaine increases blood pressure and pulse and induces constriction of small vessels, and in the central nervous system, where it induces its psychological effects. The addictive properties of cocaine are believed to be related to its effects on dopamine pathways in the brain that are involved in reward and reinforcement (Johanson & Fischman, 1989; see also Fibiger & Phillips, 1988). In animals, chronic administration of cocaine induces compen-satory changes at the neuronal level, including the downregulation of presynaptic transmitter activity and supersensitivity of postsynaptic target sites (Dackis & Gold, 1987), although these changes do not appear to endure much beyond cessation of drug administration.

Cocaine can be taken into the body by several routes, the most common being nasal inhalation ("snorting"), smoking ("free-base" or "crack"), and intravenous injection. Intranasally administered cocaine reaches peak blood concentration levels approximately 30 minutes after inhalation, whereas peak levels occur almost immediately after smoking or injecting cocaine. Regardless of route, cocaine is readily converted into inactive metabolites by the body. The eliminative *half-life* is approximately 40–60 minutes under usual circumstances (Johanson & Fischman, 1989). Thus, the period of intoxication is directly proportional to drug dosage. In this regard, it should be noted that crack cocaine preparations are frequently as much as 95% pure cocaine, compared to approximately 50% pure in most powder preparations. Thus, it is easier for users to obtain higher doses and thus peak blood levels of cocaine using crack.

In 1988, an estimated 21 million Americans had tried cocaine; of those, some 2–3 million had tried crack (NIDA, 1989). Over two million people continue to use cocaine at least once a month. These figures, alarmingly high, seem to indicate a decline from the levels observed as recently as 1985, when an estimated 5 million Americans used cocaine on a regular basis. Up to 1985, cocaine use was seen most commonly in white, middle-income individuals, more often male; by 1987 the demographic characteristics of cocaine use had undergone a transformation, spreading to lower income individuals, minority groups, and more women (Washton & Gold, 1987, cited by Johanson & Fischman, 1989). This change was paralleled by a shift from cocaine inhalation towards the smoking of crack cocaine.

Brain damage due to cocaine use usually occurs as a result of the drug's effects on cerebral blood vessels. Hemorrhagic strokes have been observed following both inhaled (Schwartz & Cohen, 1984; Lowenstein, Massa, Rowbotham, Collins, McKinney, & Simon, 1987) and smoked cocaine (Lowenstein et al., 1987; Levine, Washington, Jefferson, Kieran, Moen et al., 1987; Golbe & Merkin, 1986). Cerebral hemorrhage frequently occurs in the presence of a preexisting vascular abnormality, such as aneurysms and arteriovenous malformations (Jacobs, Rozler, Kelly, Klein, & Kling, 1989), but may also occur in their absence. Cocaine use has also been associated with episodes of cerebral *ischemia* that may injure brain tissue but not lead to complete infarction (Jacobs et al., 1989). Cocaine-related damage may occur in any part of the brain, and the size of the involved area may vary considerably; multiple concurrent strokes have been observed. The degree of dysfunction and disability in each case is a function of the areas of the brain involved in the stroke, but symptoms that bring cocaine users to medical attention commonly include gross motor and sensory deficits. It should be kept in mind, however, that subtler deficits may often be overshadowed, and cocaine users who experience less notable deficits may not present themselves for treatment.

The most likely mechanism for cocaine-induced cerebral hemorrhage is via increase in systemic blood pressure and subsequent rupture of weaker points in the cerebral vasculature. Ischemic episodes, on the other hand, may result from cocaine's ability to provoke vasospasm either directly through its action on vessel-wall tissue (Levine et al., 1987) or indirectly as a local response to systemic hypertension. It has been suggested that cocaine may also contribute to *vasculitis* (Kaye & Fainstat, 1987), although there is disagreement in the literature on this point (Levine & Brust, 1988).

Documentation concerning CVAs in cocaine users has had to rely upon the close temporal association between cocaine use and subsequent onset of symptoms. For ethical reasons, a more convincing causal relationship may never be demonstrated in humans, but animal studies may provide more evidence in the future. Another weakness of this literature, as mentioned earlier, concerns the relative rate of occurrence of CVAs in cocaine users compared to nonusers. In a chart review, Jacobs et al. (1989) identified only 13 patients with neurological deficits attributable to cocaine-induced CVAs out of a population of 3,712 drug abusers seen for medical consultation. Similarly, in a review of 1,275 charts of patients seen for complications of cocaine use, only eight exhibited symptoms indicating cerebrovascular origin (Lowenstein et al., 1987). Unfortunately, the number of cocaine users who did not experience neurologic complications was not known for either general population concerned. Nonetheless, the rate of CVAs in young and generally healthy individuals is presumed to be quite low.

Another neurologic complication associated with cocaine use is epileptic seizures during the period of intoxication. Cocaine's epileptogenic quality is attributed to its action as a general nervous system stimulant. The seizures are usually global (Myers & Earnest, 1984) and may be prolonged (Merriam, Medalia, & Levine, 1988). No relationship has been observed between seizures and amount of prior cocaine use; seizures have been documented in both first-time users and in chronic addicts (Lowenstein et al., 1987). A survey of 279 adolescent cocaine users revealed that drug-associated seizures were rare among those who snorted cocaine, but occurred in approximately 10% of those who had smoked crack (Schwartz, 1989). This difference may be due to the greater purity, and higher peak blood levels, associated with crack cocaine. Epileptic seizures do not necessarily result in damage to neural tissue, but prolonged excitation of cells will eventually cause cell death. Cocaine-induced seizures on occasion have proven to be difficult to control medically, resulting in lasting cerebral impairment (Alldredge, Lowenstein, & Simon, 1989). In one case, uncontrollable seizures resulted in marked cerebral atrophy, appearing within three days of hospital admission, and significant functional impairment (Rowbotham, 1988).

To date, no neuropsychological evaluation of cocaine users, other than as polydrug abusers, has been published. The more subtle neurological effects of cocaine have also not been well studied. One important exception is an examination of cerebral blood flow in 20 cocaine abusers using positron emission tomography (PET) by Volkow, Mullani, Gould, Adler, and Krajewski (1988). Investigators examined subjects within 72 hours of hospitalization (for drug-induced delirium) and then again 10 days later. Compared to normal control subjects, cocaine abusers demonstrated patchy regions of abnormal blood flow and decreased relative flow in the prefrontal cortex. Reduced prefrontal blood flow remained after 10 days of cocaine abstinence. Given the range and importance of abilities attributed to prefrontal cortex, cocaine-induced prefrontal abnormalities may have profound effects. However, because the study was not prospective, the possibility cannot be ruled out that the observed abnormalities preceded cocaine use, or were due to some unidentified cause common to cocaine users.

STIMULANTS

In the present context, stimulants ("speed") refers to amphetamine compounds, a class of closely related chemicals[1] that act as a nervous system stimulant by causing the release of the brains own transmitters, particularly norepinephrine and to a lesser extent dopamine, as well as by direct stimulation of postsynaptic receptor sites. Thus, both cocaine and amphetamines stimulate the same transmitter systems within the brain, albeit by different mechanisms. For this reason, neurologic problems associated with amphetamine use are much the same as those associated with cocaine use, and the proposed mechanisms of brain damage share much in common.

Amphetamines can be taken orally or via intravenous injection. Amphetamine compounds undergo little breakdown once entering circulation. Moreover, many metabolites of amphetamines are themselves stimulants with similar mechanisma of action. Compared to cocaine, amphetamine compounds are eliminated from the body slowly, with eliminative *half-lives* around 10 hours (Vree & van Rossom, 1970).

An estimated 14 million Americans have used illicit stimulants other than cocaine, and 1-2 million have used these drugs within the past 30 days (NIDA, 1989).

As with cocaine, numerous cases of cerebral hemorrhage and ischemia closely following amphetamine use have been reported (Delaney & Estes, 1980; D'Souza & Shraberg, 1981; Cahill, Knipp & Moser, 1981; Shukla, 1982; Harrington, Heller, Dawson, Caplan, & Rumbaugh, 1983; Ng, Hamilton & Chalmers, 1986; and Conci, D'Angelo, Tampier, & Vecchi, 1988; also see Delaney & Estes for review of cases before 1980). Cerebral vasculitis associated with amphetamine use has received considerably more support than has vasculitis associated with cocaine use (Wooten, Khangure, & Murphy, 1983; Matick, Anderson, & Brumlick, 1983), although questions remain. Specifically, vasculitis is diagnosed on the basis of abnormalities ("beading") seen by angiographic examination of cerebral vessels; however, beading can indicate vascular injury due to a variety of causes

---

[1]For example, levoamphetamine, dextroamphetamine, methamphetamine, ephedrine, polyhexedrine.

(Nadeau, 1984). Regardless, angiographic abnormalities observed in amphetamine users have been associated with strokes and significant brain damage (Wooten et al., 1983, Cahill et al., 1981; and Conci et al., 1988). CVAs have occurred following intravenous, oral, and inhaled (crystalline) amphetamine use (Rothrock, Rubenstein, & Leiden, 1988). Two cases have been reported of persistent neurologic symptoms following injection of a preparation made from a nasal decongestant containing ephedrine ("stove top speed") into the neck veins (Fornazzari, Carlen, & Kapur, 1986). Amphetamine use has also been associated with seizures (Cahill et al., 1981).

As with cocaine, the ability of amphetamine use to cause CVAs is inferred from its close temporal association with the onset of symptoms. However, unlike cocaine, animal studies have carefully documented cerebral vascular changes and ischemic damage following the administration doses similar to those used by amphetamine addicts (Rumbaugh, Bergeron, Scanlan, Teal, Segall, Fang, & McCormick, 1971).

Another important difference between cocaine and amphetamine is the existence of evidence that suggests permanent alterations in neuronal function following the use of certain amphetamine compounds, in particular methamphetamine (methylamphetamine). Experimental monkeys given repeated doses of methamphetamine display reductions in dopamine levels in the basal ganglia, and norepinephrine levels in the frontal cortex, six months after treatment (Seiden, Fischman, & Schuster, 1975/76). Deficits in dopamine levels have been observed as long as four years following methamphetamine treatment of primates (Seiden & Ricaurte, 1987). Further studies using rats have found that repeated doses of methamphetamine, as well as of amphetamine, can act in a dose-dependent manner as a selective neurotoxin by damaging cells belonging to the dopamine system with which it interacts (Wagner, Ricaurte, Johanson, Schuster, & Seiden, 1980; Ricaurte, Seiden, & Schuster, 1984). Similar results have been obtained in monkeys and rats using high doses of dextroamphetamine, but not the stimulant methylphenidate (Ritalin; Wagner, Ricaurte, Johanson, Schuster, & Seiden, 1980). Methamphetamine has been shown to also affect serotonin and acetylcholine transmitter systems, although these effects may not be long lasting. Some investigators have reported a return to normal neurochemical values within seven days (McCabe, Gibb, Wamsley, & Hanson, 1987) while others have not (Ricaurte, Schuster, & Seiden, 1980).

The neurotoxic effects of methamphetamine on dopamine systems are observed less in mice, more in rats, more so in cats, and to a great degree in primates, suggesting species sensitivity (Seiden & Ricaurte, 1987). Given our great similarity to other primates, humans may well be at considerable risk. Given amphetamine's neurotoxic effects on dopamine systems in the basal ganglia, it might be expected that amphetamine addicts would eventually display extrapyramidal motor signs as a consequence of damage to this system. Lundh and Tunving (1981) present four case studies in which this association was found. In most of their cases, the observed choreiform (writhing) movement disorders gradually faded after discontinuation of drug use, but in one case symptoms persisted for at least three years after discontinuation of use. Aside from the study above, and in contrast to the extensive documentation linking chronic amphetamine use to neural damage in experimental animals, there have been almost no investigations of the subtler neurological and neuropsychological deficits that may be expected to follow selective brain cell loss in humans. Whether amphetamine abuse results in significant cell death, and to what degree any cell loss is compensated for remain important questions.

Even as crack cocaine continues in popularity, there are reports of a new form of smokable crystalline methamphetamine, known as "ice," that may rival crack (Cho, 1990). With both drugs, it is the immediacy of the high following administration that gives the drug its highly addictive quality. As with crack, it is possible to achieve high blood levels quickly using ice, and this may increase the likelihood of neurological complications of amphetamine abuse.

MDMA AND MDA

Two compounds closely related to amphetamine group deserve separate attention. Both methylenedioxymethamphetamine (MDMA, or "ecstasy") and methylenedioxyamphetamine (MDA) represent modifications of the amphetamine parent molecule that produce hallucinogenic as well as the usual stimulant effects. Both have been used as recreational drugs, and there is evidence indicating that both have neurotoxic properties.

Whereas other amphetamine compounds appear to be toxic to dopamine cells, both hallucinogenic amphetamines appear to cause selective damage to neurons that use serotonin as their neurotransmitter. Using rats as subjects, investigators have shown that a 4-day regimen of either MDMA or MDA results in reductions in serotonin activity two weeks later, but has no appreciable effect on indicators of dopamine and norepinephrine activity (Battaglia, Yeh, O'Heran, Molliver, Kuhar, & DeSouza, 1987; Ricaurte, Bryan, Strauss, Seiden, & Schuster, 1985; Mathews, Champney, & Frye, 1989). Similar studies using primates have documented selective deficits in serotonin neurochemistry as long as 14 weeks following drug treatment (Insel, Battaglia, Johannsen, Marra, & DeSouza, 1989). Lower doses primarily affect the hippocampus and frontal cortex, whereas effects in the corpus striatum are seen only at higher doses (Ricaurte et al., 1985; Slikker, Holson, Ali, Kolta, Paule, et al., 1989). Yet even at higher doses, drug-treated rats could not be distinguished from normal animals by observation (Ricaurte et al., 1985) or behavioral tests (Slikker et al., 1989) after two weeks of recovery. In primates, however, changes in behavior have been seen under casual observation, and have been interpreted as reflecting depletion of serotonin (Ricaurte, quoted by Barnes, 1988).

The relative absence of gross behavioral changes in animals following drug-induced cell damage may help explain why MDA and MDMA have long been considered safe drugs. As late as 1986, some people believed that these drugs, particularly MDMA, were benign drugs, reliably producing pleasant alterations of consciousness (Downing, 1986). In fact, several psychiatrists at that time suggested that MDMA might serve as a useful adjunct to psychotherapy by facilitating insight and awareness (Barnes, 1988). MDMA was thought to have little potential for toxic reactions. More recently, however, life-threatening reactions have been documented as a consequence of large doses of MDMA (Brown & Osterloh, 1987). As with amphetamine's effects on dopamine systems, the neurotoxic effects of hallucinogenic amphetamines on serotonin cells appears to result at lower doses in primates in comparison to rodents. Indeed, neurotoxic effects in monkeys have been observed at doses (5 mg/kg) close to those typically used by humans (1.7-2.7 mg/kg) (Ricaurte, 1989). It remains to be seen if MDMA use may be linked to neurochemical and neuropsychological deficits in humans. Another possible reason why MDMA-induced deficits may be overlooked is that, while serotonin is widespread throughout the brain, it tends to play a modulatory and inhibitory role, such that neurotoxic effects would not be seen as an absolute deficit or lack of an ability.

LSD

Lysergic and diethylamide (LSD, or "acid") is the prototypical hallucinogen in many regards. One of the earliest hallucinogens known to modern science, it has also been one of the best studied. Partly as a result of this scrutiny, it is generally believed that the hallucinogenic properties of many other drugs (such as MDMA, mescaline, and psilocybin) are due to their interaction with serotonin systems within the brain. LSD appears to act mainly by depressing the activity of cells which release serotonin, most likely by activating the cell's own negative feedback mechanisms. The effect of serotonin on target cells is usually inhibitory, so that the net effect of LSD-like compounds is a release from normal inhibition. Continued use of LSD quickly results in tolerance to the drug's effects, so that larger doses are needed to produce the same effects.

Given the continued use of LSD, it is somewhat surprising that only a handful of older studies have examined the neuropsychological consequences of LSD use. McGlothlin, Arnold, and Freedman (1969) examined 16 subjects who had used LSD 20 or more times in a medical or therapeutic setting, but had not taken the drug in the last year. Compared to a matched control group, LSD users displayed deficits on only one out of 14 measures of cognitive functioning, several of which have been used to assess brain function. The single difference was on the Category Test, which is considered one of the most sensitive to general cerebral dysfunction. No differences were observed on another sensitive test, part B of the Trail Making Test.

Wright and Hogan (1972) compared a group of 20 young subjects reporting frequent LSD use with a matched control group on scores using the Halstead-Reitan test battery. Out of 24 measures that the investigators compared, statistically significant differences were noted on only two: the Information and Comprehension subtests of the Wechsler Adult Intelligence Scale (WAIS). Neither of these two subtests is considered a reliable indicator of neuropsychological function, in part because both subtests are heavily influenced by education and by early environmental factors and tend to resist later declines in cerebral functioning. Significant differences were not found on the Category test in this sample, nor on other measures which are sensitive to cerebral dysfunction.

In contrast with the largely negative results of the two studies discussed above, Acord and Barker (1973) observed significant differences between subjects reporting use of hallucinogens (e.g., LSD, mecaline, psilocybin) on the Category Test, Trails B, and the localization component of the Tactual Performance Test (TPT), another sensitive indicator of general cerebral function. No other tests were administered. While the mean score of LSD users on the Category Test and Trails B were still not in the impaired range, they were close to accepted cutoff values. Taken together with the poor TPT localization scores, these results do suggest the likelihood of cerebral dysfunction. An important shortcoming of this study is that the amount of drug use was not quantified, and the inclusion criterion was that the subject had taken hallucinogens "*at least once.*" It is difficult to say whether the subjects comprise a valid "drug use" group. Even more so than in the two previous studies, the current study appears vulnerable to the possibility that a confounding variable associated with occasional use of hallucinogens may explain the observed differences.

On balance it appears that the use of some hallucinogens such as LSD present less of a risk to brain function than do the hallucinogenic amphetamines such as MDMA. However, inconsistent evidence of mild neuropsychological deficits suggest the continued possibility of long-lasting consequences of LSD use. Since the end of the drug-experiment days of the late 1960s and early 1970s, virtually no research has been conducted on the effects of hallucinogens on brain function. As with most illicit drugs, it is possible to find individuals today who have taken higher doses for a longer time than previously examined. The effects of such heavy drug use cannot be confidently predicted.

PHENCYCLIDINE

Phencyclidine (PCP, or "angel dust") has been around for a number of years as an adulterant of drug preparations consisting primarily of other drugs, such as cocaine and marijuana. A number of years ago, however, PCP achieved considerable media attention for its apparent ability to provoke uncontrolled psychotic outbursts during intoxication. PCP appears to have experienced its most widespread use around 1984, mostly among black urban youths (Crider, 1986), and its use has since declined.

Pharmacologically, PCP appears to interact with opiate receptors and with excitatory glutamate receptors in the hippocampus, a brain structure associated with learning and memory. Alterations in all other major neurotransmitter systems have also been demonstrated (Marwah & Pitts, 1986), the most consistent effects involving dopamine function. Psychologically, with increasing doses, PCP appears to act, in order, as a depressant, stimulant, or hallucinogen. PCP's stimulant activity appears to be due to actions on norepinephrine and dopamine systems similar to those of both amphetamines and cocaine.

PCP users frequently report losses or gaps in memory around the time of intoxication and for some weeks following use (Burns & Lerner, 1981), prompting several investigations of memory and other cognitive functions among PCP users. Handelmann, Contreras, and O'Donohue (1987) have shown that, while PCP given to animals during learning does not interfere with the ability to learn, drug treatment does interfere with the long-term storage of learned information. Burns and Lerner (1981) failed to find significant differences between PCP users and control subjects using the Wechsler Memory Scale. Thus it may be that the effects of PCP on memory occur only during intoxication, and do not present a long-term threat to brain function.

Carlin, Grant, Adams, and Reed (1979) compared 12 PCP drug users with the same number of drug users who had not used PCP and with controls with no history of drug abuse on the Halstead-Reitan test battery. PCP users performed worse than normal controls, but better than nonPCP drug users. (Carlin et al. did not administer any specific tests of memory.) Both drug use groups scored below normal controls on the Category Test, WAIS Performance and Verbal scores, and the Rhythm Test (which assesses general cerebral and non-dominant hemisphere function). It should be noted, however, that only on the Rhythm Test did PCP subjects score in ranges which suggest neuropsychological impairment. Although the results obtained by Carlin et al. (1979) do present indications of mild cerebral impairment in half of the PCP users, this represents the same proportion of nonPCP drug users with signs of impairment. Thus, their results cannot be taken to indicate that PCP itself is a particular threat to brain function, although any damaging effects may be masked by the effects of other drug use.

Lewis and Hordan (1986) present a discussion of neuropsychological testing in PCP users, along with the data from 30 subjects on an abbreviated Halstead-Reitan battery. Theirs was not a formal study, however, and no comparison group was used. Moreover, their subjects were largely from underprivileged backgrounds, and fully 25 percent qualified as learning disabled in childhood. For these reasons, no conclusions can be drawn regarding the potential effects of PCP use.

In addition to its psychoactive properties, PCP has been shown to induce vascular spasm by direct interaction with vessel tissue (Altura, Quirion, Pert, & Altura, 1983). Not surprisingly, there have been at least two documented cases of cerebral hemorrhage, both fatal, associated with PCP use (Bessen, 1982, Boyko, Burger, & Heinz, 1987). This complication appears rare, however; and it is not clear that PCP use is associated with an increased risk of CVA. As with all case reports, it is difficult to draw conlcusions about cause and effect. PCP use has also been associated with epileptic seizures (Alldredge, Lowenstein, & Simon, 1989). Residual impairment as a result of these seizures has not been examined.

OPIATES

The most commonly abused opiates are heroin, morphine, and meperidine (Demerol). The addictive quality of opiates comes from their ability to mimic the brains own opioid transmitters (endorphins and enkephalins) and directly stimulate postsynaptic receptors, thus producing euphoria that lasts from 3 to 5 hours (Hollister, 1987). Repeated administration depletes the brain's own transmitters, and cessation of drug use is followed by the understimulation of receptor sites. The resulting withdrawal syndrome begins approximately 10 hours after last use, and is characterized by the aversive over-activation of the sympathetic autonomic nervous system (Hollister, 1987). Withdrawal may last weeks, although symptoms gradually diminish with time. Recent estimates of the number of opiate abusers in the United States place the figure near one half million (Hollister, 1987).

Neurological complications associated with heroin use include cerebral vasculits and stroke (Brust & Richter, 1976; King, Richards, & Tress, 1978). In 10 documented cases, however, the temporal association of drug use and subsequent CVA is quite loose. Moreover, since the illicit use of heroin is by intravenous injection, it is quite likely that foreign matter in the injected solution may have been the true source of infection or embolism. Computed tomographic examinations of the brains of heroin users have failed to demonstrate an association between heroin use and cortical atrophy. In a sample of 15 subjects who had used heroin for 4-14 years and who had no history of alcohol abuse, Hill and Mikhael (1979) found no signs of cortical atrophy by examining either the separation of cortical gyri or ventricular size. Strang and Gurling (1989) examined an unusual sample of older subjects who had used high doses of heroin for 29-43 years, and found few signs of atrophy using CT. It cannot be concluded whether the mild signs of atrophy noted in several subjects are linked to heroin use, because no control group was examined. All but one subject had histories of alcohol or other drug abuse lasting for periods of years. As the authors point out, that their subjects appear alert and cognitively intact on clinical examination in spite of years of heavy opiate use seems to argue that opiates present little risk of gross neurological abnormalities.

Neuropsychological studies of heroin users suggest that subtler deficits in brain function may occur. Strang and Gurling (1989) found no consistent evidence of cognitive impairment in their sample of long-term heroin users. Hill and Mikhael (1979), on the other hand, observed significant differences between heroin users and control subjects on the memory and localization components of the TPT, and on a test of fine motor speed. No statistically significant differences were observed on the Category Test, although a greater number of heroin users than controls earned scores suggestive of functional impairment. In a sample of 25 heroin users, Fields and Fuller (1975) found no evidence of neuropsychological impairment, and in fact observed a trend for drug users to perform better than matched controls on eight of nine Halstead subtests, including the Category Test. In a larger sample of 72 opiate addicts, Rounsaville, Jones, Novelly and Kleber (1982) observed the same surprising tendency for drug users to perform better than demographically matched controls on a range of neuropsychological tests. Guerra, Sole, Cami, and Tobena (1987) found that neuropsychological deficits apparent immediately following rapid opiate detoxification disappear within a few weeks. As with LSD, the data regarding the neuropsychological consequences of opiate use are equivocal. It appears that even heavy opiate use is not always associated with cerebral impairment. Further studies are needed to evaluate the degree to which IV drug injection and other aspects of illicit opiate use account for the observed deficits.

SEDATIVES

Commonly used nervous system depressants usually belong to one of two classes of pharmaceuticals. Barbiturates such as phenobarbital (Luminol) and pentabarbital (Nembutal) depress general brain activity by a variety of mechanisms which ultimately reduce the postsynaptic changes caused by many excitatory neurotransmitters. Although these effects are observed throughout the brain, pathways in the brain involved in the maintenance of arousal are particularly susceptible to the effects of barbiturates. Lethal overdose with barbiturates is not difficult. The second major class of nervous system depressants, the benzodiazepines, include such common drugs as diazepam (Valium), triazolam (Halcion) and alprazolam (Xanax). Benzodiazepines act by indirectly facilitating the activity of the inhibitory transmitter, gamma-aminobutyric acid (GABA). Cessation of either barbiturates or benzodiazepines after prolonged use results in a characteristic withdrawal syndrome, characterized by delirium, agitation and not uncommonly seizures.

Despite the marked effects that sedatives have upon brain function, there is little to suggest that their abuse causes neurological damage. Computed tomographic examination of 28 long-term benzodiazepine abusers revealed no evidence of cerebral atrophy compared to normal controls, while benzodiazepine users with a concomitant history of alcohol abuse did display signs of atrophy (Poser, Poser, Roscher, & Argyrakis, 1983). Similarly, CT evaluation of 33 patients who had abused sedatives indicated that signs of cerebral atrophy were not significantly more common than in age-matched controls (Allgulander, Borg, & Vikander, 1984). Bergman, Borg, Engelbrektson, and Vikander (1989) also failed to find an increase in the prevalence of cortical atrophy compared to controls, although they did observe a slightly higher occurrence of dilation of the third ventricle among sedative abusers.

Neuropsychological studies of sedative abusers follow the familiar pattern of revealing subtle functional deficits in the absence of gross neurological changes. An early study reporting neuropsychological deficits among sedative abusers is limited by the fact that the great majority of subjects had abused several drugs, including amphetamines, alcohol, and IV drug use (Judd & Grant, 1975). For this reason, the observed deficits cannot be convincingly attributed to sedative abuse. Another study, one which examined cognitive deficits among patients prescribed benzodiazepines for a year or more, is limited because the drug use subjects were previously diagnosed as having anxiety disorders, whereas the control subjects were not (Golombok, Moodley, and Lader, 1988). It is possible that the observed deficits in visual-spatial ability and sustained attention reflect some aspect of the pathology underlying anxiety disorders and not the effects of benzodiazepine use. When subjects' scores were analyzed as two groups, consisting of those still taking medication and those who had withdrawn, performance deficits were observed only in the group currently medicated. This suggests that at medically prescribed doses, benzodiazepines may present little risk for long-term neuropsychological impairment.

The same does not appear to be true for the abuse of illicit sedatives. Bergman, Borg, and Holm (1980) examined 55 patients being treated for sedative abuse who had no history of alcohol or other drug abuse. Compared to matched control subjects, drug users were found to perform poorly on several tests of reasoning, visuospatial ability (as assessed by Block Design), visual memory, and executive functions (as assessed by the Trail Making Test, part B). Significantly more of the drug users were judged to show signs of cognitive impairment (54% versus 16% of controls). Follow-up examination of thirty of the subjects four to six years later revealed little improvement (Bergman, Borg, Engelbrektson, & Vikander, 1989). Approximately the same proportion of sedative users (47%) showed signs of cerebral impairment at follow-up. Interestingly, those patients who failed to recover from their addiction, as indicated by continued abuse of sedatives and the emergence of alcoholic symptoms, performed worse than recovering patients on Block Design and Trails B, during both the initial evaluation and subsequent follow-up.

INHALANTS

The range of abused volatile substances is wide. People in search of a high have turned to the inhalation of glues, solvents, adhesives, paints and thinner, aerosol propellant, cleaning fluid, nail polish, gasoline, nitrous oxide, and typewriter correction fluid, to name but a few. The most common methods of inhalation include breathing fumes out of a bag held over the face, and sniffing from a soaked rag held against the face, a practice known as "huffing." Unlike many other drugs of abuse, volatile substances are obtained from a variety of cheap and readily available household products. As an unfortunate result, inhalant abuse is common among the poor, children, and in many less-developed countries. In the United States, an estimated 11 million people have abused inhalants of various kinds (NIDA, 1989). More alarmingly, an estimated 1 to 1½ million Americans have used inhalants within the past month, one-third of them between 12 and 18 years of age.

The active ingredients found among abused inhalants are many, but the organic solvent toluene (methyl benzene) appears to be the most common. Consequently, toluene abuse has received the most attention. Like most abused inhalants, toluene is fat-soluble, and consequently enters the blood supply and the brain readily. Blood concentrations reach 60% of their maximum level within 10 to 15 minutes of exposure; toluene is just as readily eliminated from the body, and is difficult to detect in the body 6–8 hours after last exposure (Ron, 1986). The effects of inhalant use are similar to those caused by alcohol intoxication. They include poor coordination, slurred speech, impaired judgement, lethargy, often followed by nausea and tremors. These psychomotor effects usually last for 30–45 minutes after last exposure (Ron, 1986).

The harmful effects of solvents in occupational settings have received considerable documentation (see Hartman, this volume), but there is reason to examine inhalant abuse separately. The occupational exposure to solvents usually consists of chronic, low-level exposure. In contrast, inhalant abuse results in discrete episodes of high-level exposure, wherein peak concentrations of substances within the brain may exceed occupational levels by a factor of ten or a hundred. In addition, the likelihood of oxygen deprivation, which may cause damage to brain tissue by itself, is greater in cases of abuse than occupational exposure.

Inhalant abuse has been associated with a variety of peripheral nervous system abnormalities, such as limb weakness and sensory loss. There is considerable evidence linking the abuse of solvents to central nervous system abnormalities as well (see review by Lolin, 1989). Associated neurological complications include motor dysfunction associated with cerebellar damage (King, 1982; Escobar & Aruffo, 1980), atrophy of the cerebellum (Lazar, Ho, Melen, & Gaghestani, 1983; Hormes, Filley, & Rosenberg, 1986; Rosenberg, Kleinschmidt-DeMasters, Davis, Dreisbach, Hormes, & Filley, 1988), and atrophy of the cerebral cortex (Escobar & Arrufo, 1980; Schikler, Seitz, Rice, & Strader, 1982; Lazar et al., 1983; Hormes et al., 1986; Rosenberg et al., 1988). Among the eleven subjects examined by

Schikler et al. (1982), CT examination revealed signs of cerebral atrophy in all six cases in which solvent abuse had lasted more than 10 years, and did not reveal atrophy in the five cases in which abuse had lasted for less time.

Epileptic seizures have also been seen in inhalant abusers. Allister, Lush, Oliver, and Watson (1981) report a case of a 15-year-old male with laboratory-confirmed toluene intoxication who experienced the onset of repeated seizures despite anti-epileptic medication. Although the patient seemed to recover steadily in the following weeks, comparison of CT images taken upon admission and 10 weeks later revealed the appearance of ventricular dilation and several small tissue lesions. Somewhat surprisingly, upon examination 2 years later the patient showed no focal neurologic signs or psychometric deficits. The type of tests administered to the patient were not reported.

Not all evidence indicates that inhalant abuse causes cerebral atrophy. One study found no signs of abnormalities on CT scans, although only seven subjects were examined (Devathasan, Low, Tech, Wan, & Wong, 1984). In virtually every case in which abnormalities have been found, the subjects came to medical attention because of various neurological complaints, including confusion, ataxia, gait disturbances, and memory loss. It is not surprising that subjects with such symptoms should show neurological abnormalities. As with cocaine and CVAs, it remains to be shown that degenerative abnormalities occur with significantly greater frequency among solvent abusers. Given the rarity of such disorders, especially among the young, it is reasonable to expect that epidemiological investigation will confirm the greater rate of cerebral abnormalities among solvent abusers.

One study deserves particular attention because it suggests the mechanisms by which solvent abuse may cause encephalopathy. Rosenberg et al. (1988) used magnetic resonance imaging (MRI) to examine the brains of six former solvent abusers who had abstained from its use for at least 2 weeks. They observed marked changes in the consistency of the white matter of the brain underlying the cerebral cortex. These changes were interpreted to indicate an increase in the water content, to which MRI is particularly sensitive, within the white matter. This is particularly relevant because white matter consists primarily of the axons of neurons surrounded by fatty myelin sheaths. Because most abuse solvents act particularly upon fatty tissue, this finding suggests that the brain's white matter is directly subject to the damaging effects of solvent abuse. By damaging the fibers that interconnect the entire cerebral cortex, profound functional deficits may be expected to result.

Studies that have examined the neuropsychological functioning of inhalant abusers have observed a variety of deficits. Deficits have been found on tests of memory (Allison & Jerrom, 1984), Verbal and Performance intelligence tests (Korman, Mathews, & Lovitt, 1981; Trites et al., 1976, cited by Chadwick & Anderson, 1989; Berry et al., 1978, cited by Chadwick & Anderson, 1989; Mahmood, 1983), as well as on a variety of neuropsychological measures (Bigler,

1979; Korman et al., 1981; Trites et al., 1976; Berry et al., 1978). Deficits appear to be found most reliably using the Tactual Performance and Trail Making tests, and on measures of fine sensorimotor function. In one study, these deficits were observed even when inhalant abusers were compared to a sample of polydrug abusers who had not used inhalants (Korman, Mathews, & Lovitt, 1981).

Chadwick and Anderson (1989) have criticized these studies for a variety of methodological reasons, including small sample size, inadequate control of acute intoxication, and the possibility that control groups were not appropriate. Although not ruling out the possibility that inhalant abuse causes neuropsychological impairment, Chadwick and Anderson suggest that various environmental factors, such as poor education and motivation, may have contributed to the results. They note that there has been a tendency to observe greater deficits when comparing Verbal intelligence scores than when comparing Performance scores. Generalized cerebral impairment usually produces the reverse association, whereas the observed pattern is common among juvenile delinquents and the educationally handicapped. Mahmood (1983) also raised this possibility, by suggesting that greater deficits are observed on acquired abilities than on "potential" abilities.

Given the strong evidence for diffuse cerebral damage on the one hand and the less conclusive evidence of neuropsychological deficits on the other, some speculation seems in order. Most cases in which neurological abnormalities have been found came to medical attention because of outward signs of neurological problems, whereas the subjects in neuropsychological cases were usually drawn from treatment or rehabilitation settings. The two kinds of studies may be sampling from different subpopulations within inhalant abusers. Once again, a study that samples broadly from the population of inhalant abusers is needed to clarify this issue.

SUMMARY AND CONCLUSIONS

Critical review of the literature examining the neurological and neuropsychological consequences of drug use reveals numerous shortcomings. Many studies contain methodological flaws that make it difficult to accept fully the conclusions that are reached. One is forced to engage in a kind of informal meta-analysis of the various studies in order to evaluate the risks presented by abuse of a particular drug. Virtually all of the studies presented here are subject to one confounding variable: Subjects were not randomly assigned to the drug use group. It remains a possibility that preexisting cognitive deficits or neurological vulnerabilities explain some of the observed differences. Nonetheless, it is our opinion that provisional conclusions can be reached while the results of further investigation are awaited.

Among those drugs that present the greatest danger to the brain one has to include cocaine and the amphetamines. It seems certain that both kinds of stimulants contribute to CVAs (and to secondary systemic effects that may produce brain injury), although the size of the increase in risk cannot be determined. To date, there has been an unfortunate lack of empirical evidence concerning the neuropsychological consequences of cocaine use by humans. It is not known whether cocaine has harmful effects on the brain, other than via its effects on cerebral blood vessels. The hallucinogenic amphetamines, MDMA and MDA, as well as high doses of amphetamines in general, appear to be reliably toxic to certain brain cells. Once again, neuropsychological documentation is lacking in this area. Designer drugs such as the opiate-analog MPTP must be included among those drugs that present the greatest danger to brain function, due to its reliably neurotoxic effects. From studies examining poly-drug abusers as well as from those examining sedative abuse in particular, data have accumulated that suggest that the abuse of central nervous system depressants presents risks for neuropsychological functioning.

The evidence is less clear for cannabis and marijuana. In both cases, there is evidence indicating cognitive impairment and evidence indicating a lack of impairment. Neuropsychological data regarding the classic hallucinogen LSD and the opiates are also equivocal. For each of these classes of drugs, however, gross neurological changes such as cerebral atrophy appear not to occur.

Several drugs of abuse are not reliably associated with signs of cerebral atrophy. Upon reflection, this result is not surprising. If a drug such as marijuana or heroin were to result in such profound changes, the corresponding neurological and neuropsychological changes would be dramatic and consistent. Instead, most drugs of abuse appear to have subtler effects, which impair mainly the higher aspects of neuropsychological function, such as abstract problem solving and fine motor control—effects that can most easily be confused with the effects of drug intoxication itself. The main exception to this rule is the inhaled solvents. These substances, in their varied and widespread forms, are undeniably toxic to neural tissue, both in the peripheral and central nervous systems. Although inhalant abuse represents one of the greatest risks to brain function, it has received far less attention than many drugs. It is perhaps concerning the dangers of inhalant abuse that education efforts may serve the greatest need.

Is a brain on drugs to be likened to an egg in a frying pan? The answer appears to be yes and no. Although some drugs present clear dangers to brain function, the permanent effects of other drugs appear to be small. Because neuropsychological effects are more reliably observed following prolonged use of drugs, it is reasonable to conclude that infrequent drug use does not result in long-term neuropsychological impairment in most cases. If there is a silver lining to the cloud of drug abuse, this is it; and this underscores the hope that the rehabilitated drug abuser may not suffer permanent brain damage if treated in time.

REFERENCES

Acord, L. C., & Barker, D. D. (1973). Hallucinogenic drugs and cerebral deficit. *Journal of Nervous and Mental Disorders, 156,* 281-283.

Adams, K. M., Rennick, P. M., Schoof, K. G., & Keegan, J. F. (1975). Neuropsychological measurement of drug effects: Polydrug research. *Journal of Psychedelic Drugs, 7,* 151-160.

Allcott, J. V., Barnhart, R. A., & Mooney, L. A. (1987). Acute and lead poisoning in two users of illicit methamphetamine. *Journal of American Medical Association, 258,* 510-511.

Alldredge, B. K., Lowenstein, D. H., & Simons, R. P. (1989). Seizures associated with recreational drug abuse. *Neurology, 39,* 1037-1039.

Allgulander, C., Borg, S., & Vikander, B. (1984). A 4-6-year follow-up of 50 patients with primary dependence on sedative and hypnotic drugs. *American Journal of Psychiatry, 141,* 1580-1582.

Allison, W. M., & Jerrom, D. W. A. (1984). Glue sniffing: A pilot study of the cognitive effects of long-term use. *International Journal of Addiction, , 19,* 453-458.

Allister, C., Lush, M., Oliver, J. S., & Watson, J. M. (1981). Status epilepticus caused by solvent abuse. *British Medical Journal (Clinical Research), 283,* 1156.

Altura, B. T., Quirion, R., Pert, C. B., & Altura B. M. (1983). Phencyclidine ("angel dust") analogs and sigma opiate benzomorphans cause cerebral arterial spasm. *Proceedings of the National Academy of Science U.S.A., 80,* 865-869.

Ballard, P. A., Tetrud, T. W., & Langston, J. W. (1985). Permanent human parkinsonism due to 1-methyl-4-phenyl-1,2,3,6-tetrahydropyridine (MPTP): Seven Cases. *Neurology, 35,* 949-956.

Barnes, D. M. (1988). New data intensify the agony over ecstasy. *Science, 239,* 864-866.

Battaglia, G., Yeh, S. Y., O'Hearn, E., Molliver, M. E., Kuhar, M. J., & DeSouza, E. B. (1987). 3,4-methylenedioxymethamphetamine and 3,4-methylenedioxyamphetamine destroy serotonin terminals in rat brain: Quantification of neurodegeneration by measurement of [^{3}H]paroxetine-labeled serotonin uptake sites. *Journal of Pharmacology and Experimental Therapeutics, 242,* 911-916.

Bergman, H., Borg, S., Engelbrektson, K., & Vikander, B. (1989). Dependence on sedative-hypnotics: neuropsychological impairment, field dependence and clinical course in a 5-year follow-up study, *British Journal of Addiction, 84,* 547-553.

Bergman, H., Borg, S., & Holm, L. (1980). Neuropsychological impairment and exclusive abuse of sedatives or hypnotics. *American Journal of Psychiatry, 137,* 215-217.

Bessen, H. A. (1982). Intracranial hemorrhage associated with phencyclidine abuse. *Journal of the American Medical Association, 248,* 585-586.

Bigler, E. D. (1979). Neuropsychological evaluation of adolescent inpatients hospitalized with chronic inhalant abuse. *Clinical Neuropsychology, 1,* 8-12.

Bigler, E. D. (1988). *Diagnostic clinical neuropsychology.* rev. ed. Austin, Texas: University of Texas Press.

Bigler, E. D., & Ehrfurth, J. W. (1980). Critical limitations of the Bender-Gestalt test in clinical neuropsychology: Response to Lacks. *Clinical Neuropsychology, 2,* 88-90.

Boor, J. W., & Hurtig, H. I. (1977). Persistent cerebellar ataxia after exposure to toluene. *Annals of Neurology, 2,* 440-442.

Boyko, O. B., Burger, P. L., & Heinz, E. R. (1987). Pathological and radiological correlation of subarachnoid hemorrhage in phencyclidine abuse. Case report. *Journal of Neurosurgery, 67,* 446-448.

Brandt, J., & Doyle, L. F. (1983). Concept attainment, tracking and shifting in adolescent polydrug abusers. *Journal of Nervous and Mental Disorders, 171,* 559-563.

Bruhn, P., & Maage, N. (1975). Intellectual and neuropsychological functions in young men with heavy and long-term patterns of drug abuse. *American Journal of Psychiatry,* *132,* 397-401.

Brust, J. C. M., & Richter, R. W. (1976). Stroke associated with addiction to heroin. *Journal of Neurology and Neurosurgical Psychiatry, 39,* 194-199.

Burns, R. S., & Lerner, S. E. (1981). The effects of phencyclidine in man: A review. In E. F. Domino (Ed.), *PCP (phencyclidine): historical and current perspectives.* Ann Arbor: NPP Books.

Cahill, D. W., Knipp, H., & Mosser, J. (1981). Intracranial hemorrhage with amphetamine abuse [Letter]. *Neurology, 31,* 1058-1059.

Campbell, A. M. G., Evans, M., Thompson, J. L. G., & Williams, M. J. (1971). Cerebral atrophy in young cannabis smokers. *Lancet, 2,* 1219-1224.

Caplan, L. R., Hier, D. B., & Banks, G. (1982). Current concepts of cerebrovascular disease—stroke: Stroke and drug abuse. *Stroke, 13,* 869-872.

Carlin, A. S., Grant, I., Adams, K. M., & Reed, R. (1979). Is phencyclidine (PCP) abuse associated with organic mental impairment? *American Journal of Drug and Alcohol Abuse, 6,* 273-281.

Carlin, A. S., & Trupin, E. W. (1977). The effect of long-term chronic marijuana use on neuropsychological functioning. *International Journal of Addiction, 12,* 617-624.

Chadwick, O. F. D., & Anderson, H. R. (1989). Neuropsychological consequences of volatile substance abuse: A review. *Human Toxicology, 8,* 307-312.

Cho, A. K. (1990). Ice: a new dosage form of an old drug. *Science, 249,* 631-634.

Co, B. T., Goodwin, D. W., Gado, M., Mikhael, M., & Hill, S. Y. (1977). Absence of cerebral atrophy in chronic cannabis users evaluation by computerized transaxial tomography. *Journal of the American Medical Association, 237,* 1229-1230.

Conci, F., D'Angelo, V., Tampieri, D., & Vecchi, G. (1988). Intracerebral hemorrhage and angiographic beading following amphetamine abuse. *Italian Journal of Neurological Science, 9,* 77-81.

Crossman, A. R., Clarke, C. E., Boyce, S., Robertson, R. G., & Sambrook, M. A. (1987). MPTP-induced parkinsonism in the monkey: Neurochemical pathology, complications of treatment and pathophysiological mechanisms. *Canadian Journal of Neurological Science, 14,* 428-435.

Delaney, P., & Estes, M. (1980). Intracranial hemorrhage with amphetamine abuse. *Neurology, 30,* 1125-1128.

Devane, W. A., Dysarz, F. A., Johnson, M. R., Melvin, L. S., & Howlett, A. C. (1988). Determination and characterization of a cannabinoid receptor in the rat brain. *Molecular Pharmacology, 34,* 605-613.

Devathasan, G., Low, D., Teoh, P. C., Wan, S. H., & Wong, P. K. (1984). Complications of chronic glue (toluene) abuse in adolescents. *Australia and New Zealand Journal of Medicine, 14,* 39-43.

Downing, J. (1986). The psychological and physiological effects on MDMA on normal volunteers. *Journal of Psychoactive Drugs, 18,* 335-340.

D'Souza, T., & Shraberg, D. (1981). Intracranial hemorrhage associated with amphetamine use [Letter]. *Neurology, 31,* 922-923.

Elsworth, J. D., Deutch, A. Y., Redmond, D. E., Taylor, J. R., Sladek, J. R., & Roth, R. H. (1989). Symptomatic and asymptomatic 1-methyl-4-phenyl-1,2,3,6-tetrahydropyridine-treated primates: Biochemical changes in striatal regions. *Neuroscience, 33,* 323-331.

Escobar, A., & Aruffo, C. (1980). Chronic thinner intoxication: clinicopathologic report of a human case. *Journal of Neurology and Neurosurgical Psychiatry, 43,* 986-994.

Ezrin-Waters, C. (1987). Nonconvulsive status epilepticus and barbiturate abuse [Letter]. *Neurology, 37,* 1268.

Fibiger, H. C., & Phillips, A. G. (1988). Mesocorticolombic dopamine systems and rewards. *Annals of the New York Academy of Science, 537,* 206–215.

Fields, S., & Fullerton, J. (1975). Influences of heroin addiction on neuropsychological functioning. *Journal of Consulting and Clinical Psychology, 43,* 114.

Fornazzari, L., Carlen, P. L., & Kapur, B. M. (1986). Intravenous abuse of propylhexedrine (Benzedrex) and the risk of brainstem dysfunction in young adults. *Canadian Journal of Neurological Science, 13,* 337–339.

Golbe, L. I., & Merkin, M. D. (1986). Cerebral infarction in a user of freebase cocaine ("crack"). *Neurology, 36,* 1602–1604.

Golombok, S., Moodley, P., & Lader, M. (1988). Cognitive impairment in long-term benzodiazepine users. *Psychological Medicine, 18,* 365–374.

Grant, I., Adams, K. M., Carlin, A. S., Rennick, P. M., Judd, L. L., & Schoof, K. (1978). The collaborative neuropsychological study of polydrug users. *Archives of General Psychiatry, 35,* 1063–1074.

Grant, I., & Judd, L. L. (1976). Neuropsychological and EEG disturbances in polydrug users. *American Journal of Psychiatry, 133,* 1039–1042.

Grant, I., Mohns, L., Miller, M., & Reitan, R. M. (1976). A neuropsychological study of polydrug users. *Archives of General Psychiatry, 33,* 973–978.

Gupta, M., Felten, D., & Gash, D. M. (1984). MPTP alters central catecholamine neurons in addition to the nigrostriatal system. *Brain Research Bulletin, 13,* 737–742.

Hall, D. M. B., Ramsey, J., Schwartz, M. S., & Dookun, D. (1986). Neuropathy in a petrol sniffer. *Archives of Disease in Childhood, 61,* 900–916.

Handelmann, G. E., Contreras, P. C., & O'Donohue, T. L. (1987). Selective, memory impairment by phencyclidine in rats. *European Journal of Pharmacology, 140,* 69–73.

Harrington, H., Heller, H. A., Dawson, D., Caplan, L., & Rumbaugh, C. (1983). Intracerebral hemorrhage and oral amphetamine. *Archives of Neurology, 40,* 503–507.

Hendler, N., Cimini, C., Ma, T., & Long, D. (1980). A comparison of cognitive impairment due to benzodiazepines and to narcotics. *American Journal of Psychiatry, 137,* 828–830.

Hill, S. Y., & Mikhael, M. A. (1979). Computerized transaxial tomographic and neuropsychological evaluations in chronic alcoholics and heroin abusers. *American Journal of Psychiatry, 136,* 598–602.

Hormes, J. T., Filley, C. M., & Rosenberg, N. L. (1986). Neurologic sequelae of chronic solvent vapor abuse. *Neurology, 36,* 698–702.

Howlett, A. C. (1985). Cannabinoid inhibition of adenylate cyclase. Biochemistry of the response in neuroblastoma cell membranes. *Molecular Pharmacology, 27,* 429–436.

Howlett, A. C., Johnson, M. R., Melvin, L. S., & Milne, G. M. (1988). Nonclassical cannabinoid analgesics inhibit adenylate cyclase: Development of a cannabinoid receptor model. *Molecular Pharmacology, 33,* 297–302.

Insel, T. R., Battaglia, G., Johannssen, J. N., Marra, S., & DeSouza, E. B. (1989). 3,4-Methylenedioxymethamphetamine ("ecstasy") selectively destroys brain serotonin terminals in rhesus monkeys. *Journal of Pharmacology and Experimental Therapeutics, 249,* 713–720.

Jacobs, I. G., Roszler, M. H., Kelly, J. K., Klein, M. A., & Kling, G. A. (1989). Cocaine abuse: Neurovascular complications. *Radiology, 170,* 223–227.

Johanson, C., & Fischman, M. (1989). The pharmacology of cocaine related to its abuse. *Pharmacological Reviews, 41,* 3–38.

Judd, L. L., & Grant, I. (1975). Brain dysfunction in chronic sedative users. *Journal of Psychedelic Drugs, 7,* 143–149.

Kaelan, C., Harper, C., & Vieera, B. I. (1986). Acute encephalopathy and death due to petrol sniffing: neuropathological findings. *Australian and New Zealand Journal of Medicine, 16,* 804–807.

Karacan, I., Fernandez-Salas, A., Coggins, W. J., Carter, W. E., Williams, R. L., Thornby, J. I., Salis, P. J., Okawa, M., & Villaume, J. P. (1976). Sleep electroencephalographic-electrooculagraphic characteristics of chronic marijuana users. Part I. *Annals of the New York Academy of Science, 282,* 348-374.

Kaye, B. R., & Fainstat, M. (1987). Cerebral vasculitis associated with cocaine abuse. *Journal of the American Medical Association, 258,* 2104-2106.

King, M. D. (1982). Neurologic sequelae of toluene abuse. *Human Toxicology, 1,* 281-287.

King, M. D., Day, R. E., Oliver, J. S., Lush, M., & Watson, J. M. (1981). Solvent encephalopathy. *British Medical Journal (Clinical Research), 283,* 663-665.

Korman, M., Matthews, R. W., & Lovitt, R. (1981). Neuropsychological effects of abuse of inhalants. *Perceptual and Motor Skills, 53,* 547-553.

Kuehnle, J., Mendelson, J. H., Davis, K. R., & New, P. F. J. (1977). Computed tomographic examination of heavy marijuana smokers. *Journal of the American Medical Association, 237,* 1231-1232.

Langston, J. W., Ballard, P., Tetrud, J. W., & Irwin, I. (1983). Chronic parkinsonism in humans due to a product of meperidine-analog synthesis. *Science, 219,* 979-980.

Lazar, R. B., Ho, S. U., Melen, O., & Daghestani, A. N. (1983). Multifocal central nervous system damage caused by toluene abuse. *Neurology, 33,* 1337-1340.

Levine, S. R., Washington, J. M., Jefferson, M. F., Kieran, S. N., Moen, M., Feit, H., & Welch, K. M. A. (1987). "Crack" cocaine-associated stroke. *Neurology, 37,* 1849-1853.

Levine, S. R., Welch, K. M. A., & Brust, J. C. (1988). Cerebral vasculitis associated with cocaine abuse or subarachnoid hemmorrhage? [Letter]. *Journal of the American Medical Association, 259,* 1648.

Lewis, J. E., & Hordan, R. B. (1986). Neuropsychological assessment of phencyclidine abusers. *NIDA Research Monograph, 64,* 190-208.

Lezak, M. D. (1983). *Neuropsychological Assessment.* 2nd ed. New York: Oxford University Press.

Lolin, Y. (1989). Chronic neurological toxicity associated with exposure to volatile substances. *Human Toxicology, 8,* 293-300.

Lowenstein, D. H., Massa, S. M., Rowbotham, M. C., Collins, S. D., McKinney, H. E., & Simon, R. P. (1987). Acute neurologic and psychiatric complications associated with cocaine abuse. *American Journal of Medicine, 83,* 841-846.

Lundh, H., & Tunving, K. (1981). An extrapyramidal choreiform syndrome caused by amphetamine addiction. *Journal of Neurology and Neurosurgical Psychiatry, 44,* 728-730.

Mahmood, Z. (1983). Cognitive functioning of solvent abusers. *Scott Medical Journal, 28,* 276-280.

Marwah, J., & Pitts, D. K. (1986). Psychopharmacology of phencyclidine. *NIDA Research Monograph, 64,* 127-133.

Matick, H., Anderson, D., & Brumlik, J. (1983). Cerebral vasculitis associated with oral amphetamine overdose. *Archives of Neurology, 40,* 253-254.

Matsuda, L. A., Lolait, S. J., Brownstein, M. J., Young, A. C., & Bonner, T. I. (1990). Structure of a cannabinoid receptor and functional expression of the cloned cDNA. *Nature, 346,* 561-564.

McCabe, R. T., Gibb, J. W., Wamsley, J. K., & Hanson, G. R. (1987). Autoradiographic analysis of muscarinic cholinergic and serotonergic receptor alterations following methamphetamine treatment. *Brain Research Bulletin, 19,* 551-557.

McGlothlin, W. H., Arnold, D. O., & Freedman, D. X. (1969). Organicity measures following repeated LSD ingestion. *Archives of General Psychiatry, 21,* 704-709.

McGrath, J. (1986). Petrol "sniffing" and lead encephalopathy. [Letter]. *Medical Journal of Australia, 144,* 221.

Mendhiratta, S. S., Varma, V. K., Dang, R., Malhotra, A. K., Das, K., & Nehra, R. (1988). Cannabis and cognitive functions: a re-evaluation study. *British Journal of Addiction*, *83*, 749–753.

Merriam, A. E., Medalia, A., & Levine, B. (1988). Partial complex status epilepticus associated with cocaine abuse. *Biological Psychiatry*, *23*, 515–518.

Miller, L. (1985). Neuropsychological assessment of substance abusers: Review and recommendations. *Journal of Substance Abuse Treatment*, *2*, 5–17.

Mody, C. K., Miller, B. L., McIntyre, H. B., Cobb, S. K., & Goldberg, M. A. (1988). Neurologic complications of cocaine abuse. *Neurology*, *38*, 1189–1193.

Murray, J. B. (1986). Marijuana's effects on human cognitive functions, psychomotor functions and personality. *Journal of General Psychology*, *113*, 23–55.

Myers, J. A., & Earnest, M. P. (1984). Generalized seizures and cocaine abuse. *Neurology*, *34*, 675–676.

Nadeau, S. E. (1984). Intracerebral hemorrhage and vasculitis related to ephedrine abuse. *Annals of Neurology*, *15*, 114–115.

National Academy of Science, Institute of Medicine. (1982). *Marihuana and health: report of a study by a committee of the Institute of Medicine*. Washington DC: National Academy of Science.

National Institute of Drug Abuse. (1989). *National household survey on drug abuse: population estimates 1988*. Rockville, MD.

National Institute of Drug Abuse. (1987). *NIDA capsules: high school senior drug use, 1975–1986*. Rockville, MD.

Ng, L. L., Hamilton, D. V., & Chalmers, T. M. (1986). Intra-cranial hemorrhage from drug abuse. *British Journal of Clinical Practice*, *40*, 255–256.

Ohlsson, A., Lingren, J. E., Wahlen, A., Agurell, S., Hollister, L. E., & Gillespie, H. K. (1980). Plasma delta-9-tetrahydrocannabinol concentrations and clinical effects after oral and intravenous administration and smoking. *Clinical Pharmacological Therapeutics*, *28*, 409–416.

Petursson, H., Gudjonsson, G. H., & Lader, M. H. (1983). Psychometric performance during withdrawal from long-term benzodiazepine treatment. *Psychopharmacology*, *81*, 345–349.

Poser, W., Poser, S., Roscher, D., & Argyrakis, A. (1983). Do benzodiazepines cause cerebral atrophy? [Letter]. *Lancet*, *1*, 715.

Ray, R., Prabhu, G. G., Mohan, D., Nath, L. M., & Neki, J. S. (1979). Chronic cannabis used and cognitive functions. *Indian Journal of Medical Research*, *69*, 996–1000.

Ricaurte, G. A. (1989). Studies of MDMA-induced neurotoxicity in nonhuman primates: A basis for evaluating long-term effects in humans. *NIDA Research Monograph*, *94*, 306–322.

Ricaurte, G., Byran, G., Strauss, L., Seiden, L., & Schuster, C. (1985). Hallucinogenic amphetamine selectivity destroys brain serotonin nerve terminals. *Science*, *229*, 986–988.

Ricaurte, G. A., Schuster, C. R., & Seiden, L. S. (1980). Long-term effects of repeated methylamphetamine administration on dopamine and serotonin neurons in the rat brain: A regional study. *Brain Research*, *193*, 153–163.

Ricaurte, G. A., Seiden, L. S., & Schuster, C. R. (1984). Further evidence that amphetamines produce long-lasting dopamine neurochemical deficits by destroying dopamine nerve fibers. *Brain Research*, *303*, 359–364.

Rischbieth, R. H., Thompson, G. N., Hamilton-Bruce, A., Purdie, G. H., & Peters, J. H. (1987). Acute encephalopathy following petrol sniffing in two aboriginal patients. *Clinical and Experimental Neurology*, *23*, 191–194.

Rodin, E. A., Domini, E. F., & Porzak, J. P. (1970). The marihuana-induced "social high." *Journal of the American Medical Association*, *213*, 1300–1302.

Ron, M. A. (1986). Volatile substance abuse: A review of possible long-term neurological, intellectual and psychiatric sequelae. *British Journal of Psychiatry*, *148*, 235–246.

Rosenberg, N. L., Kleinschmidt-DeMasters, B. K., Davis, K. A., Hormes, J. T. & Filley, C. M. (1988). Toluene abuse causes diffuse central nervous system white matter changes. *Annals of Neurology*, *23*, 611–614.

Ross, C. A. (1982). Gasoline sniffing and lead encephalopathy. *CMA Journal*, *127*, 1195–1197.

Rothrock, J. F., Rubenstein, R., & Lyden, P. D. (1988). Ischemic stroke associated with methamphetamine inhalation. *Neurology*, *38*, 589–592.

Rounsaville, B. J., Jones, C., Novelly, R. A., & Kleber, H. (1982). Neuropsychological functioning in opiate addicts. *Journal of Nervous and Mental Disorders*, *170*, 209–216.

Rowbotham, M. C. (1988). Neurologic aspects of cocaine abuse [Medical Staff Conference]. *Western Journal of Medicine*, *149*, 442–448.

Rumbaugh, C. L., Bergeron, R. T., Scanlan, R. L., Teal, J. S., Segall, H. D., Fang, H. C. & McCormick, R. (1971). Cerebral vascular changes secondary to amphetamine abuse in the experimental animal. *Radiology*, *101*, 345–351.

Satz, P., Fletcher, J. M., & Sutker, L. S. (1976). Neuropsychologic, intellectual, and personality correlates of chronic marijuana use in native Costa Ricans. *Annals of the New York Academy of Science*, *282*, 266–306.

Schaeffer, J., Andrysiak, T., & Ungerleider, J. T. (1981). Cognitive and long-term use of ganja (cannabis). *Science*, *213*, 465–466.

Schikler, K. N., Seitz, K., Rice, J. F., Strader, T. (1982). Solvent abuse associated cortical atrophy. *Journal of Adolescent Health Care*, *3*, 37–39.

Schwartz, K. A., & Cohen, J. A. (1984). Subarachnoid hemorrhage precipitated by cocaine snorting [Letter]. *Archives of Neurology*, *41*, 705.

Schwartz, R. H. (1989). Seizures associated with smoking 'crack'—a survey of adolescent 'crack' smokers [Letter.] *Western Journal of Medicine*, *150*, 213.

Seiden, L. S., & Ricaurte, G. A. (1987). Neurotoxicity of methamphetamine and related drugs. In H. Y. Meltzer (Ed.), *Psychopharmacology: the third generation of progress* (pp. 359–366). New York: Raven Press.

Shukla, D. (1982). Intracerebral hemorrhage associated with amphetamine use [Letter]. *Neurology*, *32*, 917–918.

Slikker, W., Holson, R. R., Ali, S. F., Kolta, M. G., Paule, M. G., Scallet, A. C., McMillan, D. E., Baily, J. R., Hong, J. S., & Scalzo, F. M. (1989). Behavioral and neurochemical effects of orally administered MDMA in the rodent and nonhuman primate. *Neurotoxicology*, *10*, 529–542.

Stefanis, C., Dornbush, R., & Fink, M. (Eds.) (1977). *Hashish: studies of long-term use*. New York: Raven Press.

Stern, Y., Tetrud, J. W., Martin, W. R. W., Kutner, S. J., & Langston, J. W. (1990). Cognitive change following MPTP exposure. *Neurology*, *40*, 261–264.

Stiglick, A., & Kalant, H. (1982). Learning impairment in the radial-arm maze following prolonged cannabis treatment in rats. *Psychopharmacology*, *77*, 117–123.

Strang, J., & Gurling, H. (1989). Computerized tomography and neuropsychological assessment in long-term high-dose heroin addicts. *British Journal of Addiction*, *84*, 1011–1019.

Tetrud, J. W., Langston, J. W., Garbe, P. L., & Ruttenber, A. J. (1989). Mild parkinsonism in persons exposed to 1-methyl-4-phenyl-1,2,3,6,-tetrahydropyridine (MPTP). *Neurology*, *39*, 1483–1487.

Valpey, R., Sumi, S. M., Copass, M. K., & Goble, G. J. (1978). Acute and chronic progressive encephalopathy due to gasoline sniffing. *Neurology*, *28*, 507–510.

Volkow, N. D., Mullani, N., Gould, K. L., Adler, S., & Krajewski, K. (1988). Cerebral blood flow in chronic cocaine users: A study with positron emission tomography. *British Journal of Psychiatry, 152,* 641–648.

Vree, T. B., & van Rossom, J. M. (1970). In E. Costa & S. Garattini (Eds.), *Amphetamines and related compounds* (pp. 165–190). New York: Raven Press.

Wagner, G. C., Ricaurte, G. A., Johansen, C. E., Schuster, C. R., & Seiden, L. S. (1980). Amphetamine induced depletion of dopamine and loss of dopamine uptake sites in caudate. *Neurology, 30,* 547–550.

Wert, R. C., & Raulin, M. L. (1986). The chronic cerebral effects of cannabis use. I. methodological issues and neurological findings. *International Journal of Addiction, 21,* 605–628.

Wert, R. C., & Raulin, M. L. (1986). The chronic cerebral effects of cannabis use. II. Psychological findings and conclusions. *International Journal of Addiction, 21,* 629–642.

Wolf, S. L., & Mikhael, M. A. (1979). Computerized transaxial tomography and neuropsychological evaluations in chronic alcoholics and heroin abusers. *American Journal of Psychiatry, 136,* 598–602.

Wolters, E. C., Van Wijngaarden, G. K., Stam, F., Rengelink, H., Lousberg, R. J. Schipper, M. E. I., & Verbeeten, B. (1982). Leucoencephalopathy after inhaling "heroin" pyrolysate. *Lancet, 2,* 1233–1236.

Wooten, M. R., Khangure, M. S., & Murphy, M. J. (1983). Intracerebral hemorrhage and vasculitis related to ephedrine abuse. *Annals of Neurology, 13,* 337–340.

Wright, J. M., Wall, R. A., Perry, T. L., & Paty, D. W. (1984). Chronic parkinsonism secondary to intranasal administration of a product of meperidine-analogue synthesis [Letter]. *New England Journal of Medicine, 310,* 325.

Wright, M., & Hogan, T. P. (1972). Repeated LSD ingestion and performance on neuropsychological tests. *Journal of Nervous and Mental Disorders, 154,* 432–438.

CHAPTER 13

NEUROPSYCHOLOGICAL CONSEQUENCES OF MALNUTRITION

Rik Carl D'Amato, Mary Mathai Chittooran, and Janice D. Whitten

It has been well established that both heredity and environment contribute to each human's ability to function. When individuals receive the necessary physical and psychological sustenance, they are able to grow and develop maximally. However, development can be, and frequently is, obstructed by significant environmental factors such as undernutrition. The focus of this chapter is on the neuropsychological correlates of malnutrition in children. Following a general overview, critical periods of brain growth and development are reviewed and a section on maternal malnutrition is presented. The chapter then reviews concurrent, intermediate, and long-term neuropsychological consequences of malnutrition, followed by a summary portraying prevention as the key to solving nutritional problems.

OVERVIEW

Historically, research has suggested that the effects of malnutrition were transient and remediated simply by supplying sufficient nutrients (Cravioto & Arrieta, 1983). More recently, research has indicated that developing organisms who suffer undernutrition display serious and often permanent consequences (Galler, 1984). Malnutrition can occur during prenatal development, postnatal development, or both periods.

Prenatal Malnutrition

Prenatal undernutrition is usually the effect of maternal malnutrition, which refers to mothers who serve as inadequate sources of nutrition for their unborn children. When mothers themselves are undernourished, fetal development is often affected. This malnutrition can result in low birth weight, premature births, general fetal growth retardation, and growth failure of specific organs, as well as a variety of other behavioral and developmental problems that are unmasked after the child is born (Galler, 1984).

Postnatal Malnutrition

Physical growth in well-nourished children is phenomenal. Average infants usually double their weight in the first 4–5 months of life and triple their weight by age 1; height is just as remarkable, with children on average increasing from birth to the first year of life by at least 50% (Pantell, Fries, & Vickery, 1984). In fact, although a bit less noteworthy, head size is about 60% developed at birth, and by age 3 is almost 90% of the adult size (Pantell et al., 1984). These averages, of course, stem from data on children who received normal amounts of nutrients both before and after birth.

Relative to body size, caloric intake requirements for children are greater than for adults, since infants need to grow and adults need only to maintain. Malnutrition can and does halt the body's achievement of normal growth and development; with this general tenet in mind, "the earlier the malnutrition, the worse its effects" (Lerner & Hultsch, 1983, p. 102). A deviation from normal development can be noticed, such as changes in a child's appearance (e.g., skin color, body size) and body functioning (e.g., diarrhea), or can be difficult to detect such as changes in a child's behavior (e.g., apathy, memory problems). Moreover, a variety of neurological correlates such as school performance problems and impaired perception have been related to nutritional deprivation. Some correlates, like reduced head circumference, have a great deal of face validity. Indeed, reduced head circumference in malnourished children has been seen as implying reduced brain weight (Galler, 1984). However, since development of the brain occurs during certain critical periods, the specific type of damage appears most related to the age when malnutrition occurs (Dobbing, 1970; Monckeberg, 1975).

Kwashiorkor and Marasmus

The generic term "protein-caloric malnutrition" is commonly used to refer to children who do not receive enough food or to children who eat enough, but do not receive adequate amounts of protein. In an attempt to offer greater specificity, children suffering from postnatal malnutrition have been classified into one of two clinical categories of what has been seen as a single human-induced syndrome. The first, known as "kwashiorkor," is due to a protein deficiency alone. The second, marasmus, is due to insufficient intake of food including calorie and protein deficiencies. These differences in deficient intake of nourishment are often related to the age of the child, since certain periods can be especially problematic such as when the child is fully weaned to a less than adequate diet (Cravioto & Arrieta, 1983). Kwashiorkor usually occurs between the ages of 1 and 3 years, and is often associated with the child being transferred from breast milk to a starchy diet; marasmus frequently occurs in children under 1 year of age who are weaned early (Galler, 1984). So too, Cravioto and Arrieta (1983) argue that marasmus predominates in urban settlements and kwashiorkor prevails in rural areas, with kwashiorkor replaced by marasmus as breast feeding declines.

"Kwashiorkor" is an African term meaning displaced child. The term typically refers to infants who breast feed but do not get enough milk to sustain growth (Engel, 1956). The clinical picture is of a child with general growth failure, muscle wasting, and diarrhea. The child may have patchy skin or lesions, frequently with areas of depigmentation; the child's hair, if present, may be soft, brittle, dry, and pale. A bulging abdomen and liver enlargement associated with fatty infiltration are also common, as well as other medical abnormalities (Galler, 1984). The following distinctive behavioral features have been reported by Trowell, Davies, and Dean (1954):

> Even those children who are not severely ill are remarkable silent and still. They sit where they are put, and although they may be well able to walk, never seem to want to do so. They have lost all the normal curiosity and desire for exploration that is natural to a child. If their general condition is worse, they are hopelessly apathetic. They lie in wet and dirty beds without protest. They resent any disturbance with an intensity that makes them come suddenly alive; they cry if they are strong enough, or moan if they are weak. A renewal of interest is one of the most obvious signs of improvement and the child who smiles is well on the way to recovery. (cited in Engel, 1956, p. 489)

The clinical picture for marasmus is similar to kwashiorkor and includes general growth failure, muscle wasting, reduced body weight for age, and reduced body length. Diarrhea is typical, and children are more often irritable than apathetic (Galler, 1984). For both disorders, the severity of the malnutrition affects not only the rate of recovery, but determines whether recovery is possible. It is not uncommon for hospitalized children to die, and differentiation of who will survive in the hospital is related to the severity of the disorder.

Although some argue that differentiation between subtypes of undernutrition is problematic and of little value, malnourished children often display distinctive characteristics that allow them to be identified as suffering from kwashiorkor or marasmus (Monckeberg, 1975). Although these labels are used most frequently in literature from the United States and the British Commonwealth, the underlying biochemical and clinical features of malnutrition do not appear to change as a function of geographical location. However, differences that relate to patterns of weaning, and limited treatment of medical problems, may modify the clinical features in certain regions of the world (Cravioto & Arrieta, 1983). It is also difficult to tease out the singular effects of malnutrition since it is part of a total system, growing out of a segment of society that suffers universal disadvantages such as unemployment, limited mobility, lack of education, inadequate sanitation, overcrowding, poor medical treatment, and little or no attention paid to child stimulation and development.

Issues in the Evaluation of Malnutrition

Malnutrition at young ages can be evaluated by reviewing developmental and anthropological measures such as height for age, weight for age, weight for height for age, skin fold thickness, and arm circumference; in addition to these indices, older children are often evaluated with neuropsychological measures as well (Galler, 1984). However, informal visual observations of children's body weight can be deceiving due to body bloating.

Malnutrition can result in deficiencies that lie along a continuum, with substantial damage at one end and little or no damage at the other. Since it has been established (Cravioto & Arrieta, 1983; Lezak, 1983) that substantial damage to the brain is needed to cause alterations in simple reflexes, and nominal damage is more likely to relate to difficulty in complex neuropsychological processes, it seems most appropriate to consider malnutrition from a neuropsychological view. Indeed, neuropsychology, the study of brain-behavior relationships, has been offered as a tool to help diagnose brain dysfunction, chart the course of a disorder, and offer data to plan a rehabilitation program (D'Amato, 1990; Lezak, 1983). So too, since neurodevelopment continues into late adolescence and early adulthood, the effects of malnutrition cannot be adequately understood until that time. Another difficulty in understanding the effects of inadequate nutrition relates to the fact that underdeveloped countries have higher rates of malnutrition and are less sophisticated both medically and psychologically in understanding the consequences of this disorder. Since development has been shown to be culturally related, the very measures we use to consider developmental differences in children must be carefully considered from a cross-cultural perspective (Galler, 1984).

Research indicates that if a child is hospitalized for severe malnutrition, this identifies all children in the family as at risk and suggests that the potential for malnutrition exists for siblings as well (Cravioto & Arrieta, 1983). This may be related to parental patterns of childrearing, which may result in unsuccessful coping in general, and malnutrition in particular, being passed on from generation to generation. When poverty is extreme within the family unit, relationships between children and adults are usually diminished. There seems to be verly little activity at any level, which leads to familial interaction insufficient for the child's overall development (Monckeberg, 1976). The impoverished and malnourished mother is often unable to care for even herself. However, on the positive side, mothers who break away from traditional patterns by listening to the radio or using a national language over a local dialect are more apt to have children who are not undernourished (Cravioto & Arrieta, 1983).

Epidemiological Estimates

The prevalence of protein-calorie malnutrition is not clearly understood due to the insidious ease with which malnutrition can develop in children. Caretakers may not realize undernutrition is taking place, or they may understand, but be unable to provide nutritious food. For children below the age of 5, estimates of severe malnutrition vary from 0.5% to 7.5% in preindustrial regions of the world (Cravioto & Arrieta, 1983). About 10 million Latin American children less than 5 years of age experience various degrees of malnutrition. Data from Mexico suggest about 7.5% of preschool children in central regions experience malnutrition (Cravioto & Arrieta, 1983). Postnatal undernutrition has been seen as the most common cause of substandard health in the world, with 60% of all children suffering from it to some degree (Chase, Cipriano, Canosa, Dabiere, Welch, & O'Brien, 1974; Monckeberg, 1976). With minor exceptions, malnutrition is more prevalent in countries that have experienced, or are experiencing famine, like Bangladesh, India, and parts of Africa and Latin America (Mata, 1976).

CRITICAL PERIODS OF BRAIN DEVELOPMENT

There is currently considerable evidence that malnutrition, especially during critical periods of brain development, can prohibit brain growth and culminate in lower levels of neuropsychological functioning (Chase et al., 1974; Monckeberg, 1975). Once conception is achieved, the brain develops according to its genotypically ordained schedule irrespective of nutritional status, unless undernutrition is so severe that the fetus dies. Therefore, it is incorrect to consider a malnourished brain to be retarded in its growth—rather, its growth has been prohibited (Dobbing, 1970). Studies have suggested that any substance or lack thereof that can produce an effect, however transient, upon neuropsychological abilities may have profound effects during critical periods of embryonic development (Kalat, 1984; Lytle, Whitacre, & Nelson, 1984; Pryor, 1975; Winick & Rosso, 1969). The consequences of brain damage in infancy may be cumulative as well, since the formation of developing structures appears to be dependent upon the functional integrity of earlier developmental processes. There is also evidence that malnutrition sustained during gestation or early in life may not become neuropsychologically apparent until much later in development (Cravioto & Arrieta, 1983; Galler, 1984; Lytle et al., 1984). Therefore, the timing of malnutrition, in relationship to the stage of maturation of the brain, appears to be as significant to future behavioral outcomes as the nature of the nutritional deficit itself.

Human as well as animal studies suggest that the impact of nutritional deficits is greatest within the fastest growing portion of the nervous system (Brasel & Winick, 1972; Monckeberg, 1975; Lytle et al., 1984). Although available nutrients are used by the nervous system first, often stunting growth in other parts of the body (e.g., the liver), when the deficit affects the brain it will affect the fastest growing area of the brain first and most profoundly. Thus, the time when certain parts of the brain grow and develop most rapidly, are seen as critical periods of development.

Brain Development

Development of the nervous system begins at about the ninth day of embryonic development and culminates in a system composed of many cell types, arranged in a species-specific manner (Volpe, 1987). After the child is born, the brain gains weight at the rate of approximately 2 milligrams per minute (Cravioto, 1966; Cravioto & Arrieta, 1983). Studies have defined some of the processes of brain development and their critical periods of rapid growth, in terms of the developmental pattern of the nervous system (Pryor, 1975). These neurodevelopmental processes are seen as (a) neurulation, (b) histogenesis, (c) cell migration, (d) synapse formation, (e) myelination, and (f) neurotransmission (Volpe, 1987). Actually, neurotransmission is not a growth process but the culmination of the other five stages; it is the process whereby cells within the nervous system communicate with one another. This process is accomplished by electrochemical transmission, which is impacted by the nutritional milieu of the brain. Malnutrition may upset the delicately balanced nature of neurotransmission and could therefore account for the late onset of certain neuropsychological disabilities. Because of the complex nature of neurotransmission, which changes through the life-span, early insult may not be apparent until puberty or until highly abstract thought is necessary for adaptation.

The first stage, neurulation is the process whereby the fetus begins to produce neural cells (Volpe, 1987). The critical period for neurulation typically takes place during the first 3-4 weeks of gestation. Histogenesis, the second stage, is the process whereby neural cells divide and differentiate into the different types of neurons found in the mature nervous system. This critical period is accomplished within the first 2-4 months of gestation (except for the formation of glial cells, which differentiate just prior to cell migration and continue to about 3 years of age). When malnutrition is present, cell division during histogenesis has been shown to be curtailed and the resulting brain to contain fewer cells than normal (Winick & Rosso, 1975). Interruption of neuronal development in these two earliest stages of prenatal brain development, whether by lack of adequate nutrition or other means can be lethal; with the few surviving infants exhibiting devastating neurologic deficits (e.g., spina bifida) (Volpe, 1987).

Malnutrition has been shown to permanently affect cell migration, the third neurodevelopmental stage (Winick & Rosso, 1975). The critical period for cell migration is from 3 to 5 months after conception. Neurons must often move quite far in extremely intricate pathways before they reach their functional sites. Defects in this migratory pattern can lead to improper neuronal connections in the mature brain (Freeman, 1985). Although the precise nature of the chemical factors directing cell migration is not known, glial cells appear to mediate the process. Defects in migration have been shown to lead to aberrations in neuronal development resulting in important functional and behavioral consequences (e.g., problems in intellectual and motor development) both immediately and later in development (Hoorweg & Stanfield, 1976).

Because of the lethal nature of early prenatal nutritional deficits, the long-term effects of malnutrition appear to occur during the final 3 stages of development within the nervous system. It is during these processes (cell migration, synapse formation, and myelination), that the fetus typically survives and yet has varying degrees of neuropsychological dysfunction (Volpe, 1987). Undernutrition in late prenatal or early postnatal stages of development has been shown to produce a continuum of disorders ranging from severe pathologies to an undetectable rerouting of neurological functioning (Kalat, 1984).

The critical period for synapse formation, the fourth stage, begins at about 6 months after conception and continues for several years postnatally. Synapses continue to be formed throughout the lifetime but at a much slower rate, which appears to be controlled by environmentally induced experience (Volpe, 1987). During the critical period for synapse formation, neurons begin to grow, branch, and become functional. The physical arrangement of synapse formation is specific to the type and function of each neuron. Alteration of these geometric factors would be expected to drastically disrupt the function of the neuron. Undernourished children have been shown to have smaller, less branched synapses, which in turn have been shown to lead to lowered mental abilities (Winick & Rosso, 1975). The specific mechanisms of synapse formation are not well understood; however, since 60-70 proteins have been postulated as candidates for involvement in various ways (Carlson, 1986).

Myelination is the final stage in physical neuronal development and is typically not complete until 3-6 years of age. The critical period for this process begins at birth and continues for up to 3 years. Myelination is the process whereby specialized glial cells form a protective covering around the axons of neurons. Disruptions in myelination have been shown to affect higher order arousal, alerting cognitive communication and emotional functions of the brain without affecting the lower autonomic functions (Volpe, 1987). Not surprisingly, myelination has also been shown to be reduced in malnourished children (Winick & Rosso, 1969).

Lastly, communication within the nervous system is controlled by neurotransmitters, protein molecules used to transfer messages within the system. The process of neurotransmission provides the chemical code for the development and subsequent behavior of the child. Although the exact type and configuration of the neurotransmitters used may change throughout the growth process, the need for the primary protein precursors and trace minerals remains fairly constant, since the overall level of protein synthesis remains fairly stable (Lytle et al., 1984).

Alterations in nutritional status might influence neurotransmission at any of the major steps involved in the neurotransmission process (by altering uptake or synthesis, storage, release, receptor interaction, or inactivation) (Lytle et al., 1984). Since all of the neurotransmitters isolated so far are nutrient components of common foods or their metabolic byproducts, it would appear likely that these process can be affected by nutrition. It also follows that nonavailability of these nutrients or their metabolic precursors at critical times in development could lead to prohibited brain development (Freeman, 1985). In fact, many studies have been completed which support this premise (Galler, 1984).

In sum, malnutrition has been shown to relate to structural and functional changes in the brain, including decreased myelinization, decreased numbers of neurons, and glial cells, reduction in synaptic connections, and decreased velocity of impulse conduction. Moreover, lowered encephalogram alpha and beta wave activity have also been documented (Engel, 1956). This brief review of development from the perspective of the nutritive requirements of the developing child suggests the importance of nutrition as providing the building blocks for neurodevelopment. The later stages of development, between the ages of 18 weeks prior to birth until 18 months after birth has been argued to be the most critical period of brain growth because the overall mass of the brain increased faster than at any other period, although the child acquires very few new cells at that time (Dobbing, 1970; Pryor, 1975).

PRENATAL MALNUTRITION

As indicated, much of the development of the brain is accomplished during gestation. All organs are in a stage of geometric growth during fetal development, and are therefore susceptible to damage due to nutritional insult. Insults due to malnutrition during periods of individual cell growth and neurotransmission appear to be reversible, when sufficient nutrients become available. However, insults during periods of neurulation, histogenesis, cell differentiation, and synapse formation do not appear to be reversible. At these times of critical brain development, the nutrients necessary for growth of the fetus are provided by the mother. Therefore, it logically follows that maternal nutrition is important to fetal brain development.

By the time pregnancy is first diagnosed most women beginning prenatal care have already passed the first two critical stages of brain development, neurulation and histogenesis. Women have missed at least one and usually two menses before gynecologists routinely conduct pregnancy tests or schedule an initial obstetrical visit. As detailed earlier, during the first 8 weeks the fetus is quite vulnerable to damage (Freeman, 1985). This vulnerability is, incredible as it sounds, the result of doctors' orders in western culture since early obstetrical appointments are not encouraged. Many other mothers, especially those living in third world countries, never see a doctor and are assisted with delivery by other women in their village. Research in underdeveloped countries suggest that 8-15% of newborns worldwide show evidence of prenatal malnutrition and that 1-3% of children experience malnutrition during the first months of life (Monckeberg, 1976). These are the critical periods for a large portion of the neural processes responsible for brain development.

Unborn children, although living in a comparatively comfortable, well-protected environment, are not totally immune to the larger environment surrounding the mother. There are some well-documented ways in which this environment can and does affect the unborn child. Since the mother's general health can affect the overall prenatal development of the child, including the nervous system, maternal malnutrition is a prominent concern. Certain diseases are known to disrupt physical development of the child, including the physical development of the brain. For example, German measles contracted by the mother during the first 3 months of gestation has been shown to result in mental retardation in infants (Yussen & Santrock, 1982). Diabetes has also been found to affect fetal development. This is important from a nutritional perspective since several studies have shown that children born to mothers with inadequate diets are more likely to contract diseases during infancy (Yussen & Santrock, 1982). In fact, malnutrition—particularly protein deficiency—may be linked to mental retardation because of the importance of protein in brain development.

Throughout history, special attention has been directed toward the diets of pregnant women (Pantell et al., 1984). Dietary restrictions as well as supplements have been fashionable in western culture, while general malnutrition is prevalent over much of the underdeveloped world. Nutrition studies usually take maternal weight gain as an index of maternal and fetal nutrition. This may not be an adequate measure since protein and trace minerals, such as copper and manganese have been shown to be more critical than calories in development of the nervous system in animals (Lytle et al., 1984). It is clear from this review that maternal nutrition is as imperative as the nutrition of children in the world. The environment created by mothers for their offspring can alter that child's biologically based abilities. Mothers need to be educated and provided with the means to secure an adequate nutritional environment for themselves and the development of their unborn children.

CONSEQUENCES OF MALNUTRITION

Issues in Determining Effects

One of the difficulties involved in assessing the consequences of malnutrition in children is philosophical in nature: One cannot, with impunity, and without regard for ethical implications, manipulate children's diets merely to study malnutrition and its correlates. In light of such objections, researchers (e.g., Dobbing, 1970; Sinnett, 1983) have resorted to using animal models to explain the effects of starvation or nutrient deprivation. This is a procedure of limited utility in that generalizations about corresponding effects in humans cannot be assumed.

Methodological problems have further hindered the acquisition of knowledge about malnutrition and its effects. For example, much of the existing information on malnutrition in humans is based upon postmortem analyses, studies of children admitted to hospitals, or referred for medical care subsequent to prolonged periods of nutrient deprivation. The literature is replete with studies that have employed small samples of convenience, poor randomization procedures, and inadequate controls. A related concern has to do with the reliability and validity of tests used to measure neuropsychological development, mental abilities, and other behavioral functions in children (Lezak, 1983). Most of these measures were not designed for, nor standardized on, the populations where malnutrition may be severe and, therefore, in most need of study (Cravioto & Arrieta, 1983). Such deficiencies warrant a conservative interpretation of results obtained with these groups.

As mentioned earlier, it is difficult to separate out and, therefore, to assess the detrimental effects of malnutrition because it tends to accompany other unfavorable circumstances, such as substandard living conditions, poor hygiene and medical care, and disease (Cravioto & Arrieta, 1983). The entire ecological system contributes to growth and developmental deficiencies in children, so that the isolation of the effects of current or previous malnutrition becomes a complicated matter, at best.

Many intellectual, neuropsychological, and academic functions are not immediately sensitive to changes in nutritional status. This is particularly true in the assessment of changes resulting from undernutrition during infancy and the preschool years (Cravioto & Arrieta, 1983; Galler, 1984). Therefore, answers about the effects of malnutrition can only be provided when an adequate interval is allowed to elapse between the time of primary risk and the time during which these functions may be adequately measured. In general, however, there is a significant probability that such functions may never be fully measured, given the relatively unsophisticated measures at our disposal (Lezak, 1983). It is unfortunate that our knowledge of malnutrition is limited by the fact that many studies in this area have followed individuals only through adolescence (Galler, 1984). Concrete evidence concerning effects that appear in, or are maintained through adulthood are singularly lacking. However, preadulthood behavioral patterns that modify the child's response to his or her environment can often be used as predictive indices of later performance.

Several authors studying malnutrition have differentiated between its effects on the basis of type and severity. Galler (1984) has provided an efficient three-pronged classification that has proven particularly useful in understanding both the breadth, as well as the implications of malnutrition. First, are the concurrent effects, or those that occur along with the acute phase of malnutrition. Second, are the intermediate effects—those that occur once the period of malnutrition is over, and which may be manifested for 2–3 years during the recovery period. Third, are the long-term effects that may persist many years after the initial period of malnutrition. These major classes of effects will be reviewed in the following three sections.

Concurrent Effects of Malnutrition

A number of studies have indicated that neurological changes tend to occur concurrently with severe malnutrition such as marasmus. Several studies (Monckeberg, 1975; Rozovski, Novoa, Abbarzua, & Monckeberg, 1970) have indicated that malnourished children show reduced head circumference and, by implication, a corresponding reduction in brain size. Corroborating evidence was garnered on Ugandan children who died of malnutrition; these children's brains did indeed weigh less than those of children who had died of other causes (Brown, 1965). Research completed with other South American and African populations (Chase et al., 1974; Engsner, Hable, Stogren, & Vahlquist, 1974; Winick & Rosso, 1969) revealed a reduction in brain cell number as well as in cell size. Dobbing (1974) hypothesized that such brain changes were the result of lowered levels of dendritic branching, which therefore reduced the number of connections between brain nerve cells.

Until relatively recently, the brain was thought to be invulnerable to starvation or nutrient deprivation; however, Dobbing and Kersley (1963) showed conclusively that the immunity to starvation enjoyed by the adult brain did not hold true for the developing brain. Again, if the brain is deprived, even temporarily, of essential nutrients during certain critical periods of development, its development can be irreversibly affected (Cravioto, DeLicardie, & Birch, 1966; Winick, 1969). Severe nutritional deficiencies could conceivably result in up to 40% deficit in the number of brain cells (Patton, Payne, & Beirne-Smith, 1990; Resnick, 1988). In a similar vein, Coulter (1988) hypothesized that intellectual deficits attributable to sociocultural influences were the result of hypoconnection syndrome. Specifically, sociocultural influences such as inadequate diet and medical care, which result in diffuse environmental deprivation, might cause a deficiency or abnormality of neuronal connections throughout the brain, especially if they occurred during critical periods of development.

Electrophysiological studies of the brain (e.g., Barnet, Weiss, Sotillo, Ohrlich, Sakurovich, & Cravioto, 1978; Engel, 1956; Nelson & Dean, 1959) have also shown clear evidence of cerebral dysfunction in electroencephalograms (EEGs) obtained with undernourished children. Other concurrent effects of malnutrition have included apathy, passivity, reduced motor activity, and inadequate or absent interpersonal interactions (Galler, 1984). Language and verbal abilities, because of their intimate relation to intellectual abilities, are thought to be particularly sensitive predictors of cerebral dysfunction (Galler, 1984; Lezak, 1983). For example, a number of studies of malnourished children have reported marked depression in verbal responses and overall language scores on the Bayley and the Gesell Scales (Cravioto & DeLicardie, 1972; Cravioto & Robles, 1965; Guthrie, Masangkay, & Guthrie, 1976).

Rate of cardiac habituation (or adaptation) to unfamiliar auditory or visual stimuli is another promising area of research. Unlike normal children, whose heart rates rapidly increase and then return to baseline levels upon presentation of a novel auditory or visual stimulus. Lester (1975, 1976) found that malnourished children exhibited a slower rate of habituation. Such changes in heart rate are felt to occur partially as a result of the individual's attention to, and concentration on relevant patterns of stimuli. Since these tasks are considered to be important indicators of adequate neuropsychological functioning (Lezak, 1983), it is evident that the rate of cardiac habituation has neuropsychological implications. Lower responsiveness to sounds (Lester, 1976) and abnormalities in crying patterns (Juntunen, Siroio, & Michelsson, 1978) have also been identified in malnourished children; these findings have led researchers to speculate that crying patterns, along with response to external stimuli, may provide valuable information on the extent of brain damage resulting from malnutrition.

It is clear that malnutrition can result in a dismaying array of problems occurring during the acute phase of the disorder. Malnourished children have consistently exhibited physical, behavioral, and neuropsychological deficiencies that affect functioning, inhibit adequate interactions with the environment, and frequently foreshadow problems of a more serious nature.

Intermediate Effects of Malnutrition

Many children do survive the acute phase of malnutrition; for those who do, aggressive intervention efforts such as the establishment of new feeding patterns, treatment of metabolic problems, and improvement of medical care may help reverse many of the deleterious effects of the disorder. Other effects, however, linger to form the basis of more persistent deficits, which may manifest themselves in the 2–3-year recovery period following the malnutrition episode. One of the most obvious intermediate effects is the reversal of apathy and passivity that are the hallmarks of the severely malnourished child. The listlessness and functional isolation usually disappear shortly after intervention efforts are undertaken. As children recover, curiosity and exploratory behavior begin to show a marked turn for the better, and motor activity tends to increase concomitantly with other abilities.

Regardless of these positive effects, Ashem and James (1978) reported lower overall intellectual performance on the McCarthy Scales of Children's Abilities in severely malnourished children from poor urban and rural environments; the more serious the previous level of nutritional deficit, the poorer the performance. Grantham-McGregor, Powell, Stewart, and Schofield (1982) compared children 3-5 years old, who had a history of hospitalization for malnutrition, with children who had been hospitalized for other reasons. Significant deficits in intellectual development, as measured by the Griffiths Mental Development Scales, were found with previously malnourished children. These results were consistent not only at the time of discharge from the hospital, but up to 3 years later. Differences between the groups were maintained even when the authors controlled for the possibility of differential effects arising from the quality of subsequent home environments.

Longitudinal studies of intellectual development with small groups of previously malnourished children (e.g., Botha-Antoun, Babayan, & Harfouche, 1968; DeLicardie & Cravioto, 1973; McLaren, Yaktin, Kanawati, Sabbagh, & Kadi, 1973, 1975) have all shown reduced performance on intelligence tests. However, the fact that none of these studies employed a control group makes it difficult to draw definitive conclusions about the reason for depressed performance. Lloyd-Still, Hurwitz, Wolff, & Shwachman, (1974) also reported deficits in intellectual abilities among children who were compared with their siblings, 1-6 years after infantile malnutrition. Chase and Martin (1970) showed that previously malnourished children continued to exhibit lowered language and verbal performance well after the acute period of the disease was over. In related neruopsychological studies, Barnet et al. (1978) noted abnormal responses to auditory evoked potentials in 26 infants with marasmus; this pattern of responses was maintained up to 1 year later. An early study by Engel (1956) examined 25 children who had suffered from kwashiorkor between the ages of 8 months and 5 years. These children's diets were significantly improved during the recovery period, and results indicated that EEGs appeared to be within normal limits.

The research on the intermediate effects of malnutrition is sadly lacking; this may be due to the failure of researchers to follow up on previously malnourished children and the difficulty of obtaining samples for study. Regardless of the dearth of information in this area, it is evident that even 2 or 3 years after suffering malnutrition, children display negative effects in intellectual, behavioral, and neuropsychological functioning.

Long-Term Effects of Malnutrition

In spite of intervention efforts aimed at combating malnutrition, many of its effects do persist—some, into the recovery period, yet others into the next few years, perhaps even into adulthood or subsequent generations (Galler, 1984). A few effects may not become apparent until the individual's development requires new responses to his or her environment, for example, child bearing or complex planning abilities (Galler, 1984; Lezak, 1983). These long-term effects are often the result of months or even years of inadequate diets and insufficient nutrients.

A seminal study conducted by Baird (1947) examined 200,000 births in Scotland, in order to identify the sociobiological factors contributing to a woman's childbearing history. Mothers whose heights were in the lowest percentiles—and it was speculated that undernutrition played a role in their stature—were more likely to give birth to smaller babies who exhibited lowered intellectual performance as they matured. Evidently, a woman's nutritional background can play a significant part in her future, as well as those of the children she bears.

A number of studies have examined the physical correlates of brain functioning in children with marasmus and kwashiorkor (Birch & Richardson, 1972; Hoorweg & Stanfield, 1976; Stoch & Smythe, 1976). It has generally been found that early incidence of marasmus leads to significantly reduced adult head circumference with reduced brain size (Branko, 1979). As indicated previously, other structural and functional changes in the brain have been described as decreased myelinization, decreased number of neurons and glial cells, reduction in synaptic connections, and decreased velocity of peripheral nerve conduction (Lozoff, 1989). Most studies of children who had suffered malnutrition early in life did not reveal abnormal electroencephalograms in later life (Galler, 1984). However, a study by Bartel, Griesel, Freiman, Rosen, and Geefhuysen (1979) of EEG patterns among low-socioeconomic-status children ages 6–12, with histories of kwashiorkor, found lower alpha activity and increased slow wave activity. Lozoff (1989) also reported slowing of dominant EEG frequencies in sleep and waking states. Findings such as these suggest reduced arousal as a significant long-term effect of malnutrition, although it has been cautioned that more sophisticated computer analyses of electrophysiological functioning are necessary before valid conclusions can be drawn (Galler, 1984).

A particularly interesting facet of research in the area of long-term effects relates to changes in intellectual status as a result of early nutritional deficiencies. One comparative study (Lien, Meyer, & Winick, 1977; Winick, Meyer, & Harris, 1975) followed 240 Korean children who had been adopted by American families when they were about 2 years of age, and who were, at the time of the study, between 7 and 15 years of age. The children who were previously malnourished showed a significant reduction in performance on several intelligence tests. They also performed less well on tests of academic achievement, with lowest levels being reported among those who had been the oldest when they were adopted. Similarly, Monckeberg (1975) found that infants seen 4–7 years after an acute period of malnutrition showed intelligence levels in the mentally retarded range and did poorly on developmental scales.

Long-term studies of intelligence in previously malnourished children found similar results relating to depressed intellectual performance (Birch, Pineiro, Alcalde, Toca, & Cravioto, 1971; Galler, Ramsey, Solimano, Lowell, & Mason, 1983; Pereira, Sundararaj, & Begum, 1979). Although these studies correlated malnourishment with lowered intellectual abilities, other studies (Hoorweg & Stanfield, 1976; Richardson, 1972) have concluded that intellectual deficits and behavioral problems may stem from concurrent factors other than malnutrition.

Other studies of the persistent effects of malnutrition have dealt with inter-sensory integration, hyperactivity, attention span, memory, and reduced socialization (Hoorweg & Stanfield, 1976; Galler, 1984). All of these studies tended to show depressed performance many years after the acute phase of the disease; however, once again, small samples and poor research design may have contributed to spurious results.

An important longitudinal study of 129 Barbadian boys and girls ages 5–11 years was conducted by Galler (1984) to determine the effects of malnutrition on various indices such as intelligence, neuropsychological functioning, family background, behavior, and school performance. All children had been hospitalized for severe malnutrition (marasmus) within the first year of life. The sample excluded those with significant fetal retardation, prenatal or perinatal complications, and neurological problems. These children were matched on variables of age, gender, and handedness with 129 classmates of similar social backgrounds who had no history of malnutrition. The two groups of children (a total of 258) were studied 11–16 years after hospitalization. Results indicated that previously malnourished children exhibited difficulty demonstrating a variety of soft neurological signs such as finger tapping, successive finger movements, hand-patting, toe-tapping, and heel-toe rocking (Galler, 1984). Results also indicated that on the Wechsler Intelligence Scale for Children–Revised (WISC-R), previously malnourished children obtained intelligence scores that were 12 points lower than those of control group children, with the greatest differences being seen among girls.

Furthermore, Galler (1984) found that a number of the previously malnourished children were achieving below expected grade level in school, and were generally doing relatively poorly in language arts, mathematics, and general science when compared to control group children. Intelligence test scores were significantly related to classroom achievement scores for both groups. In terms of classroom behavior, previously malnourished children exhibited impaired performance in the areas of attention span, memory, cooperativeness, and motor activity. The previously malnourished and control group children could also be differentiated in terms of family background, with the former group's mothers being more depressed, less educated, and less apt to socialize than mothers of the control group children. The results of this study indicated significant differences in a variety of areas, between previously malnourished children and those with no history of malnutrition.

Authors such as Pereira et al. (1979) have suggested that malnutrition can have long-term effects in other areas. For example, they reported that previously malnourished children did significantly worse on tests of visual perception and intersensory integration. Galler (1984) noted that previously malnourished children with attention deficit disorder, who were followed up almost 18 years later, continued to exhibit significant attention and distractibility problems. In terms of emotional stability and social skills, once again previously malnourished children were found to have poorer performance than children with no history of malnutrition.

Although the majority of long-term studies have mentioned the negative repercussions of malnutrition, other studies have reported more optimistic results; for example, Grantham-McGregor, Schofield, and Powell (1987) found that 6 years after the initial malnutrition episode, children showed increases in performance on the Stanford-Binet.

The information on long-term effects of malnutrition is mixed. It is uncertain whether later negative effects are the result of malnutrition alone, or a combination of nutritional and emotional deprivation. Some authors (e.g., Eckholm & Record, 1976; Lozoff, 1989) have suggested that malnourished children are apathetic and tend not to seek the social and cognitive stimulation needed for adequate development. Consequently, a vicious cycle is set in motion, with levels of functioning becoming lower as stimulation decreases. However, undernourished children adopted into families with improved environmental conditions have shown near normal academic, intellectual, and behavioral performance. This suggests either that environmental advantages can allow individuals to compensate for early damage or that measures of performance are not sensitive enough to evaluate deficits arising from malnutrition.

Most of the malnourished children in the world are under the age of 2, and it is this population that has been studied most extensively and about whom we have the most information. Still lacking, is a comprehensive body of knowledge about the effects of malnutrition in adolescence and beyond. However, with increasing research sophistication and interest in the field, a clearer understanding of the implications of malnutrition should be forthcoming. Since understanding is generally a precursor to informed action, it is hoped that this increase in knowledge will lead to serious efforts to combat the insidious effects of malnutrition, and to start making a difference in the lives of affected children.

SUMMARY

The consequences of malnutrition are grave. The effects of nutrient deprivation appear to range from simple transient behavioral difficulties to complex permanent neuropsychological deficits and can occur before birth, after birth, or both prenatally and postnatally. Perhaps the most distressing characteristic of malnutrition relates to the fact that it is a human-induced disorder. Unlike many diseases that have unidentifiable causes and therefore elusive cures, both the cause and the cure of malnutrition are well understood. Indeed, the remedy is simple—provide adequate nutrition. Unquestionably then, the solution to this grim problem lies in proactive planning and prevention. Lozoff (1989) argues, "thus, prevention rather than treatment of nutritional deficiencies holds greater promise for eliminating behavioral and developmental ill effects. These observations suggest that prevention of nutritional problems deserves the highest priority in terms of public health policies" (p. 236). This raises the question of why we need to deal with the numerous, serious effects of malnutrition at all, when simply providing adequate food to the undernourished can completely extinguish the undernutrition cycle.

However, this solution becomes a complicated process due to the cost and location of available food, and the geographical area where the need for food is prevalent. In fact, from this view, the problem has been seen as political (Field & Levinson, 1976). Whatever the reason, children this very day are starving in most, if not all, countries of the world. In an effort to evaluate the reasons behind malnutrition, Cravioto and Arrieta (1983) report that malnutrition is a multi-faceted problem which is:

> characteristic of the poorer segments of society, particularly of pre-industrial societies, where the social system consciously or unconsciously creates malnourished individuals, generation after generation, through a series of social mechanisms that includes limited access to goods and services, limited social mobility, and restricted experiential opportunities at crucial points in the lives of children. (p. 32)

Although the cure for malnutrition is simple, making it a reality is a complex undertaking. The first step in combating malnutrition, of course, would be to make such a solution an international priority. Only when individuals from all countries, in all walks of life, direct their combined efforts toward solving this perplexing problem, will progress be made in feeding the hungry children of the world.

REFERENCES

Ashem, B., & James, M. D. (1978). Deleterious effects of chronic undernutrition on cognitive abilities. *Journal of Child Psychology and Psychiatry, 19*, 23–31.

Baird, D. (1947). Social class and foetal mortality. *Lancet, 253*, 531–535.

Barnet, A. B., Weiss, I. P., Sotillo, M. V., Ohrlich, E. S., Sakurovich, Z. M., & Cravioto, J. (1978). Abnormal auditory evoked potentials in early infancy malnutrition. *Science, 201*, 450–452.

Bartel, P. R., Griesel, R. D., Freiman, I., Rosen, E. U., & Geefhuysen, J. (1979). Long-term effects of kwashiorkor on the electroencephalogram. *American Journal of Clinical Nutrition, 32,* 753–757.

Birch, H. G., Pineiro, C., Alcalde, E., Toca, T., & Cravioto, J. (1971). Relation of kwashiorkor in early childhood and intelligence at school age. *Pediatric Research, 5,* 579–585.

Birch, H. G., & Richardson, S. A. (1972). The functioning of Jamaican school children severely malnourished during the first two years of life. In *Nutrition, the nervous system, and behavior* (pp. 64–72). Proceedings of the Seminar on Malnutrition in Early Life and Subsequent Mental Development. Washington, DC: Pan American Health Organization Scientific publication no. 251.

Botha-Antoun, E., Babayan, S., & Harfouche, J. K. (1968). Intellectual development related to nutritional status. *Journal of Tropical Pediatrics, 14,* 112–115.

Branko, Z. (1979). Height, weight, and head circumference in survivors of marasmus and kwashiorkor. *American Journal of Clinical Nutrition, 32,* 1717–1727

Brasel, J. A., & Winick, M. (1972). Maternal nutrition and prenatal growth. *Archives of Disease in Childhood, 47,* 479–485.

Brown, R. E. (1965). Decreased brain weight in malnutrition and its implications. *East African Medical Journal, 42,* 584–595.

Carlson, N. R. (1986). *Physiology of behavior.* 3rd ed. Boston: Allyn Bacon.

Chase, H. P., Cipriano, A., Canosa, C. A., Dabiere, C. S., Welch, N. N., & O'Brian, D. (1974). Postnatal undernutrition and human brain development. *Journal of Mental Deficiency Research, 18,* 355–366.

Chase, H. P., & Martin, H. P. (1970). Undernutrition and child development. *New England Journal of Medicine, 282,* 933–939.

Coulter, W. A. (1988). The neurology of mental retardation. In F. J. Menolascino & J. A. Stark (Eds.), *Preventive and curative intervention in mental retardation* (pp. 113–152). Baltimore: Paul H. Brookes.

Cravioto, J. (1966). Malnutrition and behavioral development in the preschool child. In *Preschool Child Malnutrition* (pp. 74–84). Washington, DC: National Academy of Science publication number 1282.

Cravioto, J., & Arrieta, R. (1983). Malnutrition in childhood. In M. Rutter (Ed.), *Developmental neuropsychiatry* (32–51). New York: Guilford.

Cravioto, J., & DeLicardie, E. (1972). Environmental correlates of severe clinical malnutrition and language development in survivors from kwashiorkor or marasmus. In *Nutrition, the Nervous System, and Behavior* (pp. 73–94). Proceedings of the Seminar on Malnutrition in Early Life and Subsequent Mental Development. Washington, DC: Pan American Health Organization publication number 251.

Cravioto, J., DeLicardie, E. R., & Birch, H. G. (1966). Nutrition, growth, and neurointegrative development: An experimental and ecologic study. *Pediatrics, 38,* 319–372.

Cravioto, J., & Robles, B. (1965). Evolution of adaptive and motor behavior during rehabilitation from kwashiorkor. *American Journal of Orthopsychiatry, 35,* 449–464.

D'Amato, R. C. (1990). A neuropsychological approach to school psychology. *School Psychology Quarterly, 5,* 141–160.

DeLicardie, E. R., & Cravioto, J. (1973) Behavioral responsiveness of survivors or clinically severe malnutrition to cognitive demands. In J. Cravioto, L. Hambreau, & B. Vahlquist (Eds.), *Early malnutrition and mental development* (pp. 134–154). Uppsala: Almquist and Wiskell.

Dobbing, J. (1970). Undernutrition and the developing brain: The relevance of animal models to the human problem. *American Journal of Diseases of Children, 120,* 411–415.

Dobbing, J. (1974). The later development of the brain and its vulnerability. In J. A. Davis & J. Dobbing (Eds.), *Scientific foundations of pediatrics* (pp. 565–577). Philadelphia: W. B. Saunders.

Dobbing, J., & Kersley, J. B. (1963). The vulnerability of the developing brain. *Journal of Physiology, 166,* 134.

Eckholm, E., & Record, F. (1976). *The two faces of malnutrition.* New York: Worldwatch Institute.

Engel, R. (1956). Abnormal brain wave patterns in kwashiorkor. *Electroencephalography Clinical Neurophysiology, 8,* 489–500.

Engsner, G., Hable, D., Stogren, I., & Vahlquist, B. (1974). Brain growth in children with kwashiorkor. *Acta Paedatrica Scandinavica, 63,* 687–694.

Field, J. O., & Levinson, F. J. (1976). Nutrition and development: The dynamics of commitment. In N. S. Scrimshaw & M. Behar (Eds.), *Nutrition and agricultural development: significance and potential for the tropics* (pp. 13–23). New York: Plenum.

Freeman, J. M. (Ed.). (1985). *Prenatal and perinatal factors associated with brain disorders.* Washington, DC: U.S. Department of Health and Human Services, Public Health Service, National Institutes of Health, Publication no. 85-1149.

Galler, J. R. (1984). Behavioral consequences of malnutrition in early life. In J. R. Galler (Ed.), *Human nutrition: a comprehensive treatise: vol 5. Nutrition and behavior* (pp. 63–117). New York: Plenum.

Galler, J. R., Ramsey, F., Solimano, G., Lowell, W. E., & Mason, E. (1983). The influence of early malnutrition on subsequent behavioral development. *Journal of Child Psychiatry, 22,* 8–15.

Grantham-McGregor, S. M., Powell, C., Stewart, M. E., & Schofield, W. N. (1982). Longitudinal study of growth and development of young Jamaican children recovering from severe malnutrition. *Developmental Medicine and Child Neurology, 24,* 321–331.

Grantham-McGregor, S. M., Schofield, W., & Powell, C. (1987). Development of severely malnourished children who received psychosocial stimulation: Six-year follow-up. *Pediatrics, 79,* 247–254.

Grantham-McGregor, S. M., Stewart, M. E., & Desaix, P. (1978). A new look at the assessment of mental development in young children recovering from severe malnutrition. *Developmental Medicine and Child Neurology, 20,* 773–778.

Guthrie, G. M., Masangkay, A., & Guthrie, H. A. (1976). Behavior, malnutrition, and mental development. *Cross-Cultural Psychology, 7,* 169–180.

Hoorweg, J., & Stanfield, J. P. (1976). The effects of protein energy malnutrition in early childhood on intellectual and motor abilities in later childhood and adolescence. *Developmental Medicine and Child Neurology, 18,* 330–350.

Juntunen, K., Siroio, P., & Michelsson, K. (1978). Cry analysis in infants with severe malnutrition. *European Journal of Pediatrics, 128,* 241–246.

Kalat, J. W. (Ed.). (1984). *Biological psychology.* 2nd ed. Philadelphia: Wadsworth.

Lerner, J. S., & Hultsch, C. E. (1983). *Human development: a life-span perspective.* New York: McGraw Hill.

Lester, B. M. (1975). Cardiac habituation of the orienting response to an auditory signal in infants of varying nutritional status. *Developmental Psychology, 11,* 432–444.

Lester, B. M. (1976). Spectrum analysis of the cry sounds of well-nourished and malnourished infants. *Child Development, 47,* 237–241.

Lezak, M. D. (1983). *Neuropsychological assessment.* 2nd ed. New York: Oxford University.

Lien, N. M., Meyer, K. K., & Winick, M. (1977). Early malnutrition and "late" adoption: A study of their effects on the development of Korean orphans adopted into American families. *American Journal of Clinical Nutrition, 30,* 1734–1739.

Lloyd-Still, J. D., Hurwitz, I., Wolff, P. H., & Shwachman, H. (1974). Intellectual development after severe malnutrition in infancy. *Pediatrics, 43,* 306–311.

Lozoff, B. (1989). Nutrition and behavior. *American Psychologist, 44,* 231–236.

Lytle, L. D., Whitacre, C. S., & Nelson, M. F. (1984). Mechanisms of nutrient action on brain function. In J. R. Galler (Ed.), *Human nutrition: A comprehensive treatise: Vol 5. Nutrition and behavior* (pp. 223–258). New York: Plenum.

Mata, L. J. (1976). The environment of the malnourished child. In N. S. Scrimshaw & M. Behar (Eds.), *Nutrition and agricultural development: significance and potential for the tropics* (pp. 45–59). New York: Plenum.

McLaren, D. S., Yaktin, U. S., Kanawati, A. A., Sabbagh, S., & Kadi, Z. (1973). The subsequent mental and physical development of rehabilitated marasmic infants. *Journal of Mental Deficiency Research, 17,* 273–281.

McLaren, D. S., Yaktin, U. S., Kanawati, A. A., Sabbagh, S., & Kadi, Z. (1975). The relationship of severe marasmic protein-energy malnutrition and rehabilitation in infancy to subsequent mental development. In R. E. Olson (Ed.), *Protein-calorie malnutrition* (pp. 107–112). New York: Academic Press.

Monckeberg, F. (1975). The effect of malnutrition on physical growth and brain development. In J. W. Prescott, M. S. Read, & D. B. Coursin (Eds.), *Brain function and malnutrition: neuropsychological methods of assessment* (pp. 15–39). New York: Wiley.

Monckeberg, F. (1976). Definition of the nutrition problem-poverty and malnutrition in mother and child. In N. S. Scrimshaw & M. Behar (Eds.), *Nutrition and agricultural development: significance and potential for the tropics* (pp. 13–23). New York: Plenum.

Nelson, G. K., & Dean, R. F. (1959). The electroencephalogram in African children: effects of kwashiorkor and a note on the newborn. *Bulletin of the World Health Organization, 21,* 779–782.

Pantell, R. H., Fries, J. F., & Vickery, D. M. (1984). *Taking care of your child: A parent's guide to medical care.* rev. ed. Reading, MA: Addison-Wesley.

Patton, J. R., Payne, J. S., & Beirne-Smith, M. (1990). *Mental retardation.* 3rd. ed. Columbus, OH: Merrill Publishing.

Pereira, S. M., Sundararaj, R., & Begum, A. (1979). Physical growth and neurointegrative performance of survivors of protein-energy malnutrition. *British Journal of Nutrition, 42,* 165–171.

Pryor, G. (1975). Malnutrition and the critical period hypothesis. In J. W. Prescott, M. S. Read, & D. B. Coursin (Eds.), *Brain function and malnutrition: neuropsychological methods of assessment* (pp. 103–112). New York: Wiley.

Resnick, O. (1988). Nutrition, neurotransmitter regulation and developmental pharmacology. In F. J. Menolascino & J. A. Stark (Eds.), *Preventive and curative intervention in mental retardation* (pp. 161–176). Baltimore: Paul H. Brookes.

Richardson, S. A. (1972). Ecology of malnutrition: Non-nutritional factors influencing intelligence and behavioural development. *Pan American Health Organization Scientific Publication, 251,* 101–110.

Rozovski, J., Novoa, F., Abbarzua, J., & Monckeberg, F. (1970). Cranial transillumination in early severe malnutrition. *British Journal of Nutrition, 24,* 107–111.

Stinnett, J. D. (1983). *Nutrition and the immune response.* Boca Raton, FL: CRC Press.

Stoch, B. M., & Smythe, P. M. (1976). 15-Year developmental study on effects of severe undernutrition during infancy on subsequent physical growth and intellectual functioning. *Archives of the Disabled Child, 51,* 327–336.

Trowell, H. C., Davies, J. N. P., & Dean, R. F. A. (1954). *Kwashiorkor.* London: Edward Arnold.

Volpe, J. J. (1987). *Neurology of the newborn.* 2nd ed. Philadelphia: Saunders.

Winick, M. (1969). Malnutrition and brain development. *Journal of Pediatrics, 75,* 667–679.

Winick, M., Meyer, K. K., & Harris, R. C. (1975). Malnutrition and environmental enrichment by early adoption. *Science, 190,* 1173–1175.

Winick, M., & Rosso, P. (1969). Head circumference and cellular growth of the brain in normal and marasmic children. *Journal of Pediatrics*, 74, 774–778.

Winick, M., & Rosso, P. (1975). Malnutrition and central nervous system development. In J. W. Prescott, M. S. Read, & D. B. Coursin (Eds.), *Brain function and malnutrition: Neuropsychological methods of assessment* (pp. 41–51). New York: Wiley.

Yussen, S. R., & Santrock, J. W. (1982). *Child development: an introduction*. 2nd ed. Dubuque, IA: Brown.

CHAPTER 14

CONCLUSION: STRATEGIES FOR PREVENTION

Donald I. Templer, Lawrence C. Hartlage, and W. Gary Cannon

As has been shown in the preceding chapters, there are a large number of phenomena by which brains can be harmed. Interestingly, however, almost all of the sorts of brain damage discussed in this book are either directly or indirectly caused by humans and are therefore preventable. People do have control over their brain health to a greater extent than the health of most other organs and systems of their body. As an example, cancer is probably more determined by heredity and other factors presently outside of human control than brain abnormalities. Brain health appears to be very much a matter that could be and should be improved by public health education and intervention.

The recommendations for prevention here given are to some extent an extension of those recommended in the individual chapters and to some extent a synthesis. In this synthesis, a distinction is made between impact damage and chemical damage. One difference between impact damage and chemical damage is that the former may be observable and the latter is usually unseen. A related difference is that impact damage is usually instantaneous and the chemical damage is more likely to be insidious and occurring over a period of time. Chemical damage is usually diffuse, and impact damage has more comparative likelihood of focal components. More important to the focus of this final chapter is that the human element is different. Impact damage is more likely than chemical damage to be the result of intended aggression such as in assaults, fights, and contact sports. The aggressor wants to harm or subdue the other person but usually does not have brain damage as a central intent of the attack.

In chemical damage, the perpetrator is usually oneself or an institution or group of persons rather than one other person. Also chemical damage can ordinarily be attributed to more passive causes such as ignorance or irresponsibility.

PREVENTING IMPACT DAMAGE

Classification of brain damage prevention initiatives can be done on a threefold basis, including protective headgear, public health education, and legislation (and associated law enforcement). Public health education for impact damage should be directed by the media to the general population, especially toward those persons at high risk. Impact damage information should also be highly directed toward those segments of the general population that have the responsibility of preventing damage such as parents, grade school and high school teachers and athletic coaches, law enforcement officials, and college and university administrators and athletic coaches. As an example, in regard to legislation and law enforcement, child abuse and spousal abuse could be deterred by penalties at least as severe as those for assault to a stranger. As another related example, fighting could be treated as a crime almost as serious as assault. Too often, fighting between two voluntary combatants is regarded as a personal and minor matter that should not be brought to police attention. However, fighting can cause very serious injury to the brain.

A strong recommendation is the greater use of protective headgear in industry and sports, and by drivers and passengers of motor vehicles.

One radical and unquestionably controversial possibility is that both drivers and passengers of motor vehicles, as well as bicycles be required to wear helmets.

Perhaps a less radical possibility includes a requirement that adequate headgear should be worn in almost all relevant sports, professional or amateur, as played by children, adolescents, and adults. This would include such sports as wrestling and even a number of less obvious sports. For example, people are hit in the head by golf balls, as well as golf clubs. Recall the publicity surrounding a former President's golf ball hitting a spectator in the head! Mountain climbers and skiers would also be acting prudently if they wore protective helmets.

We recommend vigorous public education about the danger of head injuries and other brain assaults. Children should be taught precautions, such as wearing helmets in sports, just as they are taught to brush their teeth after eating and to stay away from potential molesters. On the adult level, the public should be informed about the risks of brain pathology just as they are about the risks associated with cigarette smoking.

The authors laud the public education carried out by subgroups as the National Head Injury Foundation (NHIF), the National Brain Injury Research Foundation (NBIRF), and the JMA Foundation. Membership in these foundations is open to brain-damaged individuals, their families, and professional persons. Although these groups are more focused upon rehabilitation than prevention, they do devote some attention to the former. The NHIF provides many booklets, books, pamphlets, cassettes, and videotapes that are quite understandable for the lay person. A more detailed description of these publications is contained in the

NHIF Catalog of Educational Material. NHIF's address is 333 Turnpike Road, Southboro, Massachusetts 01772. This address may also be used for the NHIF Newsletter. The newsletter contains news about both the national and state NHIF organizations. The JMA Foundation and the NBIRF produce magazines and journals oriented toward both lay and professional audiences.

Persons who have had a prior injury in sports or in other endeavors should be monitored closely, and any subsequent participation with risk for head injury should be monitored *very* closely. Any subsequent participation should not occur until after a return to normalcy. Neuropsychological testing would likely be helpful in such a determination. A related recommendation is that persons who could be accumulating mini-assaults such as boxers should be regularly tested before proceeding with relevant activities. Indeed, the California Boxing Commission has recently instituted such a program, and one of us (L.C.H.) is a consultant to that program.

Indeed, boxing provides such opportunity for illustrating how a number of prevention strategies can be implemented that it may be worthwhile to elaborate on one of these as a model for conceptualization and organized strategies for prevention. There have been recommendations, short of abolition, directed toward a lessening of the risk of brain damage. The research of Drew et al. (1986) found that the number of professional bouts, but not number of amateur bouts, was associated with degree of neuropsychological impairment. Does this suggest that making the professional rules similar to amateur rules would lessen the risk of brain damage? Let us now examine these and other recommendations for modification of boxing rules and regulations.

1. Decreasing the number of rounds is one such change that has been proposed. Common sense tells us that fewer rounds mean fewer punches and that fewer punches mean less brain damage. Also, the chances of a boxer being too dazed to protect himself are decreased. Nevertheless, our common sense also tells us that fewer rounds mean less brain damage rather than no brain damage. It would be like going from three packages of cigarettes to two packs of cigarettes in an attempt to avoid lung cancer and other respiratory disorders.

2. Decreasing the length of rounds has also been recommended. The advantages and limitations of such are essentially the same as in regard to number of rounds.

3. It has been suggested that boxers be examined and closely monitored so that a subsequent fight cannot be scheduled if the boxer's neurological and neuropsychological status are unfavorable or questionable. This is obviously a step in the right direction. However, in a sense it is like closing the barn door after the horse has run out. To give a human example, it is like going to the dentist *after* rather than *before* one's tooth starts hurting.

4. A recommendation is that a computer system for exchange of information among various states and countries be set up. Currently one could be forbidden

to box in one state, but allowed to box in another; or allowed to box in one country, but not in another. In 1979, Willie Classen was knocked unconscious in a bout in New York and died 5 days later. He had been under an indefinite medical suspension of the New York State Athletic Commission, but was cleared to fight when he lied about a fight in London 3 weeks earlier when he was knocked down three times and later complained of double vision. Fortunately, Classen's death did result in improvement in the New York State Athletic Commission's rules and practices that include increasing suspension after a knock-out from 30 to 90 days, recording amount of punishment a fighter absorbs in each bout, and postfight neurological tests, including computed axial tomography (CAT) scans.

5. It has been recommended that the matter of selecting ringside physicians should be reassessed. Currently, the physician is ordinarily hired by the promoter. This could result in a conflict of interest between the doctor's need to protect his patient and the business need to please the crowd (Moore, 1980).

6. Referees need better training in detecting when brain injury appears imminent, and they should be encouraged to have a conservative attitude. If in doubt, it is better to have the crowd be bored and go home disappointed than to have the boxer go home with a battered brain or to have a visit to the coroner's office.

7. The recommendation of disallowing blows to the head would certainly prevent head injury. Although it is certainly reasonable, the present authors would have reservations about a sport in which one person strikes another even in the torso. However, the relative dullness of such fights would hopefully cause a decrease in public boxing interest.

8. A modification of the boxing gloves has been recommended. It is generally believed that larger gloves provide greater protection. However, La Cava (1983) in arguing for lighter and thinner gloves stated: "Chronic injuries, much more frequent since the introduction of big gloves, are caused quite differently. It is well known that when the impact zone is limited, the force of the blow is *totally concentrated in that specific area*. When the impact zone is bigger the force is dissipated over a wider area. In this case, even if the impact is too small to cause a knock-out, repeated punches of this kind have a cumulative effect. The simple laws of physics discussed above explain why injuries increased after the introduction of bigger, heavier gloves. The big gloves prevent the more visible facial injuries, but cause much more injuries inside the cranium" (pp. 361–362).

High-risk persons, in general, should be encouraged to take appropriate precautions. Occupation and recreation are two variables obviously related to risks. Two demographic variables that are also clearly related to risk are gender and age. Young men tend to be accident prone and violence prone.

Although when we think of vehicle accidents we usually think of motor vehicles, both bicycle accidents involving a motor vehicle and those not involving such are common occurrences. The authors on numerous occasions have seen grade school children riding their bicycles after dark wearing dark clothes, with no lights and no reflectors. We urge both the rigorous enforcement of bicycle safety laws and the enactment of strict laws where they do not exist.

In California, we have the good fortune of having police officers who for the most part are well trained and who are very professional. Nevertheless, it is possible that all police departments are not as well endowed with well-trained officers. Police should be taught to strike a combative person on the head only if it is absolutely necessary.

PREVENTING CHEMICAL DAMAGE

Our two major recommendations for chemical damage prevention are (a) health education of the general public and especially those at high risk, and (b) legislation and associated law enforcement. Perhaps the legislation and law enforcement may even be more important than health education. We say this because some of the high-risk persons such as alcoholics and drug abusers may be unable to control their craving and unable to control the pressure from their environment. Many agricultural workers can do very little to prevent the pesticide toxicity. Starving children and adults in Ethiopia can do very little about the military and political situation there. Those persons who own and manage factories and farms must make a profit to survive the competition. However, if their competitors are also forced to better control their use of toxic chemicals, the competition can be better survived. The attempts of the federal, state, and local governments to control illegal drug use are not entirely unsuccessful. The same can be said about laws that prevent the sale of ethyl alcohol and the sale of certain solvents to minors.

In 1990, the April 23rd issue of *Time* (Planton, 1990) devoted considerable space to "Earth Day" activities related to improvement of the environment throughout the world. Among the recent environmental accomplishments described are imposing special taxes on carbon-dioxide emissions, toughening fuel-efficiency standards, and a ban on ozone-destroying chlorofluorocarbons by the end of the century. Concern for the environment is far from being a phenomenon confined to "Western" countries. A recent poll in Czechoslovakia revealed that 83% of respondents believed that environmental improvement should be the first priority of the new government.

Nevertheless, the authors do maintain that public health education in regard to chemical damage does have merit. In fact, one considered recommendation with both public health and legislation components is that all purchased containers of alcoholic beverages state that ethyl alcohol can be a danger to one's health, including the health of the brain. Also in regard to the substance abuse domain, it is recommended that the public be well informed of the short-term effects to the brain from alcohol and illegal drugs and some prescription drugs—along with the long-term effects, and the effects to the child from consumption by mothers during pregnancy. The basics of nutrition should be presented to the public much more than is currently the situation.

We applaud the efforts being made to educate high-risk groups about the brain damaging and other effects of Acquired Immune Deficiency Syndrome (AIDS). We are pleased that many high-risk persons are engaging in fewer high-risk activities. We are also concerned by the fact that some high-risk persons have not made changes in their high-risk activities.

The general public should be taught not only about the bad effects to the brain of chemical damage, but the apparent partial reversibility of some of this damage. This could provide hope that increases motivation for a more healthful lifestyle. Perhaps we assume damage is permanent too easily. As an example, for many years, there have been research reports (Fitzhugh, Fitzhugh, & Reitan, 1960; Fitzhugh, Fitzhugh, & Reitan, 1965; Goldstein & Chotlos, 1965) in which hospitalized alcoholics who had been abstinent about 2 weeks were significantly inferior to control subjects on the Trail Making Test, a task of perceptual-motor ability. However, in a subsequent study (Ayers, Templer, Ruff, & Barthlow, 1978), the performance of control subjects and members of Alcoholics Anonymous who had been abstinent at least a year were almost identical. Furthermore, a reversal of cortical atrophy observed on computerized tomography has been found after a rather short-term abstinence from alcohol.

Related to the ray of hope generated by partial reversibility is the "silver lining to the cloud of drug abuse" suggested by Lilliguist and Bigler. They appropriately reasoned that since research shows the permanent effects of some drugs upon the brain are often small or inconsistent, much emphasis should be placed upon rehabilitation at the early stage of drug abuse.

Thomas Robert Malthus, British economist (1766–1834), had a theory in which food played an important part. He maintained that the population of the world always increases at a faster rate than the necessities of life and that, generally speaking, people always live at the level of subsistence. Factors limiting population growth are famine, disease, and war. Malthus also blamed the lack of foresight of the poor. Was Malthus right or wrong? The present prosperity of North America and Europe do not appear congruent with his theory. In contrast, much of Africa and Asia do make Malthus' contentions sound reasonable. We contend that the starvation in the world can be attributed to both scarcity of resources and to human behavior. However, we maintain that the undesirable human behavior is more a function of economic and political systems, mismanagement, and to the greed of the wealthy and powerful, than to character defects of the poor.

Lappe and Collins (1986) challenged some of what they referred to as "myths" that might seem to indicate that growing more food would solve the world hunger problem. One of the "myths" is that there is not enough food. Lappe and

Collins said that enough grain alone is produced to provide all persons in the world 3,600 calories a day. They maintained that increases in food production in the past quarter century have outstripped the world's unprecedented population growth by about 16%. Although as many as 300 million Indian citizens go hungry, India remains near the top as a third world agricultural exporter, with an actual surplus of 24 million tons of wheat and rice. When the Sahelian countries of West Africa were suffering from severe drought and famine in the early 1970s, the value of their agricultural exports was three times that of their imports. Lappe and Collins stated that in South Africa 50,000 black children starve to death every year. Yet, South Africa's agricultural imports are exceeded by its exports. Most African governments spend less than 10% of their budgets on agriculture, with much larger expenditures for their military and police. Another "myth" Lappe and Collins attempted to discredit is that nature is to blame. In the well publicized 1985 drought in Ethiopia, only about 30% of the country's farm land was affected. The mainly conscripted army of 300,000 drained the availability of able-bodied people needed for heavy agricultural work. The government forcibly relocated over 200,000 peasants thought to be sympathetic to rebel forces. The worst starvation was found in areas where military forces burned the fields.

In regard to malnutrition in the United States, we do recommend more nutritional education, both in schools for children and through the public media of communication, for the general population, especially for those segments of the population that are at higher risk for malnutrition—persons with low income and with limited education. However, the problem with low income persons is not only a matter of knowledge. It is also a matter of allocation of resources. As Belden (1986) has pointed out, there are many people in the United States who are in poverty but, because of policies, regulations, and restrictions, are not eligible for food stamps. The same thing is true with programs for poor youngsters to receive free or reduced price breakfasts and lunches at school. Also, these meals at school often are less than optimal with respect to nutritional needs. Only half of impoverished persons over the age of 60 are eligible for the nutritional programs for the elderly.

It is possible that a vicious cycle exists in which poverty and ignorance lead to compromised brains; and malnourished brains and bodies are less capable of coping with and improving the limited resources in the environment. It is our opinion that intervention should target both the causes of malnutrition and the effects of malnutrition.

Space considerations did not permit a separate chapter on prenatal damage. The clinical and research literature, however, amply document the alarming incidence and severity of the fetal alcohol syndrome. This syndrome includes mental retardation, prenatal and postnatal growth retardation, distinctive abnormal facial features, and reduced head circumference. A number of different drugs, both illegal and legal, cause prenatal brain damage. Methadone-exposed children have more severe withdrawal symptoms both in utero and in the neonate than heroin-exposed children. Later in childhood, methadone-exposed in utero youngsters were found to have more neuropsychological deficits and behavioral problems than heroin-exposed children (Davis & Templer, 1988).

A final recommendation is that medical students, nursing students, physical education students, clinical, counseling and school psychology graduate students, and pharmacy students, should have a greater amount of material in their respective curricula on the prevention, recognition and treatment of brain damage.

Although this book has dealt with research that has not always permitted unequivocal inferences, and although technical material in a variety of areas has been presented, we are ending this book with a variety of simple rules for good brain health as illustrative of what could be presented to the general public.

RULES FOR GOOD BRAIN HEALTH

1. Wear adequate head protection gear for transportation, work, sports, and other recreation.
2. Wear seat belts in cars, trucks, buses, trains, and planes. Consider purchasing a car with air bags.
3. With contact sports, at least weigh the benefits against the risks.
4. Do not consume excessive amounts of alcohol.
5. Use no "street" drugs.
6. Only take drugs with the approval of your physician or, for over-the-counter drugs, your pharmacist.
7. Avoid any unsafe sexual behavior that could result in sexually transmitted diseases with potential neurological sequelae.
8. Avoid places where there is risk of assault, e.g., "rough" bars.
9. Take good care of your general health, especially your cardiovascular system.
   a. Have blood pressure monitored regularly, especially if hypertensive.
   b. Take high blood pressure medication regularly if prescribed by physician.
   c. Avoid obesity, or diet under the consultation of a physician if already obese.
   d. Do not consume excessive cholesterol or fats.
10. If pregnant, follow physician's advise to the letter especially in regard to drugs and alcohol.
11. In consideration of family planning, explore the possibility of familial neurological disorders with high heritability.
12. If recent head injury received, be extremely careful not to reinjure.
13. Do not drive under the influence of alcohol or drugs.
14. Be cautious about consenting to electroconvulsive therapy.
15. Monitor closely a high body temperature in yourself and your children.
16. If epileptic, regularly take medication to avoid seizures.

17. All persons who have seizures or syncope with no previous history of such should see a physician.
18. See physician for serious or lingering ear infections.
19. If diabetic, closely follow your physician's orders concerning both medication and diet.
20. Educate your children in brain health and safety.
21. Follow rules of brain safety at work. If needed rules are not in place, attempt to have them implemented.
22. Bear in mind that psychotropic medication could produce brain abnormality.
23. Hesitate to consent to psychosurgery without a second opinion.
24. Use extreme caution if riding a motorcycle, and do not permit your children to ride motorcycles until they are highly proficient. Do not ride as a passenger on a motorcycle without the person at the controls being a proficient rider. Always use a helmet when on a motorcycle.
25. Guard against heat stroke.
26. Avoid electrical injuries.
27. Do what you can to clean up and improve your environmental neurotoxin situation.
28. Report child abuse.
29. Discipline your own child with caution and restraint, avoiding physical means. Even mild shaking can damage a child's brain.

REFERENCES

Ayers, J. L., Templer, D. I., Ruff, C. F., & Barthlow, V. L. (1978). Trail making test improvement in abstinent alcoholics. *Quarterly Journal of Studies on Alcohol, 39*, 1627-1629.

Davis, D. D., & Templer, D. I. (1988). Neurobehavioral functioning in children exposed to narcotics in utero. *Addictive Behaviors, 13*, 275-283.

Drew, R. H., Templer, D. I., Schuyler, B. A., Newell, T. G., & Cannon, W. G. (1986). Neuropsychological deficits in active licensed professional boxers. *Journal of Clinical Psychology, 42*, 520-525.

Fitzhugh, L. C., Fitzhugh, K. B., & Reitan, R. M. (1960). Adaptive abilities and intellectual functioning in hospitalized alcoholics. *Quarterly Journal of Studies on Alcohol, 21*, 414-423.

Fitzhugh, L. C., Fitzhugh, K. B., & Reitan, R. M. (1965). Adaptive abilities and intellectual functioning of hospitalized alcoholics; further considerations. *Quarterly Journal of Studies on Alcohol, 26*, 402-411.

Goldstein, G., & Chotlos, J. W. (1965). Dependency and brain damage in alcoholics. *Perceptual and Motor Skills, 21*, 135-150.

La Cava, G. (1983). Prevention in boxing. *Journal of Sports Medicine, 23*, 361-363.

Lappe, F. M., & Collins, I. (1986). *World Hunger: Twelve Myths. A Food First Book.* Grove Press, Inc. New York.

INDEX

INDEX

INDEX

ATVs (All-terrain vehicles), 41, 52
Accidental injuries of children, 41–57
  and all-terrain vehicles (ATVs), 52–53
  and bicycles, 50
  epidemiology of, 41–43
  from falls, 43, 47–48
  incidence of, 41–43
  and motor vehicle accidents, 48–50
  as pedestrians, 48–50
  prevention of, 47
  risk for second injury, 46–47
  severity of, 42–44
Acetylcholine: and cannabis, 168
Affective disorders
  and ECT, 99
  and psychosurgery, 82
Age: neurotoxicity and aging, 139–141
  and risk of ECT induced brain
    damage, 104
  and risk for motor vehicle accident, 4
Aggression: and serotonin, 62
Agricultural neurotoxic substances, 132–160
  alternatives to pesticides, 141
  domestic exposure to pesticides, 137–
    138
  effects of chronic exposure to
    pesticides, 138–139
  exposure of agricultural workers to, 136
  neurotoxic pesticides, 132, 136–137
  prevention of occupational
    neurotoxicity, 141–143
  and senile dementia, 139–141
  symptoms of neurotoxicity, 133–136
Airbags, 9–11, 47
Air encephalographic studies, 18–19
Alcohol-induced brain damage, 146–157
  and benzodiazepine abuse, 181
  and bicycling accidents, 36–37
  children at risk of developing

alcoholism, 156
and cognitive rehabilitation, 150–153
and drowning, 34
and drug abuse, 163
evaluation of, 153–155
four stages of chronic substance abuse, 155
and heroin, 179
impairments of, 146
incidence of, 146
Korsakoff vs. NonKorsakoff, 147–150,
  152–153
and motor vehicle accidents, 10
prevention of, 155–156
solvent toxicity, 122, 126
treatment of, 153–155
American Academy of Pediatrics, 52
All-terrain vehicles, 41, 52
Amnesia; see Memory deficits
Amphetamines, 173–175
Amygdala
  and lead exposure, 116
  and psychosurgery, 80
Angel dust, 177–179
Anterior cingulum
  and psychosurgery, 80
Anticonvulsant medication
  and ECT, 102
  post-psychosurgery, 87–88
  see also Seizures
Anxiety disorders and psychosurgery, 82–83
Aquatic sports, 34
Armstrong, G., 101
Arsenic neurotoxin exposure, 114; see also
    Industrial toxins
Assault, 72–79
  and family violence, 77–78
  incidence of head injuries, 72–73
  misrepresented on TV, 72
  police brutality, 76–77

Assault (*continued*)
  torture, 73–74
  war, 74–76
Ataxia: and manganese exposure, 119
  and mercury exposure, 120
  and solvent toxicity, 122–124
Atrophy; *see* Cerebral atrophy
Attention deficit disorder, 207–208
Axonal injury
  and motor vehicle accidents, 6–8
  and mountain climbing, 32
  and solvent toxicity, 123

Barbiturates, 180–181
Bayley scales: and malnutrition, 204
Behavioral effects of brain damage, 46,
    62–63
  and child abuse, 61–62
  and malnutrition, 194–195, 199, 204
  and mercury exposure, 120
  and motor vehicle accidents, 5, 8
  and psychosurgery, 83
  and torture, 74
  see also Child Behavior Checklist,
    Vineland Adaptive Behavior Scales
Bender-Gestalt, 84, 100–101
Bender Visual Motor Gestalt test, 169
Benton Visual Retention Test, 100–101
Benzodiazepines, 180–181
Bicycling, 35–37, 50–52
Biomechanics and severity of injury
    estimates, 6
Bipolar disorder, 82, 99
Blood clots in brain
  and amphetamines, 173–174
  and cocaine, 171
  and drug abuse, 162
  and falls, 8
Booklet Category Test, 156
Boston Remote Memory Battery, 148
Boxing, 15–23
  brain damage assessment, 19–21, Frank
    Bruno, 15
  changes to sport, 15–16, 19
  medical precautions, 18–20
  neurological damage and symptoms,
    16–21
  punch drunk syndrome, 15–16, 19
Brain Age Quotient, 154
Brain development, 198–200
Bruno, Frank, 15

CT; *see* Computerized Tomography
CVAs; *see* Cerebrovascular accidents
Campbell, A. M. G., 168
Cannon, W. G., 21–22
Carbamate pesticide, 136–137
Carbon disulfide, 111, 123–124
Car seat, 49
Category Tests
  and alcoholics, 148
  and drug abusers, 162
  and heroin, 180
  and LSD, 176–177
  and polydrug abuse, 165–166
Cavum septi pellucidi, 17–18
Cerebral atrophy
  and benzodiazepine, 181
  and boxing, 16–21
  and cocaine, 172
  and drug abuse, 162, 168
  and ECT, 98–100
  and epileptics, 101
  and heroin, 179
  and inhalants, 182–183
  and Korsakoff and NonKorsakoff
    patients, 148
  and motor vehicle accident injuries,
    8
  and war injuries, 74
  see also Ventricle size
Cerebrovascular accidents (CVAs)
  and amphetamines, 174, 185
  and cocaine, 171–172, 185
  and drug abuse, 162
  and opiates, 178
Child abuse, 58–63
  and brain impairment, 59
  cycle of, 62–63
  diagnosis of brain injury of, 60–61
  incidence of, 58–59
  shaken baby syndrome, 59–60
  symptoms of, 60–62
Child Behavior Checklist, 46
Children
  and motor vehicle accidents, 4–5, 9
  and risk of domestic exposure to
    pesticides, 137–138
  see also Accidental injuries of, Child
    abuse, Malnutrition
Children's Coma Scale, 43
Cingulotomy, 88
Closed head injury; *see* Concussions

Cocaine, 170–173
  action of, 170
  and brain damage, 171
  crack, 171–172, 175
Code for head injuries, 7
Cognitive deficits
  in alcoholics, 147–152, 154, 157
  and child abuse, 61
  and drug abuse, 164–165, 178–179
  in head-injured children, 45
  and lead exposure, 115–117
  and mercury exposure, 120
  and motor vehicle accident injuries, 5,
    8
  post-ECT, 103
  and psychosurgery, 83, 89
  and solvent toxicity, 123–126
  as symptom of chronic neurotoxicity,
    133–134
Cognitive rehabilitation
  and alcoholics, 151–153
  and child abuse victims, 61
Color Sorting, 84
Coma
  and children, 42
  and aquatic sports, 34
  duration of, 5
  Glasgow Coma Scale, 9
  and lead exposure, 116
  and pesticide toxicity, 137
  and solvent toxicity, 122
Computerized Tomography (CT)
  and boxing, 18–22
  and child abuse injuries, 60–61
  and drug abuse, 162, 168
  and ECT induced injury, 99–100
  and heroin users, 179
  and inhalant users, 183
  and mild head injury, 44
  and sedative users, 180–181
Concussion
  and boxing, 18, 23
  and bicycling, 36–37
  and child abuse, 59–61
  and football, 24–25
  and hockey, 26
  and horseback riding, 33
  and motor vehicle accidents, 8
  and rugby, 25
  and skiing, 35
  and soccer, 31

  and wife abuse, 66
  and wrestling, 26
Contact sports, 15–29
  boxing, 15–23
  football, 23–25
  hockey, 26
  rugby, 23–25
  wrestling, 26
  see also Noncontact sports
Consumer Product Safety Commission
    (CSPSC), 52
Continuous Recognition Memory Test, 45
Convulsion; see Seizure
Corpus striatum, 175
Cortical Impact Injury Model, 6
Crack; see Cocaine

DDT (dichlorodiphenyltrichloroethane),
    132, 137–138
Dementia
  and agricultural chemicals, 139
  and solvent toxicity, 123
Demerol (meperidine), 179
Depression
  and ECT, 96, 99
  and lead exposure, 117–118
  and mercury toxicity, 120
  and psychosurgery, 81–83
  and solvent toxicity, 123–124
Dickstein, L. J., 66
Digit Symbol Substitution Test, 150
Domestic neurotoxic substances, 132,
    137–138; see also Agricultural
    neurotoxic substances
Dopamine
  and amphetamines, 173–174
  and cocaine, 170
  and MDMA and MDA, 175–176
  and MPTP, 164–165
  and PCP, 178
Drew, R. H., 21–22
Drug abuse, 161–192
  assessment of, 161–162
  cannabis, 166–170
  cocaine, 170–173
  inhalants, 182–184
  LSD, 176–177
  MDMA and MDA, 175–176
  MPTP, 164–165
  opiates, 179–180
  phencyclidine (PCP), 177–179

Drug abuse (*continued*)
  polydrug abuse, 165–166
  research limitations, 163
  sedatives, 180–181

ECT; *see* Electroconvulsive therapy
EEG; *see* Electroencephalography
Edema
  and children's injuries, 43–44
  and methyl chloride toxicity, 124
  and motor vehicle accidents, 8
  and tin toxicity, 121
  and war injuries, 74
Elder abuse, 77–78
Electroconvulsive therapy (ECT), 95– 107
  animal studies, 97–98, 101, 104
  and CT scans, 99–100
  and epileptics, 101–102
  human autopsies and, 98
  incidence of, 82, 89, 95–96
  and Korsakoff patients, 149
  modern era vs. pre-1960, 96
  recommendations for, 104–105
  and spontaneous seizures, 102–103
Electroencephalography (EEG)
  and boxers, 18–23
  detection of child abuse injuries, 61
  and drug abusers, 162
  and malnutrition, 204–206
  and mercury exposure, 120
  and soccer injuries, 32
  and torture victims, 74
Embedded Figures Test
  and Korsakoff subjects, 147
  to monitor for neurotoxicity, 142–143
Embolism; *see* Blood clot in brain
Emotional effects of brain damage
  and child abuse, 62
  and lead exposure, 116–117
  and mercury toxicity, 120
  and motor vehicle accidents, 8
  and psychosurgery, 83
  and solvent toxicity, 123–125
  and tin toxicity, 121
Environmental toxins; *see* Industrial
    toxins
Epileptic seizures
  and cocaine, 172
  epileptics vs. ECT patients, 101–102
  and inhalants, 183
  and PCP, 178

and penetrating head injury, 74
and psychosurgery, 85–87
Estimating severity of brain injury
  and child abuse, 59–60
  of children's injuries, 42–43
  effects of malnutrition, 203–208
  and motor vehicle accidents, 6
Etiology
  of abuse, 64
  of bicycling injuries, 35, 43
  of drowning, 34
  of MVAs, 3–4
Evans, M., 168

Falls, 43, 47–48
Family violence and brain impairment,
    58–71
  child abuse, 58–63
  prevention of, 67–69
  wife abuse, 63–71
  see also Assault, Child abuse
Fatality; *see* Mortality
Fatigue, 133–134
Female risk of head injury
  and girls' accidental injuries, 42
  and motor vehicle accidents, 4
  postlobotomy, 85
  and second head injury, 47
  and soccer, 31, 47, 85
Fighting; *see* Assault
Food and Drug Administration (FDA), 138
Football, 23–25
  and incidence of injury, 23
  and postinjury recommendations, 25
  and second head injury effects, 24
  and symptoms of head injury, 24
Four Word Short Term Memory Test: and
    detoxified alcoholics, 148
Frontal lobe damage
  and amphetamines, 174
  and ECT, 98–99
  and MDMA and MDA, 175
  and methyl chloride toxicity, 124
  and motor vehicle accidents, 8
  and psychosurgery, 80–87
Frontal lobe syndrome, 83, 86

GABA
  and benzodiazepine, 180
  and cannabis, 168
Gessell scales, 204

Glasgow Coma Scale: compared to
     Children's Coma Scale, 44-45
   and motor vehicle accidents, 9
   see also Coma
Glial pathology
   and epileptics, 101
   postECT in animals, 97
   postECT in humans, 98
Goldman, H., 100
Goldstein Block Designs, 84
Golf, 35
Gomer, F. E., 100
Griffiths Mental Development Scale
   and malnutrition, 205
Gray matter damage, 7
   and boxing, 171

HSCI (National Head and Spinal Cord
     Injury Foundation), 3
Halstead-Reitan Neuropsychological
     Battery
   and boxers, 21
   and children, 45
   drug abusers, 162
   and heroin users, 180
   and lobotomy patients, 84
   and LSD, 176
   and mild head injury, 5
   and PCP, 178
Hartelius, H., 97
Headache
   and carbon disulfide neurotoxicity, 123
   and methyl chloride neurotoxicity, 124
   symptom of chronic neurotoxicity, 133,
     135
   and trichloroethylene neurotoxicity,
     126
Head protection; see Helmets
Helmets
   and bicycling, 36, 51-52
   and boxing, 27
   and horseback riding, 33
   and motorcycle accidents, 9
   and mountain climbing, 32
   recommendations regarding, 76
   and sports, 38
   and war effectiveness, 75-76
Hematoma
   and boxing, 21
   and coma, 43
   and horseback riding, 33

and motor vehicle accidents, 7-9
   and postlobotomy, 86
Hemorrhages
   and amphetamines, 173
   and boxing, 23
   and cocaine, 171
   and football, 25
   and motor vehicle accidents, 8
   and mountain climbing, 32
   and postECT, 101
   postlobotomy, 86
   and psychosurgery, 83
   and strokes and drug abuse, 162
Heroin, 179-180
Hippocampus
   and boxing, 17
   in epileptics, 101
   and lead exposure, 116
   and MDMA and MDA, 175
   and PCP, 178
Hockey, 26
Hoffman, 95
Horseback riding, 33-34
Hypotension, 8
Hypoxaemia, 8
Hypoxia
   and inhalants, 182
   and lead exposure, 116
   and mountain climbing, 32

Impact injuries, 3-14
Industrial toxins, 111-131
   incidence of exposure, 111-113
   metal neurotoxins, 112-122
   neuropsychological assessment
     recommendations, 112
   neurotoxic solvents, 112-113, 116,
     122-126
Infants, 58
Inhalants, 182-184
International Classification of Diseases
     (ICD), 7
Ischemia; see Blood clots in brain

JMA Foundation, 215-216

Kwashiorkor, 194-195, 203, 205-207

LSD (lysergic and diethylamide), 176-177
Lead toxicity, 111, 114-118
   and drug abuse, 164

Lead toxicity (*continued*)
  exposure risks, 115
  incidence of exposure, 114
  inorganic lead exposure effects, 116
  mechanism of toxicity, 115–116
  organic lead exposure effects, 115–116
  toxicity of, 111
Lesions
  and aggression, 62
  and boxing, 17
  and children, 43–44
  in epileptics, 101
  and inhalants, 183
  and mercury exposure, 120
  and motor vehicle accidents, 7
  postECT, 100–101
  and psychosurgery, 80
Leukotomy, 80; *see also* Lobotomy
Limbic system damage, 8
Lobotomy, 80–87
  bilateral prefrontal, 84–85
  declining incidence of, 80
  frontal lobe, 80
  Grantham, 84
  postsurgery studies, 83–87
  transorbital, 80
  as treatment for depression, 80
Loss of consciousness
  and child abuse, 61
  and football, 24
  and solvent toxicity, 122
  and torture victims, 72–74

MDA (methylenedioxyamphetamine),
  175–176
MDMA
  (methylenedioxymethamphetamine)
  (ectasy), 175–176
MPTP; *see* Drug abuse
MRI; *see* Magnetic resonance imaging
MVAs; *see* Motor vehicle accidents
Magnetic resonance imaging (MRI)
  and boxers, 20–21
  and inhalants, 183
  pre- and postECT, 100
Males
  accidental injuries of boys, 42
  and assault risk, 73
  and bicycle injuries, 35, 37
  and mild head injuries in boys, 44
  and risk of motor vehicle accidents, 4

and postlobotomy, 85
and second head injuries, 46
and soccer injuries, 31
and wife battering, 64
Malnutrition, 193–213
  and brain development, 197–200
  concurrent effects of, 203–204
  consequences of, 202–208
  epidemiological estimates, 197
  evaluation of, 196–197
  intermediate effects of, 204–205
  kwashiorkor and marasmus, 194–195,
    203, 205–207
  long-term effects of, 205–208
  overview, 193–197
  prenatal, 193, 200–201
  postnatal, 194
Manganese neurotoxicity, 118–119
Marasmus, 194–195, 203, 205–207
Marijuana, 166–170
Martland, H. S., 15–16
Maternal nutrition, 198–201, 206; *see also*
    Malnutrition, prenatal
McCarthy Scales of Children's Abilities, 205
Memory deficits
  alcohol induced, 149–150, 153
  and boxing, 16–19
  of children with mild head injury, 44–45
  and ECT, 96, 103
  and horseback riding injuries, 33
  and inhalant use, 183
  and Korsakoff vs. NonKorsakoff
    alcoholics, 147–148
  and lead exposure, 115–118
  and malnutrition, 207
  and manganese neurotoxicity, 119
  and mild head injury, 5
  and PCP, 178
  postpsychosurgery, 85–86, 89
  and solvent toxicity, 123
  and symptoms of neurotoxicity, 133–134
  and tin toxicity, 121
  and torture victims, 74
  and the "vanishing cues" recovery
    technique, 153
Meperidine (Demerol®), 179
Mercury neurotoxicity, 111, 119–121
  neuropsychological deficits from, 120–121
  neurotoxicity of, 111
  risk for exposure, 119
Methyl chloride neurotoxicity, 124

Methylenedioxyamphetamine (MDA),
    175–176
Methylenedioxymethamphetamine
    (MDMA), 175–176
Methyl-phenyl-tetrahydo-pyridine (MPTP),
    164–165
Michigan Eye-Hand Coordination Test
    and methyl chloride toxicity, 124
Mild head injury
    and bicycling injuries, 51
    and boxing, 21
    and child abuse, 60
    and children, 43–46
    and motor vehicle accidents, 3–6
Moderate head injury
    and children, 43, 45–46
    and horseback riding, 33
    and motor vehicle accidents, 5
    and the WRAT, 45
Morphine, 179
Mortality
    and accidental injuries of children, 42
    and battered women, 65
    and bicycling injuries, 36–37, 50–52
    and boxing, 23
    and children's falls, 47
    and criminal homicides, 72
    and football, 23–24
    and horseback riding, 33
    and motor vehicle accidents, 7–10
    and mountain climbing, 32
    and pesticide toxicity, 137
    and postECT, 98
    and postpsychosurgery, 82–89
    and sedatives, 180
    and solvent toxicity, 122, 125
    and war injuries, 74
    of wife abusers, 66
    see also Helmets
Mothers Against Drunk Driving (MADD),
    10
Motor incoordination, 133, 135–136
Motor vehicle accidents (MVAs), 3–14
    biomechanics of MVA injury, 6–7
    consequences of MVA head injuries, 4–6
    epidemiology of, 3–4, 10
    injuries of children, 43
    neurological features of MVA head
        injuries, 7–9
    prevention of MVAs and MVA head
        injuries, 7, 9–11

Mountain climbing, 32
Multiple sclerosis, 135–136
Myelin degeneration
    and boxing, 17
    and malnutrition, 198–200
    and tin toxicity, 121
    and trichlorethylene toxicity, 125–126

NHIF; see National Head Injury
    Foundation
NIOSH; see National Institute of
    Occupational Safety and Health
National Brain Injury Foundation (NBIRF),
    215–216
National Head and Spinal Cord Injury
    (HSCI) Survey, 3, 8
National Head Injury Foundation (NHIF),
    3, 215–216
National Highway Transportation Safety
    Agency (NHTSA), 10
National Institute of Aging, 139–140
National Institute of Occupational Safety
    and Health, 111, 114
National Institute on Drug Abuse, 161
Nerve gas; see organophosphate
    pesticides
Neurocognitive deficits
    and boxing, 16–23
    and lead exposure, 116
    and motor vehicle accidents, 5, 7–8
    and torture, 73–74
Neurofibrillary tangles, 17
Neuronal pathology
    and amphetamines, 174
    and epileptics, 101
    and lead exposure, 116–117
    and malnutrition, 198–200
    postECT in animals, 97
    postECT in humans, 98
Neuropsychological deficits
    and abstinent alcoholics, 150–151
    and battered women, 66
    and cannabis, 168
    of children, 44–45
    and heroin, 180
    and inhalant abusers, 183–184
    and Korsakoff vs. NonKorsakoff
        alcoholics, 148
    and lead exposure, 115–117
    and mercury exposure, 120
    and PCP, 178

Neuropsychological deficits (*continued*)
  and polydrug abuse, 165–166
  and postECT, 96
  and sedative abuse, 181
  and solvent toxicity, 122–126
  and tin toxicity, 121
Neuropsychological Impairment Scale
  (NIS), 154
Neurotoxicity Screening Survey, 141–142
Newell, T. G., 21–22
Noncontact sports, 30–40
  aquatic, 34
  bicycling, 35–37
  degree of risk, 37–38
  equestrian, 33–34
  golf, 35
  mountain climbing, 32
  safety recommendations, 37–39
  skiing, 35
  soccer, 30–32
  see also Contact sports
Norepinephrine
  and amphetaminess, 173–174
  and cocaine, 170
  and MDMA and MDA, 175
  and PCP, 178
Numbness, 133, 135

OSHA (Occupational Safety and Health
  Act), 111, 119
Obsessive-compulsive disorder
  and psychosurgery, 82–83, 85, 87
Occipital lobe
  and frontal lobe damage, 8
  and mercury exposure, 120
Occupational Safety and Health Act
  (OSHA)
  and mercury exposure, 119
  and neurotoxin exposure, 111
Opiates, 179–180
Organic solvent syndrome, 111
Organic syndrome
  and boxing, 19
  and postlobotomy, 87
  and psychosurgery, 82
Organochlorine pesticides, 132, 137
Organophosphate pesticides, 136–137

PCP (phencyclidine), 177–179
PET; *see* Positron emission tomography
Paced Auditory Serial Addition Test, 31

Paranoid, 82
Parietal lobe damage
  and frontal lobe damage, 8
  and methyl chloride toxicity, 124
  postECT, 99
  and Tactual Performance Test, 162
Parkinsonian symptoms
  and agricultural chemical exposure, 139–141
  and boxing, 17
  and MPTP, 164–165
Patient's Assessment of Own Functioning
  Inventory (PAOFI), 154
Peripheral nerve conduction velocity
  (NCV) testing, 142, 144
Personality changes and brain damage
  and methyl chloride toxicity, 124
  and lead exposure, 115–117
  and postlobotomy, 85–86, 88
  symptoms of chronic neurotoxicity,
    133–134
Phencyclidine, 177–179
Police brutality, 76–77
  etiology of, 76
  recommendations for police protection
    and training, 77
Porteus Maze test, 84
Positron emission tomography, 172
Post traumatic stress disorder (PTSD), 61
Prefrontal cortex
  and cocaine use, 172–173
  and impact injuries to the back of the
    head, 8
Preinjury status
  of head injured children, 46
  and ECTs, 104
  and motor vehicle accident induced
    head injury, 4–6
Present State Examination, 88
Prevention of brain injury, 214–222
  and chemical damage, 218
  and children, 47–53
  and impact damage, 215–218
  and motor vehicle accidents, 9–11
  and sports, 27, 36–39
Protein deficiency, 194–195
Psychosis, 133, 136
Psychosurgery, 80–94
  efficacy of, 81–82
  history of, 80
  incidence of, 80–81
  indications for, 81–82

negative consequences of, 89–90
newer era of, 87–89
primitive era of, 83–87
recommendations for, 90

Quantity Frequency Index, 154
Quick Neurological Screening Test, 21

Race
  and accidental injuries of children, 42
  and beating deaths, 72
Randt Memory Test, 21
Raven Progressive Matrices
  and sensitivity to mercury toxicity, 120
  and soccer, 31
Rey Auditory Verbal Learning Test
  and lead exposure, 118
Rey's embedded figures, 125
Rhythm Test
  and PCP, 178
Ruff, C. F., 101
Rugby, 23–25

Safety belts, 9–11, 48–49
Safety measures, 27; see also Helmets,
  Airbags, Safety belts, Prevention of
  brain injury
Schizophrenics
  and ECT treatment, 96, 101
  and psychosurgery, 82–84
Schuyler, B. A., 21–22
Sedatives, 166, 180–181
Seizures
  and amphetamines, 174
  and benzodiazepine withdrawal, 180
  and cocaine, 172
  and inhalants, 183
  and lead toxicity, 116
  and PCP, 178
  and pesticide toxicity, 137
  postECT, 98, 101–104
  postpsychosurgery, 83–89
  symptom of chronic neurotoxicity, 136
  and tin toxicity, 121
  see also Epileptic seizures
Selective Reminding Test, 45
Sensory disturbances
  as symptoms of chronic neurotoxicity,
    133, 136
Serial sevens
  and lobotomy patients, 84

Serotonin
  and aggression, 62
  and cannabis, 168
  and LSD, 176
  and MDMA and MDA, 175–176
Severe head injury
  and children, 42–46, 51
  and horseback riding, 33
  and Motor vehicle accidents, 6, 8, 9
  and the WRAT, 45
  see also Mortality
Sexual dysfunction, 133, 135
Shaken baby syndrome, 59–60; see also
  Child abuse
Shipley Hartford finger dexterity measure,
  84
Shipley Hartford finger tweezer measure, 84
Shipley test for abstraction
  and alcoholics, 84, 151
Skiing, 35
Skull fracture
  and boxing, 23
  and child abuse, 59, 61
  and children, 43
  and elder abuse, 78
  and motor vehicle accidents, 7
  and mountain climbing, 32
Sleep Disturbance, 133–134
Soccer, 30–32
Socioeconomic level
  and accidental injuries of children, 42
  and assault risk, 73
Solvent toxicity, 122–126; see also Carbon
  disulfide, Methyl chloride, Styrene,
  Toluene, Trichloroethylene
Spillane, J. D., 16–18
Sports; see Contact sports, Noncontact
    sports
Stanford Binet
  and malnutrition, 208
Stark, R., 76
Stimulants, 173–175, 178
Styrene, 124–125
Substantia nigra
  in retired boxers, 17
Symbol Digit Modalities Test, 31

THC (tetrahydrocannabinol), 167, 170
Tactual Performance Test (TPT)
  and alcoholics, 148
  and drug abusers, 162

Tactual Performance Test (*continued*)
  and heroin users, 179
  and inhalant abusers, 184
  and LSD users, 177
  and polydrug abuse, 165
Templer, D. I., 21–22, 100, 101
Temporal lobe damage
  in epileptics, 101
  and motor vehicle accidents, 8
Tetrahydrocannabinol (THC), 167
Thompson, J. L. G., 168
Time Perception Test
  and drug abuse, 169
Tin toxicity, 121–122
Toluene toxicity, 125
  and inhalants, 182
Tool Matching Test
  and drug abuse, 169
Topectomy, 89
Torture, 73–74
Tractotomy, 86–88
  bifrontal, 86–87
  stereotoxic, 87–88
  subcaudate, 88
  see also Psychosurgery
Trail Making Test
  and alcoholics, 151–152, 219
  and drug abusers, 162
  and inhalant abusers, 184
  and LSD, 176–177
  and polydrug abuse, 165–166
  and sedatives, 181
Traumatic encephalopathy; *see* Boxing,
  punch drunk syndrome
Trichloroethylene toxicity, 125–126

Unipolar disorder: and psychosurgery, 83

Vascular pathology
  and amphetamines, 173–174
  and cocaine, 171–172
  and drug abuse, 162
  and opiates, 178
  and PCP, 178
  and solvent toxicity, 123
  postECT, 97–98
Ventricle size
  and drug abuse, 162, 168
  and heroin, 179
  and inhalants, 183
  postECT, 98–100

Vineland Adaptive Behavior Scales
  and head injured children, 46

WAIS; *see* Wechsler Adult Intelligence Scale
WISC-R; *see* Wechsler Intelligence Scale
  for Children-Revised
WRAT; *see* Wide Range Achievement Test
War
  and penetrating head injuries, 74–75
Wechsler Adult Intelligence Scale (WAIS)
  and alcoholics, 151–152, 54
  and boxing, 21
  and drug abusers, 162
  and ECT patients, 101
  and inhalants, 183–184
  and lead exposure, 118
  and LSD, 177
  measure of mercury toxicity, 120
  measure of solvent toxicity, 125
  neurotoxicity monitoring, 142
  and PCP, 178
  and polydrug abuse, 165–166
  postpsychosurgery, 84, 86, 89
  and sedatives, 181
Wechsler-Bellvue Intelligence Scale, 84, 86
Wechsler Digit Span subtest, 84
Wechsler Digit Symbol subtest, 84
Wechsler Intelligence Scale for Children-
  Revised (WISC-R)
  comparing levels of head injury, 45
  and malnutrition, 207
Wechsler Memory Scale
  and alcoholics, 156
  and PCP, 178
Weigl Form Sorting, 84
White matter damage, 7
  and boxing, 21
  and heroin, 162
  and inhalants, 183
Wide Range Achievement Test, 45
Wife abuse
  and brain impairment, 65
  etiology of, 64
  incidence of, 65
  typical assault and injuries, 66
  see also Family violence
Williams, M. J., 168
Wisconsin Card Sorting, 148, 151
World Health Organization (WHO) and
  carbon disulfide toxicity, 123–124
Wrestling, 26

212-838-7426

Personality and Social Encounter

Jeffrey Parker

c. 6/10/81

Personality

and Social

Encounter

Selected Essays

by Gordon W. Allport

Beacon Press   Boston

Preface

What is human personality?

Some would say that it is an ineffable mystery—a shaft of creation, an incarnation. Since no man can transcend his own humanity, he cannot hold the full design of personality under a lens. The radical secret will ever elude us.

Others would say that personality is a product of nature. It is a nervous-mental organization, which changes and grows, while at the same time remaining relatively steadfast and consistent. The task of science is to explain both the stability and the change.

Those who hold either of these views—or both views—are right. And there are other possible answers to our question, likewise paradoxical.

Some say that personality is a self-enclosed totality, a solitary system, a span pressed between two oblivions. It is not only separated in space from other living systems, but also marked by internal urges, hopes, fears and beliefs. Each person has his own pattern, his own unique conflicts; he runs his own course, and he dies alone. This point of view is correct.

But others say that personality is social in nature, wide open to the surrounding world. It owes its existence to the love of two mortals for each other and is maintained through love and nurture freely given by others. Personality is affiliative, symbiotic, sociable. Culture cooperates with family in molding its course. "No man is an island." This view, too, is right.

The essays in this volume, I trust, give full recognition to the truth that lies in all these divergent positions. If Parts I and II favor the "self-enclosed totality," I hope Parts III, IV and V show that personality is "wide open to the world." As for the metaphysical paradox, I hold that any *valid* naturalistic approach must have open doors and clear windows, so that our chance of glimpsing ultimate philosophical and religious truth may not be blocked.

My own approach is naturalistic, but open-ended. Naturalism, as I see it, is too often a closed system of thought that utters premature and trivial pronouncements on the nature of man. But it can and should be a mode of approach that deliberately leaves unsolved the ultimate metaphysical questions concerning the nature of man, without prejudicing the solution. My essays are all psychological, and therefore naturalistic, but they have one feature in common—a refusal to place premature limits upon our conception of man and his capacities for growth and development.

A word about the selection of essays for this volume: they are neither "technical" nor "popular." They have been written either to amplify the theory of personality contained in my book *Personality: a psychological interpretation* (1937) or to express my concern with topical problems in social psychology. My belief that personality is both a self-contained system and open to the world accounts for the title of this collection, *Personality and social encounter*. Five of the papers were previously included in *The nature of personality: selected papers* (1950); but, since that collection is out of print, it seems convenient to reprint them here. Some of the chapters have been revised for the present publication.

In preparing this volume I have had helpful advice and assistance from Professor P. A. Bertocci; from my wife, Ada L. Allport; from Mr. Alan Levensohn, Mrs. Eleanor Sprague and Mrs. Katherine F. Bruner. I should like to express my gratitude to them all, as well as to Edward Darling, director of Beacon Press, who insists that my thoughts are worthy of a fresh printing.

Gordon W. Allport

CAMBRIDGE, MASSACHUSETTS
FEBRUARY 1960

Acknowledgments

I wish to acknowledge with thanks permission to reprint certain materials from the following sources:

AMERICAN JOURNAL OF ORTHOPSYCHIATRY for "The trend in motivational theory," 1953.

AMERICAN PSYCHOLOGICAL ASSOCIATION for two articles from *Journal of Abnormal and Social Psychology*: "What is a trait of personality?" 1931, and "The open system in personality theory," 1960. For three articles from *Psychological Review*: "The ego in contemporary psychology," 1943; "The psychology of participation," 1945; "Scientific models and human morals," 1947.

CRANE REVIEW for "Religion and prejudice," copyright 1959 by Crane Theological School, Tufts University.

BEACON PRESS for "A psychological approach to the study of love and hate," Chap. 5 in P. A. Sorokin (ed.), *Explorations in Altruistic Love and Behavior*, 1950; "Techniques for reducing group prejudice," Chap. 24 in P. A. Sorokin (ed.), *Forms and Techniques of Altruistic and Spiritual Growth*, 1954.

BRITISH JOURNAL OF EDUCATIONAL PSYCHOLOGY, University of Edinburgh, for "Geneticism *versus* ego-structure in theories of personality," 1946.

HARPER & BROTHERS for "Normative compatibility in the light of social science," in A. H. Maslow (ed.), *New Knowledge in Human Values*, 1959.

HOLT, RINEHART & WINSTON, INC., for "What units shall we employ?" Chap. 9 in G. Lindzey (ed.), *Assessment of Human Motives*, Rinehart, 1958.

THE PERSONALIST, School of Philosophy, University of Southern California, for "The psychological nature of personality," 1953.

PUBLIC OPINION QUARTERLY, Princeton University, for "An analysis of rumor" (with Leo Postman), 1946-1947.

SOCIETY FOR THE PSYCHOLOGICAL STUDY OF SOCIAL ISSUES, University of Michigan, for "Guidelines for research in international cooperation," *Journal of Social Issues*, 1947.

SOCIOLOGICAL REVIEW, University College of North Keele, for "Personality: normal and abnormal," 1958.

UNIVERSITY OF ILLINOIS PRESS for "The role of expectancy," Chap. 2 in H. Cantril (ed.), *Tensions That Cause Wars*, 1950.

SOCIETY OF PUBLIC HEALTH EDUCATORS, INC., Health Education Monograph Committee, for "Perception and public health," *Health Education Monograph*, 1958.

TRUSTEES OF COLUMBIA UNIVERSITY for "The limits of social service," in J. E. Russell (ed.), *National Policies for Education, Health and Social Services*, Bicentennial Conference Series, Doubleday, 1955.

Acknowledgments

I wish to acknowledge with thanks permission to reprint certain materials from the following sources:

Table of Contents

Preface   v

PART I: *An Approach to Personality*
1. Personality: a problem for science or for art?   3
2. The psychological nature of personality   17
3. The open system in personality theory   39
4. Scientific models and human morals   55

PART II: *Motivation and Structure*
              in Personality
5. The ego in contemporary psychology   71
6. The trend in motivational theory   95
7. What units shall we employ?   111
8. What is a trait of personality?   131
9. Geneticism *versus* ego-structure   137

PART III: *Normative Problems in Personality*
10. Personality: normal and abnormal   155
11. Circles of interest and the resolution of conflict   169
12. The psychology of participation   181
13. A basic psychology of love and hate   199

PART IV: *Group Tensions*
14. Prejudice in modern perspective   219
15. Techniques for reducing group prejudice   237
16. Religion and prejudice   257

PART V: *Perception and Social Programs*

17. Social service in perspective   271
18. Perception, proception and public health   295
19. The analysis of rumor (with Leo Postman)   311
20. Expectancy and war   327
21. Guidelines for research in international
        cooperation   347

    Bibliography (1921-1963)   363
    Index of Names   377
    Index of Subjects   383

PART I: *An approach to personality*

CHAPTER I

Personality: a problem for science or for art?

There are two principal approaches to the detailed study of human personality: *literature and psychology*.

Neither is "better" than the other; each has its distinctive merits and ardent devotees. Too often, however, partisans of one method heap scorn upon the other. This essay attempts a reconciliation and, in so doing, etches a scientific-humanistic frame for the study of personality.

The present essay, based on a lecture at Smith College, first appeared in the Rumanian journal *Revista de Psihologie* in 1938. Some years later the editor of this journal, Nicholas Margineanu, an able psychologist and outspoken social democrat, fell a martyr to the political ravages that swept his native land.

Readers who have a special interest in this topic will find a more extended and more technical discussion in my monograph *The use of personal documents in psychological science* (1942).

Already in the twentieth century three great revolutions have occurred in man's thinking about his own mind. These are, first, Freudian psychoanalysis, with its discovery of the depth and the emotion in mental life; second, Behaviorism, with its discovery of the accessibility of mind to objective study; and, third, Gestalt psychology, with its discovery of the essential orderliness and self-regulation of mind. It is not at all unlikely that these new modes of thought will revolutionize our ways of life during the present century, much as the natural and biological sciences revolutionized ways of life during the past century. We may well expect them to affect profoundly the morals, manners and mental health of our generation and of generations to come. Psychology, it is often said, is destined to become *the* science of the twentieth century.

Now, one of the most significant happenings in the first part of the twentieth century has been the discovery—to which Freudian, Behavioristic and Gestalt psychologies have all contributed—that human *personality* is an accessible subject for scientific probing. It is this event, above all others, I think, that is likely to have the most practical consequences for education, for ethics and for mental health.

3

But before getting into the problem of personality, I should like to dwell for a moment upon the somewhat stormy state of psychological science today. It sometimes seems to me that all the four winds of the intellectual heavens had collided in one storm center, competing for mastery, with the outcome as yet unsure.

According to a division commonly adopted, there are exactly four winds in the intellectual heavens, springing from the four basic provinces of research and learning—the natural sciences, the biological sciences, the social sciences and the humanities. Have you ever thought before that it is in the territory of psychology, and *only there*, that all these four intellectual winds collide and run a tempestuous course? I suppose it is natural enough that they should do so, for only by the aid of all the inventions and all the resources of the mind can the creative mind itself be adequately explored.

From the *natural sciences* comes the colossal impact of scientific methodology. I suppose that in the entire history of human thought there never was a case where one science has been bullied by another science as psychology is bullied by her elder sister science, physics. And I suppose no younger sister ever had so acute an inferiority complex as psychology has in relation to her well-groomed and socially correct elder sister. The desire to emulate the success of physics has led psychology to import at an increasing rate instruments of precision and mathematics into its treatment of mental life. Heaven help the psychologist nowadays who doesn't know his amplifiers and electrical circuits. It is, of course, particularly in the study of sensation that the physical sciences dominate psychology, though it is also true that their influence is felt throughout the entire structure of psychological science.

From the *biological sciences* also come high standards and exacting methods of research, as well as the evolutionary and organismal points of view without which psychology would still be scholastic in character. But the freshening winds of biology have not blown gently and with moderation; they have blown, rather, with the force of a gale, so forcefully that in many quarters they have threatened to push every vestige of humanism out, leaving psychology with a plague of rats. Today it is probably true that more rats are used in the American laboratories of psychology as subjects than men, women and children combined. Some people feel that what psychology really needs is an efficient Pied Piper.

It is, then, the impact of the natural and biological sciences upon psychology that accounts for its obsession to reach the eminence of scientific respectability. The methodological advances have indeed been considerable; but the findings from these points of approach have not as yet by any manner of means solved the problems of human personality. Their value lies chiefly in their advancement of sensory and reflex psychology—or, as someone has a bit derisively called it, "eye-ear-nose-and-throat" psychology.

In recent years the third wind has risen likewise to the force of a gale. *Social science* is causing a tornado all its own. It refuses to blend amicably with natural and biological science, but claims mind pretty much as its own province for study. Anthropologists and sociologists give no quarter. Mind, they insist, takes its form almost wholly in response to cultural demands. Language precedes the individual; so, too, do the religion, the morals, the economic system into which the individual is born. Mind, then, is a matter not for instrumental or biological study but for cultural study. A large number of psychologists have been converted, at least partially, to this view and recently have staged a rebellion within their own ranks, four hundred of them forming a society to investigate as realistically as possible the fate of mind as it is conditioned and constrained by the gigantic movements of contemporary society.

The last wind that blows in our storm center is gentler and less voracious. Yet its presence is always felt. In spite of all counter currents, it is perhaps still the prevailing wind. It is the wind of humanism. After all is said and done, it is philosophy and literature, and not the natural, biological or social sciences, that have fostered psychology throughout the ages. Only in comparatively recent years has psychology detached itself from philosophy and from art to become the storm center that it is.

Now we come to personality. One of the outstanding events in psychology of the present century has been the discovery of personality. Personality, whatever else it may be, is the substantial, concrete unit of mental life that exists in forms that are definitely single and individual. Throughout the ages, of course, this phenomenon of personal individuality has been depicted and explored by the humanities. The more aesthetic philosophers and the more philosophical artists have always made it their special province of interest.

Tardily, psychologists have arrived on the scene. One might almost say they are beginning two thousand years too late. The psychologist's work, it might seem, has been done for him, and done most brilliantly. With his scant and recent background, the psychologist looks like a conceited intruder. And so he is, in the opinion of many literati. Stephan Zweig, for example, speaking of Proust, Amiel, Flaubert and other great masters of characterization, says: "Writers like these are giants in observation and literature, whereas in psychology the field of personality is worked by lesser men, mere flies, who have the safe anchorage of a frame of science in which to place their petty platitudes and minor heresies."

It *is* true that the giants of literature make psychologists, who undertake to represent and to explain personality, seem ineffectual and sometimes a bit foolish in comparison. Only a pedant could prefer the dry collections of facts that psychology can offer regarding an individual mental life to the glorious and unforgettable portraits that the gifted novelist, dramatist or biographer can give. The literary artist creates his account; the psychologist merely compiles his. In the one case a unity emerges, self-consistent even through its subtleties of change. In the other case a ponderous accumulation of discontinuous data piles up.

One critic has put the matter crisply. Psychology, he remarks, whenever it deals with human personality, is only saying what literature has always said, and is saying it much less artfully.

Whether this unflattering judgment is entirely correct, we shall soon see. For the moment it serves at least to call attention to the significant fact that in a sense literature and psychology are competitors; they are the two methods par excellence for dealing with the personality. The methods of literature are those of art; the methods of psychology are those of science. Our question is: which approach is the more suitable for the study of personality?

Literature has had centuries of headstart, and it has been served by genius of the highest order. Psychology is young and has bred as yet few, if any, geniuses in the depiction and explanation of human personality. Being youthful, it would be becoming for psychology to learn a few basic truths from literature.

To show what it can profitably learn, let us take a concrete example. I have chosen one from ancient times in order to show clearly the maturity and ripeness of literary wisdom. Twenty-three hundred years ago, Theophrastus, Aristotle's pupil and successor at the Lyceum in Athens, wrote a number of brief characterizations of certain of his Athenian acquaintances. Thirty of his sketches have survived.

The sketch that I shall select is called "The Coward." Please note its timelessness. The coward of today is essentially the same kind of mortal as the coward of antiquity. Please note also the remarkable directness and economy of the portrait. No words are wasted. It is like a prose sonnet. No one could add or subtract a single sentence to its betterment.

THE COWARD by Theophrastus
THEOPHRASTUS

Cowardliness is a shrinking of the soul caused by fear. The Coward is this sort of person. At sea he thinks cliffs are pirates and directly the sea gets rough inquires anxiously whether all the passengers are initiated [into the mysteries of the Cabeiri]; as he looks up at the sky he asks the steersman if they are halfway and what he thinks of the weather; he tells the person next him that he has had a disturbing dream; he takes off his tunic and gives it to his slave [so that he can swim]; and finally begs to be put on shore. On active service when the infantry are going into action, he calls to the men of his deme to come and stand by him and to keep a good look-out—pretending that it is hard to distinguish who is the enemy. Then hearing the noise of battle and seeing men fall, he tells his comrades that in the hurry he has forgotten his sword; he runs back to his tent and, after getting rid of his slave by sending him out to reconnoitre, hides the sword under his pillow and wastes time in pretending to look for it. If he sees a wounded friend carried in, he rushes up, tells him to keep cheerful, holds him under the arms to support him; then he attends him, wipes the blood off and sits down by him to keep the flies away—in short, does everything except fight. The trumpets sound the charge and, as he sits in the tent, he murmurs: "Curse you! Won't you let the poor man sleep with your everlasting trumpeting!" Covered with the other man's blood he goes out to meet the returning soldiers and tells them he has saved one of his friends at the risk of his own life; and he brings to the bedside the men of his deme and tribe and explains to each visitor that he carried the wounded man to the tent with his own hands.[1]

There is one feature in this classic sketch that I should like to call particularly to your attention. You will note that Theophrastus selects two situations for recording his observations. In one the coward is traveling; in the other he is unwillingly engaged in a battle. In the first situation, seven typical episodes are depicted: the coward's illusion of seeing the cliffs as pirates, his superstitious fear lest some of the passengers might bring bad luck through having neglected a religious rite, his desire to be at least halfway on the dangerous journey, his consulting expert opinion on the weather, his fear of his own disturbing dreams, his preparations for swimming to safety and, finally, his emotional collapse in begging to be put on shore. Even more subtle are the seven telltale episodes during battle. In all there are fourteen situations described; all of them for the coward are equivalent: whatever stimulation he is exposed to arouses the same deep, dominant disposition. His separate acts are quite distinctive, yet all are equivalent in that each is a manifestation of the same dominant cowardly disposition.

In short, Theophrastus, more than two thousand years ago, used a method just now being glimpsed by psychologists—that of defining, with the aid of equivalent stimulations and equivalent responses, the major dispositions of a character.

To state the point yet more broadly: almost all the literature of character—whether sketch writing, as in the case of Theophrastus, or fiction, drama or biography—proceeds on the psychological assumption that each character has certain *traits* peculiar to himself, which can be defined through the narrating of typical episodes from life. In literature a personality is never regarded, as it sometimes is in psychology, as a sequence of unrelated specific actions. Personality is not like a water-skate, darting hither and yon on the surface of a pond, with its several fugitive excursions having no intrinsic relation to one another. Good literature never makes the mistake of confusing the personality of man with that of a water-skate. Psychology often does.

The first lesson, then, that psychology has to learn from literature is something about the nature of the substantial and enduring dispositions of which personality is composed. This is the problem of traits; and by and large, I maintain, it has been handled more successfully through the assumptions of literature than through the assumptions of psychology. More specifically, it seems to me, the concept of the equivalence of stimulation and the equivalence of response, seen so clearly in the ancient sketches of Theophrastus, may serve as a strikingly productive guide for the scientific study of personality—where equivalences may be determined with greater accuracy and greater verifiability than in literature itself. Using the resources of the laboratory and controlled observation outside, psychology might be able to establish for the single individual, far more exactly than literature can, the precise range wherein various life-situations are for him equivalent and the precise range of responses that for him have equivalent significance.

A second major lesson from literature concerns the self-consistency of its products. No one ever asked their authors to prove that the characters of Hamlet, Don Quixote, Anna Karenina, Hedda Gabler or Babbitt were true and authentic. Great characterizations by virtue of their greatness prove themselves. They are plausible; they are even necessary. Every act seems to be in some subtle way both a reflection of and a rounding out of a single, well-knit character. This adhesiveness of behavior meets the test known as self-confrontation: one bit of behavior supports another, so that the whole can be comprehended as a self-consistent, if intricate, unity. Self-confrontation is the only method of validation applied to the work of artists (except perhaps to the work of biographers, who indeed have certain requirements for external validation to contend with). But the method of self-confrontation, I think it may rightly be said, is barely beginning to be applied to the productions of psychology.

Once, in commenting on a character of Thackeray's, Gilbert K. Chesterton remarked, "She drank, but Thackeray didn't know it." Chesterton's quip springs from the demand that all good characterizations possess "systematic relevance" within themselves. Given one set of facts about a personality, other relevant facts should follow. To be sure, a deep and intimate knowledge of a character is required before these necessary inferences can be made. One must know just what the most intimate motivational traits in each case are. For this most central, and therefore most unifying, core of any personality, Wertheimer has proposed the concept of the *radix*—a root from which all stems may grow. He illustrates his conception with the case of a schoolgirl who was a zealous scholar, but at the same time addicted to vivid cosmetics. On the surface there certainly seems to be no systematic relevance here. The two lines of conduct seem to clash. But the apparent contradiction is resolved in this case by exploring beneath the surface for the basic root. In this case, it turned out that the schoolgirl had deep admiration for (a psycho-analyst might call it a fixation upon) a certain teacher who, in addition to being a scholarly woman, had a natural vivid complexion. The schoolgirl simply wanted to be like her teacher. The same facts in another case might betoken a basic desire for power, or simply a double-barreled attempt to capsize the studious boy across the aisle. Whatever the explanation in this case, the point is that with radical understanding it becomes possible to harmonize the apparent incon-sistencies in a personality.

Of course, the problem is not always so simple. Not all per-sonalities have basic unity. Conflict, changeability, even the dis-sociation of personality are common. Much of the *literature* we read exaggerates the consistency of personality; caricatures rather than characters emerge. Oversimplification is found in drama, fiction and biography. The confrontation seems to come almost too easily. The characters of Dickens are a good example of oversimplification. They never have conflicts within themselves; they are always what they are. They may, and usually do, meet unfriendly forces in the environment, but they themselves are entirely perfect in consistency and devoid of inner conflict.

But, if literature often errs through its selectivity in exaggerating the unity of personality, psychology—through its lack of interest and restricted techniques—generally fails to discover or to explore such consistency as does exist.

The greatest failing of the psychologist at the present time is his inability to prove what he knows to be true. No less than the literary artist, he knows that personality is an intricate, well-proportioned and more or less consistent mental structure—but he can't prove it. He makes no use, as the writer does, of the obvious method of self-confrontation of facts. Instead of emulating the artist in this matter, he usually takes safe refuge in the thickets of statistical correlation.

One investigator, thinking to study the virility of his subjects, for a whole population of people, correlates the width of hips and shoulders with interests in sports; another, to find the bases of intelligence, carefully compares the IQ in childhood with the ossification of the wrist bones; a third compares phosphorous per body weight with good-naturedness or with leadership. Investigations such as these, though they are the fashion in research on personality, run their course entirely on a subpersonal level. Devotion to the microscope and to mathematics has led the investigators to shun complex, patterned forms of behavior and thought, even though it is only in these complex forms that personality can be said to exist at all. Bullied by the instruments of physics, many psychologists neglect the most delicate recording instrument ever devised for the relating and proper clustering of facts—namely, their own minds.

Psychology, then, needs techniques of self-confrontation—techniques whereby the togetherness of a personality can be determined. Only a few rudimentary attempts in this direction have been made.[2]

One study employed the English themes of seventy college students. Nine themes were gathered from each student—three in October, three in January and three in May. The topics for the themes were prescribed and were uniform for all students. After the themes were typed and divested of all identifying signs, two experimenters attempted to sort them carefully so that they might, from style alone, group all the themes written by the same student. For both experimenters the results were strikingly positive, well above chance.

The point of interest here is the method by which successful matchings were made. Occasionally, to be sure, some striking mechanical feature caught the eye and aided in identification. Addiction to semicolons would mark the writing of one student, or some other oddity of punctuation or spelling. But most of the identifications were made not on this basis but through a diagnosis of the *personal traits* of the writers. "The investigators found themselves searching for a form-quality of the individual." They felt in each production a reflection of certain complex qualities in the writer himself. These qualities were different in each case and difficult for the experimenter to reduce to words.

In spite of the difficulty of expressing these hypotheses of "form-quality" in words, the fact remains that they were ordinarily the basis of judgment and likewise that the judgments were to a significant degree successful.

It is of interest to note some of the bases upon which this matching proceeded. The production of one student, for example, would be felt always to reflect "a feeling for atmosphere; a well-balanced sense of humor; a quiet, amused tolerance of social relations and situations." Another showed in all his themes "a positive self-assurance; definite, but neither prejudiced nor opinionated; sense of humor." A third was "constantly bored. Looks at life as a monotonous experience in which one follows the easiest course of action." A fourth had a "simple, optimistic attitude toward life and people; simple, direct, declarative sentences."

III   There is yet another major lesson for psychologists to learn from literature—namely, how to keep a sustained interest in one individual person for a *long* period of time. It was said of a certain famous English anthropologist that although he wrote about savages, he never actually had seen one. He admitted the charge, and added: "And I hope to Heaven I never shall." A great number of psychologists in their professional capacity have never really *seen* an individual; and many of them, I regret to say, hope they never will.

Following the lead of the older sciences, they assume that the individual must be brushed aside. Science, they insist, deals only with general laws. The individual is a nuisance. What is wanted are <u>uniformities</u>. This tradition has resulted in the creation of a vast, shadowy abstraction in psychology called <u>the generalized-adult-human-mind</u>. The human mind, of course, <u>exists in no such form;</u> <u>it exists only in concrete, intensely personal forms.</u> There is no generalized mind. The abstraction that the psychologist commits in measuring and explaining a non-existent mind-in-general is an abstraction that no literary writer ever commits. The literary writer knows perfectly well that mind exists only in singular and particular forms.

Here, of course, we are facing the basic opposition between science and art. <u>Science,</u> it is said, <u>always deals with the general</u>, <u>art always with the particular</u>. But, if this distinction is true, what are we to do about personality? Personality is never general; it is always particular. Must it then be handed over wholly to the arts? Can psychology do nothing about it? I am sure that very few psychologists would accept this solution. Still, it seems to me that the dilemma is inexorable. Either we must give up the individual or we must learn from literature to dwell longer upon him, modifying as is necessary our conception of the scope of science so as to accommodate the single case more hospitably than heretofore.

You may have remarked to yourself that the psychologists you have known, in spite of their profession, are no better than anyone else in understanding people. They are not exceptionally shrewd, nor are they always able to give advice on problems of personality. This observation, if you have made it, is certainly sound. I should go further and say that, because of their habits of excessive abstraction and generalization, many psychologists are actually inferior to other people in their comprehension of the *single* lives that confront them.

When I say that in the interests of a proper science of personality the psychologist should learn to dwell longer on the single case, it might seem that I am poaching upon the domain of biography, whose precise purpose is to dwell exhaustively upon one life.

In England biography began as hagiography and as a recounting of legendary deeds. Neither interest was conducive to objectivity or truthfulness. The term *biography* was first used by Dryden in 1683 and defined by him as "the history of particular men's lives." Reaching a high point in Boswell's *Life of Johnson,* and again in Lockhart's *Life of Scott,* and for a third time in Edmund Gosse's *Father and son,* English biography has had a career of ups and downs. Some biographies are as flat and lifeless as eulogies upon a gravestone; others are sentimental and false.

Increasingly, however, biography is becoming rigorous, and objective, and even heartless. For this trend, psychology has no doubt been largely responsible. Biographies more and more are coming to resemble scientific *autopsies,* performed for the sake of understanding rather than for inspiration or acclaim. There are now psychological and psychoanalytic biographies, and even medical and endocrinological biographies.

The influence of psychological science is felt in autobiography as well. There have been many experiments in objective self-depiction and self-explanation, with improvement upon the disingenuous confessions of Casanova, Rousseau or Barbellion. Two fascinating examples, illustrating the direct influence of psychology, are the *Experiment in autobiography* by H. G. Wells (1935) and *The locomotive god* by W. E. Leonard (1927). But for all their enhanced warmth and intimacy, autobiographers suffer one disadvantage compared with biographers. The autobiographer as a rule cannot bear to disparage himself, and the reader cannot bear to read his praise of himself. Perhaps in time writers may learn how to control their powerful impulse to justify their deeds in the telling, and readers may learn correspondingly to be less suspicious of virtue when it is self-disclosed.

— SUMMARY —

I have mentioned three lessons that the psychologist may learn from literature for the improvement of his own work. The first is the conception held universally in all of literature concerning the nature of traits. Each literary artist proceeds on the assumption that his characters have broadly organized inner dispositions that can be identified and defined. The method that literature uses in identifying and defining traits—namely, the study of equivalent fields of stimulation and equivalent fields of response—needs urgently to find its way into the psychologist's store of methods. The second lesson concerns the test of self-confrontation, which good literature always meets and psychology nearly always avoids meeting. Owing to their neglect of this basic principle of literary validation, psychologists generally fail to find the style and coherence of the personalities that they study. The third lesson calls for more sustained interest in the single case, through longer periods of time. The psychologist should dwell upon one life more exhaustively than he does, no matter if in so doing he sacrifices his impulse to make broad (and usually premature) generalizations about the abstract, nonexistent, average human mind.

In presenting these three advantages of the literary method, I have said little about the distinctive merits of psychology. In conclusion I ought to add at least a few words in praise of my profession. Otherwise you might infer that I am willing and even eager to sell psychology down the river in return for a copy of *Madame Bovary* and a free pass to the Athenaeum.

Psychology has a number of potential advantages over literature. Its disciplined character offsets the subjective dogmatism inherent in imaginative writing. Sometimes literature passes the test of self-confrontation of facts too easily. For example, in one comparative study of biographies of the same person it was found that each version of the life seemed plausible enough but that only a small percentage of the events and interpretations given in one biography were to be found in the others. No one could know which, if any, was the *true* portrait.

It is not necessary for good writers to agree in their observations and in their explanations to anything like the same extent that all good psychologists must agree. Biographers can give vastly different interpretations of a life without discrediting the literary method, whereas psychology is ridiculed when its experts fail to agree with one another.

A psychologist is properly troubled by the arbitrary metaphors of literature. The implication of many metaphors is often grotesquely false, yet they are seldom challenged. In literature one may find, for example, that the docility of a certain character is explained by the fact that "he had menial blood in his veins," the fieriness of another character by the fact that "his temperament he shared with all other redheads" and the intellectuality of a third by the "height of his massive brow." A psychologist would be torn limb from limb if he made any such fantastic assumptions concerning cause and effect.

The artist, furthermore, is permitted and encouraged to be entertaining and engaging, to communicate his own images, to express his own biases. His success is measured by the responsiveness of his readers, who often demand nothing more than that they may languidly identify themselves with a character and escape from their immediate worries. The psychologist, on the other hand, is never permitted to entertain his reader. His success is measured by sterner criteria than the reader's applause.

In gathering his material, the writer draws from his casual observations of life, elides his data and discards troublesome facts at will. The psychologist is held by requirements of fidelity to fact, to *all* facts; and he is expected to secure his facts from controlled and verifiable sources. He must prove his inferences step by step. His terminology is standardized, and he is deprived almost entirely of the use of seductive metaphor. These restrictions surrounding the psychologist make for reliability, verifiability, lessened bias and relative freedom from self-projection into the products of his work.

Psychologists who study personality are, I agree, essentially striving to say what literature has always said, and they are of necessity saying it much less artfully; but as far as they have gone—and it is not very far—they are striving to speak more exactly and, from the point of view of human progress, more helpfully.

The title of this essay, like the titles of many essays, is idly stated. Personality is not a problem for science or a problem for art exclusively, but for both together. Each approach has its merits, but both are needed for even an approximately complete study of the infinite richness of personality.

If in the interests of good pedagogy I am expected to conclude with one pointed bit of advice, it would be this: If you are a student of psychology, read many, many novels and dramas of character, and read biography. If you are *not* a student of psychology, read these too, but *read psychology as well*.

REFERENCES

1. R. Aldington, *A book of characters*, London: Routledge, no date, p. 47.
2. The following experiment is described on pp. 491 ff. of my book *Personality: a psychological interpretation*, New York: Holt, 1937.

CHAPTER 2

The psychological nature of personality

The psychological analysis of human personality must come to terms not only with art but also with philosophy.

The following essay offers in compendious form a psychological theory of personality, but it does so with special reference to the tenets of so-called personalistic philosophy. Written to honor the memory of Edgar Sheffield Brightman (1884-1953), late Bowne Professor of Philosophy at Boston University, the essay appeared in abbreviated form in *The Personalist* (1953).

If you ask whether I consider myself a personalist, I would probably reply, "Does anyone like to have his thought lightly filed away under a label?" But if I am not allowed to evade the question, I would say, "In so far as I am person-centered, yes, I am a personalist." But, as this essay explains, there are areas of serious disagreement.

Readers who are not especially interested in the philosophical issues will still find in this chapter the framework of a strictly psychological theory of personality.

Personalism, says Brightman, is the theory that only persons are real.[1] Thus defined, personalism is basically a metaphysical doctrine. Since a psychologist has no professional competence to argue an ontological position, he could not, as a psychologist, be a personalist —or any other brand of metaphysician.

Having made this pious disclaimer, let us hasten to admit that, whether he knows it or not, every psychologist gravitates toward an ontological position. Like a satellite he slips into the orbit of positivism, naturalism, idealism, personalism. One of these, or some other explicit philosophy, exerts a pull upon his own silent presuppositions, even though he may remain ignorant of the affinity that exists. It is shortsighted of him to deny the dependence—or to refuse to articulate, as best he can, his own thinking about human nature with that brand of philosophy with which it is most closely allied.

In the old days every major philosopher was also a psychologist. His metaphysics and his science of mind were all of a piece. At the present time specialization has reached a point—owing chiefly to the growing dominance of scientific method in psychology—where completely congruent philosophical-scientific views of human nature are exceedingly difficult to achieve.

Take the theory of the person. Within the present century, psychologists have accumulated vast stores of research and insight. But unless I am mistaken, philosophical personalists have not used these findings to any great extent as a testing ground for their own theories. And, vice versa, nearly all of this psychological cumulation has taken place without benefit of the hard thinking of those philosophers who have centered their attention to an equal degree upon the person. It seems as though two separate disciplines have evolved around the same subject matter, each with a distinctive contribution but scarcely aware of the other's existence. The problem is to bring about a more coherent view of the person while respecting the dual approach.

William Stern saw the issue clearly when he proposed that *personalism* be regarded exclusively as a philosophical doctrine and that the portion or type of psychology relevant to the issues of personalism be called *personalistics*.[2] The distinction is meaningful and, up to a point, helpful. It invites the psychologist who agrees in finding personality the most absorbing and insistent topic in the world to say his say without danger of undue presumption. It invites him to collaborate in a cross-disciplinary search without committing himself to propositions beyond his range of competence.

But the distinction breaks down, verbally at least, when the adjective *personalistic*, or the noun *personalist*, is employed. A psychologist interested in personalistics—that is, in the psychology of the person—will almost certainly be labeled a "personalist," and the line of thought he represents will be called "personalistic." Hence, whether he likes it or not, he will be classified with a philosophical school whose interests he shares in part but with whose total position he may hesitate to agree. A typical ground for hesitation, for example, lies in the fact that philosophical personalism has traditionally endorsed "self-psychology" (Brightman, Calkins). Now, a "personalistic" psychologist might find himself in sympathy with the trend of philosophical personalism and yet object to being ticketed as a "self-psychologist," for self-psychology is too dependent on introspection.

It is this confusion, I believe, that has made psychologists, however person-oriented, reluctant to accept the personalistic label. It seems to overcommit them or to align them with a type of psychology they regard as inadequate. While an increasing number of psychological theorists are becoming person-centered, few of them have

as yet explicitly accepted the label *personalistic*. One recent exception is represented in the textbook written by Gardner Murphy.
He boldly declares that his view of general psychology is "personalistic." We note, however, that his position is more methodological than metaphysical: "The conception is that every psychological act is the act of a whole person, and that the first task of psychology is to focus upon the nature of the person." [3]

There is no doubt that personalistic psychology, conceived
even in this limited way, may be a valuable ally of philosophical
personalism. It may even be viewed as a necessary propaedeutic.
For if, as Brightman insists, truth is a matter of systematic coherence, then all the valid discoveries of psychology pertaining to
the nature of personality must find their place without remainder
in the philosophy of personalism. Reciprocally, the personalistic
psychologist will find the significance of his own researches deep-
ened by his acquaintance with the larger context of philosophical
personalism. *What the two disciplines have in common is their conviction that the person is altogether central in the scheme of things,
whether the scheme is explored at the psychological or at the philosophical level.*

I

With the exception of a few specialists, psychologists in the
present day nearly all deal with the problems of personality. Virtually every textbook, however nomothetically oriented—however
predisposed to universal concepts—contains a final chapter on "personality." But the final chapter is often a mere gesture. What it says
is seldom geared in with the remainder of the text. Few psychologists center their concern, as Murphy does, in acts-of-whole-persons,
nor do they regard it the central task of psychology to focus upon the
nature of the person.

Thus most psychologists who talk about personality hold theories
that have no relation whatever to a personalistic outlook. For some,
personality is an uncemented mosaic of elements, measured perhaps by scales but never vitally interrelated. For others, it is a con-
geries of "factors" mathematically determined by correlating mental
traits in a large population of people (but not in the individual person himself). For still others, it is a passive product of past experience resulting from a succession of pushes, without any contemporary motivation or "go."

It is not my purpose to review all the failures of psychology to give an adequate account of the properties of personality. Readers are already critical enough of the flatness and triviality of many of the prevailing psychological views of personality. The problem to which I wish to address myself is this: [*What attributes must a theory of personality have in order to be considered adequate to the empirical facts before us?*] If this question can be satisfactorily answered, we shall have in hand the type of theory to which personalistic philosophy—in the interests of systematic congruence—must accommodate itself.

There are, as I see the matter, at least five essential characteristics that an adequate theory of personality must possess. It must possess *all* of these, not only in order to accommodate the empirical facts as known, but also in order to avoid self-contradiction. Let me be clear. I am speaking here of the criteria of personality that appear to be mandatory to a person-centered psychologist. I also believe that the philosophical personalist is required to accept them in one form or another. I shall not object if he wishes to recast my propositions in more congenial terms, provided only that his final product leaves the substance of these criteria available for the psychologist's use in his continued researches.

An adequate theory of personality will (1) regard the human personality as integumented—that is, as centered in the organism; (2) regard the organism as replete, not empty; (3) regard motivation as normally a fact of present structure and function, not merely as an outgrowth of earlier forces; (4) employ units of analysis capable of living synthesis; and (5) allow adequately for, but not rely exclusively upon, the phenomenon of self-consciousness.

Let us now attempt to clarify these requirements.

II

Human personality has a locus—within the skin. To be sure, its imagination and memory range far and wide, but these acts are well grounded in a psychophysical matrix of some order. On another plane of existence, personality may be freed from its space-time bondage; but on the plane where the psychologist dwells, it must be viewed as an organic unity, accessible to study through its acts, its verbal report and even its reflex and physiological functioning. More than one of the body-mind solutions available to personalists would, I think, adequately meet this need. I shall not here attempt to choose among them.

The reason that I stress the criterion of integumentation is that

centered in · organism

both psychological and philosophical personalists need to rescue human personality from the clutches of those who confuse it with the impression a man makes on others, with his reputation, with his "social stimulus value." Elsewhere I have argued this "biophysical" position at length in contradiction to the view that I have called "biosocial." [4] (Neither term, I think, is well chosen; but their drift is, I hope, clear.) The "biosocial" view takes *your* personality to be what *other* people think and do about you, not what you yourself think and do. To reject this conception is not, of course, to deny that our reputations, whether true or erroneous, may have heavy impact upon others and upon ourselves. But unless we rid ourselves of all definitions that place our personalities in *other* people's minds, we shall never have a secure enough locus for a theory of personality as a system. The biophysical view, unlike the biosocial, would hold that Robinson Crusoe in solitude has "as much" personality before as after the advent of his man Friday.

Besides this crude confusion of person and reputation, there are a number of other partially biosocial views that are almost equally unacceptable. Most of these views evolved in an honest effort to recognize the indisputable fact that the individual is bound into a social context. While one must have deep sympathy with these conceptual attempts, most of them are, in effect, person-destroying. They chisel and chip away at the biophysical nature of personality until it loses its essential characteristics of locus, uniqueness and inner congruence.

For the most part, current theories of this order have to do with the recently popular subject matter in research and teaching that falls under the rubric "Personality and Culture." Two decades ago, in its effort to promote interdisciplinary investigations, the Social Science Research Council promulgated this double-barreled concept, and it was welcomed by scores of psychologists, sociologists and anthropologists. The resulting cross-fertilization of thought has been remarkably productive, not only in furthering research but also in overcoming disciplinary boundaries within universities and colleges. The resulting ferment and realignment, though undoubtedly wholesome, brought forth a number of hasty and misshapen theories.

One type of hasty formulation reduced personality wholly to a mirror-reflection of culture. "Personality is the subjective side of culture" became a popular dictum. It would be hard to imagine a more total reversal of the personalistic emphasis upon the inner coherence-maintaining and purposive properties of the individual. In fact, some writers went so far as to insist that there is no such

opposite v personalism
sociological pi v view

thing as integration within personality; the only consistency a person shows is a reflection of the orderly and patterned character of his surrounding situation.

A variant of this view is found in current "role" theory. Partisans of this concept are impressed, not by the uniqueness and integrality of the personality system, but by the diverse prescriptions laid upon this system by social expectations. A man is known, not for what he *is*, but for the *roles* he plays—as father, physician, churchman, consumer. He is a composite bundle of roles. That people *do* sometimes behave differently in various environments and in accordance with varying expectations is, of course, not to be denied. The danger with the role concept is that the personal nexus *containing* the role-habits is likely to be overlooked and, correspondingly, the orientation of the person to separate environments overstressed. One is reminded of the exuberance of William James, who declared (though he certainly didn't mean it) that a man "has as many different social selves as there are distinct groups of persons about whose opinion he cares." [5] Personality may be versatile and variable, but it is not capable of dissipation into *n* roles or *n* social selves. Nor is it a mere "equilibrium of roles." There is too much evidence that personality is highly consistent with itself from situation to situation to permit this type of reduction.[6]

A further dubious trend is seen in the currently fashionable conception of "basic" or "modal" personality. We are told that each culture tends to bring up its children according to an approved formula and that children therefore tend to develop similar traits and outlooks. Each culture has a type of personality that corresponds to its cultural pattern. While for certain gross comparisons of culture this conception may be both valid and useful, its coarseness and imprecision limit its value. For one thing, it overlooks the central fact that no single individual reflects all these traits and outlooks, and that some individuals may reflect virtually none of them. It allows not at all for the creative interweaving of cultural threads with threads that are individual and unique. To be sure, the concept does not pretend to cover the "idiosyncratic" determinants of personality; but peril lies in the tendency of certain writers to believe that, having discussed what is "basic" in this sense, they have dealt adequately with the whole subject of personality.

Much of this theoretical vertigo might have been avoided if the initial sponsors of the phrase "Personality and Culture" had changed the particle *and* to *in*. "Personality *in* Culture" poses all the legitimate problems and has the added merit of implying that their solution will be found, not by destroying the integrity of the personal system, but by studying the relation of this self-contained system to cultural and social contexts, which may in turn be regarded as systems of a different order.

In spite of my defense of integumentation, I concede that a genuine weakness in personalistic writing, both philosophical and psychological, is its tendency to sidestep the countless intersections that occur between the personality system and the social system. Even though personalists, by conviction, must ascribe primacy to the former, they can ill afford to leave unsolved the problems created by the intersection. If they persistently do so, their basic contributions will be by-passed and disregarded by advancing social science. The relation of personality to society must somehow be dealt with adequately. It is not enough to assert that a person's traits, attitudes, subjective values or other inner forces account for his conduct. *also* While this statement is true, it disregards situational variance. In spite of a prevailing consistency, one *does* vary one's behavior— within limits—according to social circumstance. To be sure, no one varies it in ways that are not already *his;* but neither is he closed off from, and independent of, the social system. He maintains his own boundaries, but those boundaries are not impermeable.

We need a theory in social science that will allow for the full integrity and primacy of the personal system while relating it adequately to boundary-maintaining social and cultural systems. Important steps in this direction have recently been taken by Parsons and others.[7]

It is Parsons' contention that the personality system is a self-contained unit exerting marked constraints upon the social system. The latter "cannot be so structured as to be radically incompatible with the conditions of function of its component individual actors as biological organisms and as personalities." [8] At the same time, the social system need not meet the needs of *all* its members, but only of a sufficient proportion to maintain its own form of organization. The social system is one in which the individual finds himself related to others in a way that tends to maintain their relationships in equilibrium.[9] The physician and the patient, for example, take certain subtly marked roles in relation to each other in order to fulfill the needs of both; nor could these needs be fulfilled unless these prescribed role relations were observed.

It would seem that this line of thought offers considerable hope for maintaining full recognition of the integral nature of the personality system, while relating it more adequately to its social context. Parsons affirms the ultimate unity of the personality system and complains that most brands of psychology do not treat personality *as* a system.[10] In short, while offering a theoretical groundwork for social science at large, this sociologist invites and welcomes a personalistic treatment of the individual.

The need for a social science that will adequately hold the assumptions of personalistic psychology is exceedingly acute. Most of the theories and trends mentioned in this section seem to veer away from personality conceived as an integumented system. They illustrate perhaps what Riesman sets forth as the most telling change in American character—the shift from "inner-directedness" to "other-directedness."[11] So great today is the demand for peer approval (children in some schools are graded not on the three R's but on "adjustment") that it seems natural for contemporary social scientists to think in terms of *basic* personality rather than *full-bodied* personality and in terms of *roles* rather than *being*. It was easier for personalism to have its say in the earlier days of "inner-directedness," when it was taken for granted that each person possessed inner purposes and inner balances. In the present day, personalistic psychology and philosophy must fight hard to breast the tide of other-directedness—the tide of the *Massenmensch*.

III

The influence of modern positivism upon the psychological study of personality is in part wholesome. Diagnostic instruments are improving; more exacting standards of evidence prevail; anecdotes and rumor are discredited; and the preference for operational definition has, in a limited way, made for more intelligible communication.

But positivism also has stultifying effects. Its devotees exclude explanations in terms of inner traits, purposes, interests; some even tell us that the nervous system can no longer be invoked in our explanatory sequences. Since nothing that occurs between the stimulus and the response is observable, no "intervening variable" is admissible. We must confine our explanatory efforts, so they say, to events that lie outside the organism. Even the *habits* of Watsonian behaviorism must go. One positivist remarked, "When we understand the properties of the stimulus, we shall not need the concept *personality*."

What lies behind this methodological craving for an empty organism? Is it an ascetic desire for scientific chastity, allowing only minimal assumptions in order to avoid the traps of subjectivism and circular reasoning? In a thousand years of chaste research built on these meager assumptions, does one hope to achieve a science of behavior having some measure of adequacy? Or could it be that this formula is from the outset an escapist device, designed to protect the harassed scientist from the pulsation of real life around him? He finds it comforting to say that "science is willingness to accept facts even when they are opposed to wishes"; yet his own wish to emulate natural scientists may lead him to reject all facts that are opposed to his wishes. Brightman has shown how the experimental scientist, however positivistic his procedure, is in fact making various silent assumptions that interpose the *self*, as an intervening variable, between the scientist's own stimuli and his own responses.[12]

While adherents of extreme positivism are relatively rare in psychology, their influence is strong enough to create a tone of apology among certain writers who timidly affirm the utility of "intervening variables," "hypothetical constructs" or "inferred tendencies"—in other words, of *traits, values, intentions, self*.

Now, it is obvious that a full-bodied psychology of personality must take precisely the opposite tack from positivism. It must assume from the outset that there is nothing scientifically shameful about postulating a well-furnished personality that *is* something and *does* something—a personality that has internal structures and substructures which "cause," or partially cause, behavior. One may, of course, gain helpful hints from positivism regarding the need for reliable criteria in establishing inferences concerning traits, habits, attitudes, needs and sentiments. Yet no psychologist concerned with personality can avoid altogether the postulation of inner dispositions within the organism to account for its consistency in conduct and for its motivation. In this connection, William McDougall has argued that "inner tendency" is the most indispensable concept in the entire science of psychology.[13] Still, the pressures emanating from positivism are all in the other direction: it is the fashion to unstock the organism, especially to strip it of dynamic power and purpose.

The same trend, to a lesser degree, is seen in what is called "field theory." While Lewin and his followers have never denied the existence of needs and attitudes within the organism, they tend to regard behavior as a function of *all* field-forces, both inner and outer. In practice, there seems to be a predilection for forces in the outer situation that exert pressure upon the individual. Thus the desires and values of the person are squeezed out of many field formulations.[14]

Gestalt psychology, too, postulates a singularly passive, if not actually empty, organism. Outer configurations impinge upon the nervous system, which, through an isomorphic type of response, yields conscious and behavioral equivalents of the stimulus pattern. This psychophysical process, as envisaged by Köhler and others, brings the organism into harmonious relations with its environment, but the organism itself seems to contribute little to the process. Stern, the personalist, felt it necessary to protest vehemently against this passive model. Mental life, he maintained, not only has the self-distributing and isomorphic properties here postulated but also shows the continuous presence of inner activity: *keine Gestalt ohne Gestalter*.

Person-centered psychologists reject the fetish of the empty organism. They cannot see why the enormous potentialities of the human cortex, energized by its own and by autonomic activity, should not allow for *dispositions* as well as for *traces*. Why should the nine billion cells in the cortex act only like iron filings in a magnetic field of force? Their combinations and their properties suggest that, while passive forms of organization (mere "traces") exist, there are also highly dynamic formations, consisting of purposes and interests, which give personality its active, urgent, directed character. We do not know precisely how mental and physical events are related; but it seems obvious that, taken together, they comprise a unified, energy-filled and boundary-maintaining system. The person, thus conceived, is alive and going places.

To be sure, person-centered psychologists do not all view this animated structure of personality in precisely the same way. Some speak of a hierarchical organization of conditioned reflexes, habits, traits and "selves." Others prefer units such as instincts, interests and sentiments. Freudians are partial to the "institutions" of id, ego and superego. While, as I shall soon show, it makes a great deal of difference just what units are chosen, it is enough for now to repeat our contention: any theory of personality pretending adequacy must be dynamic and, to be dynamic, must assume a well-stocked organism.

IV

Yet not every dynamic theory of personality is adequate. Many, indeed most of them, suffer from two shortcomings in their view of motivation: they pay too little attention to the *uniqueness* and to the *contemporaneity* of personal motives.

In their struggle to emulate nomothetic science, most theories regard the desires and intentions of individuals simply as changes rung upon a few uniform themes. These themes may be labeled *drives, instincts, needs, wishes, desires, vectors* or something else. Whatever they are called, the implication is always the same: if we could correctly classify the basic motives of men, we should be able to account for the behavior of each *individual* man. Thus the sex drive, the aggressive instinct, the need for achievement, the wish for security and the desire for dependency become variables to which all personalities may be ordered. While each motivational theory differs in some respects from all others, they have in common this heavily nomothetic bias. For certain purposes it is a defensible bias: often we *do* gain from comparing personalities according to such common categories. But a theory that is completely content with an account of abstract motives, of abstract personalities, fails to provide a foundation sound enough to bear the weight of any single full-bodied personality.

In this connection it is interesting to recall the strongly personalistic flavor of definitions of psychology offered by the founders of the science: Wundt, James and Titchener. The first wrote that psychology "investigates the total context of experience in its relations to the subject"; the second, that "psychology is the science of finite individual minds"; and the third, that "psychology is the study of experience considered as dependent on some person." None of these authors developed his account of mental life to accord with his definition. Yet some vague sense of propriety seemed to guide them in framing their definitions; they knew that mind (as a psychological datum) exists only in finite and in personal forms. Yet each, like the dynamic psychologists of the present day, spent his time exclusively in seeking the laws of mind-in-general and worried little about the concrete formations that mark minds-in-particular. (An exception to this statement is the use made by William James of case-studies in his *Varieties of religious experience*.)

The second shortcoming of current dynamic psychology has to do with its anachronistic handling of motivation. Past-reference dominates the scene. While men are busy leading their lives in the present, with much future-pointing, psychologists are busy tracing these lives backward. Let us take an example. Ask almost any psychologist (psychoanalyst or not) why the son of some famous politician is himself a politician. The answer you will receive is likely to be in terms of father identification, early slanting, conditioning and reinforcement, or something equally freighted with reference to childhood. Such answers are, of course, acceptable enough from a _historical_ point of view, but they are likely to be irrelevant and misleading in accounting for the _present_ situation. Virtually all psychologies (Freudian, Adlerian, stimulus-response) stress the initial slanting of personal development in the early years of life. While the first outlines may indeed be laid at this time, it does not follow that an adult person normally maintains this style of life for the reasons that were operative in childhood.

Returning to our example: it is indeed probable that our politician did have a father identification at the age of, say, four (most boys do); it is also likely that he was rewarded and praised for his oratorical imitations of Daddy. It is probable that he was thus slanted toward a vocation in politics. But does this bit of history explain the drive, the go, the interest of the politician fifty years later? The father is dead; times have changed; instead of rewards, he receives mostly brickbats. Tens of thousands of personal experiences have intervened, modified and reshaped the initial motivational pattern. His personality _now,_ we may say, is centered in his interest in politics, not in his father.

This confusion between the historical roots of motives and the contemporary functioning of motives has seemed to me the most stultifying of all misconceptions that mar current theories of personality. This is not the occasion to examine the damaging consequences of the fallacy or to debate the issue fully.[15] It is necessary only to insist that the forward thrusts of motivation that are so characteristic of human personality cannot adequately be accounted for by any doctrine of pushes, even a sequence of pushes, out of the past. An adequate theory must allow for the effectiveness of a current self-image and for the dynamic character of intentions, of value-orientations and of uniquely patterned psychogenic interest systems in normally healthy adults. Philosophically considered, this shift in emphasis is required in order to discover in the individual the necessary ingredients of freedom and value-orientation that would make personalism tenable.

It is only fair to say that a proper theory must allow for early fixations in personality—for infantilisms, regression and many kindred manifestations of neuroticism. It is not necessary to overlook the epochal discoveries of Freud; it is necessary only to put them in proper perspective. Even our politician _may_ be a neurotic. He may still be wistfully identified with his father, and all that he does may be an effort to fill Daddy's shoes (even, conceivably, to displace his father in his mother's affections: the Oedipus complex outlasting the death of the parents). The essential point, however, is that such a condition would be exceptional and abnormal. The Freudian view of motivation may be an acceptable model for neurotic behavior without being an acceptable model for all behavior. My own position, which goes under the designation *functional autonomy of motives*, holds that motivation may be—and in healthy people usually is—autonomous of its origins. Its function is to animate and steer a life toward goals that are in keeping with *present* structure, *present* aspirations and *present* conditions.

In recent years we observe certain marked improvements in theory, shifts in the direction of functional autonomy. What is known as neo-Freudianism shows two striking advances: a fuller recognition of the contributions of culture, and a postulation of a far more active, purposive, forward-reaching "ego." Originally Freud conceived the ego as a relatively helpless, though intelligent, rationalizer, beset by three "tyrants"—the id, the superego and external reality. More often than not, it could do nothing but repress its bitter conflicts, which would finally erupt in neurotic anxiety. Even the most orthodox psychoanalysts now say that Freud died without completing his ego theory. Nor is it customary today to regard this enlarged and improved ego as an agent only of defense; it contains mature motives approximately of the order demanded by the doctrine of functional autonomy.[16]

An equally striking development in the right direction is the revolution in theory implicit in Rogerian or "client-centered" therapy.[17] While the theoretical model underlying this movement in "non-directive counseling" is not yet fully worked out, it is certain to take a form compatible with personalistic psychology. The position, in brief, holds that the self, under proper conditions, is capable of reorganizing its perceptual field and thus of altering behavior. The therapy consists in giving the individual an opportunity to assess and rearrange his own image of his motives and circumstances, and thus to emerge a more coherent and firmly knit person.

Other contemporary movements could be cited along the same line. Whereas terms like *self* and *self-image*, *ego* and *ego-involvement*, were rarely employed by psychologists a generation ago, they are currently used with great frequency and represent emerging systematic theories of motivation free from the restraints of uniformity and past-reference, which have limited conceptual thinking heretofore.[18]

Personalists should be warned that at least one of their number does not believe that the doctrine of functional autonomy is required in an adequate theory of personality. Bertocci has argued that an instinct theory (such as McDougall's) avoids the predicament of "emergence" that is implied in the present author's position. The issue has been fully discussed in print and need not here be debated.[19] Suffice it to say that both writers agree on the need for unique and forward-pointed motives in an adequate theory of personality, whatever conceptualization is required to achieve this goal.

V

Without some units of analysis, the scientific study of personality would be impossible. The type of unit chosen is important. Person-centered psychology cannot be satisfied with the kinds of variables that are customarily isolated for study. Their weakness lies in the fact that, when synthesized, they fail to reconstitute to a satisfactory degree the personality of the individual who is the object of study. In the endeavor to make instruments (tests, questionnaires, experimental situations) standard, reliable and objective, investigators have invented variables so far removed from the structure and functioning of the particular personality that the knowledge gained often seems useless.

Take the case of vocational tests. It is sometimes assumed that a battery of tests can tell the seeker what vocation he should enter and can tell an employer which applicants to hire and which to reject. Sometimes the instruments are helpful to a degree, but, dealing as they do with "typical" variables, they tell little about the unique motivation, the patterning of skills or the underlying potentialities of the single case.

Not only in applied psychology are "typical variables" tried and found wanting; they are also deficient for the strict purposes of theoretical science. They do not yet (and they seem, in principle, unlikely to) yield a high degree of predictive power, understanding and control—the three desiderata of science. To say that John Brown scores in the eightieth percentile of the "masculinity-feminity" variable, in the thirtieth percentile on "need for achievement" and at average on "introversion-extroversion" is only moderately enlightening. Even with a more numerous set of dimensions, with an avalanche of psychometric scores, patterned personality seems to elude the psychodiagnostician.

It is for this reason that professional, especially clinical, psychologists have recourse to supplementary idiographic methods: to interviewing, life-histories, intuition. These channels of understanding are not yet scientifically "respectable"; they cause method-centered psychologists acute distress. Yet research in personalistic psychology must turn to these more patterned forms of perception if it is to improve our skills in diagnosis and help us identify the central characteristics of the individual person.

I do not mean to imply that the arsenal of painfully accumulated standard methods is worthless. Quite the contrary: for a first approximation to personality, the typical variables (especially if they are reliably scaled) have considerable value. Their strength, like their weakness, lies in their ability to order all personalities to a uniform set of variables, variously called traits, needs, attitudes, dimensions, factors or types. This comparative approach enables us to locate a subject roughly in a population of his peers. Some of the more subtle nomothetic instruments yield more than a single score and thus approach the threshold of the problem of patterning. But even the subtlest of nomothetic methods carries us only to the point where we see that the score on a certain variable is interdependent with other scores on other variables. The *personal nexus* wherein all variables are joined eludes every nomothetic approach.

Elsewhere I have spoken of this "common trait" approach and have shown that it is inferior to the more complex, but ultimately more revealing, "individual trait" approach. While the former is content with uniform variables, the latter seeks to discover the vital foci of organization within individual lives.[20]

The objection has been made that if we stress the individual trait approach, centering attention on the individuality of pattern, then "the science of human nature would come to a dead stop." [21] These generalists argue as follows: Every stone in the meadow is unique, yet the science of mineralogy wholly covers the subject; the accident of uniqueness falls, if anywhere, in the artist's province. Each manifestation of a disease is unique, but biochemistry and other constituent sciences of medicine provide the essential explanations needed. Following these models, psychology as science should seek only uniformities and leave individuality to the practitioner, the biographer or the lover. To clinch the argument, the generalists assert that, if personality is unique, so too is every moment of time during which personality runs its course—and that science cannot hope to deal with such ephemerae.

The weakness of this position, I think, lies in the fact that human personality entails an enduring psychophysical organization, whose intrinsic nature we happen to *want* to study—if we are person-centered. Since it cannot be studied adequately with uniform variables, we have no recourse but to seek the peculiar central and subsidiary trait-systems that comprise this unique datum. The effective units in personality happen to be peculiar to the individual. To acknowledge this central fact does not bring the science of human nature to a dead stop. On the contrary, it can be demonstrated that a knowledge of intra-individual patterns of consistency and congruence in behavior gives us enhanced scientific power, for such knowledge increases our comprehension, predictive ability and control over individual persons beyond the range achieved by unaided common sense or by nomothetic science. (Whether the individual *should* be scientifically "controlled" is an axiological issue that we need not here discuss. Our present debate is concerned merely with establishing the scientific respectability of research in the phenomena of uniqueness.)

To date, relatively little progress has been made in theory or research pertaining to the level of individual traits, largely because this personalistic requirement has not been admitted in traditional psychology. Yet some gains have been made. Let me mention, by way of illustration, a few directions in contemporary investigation that seem relevant and promising. Studies in expressive behavior are hopeful, for they tend to disclose the relation of overt movement to inner patterns of interest, anxiety, temperament. A few mathematical procedures are promising, especially those that attempt to deal with patterns of events within the single personality. All work that improves the preparation and use of personal documents (case records, life-histories and the like) is relevant. The process by which the human mind forms and checks its judgments of people deserves sustained study: it seems certain that inference from previous experience is not all that is involved in patterned perception. Important too are studies that fix attention upon the congruence or disconnection that exists in the motivational systems underlying a given person's acts: are his conscious and unconscious impulses of a single piece, or are they discordant? All these problems—and many more like them—require improved methods for handling pattern and individuality.[22]

While we are working out new methods for the study of individual traits and personal patterns, there is no reason, of course, to fall behind in efforts to improve nomothetic variables. Recently my colleague and critic, Henry A. Murray, on the basis of many years' labor, proposed a scheme of variables that marks a distinct advance.[23] The units are in terms of values, vectors and value-vectors. *Values* include interest in body, progeny, knowledge, freedom, affiliation and the like; *vectors* are dispositions leading to renunciation, accept-

ance, acquisition, aggression and the like; *value-vectors* ("needs")
are the more concrete dispositions to renounce, accept, acquire, construct, maintain and restore a given valued entity. This third type of
unit, I believe, since it is concrete, approaches more nearly to
adequacy, dealing as it does with the integral intentions (orientations) a person has with reference to his environment, both real and
imaginal. The scheme stops somewhat short of recognizing the ultimate manifoldness and uniqueness of each personality, for it still
presumes to order all individual patterns to a common, "typical
variable" scheme. It may, however, prove to be the most serviceable
nomothetic device yet proposed. With its aid we may find that the
personality thus analyzed can, with a higher approximation than
heretofore, be re-synthesized into its own unique structure and functioning. In so far as it succeeds, we shall have a valuable contribution to the theory and method of personality-research. In so far as it
fails, we shall have to carry our search further, pressing ever toward
the discovery of more viable units and toward improved means for
representing patterned individuality.

VI

With much that I have here written, any personalistic philosopher would, I suppose, agree. He would be bound to approve my
insistence that psychology deal adequately with personality as a
system. He may be saying: Go tell your story to the person-destroying psychologists, not to us. But we come now to a thornier criterion
—one that may call for broad concessions on the part of the philosophical personalist; if not, one that at the very least indicates the
need for a fresher basis of mutual understanding. The criterion may
be stated as follows: *An adequate psychology of personality will
allow amply for the concept of self but, unlike some philosophers,
will not employ it as a factotum.*

Let us begin by identifying the points where the philosopher and
the psychologist are in agreement concerning the properties of the
self. In the first place, they must agree that consciousness by no
means always involves self-awareness. It seems highly probable that
an animal is conscious, but also that its consciousness has no self-
reference. As Romanes put the matter, the animal knows but does
not know that it knows. Similarly, the dawn of self-awareness in the
child is now fairly securely established as a product of maturation
and learning gradually developing during the second and third
years of life. Among adults, in states of drowsiness and low vitality,

there is certainly no awareness of self. And if our criterion of self-awareness is at all exacting (that is, if we require that mental states be clearly recognized as part of a self-system), we might hazard the guess that a person can go through the entire day without being self-aware at all.

A second point of agreement lies in the fact that, despite the ephemerality of self-awareness, it remains the most certain attest we have of personal existence. It is the solid empirical core of human personality. We do not always recognize our consciousness as "owned," but the fact that we occasionally do so is basic to our sense of personal identity and of continuity.

A good deal of modern psychology is concerned with the phenomenological view of the self as datum. One popular, if fairly trivial, line of research has to do with the phenomenal localization of the self in various regions of the body.[24] A more significant interest is in the conditions under which experience is recognized as owned. Recently the topic of the self-image ("ego ideal") has come into prominence, especially in therapeutic literature. Many psychologists see that the *idea* of the self, as well as the *awareness* of the self, constitute a central pivot in the development and change of personality. In this line of work, however, the definition of self is somewhat restricted. Self is regarded only as *the individual as known to the individual.* There is as yet no explicit admission of the self as an *agent.*

But agreement does, I think, proceed further. The person-centered psychologist recognizes that the sense of self, however ephemeral, becomes a vital and active reference point for all conduct. The operation of memory—especially of recognition—brings constantly to mind the indisputable fact of personal identity. The self as anchorage point in consciousness becomes securely established after the first year or two of life, so that the child comes to locate up and down, before and behind, past and future, striving and rejection, in relation to the self he knows.

Thus conation becomes bound into the system. Especially in the second and third year of life, the child grows acutely self-aware and begins to assert himself as a "fighter for ends." (Anyone with a negativistic offspring of this age will need no further proof.) A clamorous self-centeredness sets in, which only with the passing of years becomes socialized and modified into the pursuit of values less egocentric.

Such evidence leads us to assume that, however transient the consciousness of self may be, all sensing, acting and willing are, at bottom, *owned* and that selfhood is the central presupposition we must hold in examining the psychological states of human beings. With this broad inference we agree, though one point remains troublesome. What about the baby? To say that the infant unknowingly "owns" its blurred experience establishes a self prior to the development of the capacity for self-consciousness. Personalists may insist that this is a necessary assumption, but for my part I should like to leave open the possibility that the *emergence* of selfhood in the course of early life may be a defensible proposition.

Up to this point, I assume, personalists and person-centered psychologists are in agreement. Where, then, is there crucial disagreement between them? The chief issue, to my mind, comes from the tendency of the former to overstress the function of consciousness. The tendency takes many forms, whether in connection with discussions of *self*, of *person* or of *personality*. Brightman, for example, writes: "Philosophically, then, personality is restricted to actual consciousness; psychologists will continue to interpret personality as the empirical situation in interaction with a body. This does no harm, unless one becomes confused between the given empirical situation and hypothetical entities, like bodies, which are related to it." [25] And Bertocci, another personalist, writes: "The *I*, the *self*, the *person*, the *conscious being* (all used as synonyms here) *is* the complex unity of activity which consists in sensing, thinking, wanting, imagining, willing, oughting." [26]

Confronted with such overloading of the person with consciousness, the psychologist becomes alarmed lest he be drawn into the camp of simon-pure mentalism and lest he lose the organic unity of personality functioning as he knows it. To Bertocci he would reply that many of the activities of sensing, remembering, imagining, thinking, feeling, willing and the like proceed in a unified way without full—and sometimes without any—participation of consciousness. The person, therefore, is *more* than a conscious unity. To Brightman he would say that, if, philosophically considered, personality is restricted to actual consciousness, the psychologist is talking about a different and wider entity that brooks no such arbitrary psychophysical surgery. It is reassuring to know that the problem troubles personalists themselves and that the door to understanding is not closed.

One way out of the difficulty is offered by William Stern, whose psychophysical neutrality has proved unpalatable to American personalists. Stern, in effect, offers us a *tertium quid*, neither mental nor physical, that maintains the unity and coherence—and represents the metaphysical ultimateness—that the personalist seeks. To him, "The person is living whole, individual, unique, striving toward goals, self-contained and yet open to the world around him; he is capable of having experience." [27]

We note that Stern regards all the listed attributes of the person as compulsory, excepting only "experience." While the person is endowed with the capacity for experience, the guarantee of unity lies at a deeper level. Stern's view is thus opposed to that of both Brightman and Calkins, who hold the self to be mental and to have a body. For Stern, consciousness is merely an important occasional ingredient. Experiences may be salient (*abgehoben*) or deeply imbedded, with a high, low or no degree of self-involvement. Those that are marked by greater personal relevance are of particular interest to the psychologist, but the binding principle is not self (considered either as conscious agent or as datum) but the *person*.

It is true that Stern's position seems to solve the problem by multiplying entities, offering us "neutrality" to juggle along with mind and body. I mention the view here, not with endorsement, but in order to call attention to the fact that one personalist, who was both a philosopher and a psychologist, was deeply concerned with the problem and that he could find no other solution to retain the patent unity of mind and body which here and now marks the organization and functioning of human personality. I doubt that any psychologist whose interest is truly centered in the person could work comfortably within a frame that regards unconscious processes, reflex processes and physiological processes as unintegrated, uncoordinated or less important for the unity of the person than the conscious operations of the self. All these levels of functioning are vital.

VII

In these pages I have attempted to sketch a psychological approach to human personality that seems to me to accord with the scientific evidence available. If I have intruded an unfamiliar vocabulary, and at times a controversial note, I venture to hope and believe that the direction of my argument is compatible with the broad tenets of philosophical personalism. It seems inconceivable to me that two well-intentioned disciplines, working on a common subject matter, can indefinitely remain apart.

REFERENCES

1. E. S. Brightman, *An introduction to philosophy*, rev. ed., New York: Holt, 1951, p. 334.

2. W. Stern, *Studien zur Personwissenschaft. I: Personalistik als Wissenschaft*, Leipzig: Barth, 1930.

3. G. Murphy, *Introduction to psychology*, New York: Harper, 1951, p. xvi.

4. G. W. Allport, *Personality: a psychological interpretation*, New York: Holt, 1937, especially Chap. 2.

5. W. James, *Principles of psychology*, New York: Holt, 1890, I, 294.

6. It may be well to mention some of the kinds of empirical evidence I have in mind. Nearly all "personality tests" tap behavior in *many* situations. A satisfactory "internal reliability" of such tests is *ipso facto* evidence for the inter-situational consistency of personal traits. Intensive studies of refugees whose home culture completely collapsed about their heads show that, in setting up new lives for themselves in new lands, these fugitives did so under the dominance of essentially the same traits, values and modes of adjustment. (G. W. Allport, J. S. Bruner, E. M. Jandorf, "Personality under social catastrophe: ninety life-histories of the Nazi revolution," *Char. & Pers.*, 1941, 10:1-22.) Experiments show that when the central regions of personality are aroused—in other words, when "ego-involvement" is high—the consistency of personality is especially marked. See Chapter 5 of the present volume.

7. T. Parsons and E. A. Shils, *et al.*, *Toward a general theory of action*, Cambridge: Harvard University Press, 1951. T. Parsons, *The social system*, Glencoe, Ill.: The Free Press, 1951. F. H. Allport, *Theories of perception and the concept of structure*, New York: Wiley, 1955, Chap. 21.

8. T. Parsons, *op. cit.*, p. 27.

9. *Ibid.*, p. 542.

10. *Ibid.*, p. 545.

11. D. Riesman, *The lonely crowd: a study of the changing American character*, New Haven: Yale University Press, 1951. It is well to recall in this connection that John Dewey, in *The public and its problems* (New York: Holt, 1927), raised the issue of the dismemberment of the person into mere appendages of many publics—into a taxpayer, an auto owner, a church member, a husband, a bowler, a Civic Leaguer, a dentist, ad infinitum.

12. E. S. Brightman, "The presuppositions of experiment," *Personalist*, 1938, 19:136-43.

13. W. McDougall, "Tendencies, as indispensable postulates of all psychology," *XI Congrès International de Psychologie*, Paris: Felix Alean, 1938, pp. 157-70.

14. This tendency is found in much of Lewin's writing; but in fairness to his breadth of view, it must be said that in certain portions of his work he offers an acceptable analysis of the psychological structure of personality considered as a "differentiated region." Both threads are clearly seen in his posthumous volume, *Field theory in social science* (D. Cartwright, ed.), New York: Harper, 1951. A field-theoretical work that explicitly denies inner dispositions and substitutes the concept of tendency-in-situation is W. Coutu, *Emergent human nature*, New York: Knopf, 1949.

15. See Chapters 3, 4, 6 and 9 of the present volume.

16. Representative of the neo-Freudian books here discussed are: E. Fromm, *Man for himself*, New York: Rinehart, 1947; K. Horney, *New ways in psychoanalysis*, New York: Norton, 1939; F. Fromm-Reichmann, *Principles of intensive psychotherapy*, Chicago: University of Chicago Press, 1951.

17. Cf. C. R. Rogers, *Counseling and psychotherapy*, Boston: Houghton Mifflin, 1942; *Client-centered therapy*, Boston: Houghton Mifflin, 1951; "Some observations on the organization of personality," *Amer. Psychologist*, 1947, 2:358-68.

18. Illustrative of this type of literature are: E. R. Hilgard, "Human motives and the concept of the self" (A Presidential address before the American Psychological Association), *Amer. Psychologist*, 1949, 4:374-82; D. Snygg and A. W. Combs, *Individual behavior*, New York: Harper, 1949; P. Lecky, *Self-consistency: a theory of personality*, New York: The Island Press, 1945; P. M. Symonds, *The ego and the self*, New York: Appleton-Century, 1951.

19. P. A. Bertocci, "A critique of G. W. Allport's theory of motivation," *Psychol. Rev.*, 1940, 47:501-32; G. W. Allport, "Motivation in personality: reply to Mr. Bertocci, *Psychol. Rev.*, 1940, 47:533-54. A more recent statement of Bertocci's well-considered position is found in his *Introduction to the philosophy of religion*, New York: Prentice-Hall, 1951, Chap. 8.

20. *Personality: a psychological interpretation*, op. cit. Chap. 11.

21. H. A. Murray, "Toward a classification of interactions," in T. Parsons and E. A. Shils, *op. cit.*, Part IV, Chap. 3.

22. Chapters 3-9 of the present volume deal with some of the issues here too briefly mentioned.

23. *Op. cit.*, especially pp. 463 ff.

24. Cf. E. L. Horowitz, "Spatial localization of the self," *J. Soc. Psychol.* 1935, 6:379-87.

25. E. S. Brightman, "What is personality?" *Personalist*, 1939, 20:138.

26. P. A. Bertocci, *Introduction to the philosophy of religion*, op. cit., p. 203.

27. W. Stern, *General psychology from the personalistic standpoint* (trans. by H. D. Spoerl), New York: Macmillan, 1938, p. 70. In German: *Die Person ist eine individuelle, eigenartige Ganzheit, welche zielstrebig wirkt, selbstbezogen und weltoffen ist; fähig ist zu erleben.*

CHAPTER 3

The open system in personality theory

If personality theory must come to terms with literature and with philosophy, it must also come to terms with natural and biological science. The concept of "system" is employed by many present-day psychologists in the hope that it will unify their work with that of their fellow scientists. In part their hope seems justified—provided only that the personality system is allowed to remain as open as its nature requires.

This essay was written by invitation of Division 8 (the Division of Personality and Social Psychology) of the American Psychological Association. It was delivered at the fourteenth annual meeting of the Division in Cincinnati in September 1959, and appeared in the *Journal of Abnormal and Social Psychology* (1960).

Our profession progresses in fits and starts, largely under the spur of fashion. The average duration of our fashions I estimate to be about ten years. McDougall's instinct theory held sway from 1908 to approximately 1920. Watsonian behaviorism dominated the scene for the next decade. Then habit hierarchies took command, then field theory—and now phenomenology. We never seem to solve our problems or exhaust our concepts; we only grow tired of them.

Presently it is fashionable to investigate such phenomena as response-set, coding, sensory deprivation and person perception, and to talk in terms of system-theory—a topic to which we shall soon return. Ten years ago, fashion called for group dynamics, Guttman scales and research on the unsavory qualities of the authoritarian personality. Twenty years ago it was frustration-aggression, Thurstone scales and national morale. Nowadays we watch with some consternation the partial eclipse of psychoanalysis by existentialism. And so it goes. Fortunately, most surges of fashion leave a rich residue of gain.

Fashions have their amusing and their serious sides. We can smile at the way bearded problems receive tonsorial transformation. Having tired of "suggestibility," we adopt the new hairdo known as "persuasibility." Modern ethology excites us, and we are not troubled by the recollection that a century ago John Stuart Mill staked down the term to designate the new science of human character. We like the neurological concept of "gating," conveniently forgetting that

39

American functionalism always stood firm for the dominance of general mental sets over specific. Reinforcement appeals to us but not the age-long debate over hedonism. The problem of freedom we brush aside in favor of "choice points." We avoid the body-mind problem but are in fashion when we talk about "brain models." Old wine, we find, tastes better from new bottles.

The serious side of the matter enters when we and our students forget that the wine is indeed old. Picking up a recent number of the *Journal of Abnormal and Social Psychology,* I discover that the twenty-one articles written by American psychologists confine ninety per cent of their references to publications of the past ten years, although most of the problems they investigate have gray beards. In the same issue of the *Journal,* three European authors locate fifty per cent of their references prior to 1949. What this proves I do not know, except that European authors were not born yesterday. Is it any wonder that our graduate students reading our journals conclude that literature more than a decade old has no merit and can be safely disregarded? At a recent doctoral examination the candidate was asked what his thesis on physiological and psychological conditions of stress had to do with the body-mind problem. He confessed he had never heard of the problem. An undergraduate said that all he knew about Thomas Hobbes was that he sank with the *Leviathan* when it hit an iceberg in 1912.

A Psycholinguistic Trifle

Our windows are pretty much shuttered toward the past, but we rightly rejoice in our growth since World War II. Among the many happy developments is rejuvenation in the field of psycholinguistics. (Even here, however, I cannot refrain from pointing out that the much-discussed Whorfian hypothesis was old stuff in the days of Wundt, Jespersen and Sapir.) Be that as it may, I shall introduce my discussion of open systems in personality theory by a crude Whorfian analysis of our own vocabulary. My research (aided by the kind assistance of Stanley Plog) is too cursory to warrant attempting a detailed report.

What we did, in brief, was to study the frequency of the prefixes *re-* and *pro-* in psychological language. Our hypothesis was that *re-* compounds, connoting as they do again-ness, passivity, being pushed or maneuvered, would be far more common than *pro-* compounds connoting futurity, intention, forward thrust. Our sample consisted of the indexes of the *Psychological abstracts* at five-year intervals over the past thirty years; also, all terms employing these prefixes in Hinsie and Shatzky's *Psychiatric dictionary* and in English and English's *Psychological dictionary*. In addition, we made a random sampling of pages in five current psychological journals. Combining these sources, it turns out that *re-* compounds are nearly five times as numerous as *pro-* compounds.

But, of course, not every compound is relevant to our purpose. Terms like *reference, relationship, reticular, report* do not have the connotation we seek; nor do terms like *probability, process* and *propaganda*. Our point is more clearly seen when we note that the term *reaction* or *reactive* occurs hundreds of times, while the term *proaction* or *proactive* occurs only once—and that in English's *Dictionary*, in spite of the fact that Harry Murray has made an effort to introduce the word into psychological usage.

But even if we attempt a more strict coding of this lexical material, accepting only those terms that clearly imply reaction and response on one side and proaction or the progressive programming of behavior on the other, we find the ratio still is approximately 5:1. In other words, our vocabulary is five times richer in terms like *reaction, response, reinforcement, reflex, respondent, retroaction, recognition, regression, repression, reminiscence* than in terms like *production, proceeding, proficiency, problem-solving, propriate* and *programming*. So much for the number of different words available. The disproportion is more striking when we note that the four terms *reflex, reaction, response* and *retention* together are used one hundred times more frequently than any single *pro-* compound except *problem-solving* and *projective*—and this latter term, I submit, is ordinarily used only in the sense of reactivity.

The weakness of the study is evident. Not all terms connoting spontaneous, future-oriented behavior begin with *pro*. One thinks of *expectancy, intention, purpose*. But neither do all terms connoting passive responding or backward reference in time begin with *re*. One thinks of *coding, traces, input-output* and the like. But, while our analysis leaves much to be desired, it prepares the way for our critique of personality theory in terms of systems. The connecting link is the question whether we have the verbal, and therefore the conceptual, tools to build a science of change, growth, futurity and potential; or whether our available technical lexicon tends to tie us to a science of response, reaction and regression. Our available vocabulary points to personality development from the past up to now, more readily than to its development from here on out into the future.

The Concept of System

Until a generation or so ago, science, including psychology, was preoccupied with what might be called "disorganized complexity." Natural scientists explored this fragment and that fragment of nature; psychologists explored this fragment and that fragment of experience and behavior. The problem of interrelatedness, though recognized, was not made a topic for direct inquiry.

What is called system-theory today—at least in psychology—is the outgrowth of the relatively new organismic conception reflected in the work of Von Bertalanffy and Goldstein and in certain aspects of Gestalt psychology. It opposes simple reaction theories, where a virtual automaton is seen to respond discretely to stimuli as though they were pennies in the slot. Interest in system-theory is increasing in psychology, though perhaps not so fast as in other sciences.

Now, a system—any system—is defined merely as *a complex of elements in mutual interaction.* Bridgman, as might be expected of an operationist, includes a hint of method in his definition. He writes that a system is "an isolated enclosure in which all measurements that can be made of what goes on in the system are in some way correlated." [1]

Systems may be classified as *closed* or *open.* A closed system is defined as one that admits no matter from outside itself and is therefore subject to entropy according to the second law of thermodynamics. While some outside energies, such as change in temperature and wind, may play upon a closed system, it has no restorative properties and no transactions with its environment, so that like a decaying bridge it sinks into thermodynamic equilibrium.

Some authors, such as Von Bertalanffy,[2] Brunswik[3] and Pumpian-Mindlin,[4] have said or implied that certain theories of psychology and of personality operate with the conception of closed systems. But in my opinion these critics press their point too far. We had better leave closed systems to the realm of physics where they belong (although even here it is a question whether Einstein's formula for the release of matter into energy does not finally demonstrate the futility of positing a closed system even in physics). In any event it is best to admit that all living organisms partake of the character of open systems. I doubt that we shall find any advocate of a truly closed system in the whole range of personality theory. At the same time, current theories do differ widely in the amount of openness they ascribe to the personality system.

If we comb definitions of open systems, we can piece together four criteria: (1) There is intake and output of both matter and energy. (2) There is the achievement and maintenance of steady (homeostatic) states, so that the intrusion of outer energy will not seriously disrupt internal form and order. (3) There is generally an increase of order over time, owing to an increase in complexity and differentiation of parts. (4) Finally, at least at the human level, there is more than mere intake and output of matter and energy; there is extensive transactional commerce with the environment.[5]

While all of our theories view personality as an open system in some sense, they can be fairly well classified according to the varying emphasis they place upon each of these criteria and according to how many of the criteria they admit.

Criterion 1

Consider the first criterion: material and energy exchange. Stimulus-response theory in its purest form concentrates on this criterion to the virtual exclusion of all the others. It says, in effect, that a stimulus enters and a response is emitted. There is, of course, machinery for summation, storage and delay, but the output is broadly commensurate with the intake. We need study only the two poles of stimulus and response with a minimum of concern for intervening processes. Methodological positivism goes one step further, saying, in effect, that we do not need the concept of personality at all. We focus attention on our own measurable manipulations of input and on the measurable manipulations of output. Personality thus evaporates in a mist of method.

Criterion 2

The requirement of steady states for open systems is so widely admitted in personality theory that it needs little discussion. To satisfy needs, to reduce tension and to maintain equilibrium—this comprises, in most theories, the basic formula of personality dynamics. Some authors, such as Stagner[6] and Mowrer, regard this formula as logically fitting in with Cannon's[7] account of homeostasis.[8] Man's intricate adjustive behavior is simply an extension of the principle involved in temperature regulation, balance of blood volume, sugar content and the like in the face of environmental change. It is true that Toch and Hastorf warn against over-extending the concept of homeostasis in personality theory.[9] I myself doubt that Cannon would approve the extension, for to him the value of homeostasis lay in its capacity to free man for what he called "the priceless unessentials" of life.[10] When biological equilibrium is attained, the priceless unessentials take over and constitute the major part of human activity. Be that as it may, most current theories clearly regard personality as a *modus operandi* for restoring a steady state.

Psychoanalytic theories are of this order. According to Freud, the ego strives to establish balance among the three "tyrants"—id, superego and outer environment. Likewise, the so-called mechanisms of ego-defense are essentially maintainers of a steady state. Even a neurosis has the same basic adjustive function.[11]

To sum up: Most current theories of personality take full account of two of the requirements of an open system. They allow interchange of matter and energy, and they recognize the tendency of organisms to maintain an orderly arrangement of elements in a steady state. Thus they emphasize stability rather than growth, permanence rather than change, "uncertainty reduction" (information theory) and "coding" (cognitive theory) rather than creativity. In short, they emphasize *being* rather than *becoming*. Hence, most personality theories are biologistic in the sense that they ascribe to personality only the two features of an open system that are clearly present in all living organisms.

There are, however, two additional criteria, sometimes mentioned but seldom stressed by biologists themselves, and similarly neglected in much current personality theory.

Transatlantic Perspective

Before examining Criterion 3, which calls attention to the tendency of open systems to enhance their degree of order, let us glimpse our present theoretical situation in cross-cultural perspective. In this country our special field of study has come to be called "behavioral science" (a label now firmly stuck to us with the glue of the Ford millions). The very flavor of this term suggests that we are occupied with semi-closed systems. By his very name the behavioral scientist seems committed to study man more in terms of behavior than in terms of experience; more in terms of mathematical space and clock-time than in terms of existential space and time; more in terms of response than of programming; more in terms of tension reduction than of tension enhancement; more in terms of reaction than of proaction.

Now let us leap our cultural stockade for a moment and listen to a bit of ancient Hindu wisdom. Most men, the Hindus say, have four central desires. To some extent, though only roughly, they correspond to the developmental stages of life. The first desire is for *pleasure*—a condition fully and extensively recognized in our Western theories of tension reduction, reinforcement, libido and needs. The second desire is for *success*—likewise fully recognized and studied in our investigations of power, status, leadership, masculinity and need-achievement. The third desire is to do one's duty and discharge one's responsibility. (It was Bismarck, not a Hindu, who said, "We are not in this world for pleasure but to do our damned duty.") Here our Western work begins to fade out: except for some pale investigations of parental punishment in relation to the development of childhood conscience, we have little to offer on the "duty motive." Conscience we tend to regard as a reactive response to internalized punishment, thus confusing the past "must" of learning with the "ought" involved in programming our future.[12] Finally, the Hindus tell us that for many people all these three motives pall, and they then seek intensely for a grade of understanding—for a philosophical or religious meaning—that will liberate them from pleasure, success and duty.[13] (Need I point out that most Western personality theories treat the religious aspiration in reactive terms— as an escape device, no different in kind from suicide, alcoholism and neurosis?)

Now we retrace our steps from India to modern Vienna and encounter the existentialist school of logotherapy. Its founder, Viktor Frankl, emphasizes above all the central place of *duty* and *meaning*, the same two motives that the Hindus place highest in their hierarchy of desire. Frankl reached his position after a long and agonizing incarceration in Nazi concentration camps, where, with other prisoners, he found himself stripped to naked existence.[14] In such extremity, what does a person need and want? Pleasure and success are out of the question. One wants to know the meaning of his suffering and to learn how, as a responsible being, he should acquit himself. Should he commit suicide? If so, why; if not, why not? The search for meaning becomes supreme.

Frankl is aware that his painfully achieved theory of motivation departs widely from most American theory, and he points out the implication of this fact for psychotherapy. He specifically criticizes the principle of homeostasis as implying that personality is a quasi-closed system.[15] To cater to the internal adjustments of a neurotic, or to assume that he will regain health by reshuffling his memories, defenses or conditioned reflexes, is ordinarily self-defeating. In many cases of neurosis, only a total breakthrough to new horizons will turn the trick.

Neither Hindu psychology nor logotherapy underestimates the role of pleasure and success in personality. Nor would Frankl abandon the hard-won gains reflected in psychoanalytic theory and need-theory. He says merely that in studying or treating a person we often find these essentially homeostatic formulations inadequate. A man normally wants to know the whys and wherefores. No other biological system does so; man stands alone in that he possesses a degree of openness surpassing that of any other living system.

Criterion 3

Returning now to our main argument, we encounter a not inconsiderable array of theories that emphasize the tendency of human personality to go beyond steady states and to strive for an enhancement and elaboration of internal order, even at the cost of considerable disequilibrium.

I cannot examine all of these or name all the relevant authors. One could start with McDougall's proactive sentiment of self-regard, which he viewed as organizing all behavior through a kind of "forward memory" (to use Gooddy's apt term).[16] Not too dissimilar is the stress that Combs and Snygg place on the enhancement of the phenomenal field. We may add Goldstein's conception of self-actualization as tending to enhance order in personality, as well as Maslow's theory of *growth motives* that supplement *deficiency motives*. One thinks of Jung's principle of individuation leading toward the achievement of a self—a goal never actually completed. Some theories, those of Bartlett and Cantril among them, put primary stress on the "pursuit of meaning." Certain developments in post-Freudian "ego-psychology" belong here.[17] So, too, does existentialism, with its recognition of the need for meaning and of the values of commitment. (The brain surgeon Harvey Cushing was speaking of open systems when he said, "The only way to endure life is to have a task to complete.") No doubt we should add Woodworth's recent advocacy of the "behavior primacy" theory as opposed to the "need" theory, Robert White's emphasis on "competence" and Erikson's "search for identity."

These theories are by no means identical. The differences between them merit prolonged debate. I lump them here simply because all seem to me to recognize the third criterion of open systems—

namely, the tendency of such systems to enhance their degree of order and become something more than they now are.

We all know the objection to theories of this type. Methodologists with a taste for miniature and fractionated systems complain that they do not lead to "testable propositions." [18] The challenge is valuable in so far as it calls for an expansion of research ingenuity. But the complaint is ill-advised if it demands that we return to quasi-closed systems simply because they are more "researchable" and elegant. Our task is to study what *is*, not merely what is immediately convenient.

Criterion 4

Now for our fourth and last criterion. Virtually all the theories I have mentioned up to now conceive of personality as something integumented, as residing within the skin. There are theorists (Kurt Lewin, Martin Buber, Gardner Murphy and others) who challenge this view, considering it too closed. Murphy says that we overstress the separation of man from the context of his living. Hebb has interpreted experiments on sensory deprivation as demonstrations of the constant dependence of inner stability on the flow of environmental stimulation.[19] Why Western thought makes such a razor-sharp distinction between the person and all else is an interesting problem. Probably the personalistic emphasis in Judeo-Christian religion is an initial factor; and as Murphy has pointed out,[20] the industrial and commercial revolutions further accentuated the role of individuality. Buddhist philosophy, by contrast, regards the individual, society and nature as forming the tripod of human existence. The individual as such does not stick out like a raw digit. He blends with nature, and he blends with society. It is only the merger that can be profitably studied.

Western theorists, for the most part, hold the integumented view of the personality system. I myself do so. Others, rebelling against the setting of self over against the world, have produced theories of personality written in terms of social interaction, role relations, situationism or some variety of field theory. Still other writers, such as Talcott Parsons[21] and F. H. Allport,[22] have admitted the validity of both the integumented personality system and systems of social interaction, and have spent much effort in harmonizing the two types of system thus conceived.

This problem, without doubt, is the knottiest issue in contemporary social science. It is the issue that, up to now, has prevented us from agreeing on the proper way to reconcile psychological and sociocultural science.

In this matter my own position is on the conservative side. It is the duty of psychology, I think, to study the person-system, meaning thereby the attitudes, abilities, traits, trends, motives and pathology of the individual—his cognitive styles, his sentiments, his individual moral nature and their interrelations. The justification is twofold: (1) There is a persistent though changing person-system in time, clearly delimited by birth and death. (2) We are immediately aware of the functioning of this system. Our knowledge of it, though imperfect, is direct, whereas our knowledge of all other outside systems, including social systems, is deflected and often distorted by their necessary incorporation into our own apperceptions.

At the same time, our work is incomplete unless we admit that each person possesses a *range* of abilities, attitudes and motives, which will be evoked by the different environments and situations he encounters. Hence we need to understand cultural, class and family constellations and traditions in order to know the schemata the person has probably interiorized in the course of his learning. But I hasten to warn that the study of cultural, class, family or any other social system does not automatically illumine the person-system, for we have to know whether the individual has accepted, rejected or remained uninfluenced by the social system in question. The fact that one plays the role of, say, teacher, salesman or father is less important for the study of his personality than to know whether he likes or dislikes, and how he defines, the role. But, unless we are students of sociocultural systems, we shall never know what it is the person is accepting, rejecting or redefining.

The provisional solution I would offer is the following: the personality theorist should be so well trained in social science that he can view the behavior of an individual as fitting any system of interaction; that is, he should be able to cast this behavior properly in the culture where it occurs, in its situational context and in terms of role theory and field theory. At the same time he should not lose sight—as some theorists do—of the fact that there is an internal and subjective patterning of all these contextual acts. A traveler who moves from culture to culture, from situation to situation, is none the less a single person; and within him one will find the nexus, the patterning, of the diverse experiences and memberships that constitute his personality.

Thus, I myself would not go so far as to advocate that personality be defined in terms of interaction, culture or roles. Attempts to do so seem to me to smudge the concept of personality and to represent a surrender of the psychologist's special assignment as a scientist. Let him be acquainted with all systems of interaction, but let him return always to the point where such systems converge and intersect and are patterned—in the single individual.

Hence, we accept the fourth (transactional) criterion of the open system, but with the firm warning that it must not be applied with so much enthusiasm that we lose the personality system altogether.

General Systems Theory

There are those who see hope for the unification of science in what James Miller has called *general behavior systems theory*.[23] This approach seeks formal identities between physical systems, the cell, the organ, the personality, small groups, the species and society. Critics—for example Buck[24]—complain that all this is feeble analogizing, that formal identities probably do not exist and that attempts to express analogies in terms of mathematical models result only in the vaguest generalities. As I see it, the danger in attempting to unify science in this manner lies in the inevitable approach from below—that is, in terms of physical and biological science. Closed systems or systems only partly open become our model; and if we are not careful, human personality in all its fullness is taken captive into some autistic paradise of methodology.

Besides neglecting the criteria of enhanced organization and transaction, general systems theory has an added defect. The human person is, after all, the observer and interpreter of systems. This awkward fact has recently been haunting the founder of the operational movement, P. W. Bridgman.[25] Can we as scientists live subjectively within our system and at the same time take a valid objective view thereof?

Some years ago Elkin published the case of "Harry Holzer" and invited thirty-nine specialists to offer their conceptualizations.[26] As might be expected, many different conceptualizations resulted. No theorist was able entirely to divest the case of his own preconceptions. Each read the objective system in terms of the subjective. Our theories of personality—all of them—reflect the temperament of the author fully as much as the personality of *alter*.

This sad specter of observer-contamination should not, I think, discourage us from the search for objectively valid theory. Truth, as the philosopher Charles Peirce has said, is the opinion that is fated to be ultimately agreed to by all who investigate. My point is that the opinion fated to be ultimately agreed to by all who investigate is not likely to be reached through a premature application of general systems theory or through devotion to any one partially closed theory. Theories of open systems hold more promise, though at present they are not in agreement among themselves. But somewhere, sometime, I hope and believe, we shall establish a theory of the nature of personality that all wise men who investigate, including psychologists, will eventually accept.

Some Examples

In the meantime, I suggest that we regard all sharp controversies in personality theory as probably arising from the two opposed points of view: the quasi-closed and the fully open.

The principle of reinforcement, to take one example, is commonly regarded as the cement that stamps in a response, as the glue that fixes personality at the level of past deeds. An open system interpretation is very different. Feigl, for instance, has pointed out that reinforcement works primarily in a prospective sense.[27] It is only from a *recognition* of consequences (not from the consequences themselves) that the human individual binds the past to the future and resolves to avoid punishment and to seek rewards in similar circumstances—provided, of course, that it is consonant with his interests and values to do so. Here we no longer assume that reinforcement stamps in; it is taken as one factor among many to be considered in the programming of future action.[28] What a wide difference it makes whether we regard personality as a quasi-closed or an open system!

The issue has its parallels in neurophysiology. How open is the nervous system? We know it is of a complexity so formidable that we have only an inkling as to how complex it may be. Yet one thing is certain: high level gating often controls and steers lower level processes. While we cannot tell exactly what we mean by "higher levels," they surely involve ideational schemata, intentions and generic personality trends. They are instruments for programming, not merely for reacting. In the future we may confidently expect that the neurophysiology of programming and the psychology of proaction will draw together. Until they do so, it is wise to hold lightly our self-closing metaphors of sow bug, switchboard, giant computor and hydraulic pump.

Finally, an example from motivation theory. Some years ago I argued that motives may become functionally autonomous of their origins. (And one lives to regret one's brashness.)

Whatever its shortcomings, the concept of functional autonomy succeeds in viewing personality as an open and changing system. As might be expected, criticism has come chiefly from those who prefer to view the personality system as quasi-closed. Some critics say that I am dealing only with occasional cases where the extinction of a habit system has failed to occur. This criticism, of course, begs the question, for the precise point at issue is: why do some habit systems fail to extinguish when no longer reinforced? And why do some habit systems that were once instrumental get refashioned into interests and values having a motivational push?

The common counterargument holds that "secondary reinforcement" somehow miraculously sustains all the central desires of a mature person. The scientific ardor of Pasteur, the religio-political zeal of Gandhi and, for that matter, Aunt Sally's devotion to her needlework are explained by hypothetical cross-conditioning, which somehow substitutes for the primary reinforcement of primary drives. What is significant for our purposes is that these critics prefer the concept of secondary reinforcement, not because it is clearer, but because it holds our thinking within the frame of a quasi-closed (reactive) system.

Now is not the time to reargue the matter, but I can at least hint at my present views. I would say first that the concept of functional autonomy has relevance even at the level of quasi-closed systems. There are now so many indications concerning feed-back mechanisms, cortical self-stimulation, self-organizing systems and the like[29] that I believe we cannot deny the existence of self-sustaining circuit-mechanisms, which we can lump together under the rubric *perseverative functional autonomy*.

But the major significance of the concept lies in a different direction and presupposes the view that personality is a wide open system seeking progressively new levels of order and transaction. While drive motives remain fairly constant throughout life, existential motives do not. It is the very nature of an open system to achieve progressive levels of order through change in cognitive and motivational structure. Since in this case the causation is systematic, we cannot hope to account for functional autonomy in terms of specific reinforcements. This condition I would call *propriate functional autonomy*.

Both perseverative and propriate autonomy are, I think, indispensable conceptions. The one applies to the relatively closed part-systems within personality; the other, to the continuously evolving structure of the whole.

A last example. It is characteristic of the quasi-closed system outlook that it is heavily nomothetic: it seeks similarities among all personality systems—or, as in general behavior systems theory, among *all* systems. If, however, we elect the open system view, we find ourselves forced in part toward the idiographic outlook. For now the vital question becomes: what makes the system hang together in any one person? [30] Let me repeat this question, for it is the one that more than any other has haunted me over the years: *what makes the system cohere in any one person?* That this problem is pivotal, urgent and relatively neglected will be recognized by open system theorists, even while it is downgraded and evaded by those who prefer their systems semi-closed.

Final Word

If this essay has seemed polemical, I can only plead that personality theory lives by controversy. In this country we are fortunate that no single party line shackles our speculations. We are free to pursue any and all assumptions concerning the nature of man. The penalty we pay is that, for the present, we cannot expect personality *theory* to be cumulative—although, fortunately, to some extent personality *research* can be.

Theories, we know, are ideally derived from axioms—or, if axioms are lacking (as in our field), from assumptions. But our assumptions regarding the nature of man range from the Adlerian to the Zilborgian, from the Lockean to the Leibnitzian, from the Freudian to the Hullian, from the cybernetic to the existentialist. Some of us model man after the pigeon; others view his potentialities as many-splendored. And there is no agreement in sight.

Nils Bohr's principle of complementarity contains a lesson for us. He showed that if we study the position of a particle, we do not at the same time study its momentum. Applied to our own work, the principle tells us that if we focus on reaction, we do not simultaneously study proaction; if we measure one trait, we do not fix our attention on pattern; if we tackle a subsystem, we lose the whole; if we pursue the whole, we overlook the part-functioning. For the single investigator, there seems to be no escape from this limitation. Our only hope is to overcome it by a complementarity of investigators and of theorists.

While I myself am partisan for the open system, I would shut no doors. (Some of my best friends are quasi-closed systematists.) If I argue for the open system, I plead more strongly for the open mind. Our condemnation is reserved for that peculiar slavery to fashion which says that conventionality alone makes for scientific respectability. We still have much to learn from our creative fumblings with the open system. Among our students, I trust, there will be many adventurers.

REFERENCES

1. P. W. Bridgman, *The way things are*, Cambridge: Harvard University Press, 1959, p. 188.
2. L. Von Bertalanffy, "Theoretical models in biology and psychology," in D. Krech and G. S. Klein (eds.), *Theoretical models and personality theory*, Durham, N.C.: Duke University Press, 1952.
3. E. Brunswik, "The conceptual framework of psychology," *International Encyclopedia of Unified Science*, Chicago: University of Chicago Press, 1955, Vol. I, No. 10.
4. E. Pumpian-Mindlin, "Propositions concerning energetic-economic aspects of libido theory," *Ann. N.Y. Acad. Sci.*, 1959, 76:1038-52.
5. Von Bertalanffy's definition explicitly recognizes the first two of these criteria as present in all living organisms. A living organism, he says, is "an open system which continually gives up matter to the outer world and takes in matter from it, but which maintains itself in this continuous exchange in a steady state, or approaches such steady state in its variations in time" [*Problems of life* (trans. of *Das biologische Weltbild*, 1949), New York: Wiley, 1952, p. 125]. But elsewhere in this author's writing we find recognition of the additional criteria (*Ibid.*, p. 145; "Theoretical models and personality theory," *op. cit.*, p. 34).
6. R. Stagner, "Homeostasis as a unifying concept in personality theory," *Psychol. Rev.*, 1951, 58:5-17.
7. W. B. Cannon, *The wisdom of the body*, New York: Norton, 1932.
8. In a recent review ["A cognitive theory of dynamics" (review of R. S. Woodworth, *Dynamics of behavior*), *Contemp. Psychol.*, 1959, 4:129-33], H. S. Mowrer strongly defends the homeostatic theory. He is distressed that the dean of American psychologists, Robert Woodworth (*Dynamics of behavior*, New York: Holt, 1958), has taken a firm stand against the "need-primacy" theory in favor of what he calls the "behavior-primacy" theory. With the detailed merits of the argument we are not here concerned. What concerns us at the moment is that the issue has been sharply joined. Need-primacy, which Mowrer calls a "homeostatic" theory, does not go beyond our first two criteria for an open system. Woodworth, by insisting that contact with and mastery of the environment constitute a pervasive principle of motivation, recognizes the additional criteria.
9. H. H. Toch and A. H. Hastorf, "Homeostasis in psychology," *Psychiatry*, 1955, 18:81-91.
10. W. B. Cannon, *op cit.*, p. 323.

11. When we speak of the "function" of a neurosis, we are reminded of the many theories of "functionalism" current in psychology and social science. Granted that the label, as Merton has shown (R. K. Merton, *Social theory and social structure*, rev. ed., Glencoe, Ill.: The Free Press, 1957, Chap. 1.), is a wide one, still we may safely say that the emphasis of functionalism is always on the usefulness of an activity in maintaining the steady state of a personality or social or cultural system. In short, "functional" theories stress maintenance of present direction, allowing little room or none at all for departure and change.

12. G. W. Allport, *Becoming: basic considerations for a psychology of personality*, New Haven: Yale University Press, 1955, pp. 68-74.

13. H. Smith, *The religions of man*, New York: Harper, 1958; New York: Mentor, 1959.

14. V. E. Frankl, *From death camp to existentialism*, Boston: Beacon, 1959.

15. V. E. Frankl, "Das homöestatische Prinzip und die dynamische Psychologie," Z. *Psychoth. Med. Psychol.*, 1959, 9:41-47.

16. W. Gooddy, "Two directions of memory," *J. Indiv. Psychol.*, 1959, 15: 83-88.

17. Pumpian-Mindlin (*op cit.*, p. 1051) writes, "The focus of clinical psychoanalysis on ego psychology is a direct result of the change from a closed system to an open one."

18. Cf. T. B. Roby, "An opinion on the construction of behavior theory," *Amer. Psychologist*, 1959, 14:127-34.

19. D. O. Hebb, "The mammal and his environment," *Amer. J. Psychiat.* 1955, 111:826-31. Reprinted in E. E. Maccoby, T. M. Newcomb, E. L. Hartley (eds.), *Readings in social psychology*, New York: Holt, 1958, pp. 335-41.

20. G. Murphy, *Human potentialities*, New York: Basic Books: 1958, p. 297.

21. T. Parsons, *The social system*, Glencoe, Ill.: The Free Press, 1951.

22. F. H. Allport, *Theories of personality and the concept of structure*, New York: Wiley, 1955.

23. J. G. Miller, "Toward a general theory for the behavioral sciences," *Amer. Psychologist*, 1955, 10:513-31.

24. R. C. Buck, "On the logic of general behavior systems theory," in H. Feigl and M. Scriven (eds.), *Minnesota studies in the philosophy of science*, Vol. I, 1956.

25. *Op. cit.*

26. F. Elkin, "Specialists interpret the case of Harry Holzer," *J. Abnorm. Soc. Psychol.*, 1947, 42:99-111.

27. H. Feigl, "Philosophical embarrassments of psychology," *Amer. Psychologist*, 1959, 14:117.

28. G. W. Allport, "Effect: a secondary principle of learning," *Psychol. Rev.*, 1946, 53:335-47.

29. Cf. D. O. Hebb, *The organization of behavior*, New York: Wiley, 1949; J. Olds and P. Milner, "Positive reinforcement produced by electrical stimulation of septal area and other regions of rat brain," *J. Comp. Physio. Psychol.*, 1954, 47:419-27; H. T. Chang, "The repetitive discharge of cortico-thalamic reverberating circuit," *J. Neurophysiol.*, 1950, 13:235-57.

30. Cf. J. G. Taylor, "Experimental design: a cloak for intellectual sterility," *Brit. J. Psychol.*, 1958, 49:106-16.

CHAPTER 4

Scientific models and human morals

The present chapter, like Chapter 3, is based on a talk to the Division of Personality and Social Psychology of the American Psychological Association. It was delivered as the president's address at the first annual meeting, September 1946, and was published in the *Psychological Review* (1947).

The essay expresses dissatisfaction with the root-metaphors employed in depicting human nature. It argues that theoretical systems require concepts that reflect the basic nature of conduct, goal-directed and intentional. Current fashionable models—derived from animal, child and machine—overstress the purely reactive side of personality and, in so doing, handicap the psychologist in his efforts to understand and improve the human lot.

In forming this Division of Personality and Social Psychology, we are stating our readiness to assume a certain responsibility. We are announcing, in effect, that as a group of scientists we believe we have a contribution to make in interpreting and remedying some of the serious dislocations in our society.

The test of our fitness to exist and to prosper, I submit, will be our ability to contribute substantially in the near future to the diagnosis and treatment of the outstanding malady of our time. The malady I refer to is not war, for modern warfare is but a symptom of an underlying morbid condition; it is not the threatening fission of one world into two, ominous as this threat may be; nor is it our apparent inability to control for our safety and profit the transformation of matter into atomic energy, though this crisis too is now upon us. I speak rather of the *underlying* ailment, of the fact that man's moral sense is not able to assimilate his technology.

While technological warfare, technological unemployment and the atomic age—all by-products of physical science—have overtaken us, mental and moral science have made no corresponding gains in allaying the rivalries and anxieties induced by technology, in devising methods of social control or in enhancing human cooperation and solidarity. It is, I venture to point out, precisely our own young science that has failed to keep pace with the needs of the times.

Public officials are urgently seeking the aid of psychologists.

Many of us who have been approached are embarrassed by the scarcity of scientific findings, and even of serviceable concepts and well-formulated problems, that psychology has to offer *of the type that is being sought.* What is asked for is instant help in discovering the sources and conditions of man's moral sense in order that this sense may be enlarged and brought into focus. What is asked for is aid from a science of human relationships, whose assistance Franklin D. Roosevelt likewise invoked in his last speech before his death.[1] Yet we may comb the entire file of the *Psychological Abstracts* and find very little that has any bearing upon the improvement of human relationships on an international scale.

Why have we so relatively little to offer? Is it simply that we are young? Or have we gotten off to a thoroughly bad start through our adoption of root-metaphors that lead away from, rather than toward, the problem at hand? Three generations ago psychology was commonly classified as a "moral science." Though we may not favor the aura of this term, how can we expect anything other than a science *of* moral conduct to discover the conditions that will bring the needed counterpoise to technology run wild?

In taking stock of this situation, I observe how many of us seem so stupefied by admiration of physical science that we believe psychology, in order to succeed, need only imitate the models, postulates, methods and language of physical science. If someone points out the present inutility of mechanical models in predicting any but the most peripheral forms of human behavior, we are inclined to reply: Wait a thousand years if necessary, and you will see that man is a robot and that all his mental functions can be synthesized in kind as successfully as we now synthesize table salt, quinine or a giant calculator. While we righteously scorn what one of us has called "the subjective, anthropomorphic hocus pocus of mentalism," [2] we would consider a colleague emotional and mystical should he dare speak of "the objective, mechanomorphic focus of physicalism."

Let our progress be gradual, we say. By sticking to the peripheral, visible operations, we may someday be able to approach complex problems of motivation, and then come within hailing distance of the distresses of mankind. We hope that these distresses will keep a thousand years until we are ready to cope with them and that in the meantime a free science will be permitted to linger along and take its time. But, even if such improbable conditions were fulfilled, I question whether we should endorse this counsel of patience or the premises upon which it rests.

Besides the mechanical model, there are two other currently

popular paradigms in psychology that are, in my opinion, only slightly less inept in guiding significant research or theory concerning the foundations of social morality. I refer to the phylogenetic model and to the infant mind. Although both these models during the past two generations have brought new insights and correctives into our work, they have not proved adequate to the needs of clinical, personnel and social psychology.

When any one of us undertakes a piece of research, he inevitably adopts, according to his preference, one or another of the fundamental models available to psychologists. My thesis is that now if ever we need to test our preferred model for its capacity to yield discoveries that have some sure relevance to moral nature and to social ills.

Expectancy and Intention

The machine model in psychology had its origin, not in clinical or social experience, but rather in adulation of the technological success of the physical sciences.

If I interpret the matter correctly, American psychology naturally adapted mechanical models because our culture has always been action-oriented and technological. By and large, our psychology is a motorized psychology and is only now widening its concept of action to include the ego-involved participation of the human organism in matters affecting its own destiny.[3] The earlier extreme position, represented by E. B. Holt and J. B. Watson, held personality to be essentially a battery of trigger-release mechanisms. This view paid no attention to the sustained directions of striving that are characteristic of moral behavior—to what in this essay I shall call "intentions."

This trigger-model, still preferred by a few, gave way gradually to a more purposive behaviorism. The concept of "sign-Gestalt expectancy" was introduced by Tolman and mercifully shortened by Hilgard and Marquis to "expectancy."[4] It is an interesting fact that these authors seem to regard the principle of expectancy as the most purposive of all the essentially mechanical theories derived from the multitudinous experiments on the conditioned reflex.[5] In other words, some version of the principle of expectancy is as far as many psychologists have come in their conception of the nature of personal and social conduct.

The principle holds that in the presence of certain signs the organism expects a certain goal to appear if it follows the customary behavior route. If the goal is reached, the expectation is confirmed;

if not, the organism may vary its behavior.[6] The principle, while allowing for the importance of attitude, is essentially stimulus-bound. We behave according to the cues we have learned, according to our expectancies.

In order not to complicate my argument, I shall leave out of consideration the law of effect, which, it would be easy to show, likewise ascribes behavior wholly to past experience, to learned cues and to mechanical reinforcements.[7] Both principles, so far as I can see, accord nothing to the *un*rewarded, *un*realized, yet persistive intentions of man's moral nature.

The trouble with these currently fashionable concepts, drawn from the phylogenetic model, is that while they seem to apply aptly enough to animal behavior, whence they were derived, they have only a limited or else a remote analogical bearing on the activities of human beings. We may know a person's expectancies and even his past rewards; yet we are singularly unable to predict or control his future behavior unless we know also his basic intentions, which are by no means a stenciled copy of his previous expectancies and rewards.[8]

To take an example, the sign-Gestalten today are such that we may reasonably expect future crises in our relations with Russia. Does this fact tell in any degree what we can, should or will do about it? This precise area of conflict is a novel one (as, indeed, all important situations are). The best predictive basis we have lies in our own national and personal *intentions* regarding Russia. It is our purposes, not our expectancies, that are now the issue.

As if aware of the scantiness of the expectancy principle, Tolman advises us to embrace also a "need-cathexis psychology." [9] But the situation here turns out to be parallel. Need-cathexis psychology—of course I oversimplify—holds essentially that a handful of physiological drives get attached to this, that or the other object. A man who, in Tolman's pleasing vernacular, is "raised right" meshes his drive into a socially acceptable gear. A man "raised wrong" does not. But what is so striking about human motivation is that so often a desire or aspiration is meshed into no gear. It simply reaches forward hungrily into the future like the tip of a scarlet runner bean, groping for a goal that it does not know about.

The embarrassment of the need-cathexis type of psychology is reflected in the apologetic language it uses when referring to this expansive aspect of human motivation. Accustomed to work with animals or with infants, need-cathexis psychology labels adult human intentions "secondary drives," "derived drives" or "drive conversions."

With such depreciating concepts, both the mechanical and the phylo-genetic psychologists apparently seek to dispose of those morally rele-vant desires and aspirations that are in fact so different from the drive-impelled excursions of the cozy robot or cozy rodent.[10]

My objection to the animal paradigm for personality and for social psychology is not so much that animals lack culture—a fact that Tolman in his sparkling paper first frankly admits and then amiably represses—but rather that the motivational structure of man and of lower animals seems to be in only a slight degree similar. In this respect, as with his evolutionary brain development (to quote Julian Huxley), "man stands alone."[11] Animals are demonstrably creatures of stimulus-expectancy and need-cathexis. Man, in all that is distinctive of his species, is a creature of intentions. We may well doubt that the basic equation for intentional morality, or that for intentional learning, can be written from a study of organisms that lack propositional symbols. To this point I shall return.

While I am disapproving of current models, I shall state my final grievance, this time against the rigid ontogenetic stencils that derive from Freudianism. Odd as it may appear, Freud resembles the mechanical and phylogenetic psychologists in wanting his doc-trine of motivation anchored to neuro-anatomy. I assume that this is his desire, because he refuses to see anything at all in the co-operative, socialized, affiliative undertakings of mankind except goal-inhibited sexuality. To the sex drive he adds principally the im-pulses of aggression, destruction and death. It seems obvious that Freudianism, even though eagerly adopted by many who have found the mechanical and animal models inadequate, offers an equally meager basis for a serviceable study of man's moral conduct.

The trouble lies chiefly in the excessive emphasis upon infantile experience. We are asked to believe that an individual's character-structure is, in all essentials, determined by the time his last diaper is changed. Even Suttie, who postulates as the foundation of morality an original and embracing instinct of tenderness, affection and social symbiosis, believes its fate is sealed according to the manner in which the mother handles this affiliative impulse before and after weaning.[12] If the chances for peace in the world depend to such a degree upon infant fixations, ought we not disband this Division and register as wet nurses to the mewling citizens of tomorrow?

The concept of intention, which I am here opposing to reac-tivity, expectancy and infantile fixation, is not immediately con-genial to American psychology. Yet its adoption in some form or another is necessary. With some malice aforethought I have selected the term *intention*—spiced, as it is, by an aggravating flavor of mentalism—to signify those aspects of thought and of motivation that play a leading, but now neglected, part in the complex, affiliative, moral conduct of men. I believe it is precisely the "private" worlds of desire, aspiration and conscience that must be studied if we are to succeed in the task of social engineering.

In using the term *intention,* however, I am not arguing surreptitiously for phenomenology, though in order to improve our grasp on the subtleties of man's intentions we would do well to emulate the refinement of its descriptive method.[13] Nor am I arguing for a revival of Brentano, though we have neglected unduly the central proposition of Act Psychology: that, at every moment, man's mind is directed by some intention—loving, hating, comparing, understanding, desiring, rejecting, planning or some similar mental act.

Let us define intention simply as *what the individual is trying to do.* Naïve as this definition may sound, it is in reality the product of decades of sophisticated wrestling with the problems of human motivation. In this concept influences as diversified as Brentano, Darwin, Freud, Cannon and Wertheimer are brought into focus. In essence it no longer draws the sharp distinction, advanced by both Kant and Schopenhauer, between will (or drive) on the one hand and intellect on the other. The machine, rat and infant models we have been following (though I am sure they'd be surprised and grieved to know it) preserve this irreconcilable Kantian dichotomy. They side somewhat more, however, with Schopenhauer in regarding the functions of the intellect as wholly instrumental and secondary. Without forgetting for a moment what we have learned about rationalizing and about the untrustworthiness of introspective reports on motives, we may safely declare that the opposing of motive and thought-process has gone much too far. Usually the individual is trying to do something in which his wants and his plans easily cooperate. Instead of being at opposite poles, his emotion and his reason canalize into a single endeavor. The direction of his endeavor I designate as the intention, and offer this concept as an improvement upon the one-sided irrationalistic doctrines of drive, need, instinct and cathexis.

In deference to the discoveries of psychoanalysis, we readily admit that an individual does not always know precisely what his own intentions are. *Consciously* he may misinterpret the line of his own endeavor; a neurotic frequently does so. In such cases, insight

of difference between signal and symbol, and that even his own careful system of semiotic fails adequately to bridge the gap. Though I have not actually counted the illustrations in his book, I have the impression that a majority of them refer to animal responses to signals and that relatively few deal with human responses to symbols. In any case, it is clear that Morris, like many psychologists, is enamored of the phylogenetic model.

I venture to cite another brilliant and candid passage from his book. He writes of the fact that a sign may be *iconic*—that is to say, it may itself resemble the properties of its denotatum. Thus a motion picture is highly iconic; an onomatopoeic word less so; a wholly arbitrary sign not at all iconic. He then offers this highly significant observation: "One of the dangers of the use of models in science, for instance, arises out of the temptation to ascribe to the subject matter of a theory properties of the model illustrating the theory which are not involved in the theory itself." [24]

From this warning would it not follow that an adequate theory of symbols can hardly be derived from the animal model in which *signals* alone predominate? How can we expect to understand human symbolism in terms of the phylogenetic type when, as Morris himself asserts, we are tempted to overextend the properties of our type-model and force them to serve in place of the independent theory we need to develop?

The Model We Need

To sum up: The designs we have been using in our studies of motivation, of symbol and hence of the foundations of moral behavior are not—to borrow Morris' crisp term—sufficiently iconic with our subject matter. Addiction to machines, rats or infants leads us to overplay those features of human behavior that are peripheral, signal-oriented or genetic. Correspondingly, it causes us to underplay those features that are central, future-oriented and symbolic.

What sort of a model, then, do we need? This question opens systematic vistas that lie beyond the scope of this essay. Yet, lest my numerous criticisms indicate a despair that I do not actually feel, I shall mention a few recent signs and portents that signify a newer—and, to my mind, more wholesome—outlook.

Most noteworthy is the fact that the war led many psychologists to deal directly with the integrated behavior of the GI, the factory worker, the civilian. We then learned that the interests of morale, psychotherapy, personnel placement and psychological warfare could not be pursued successfully by clinging to our threadbare models. Our inadequate root-metaphors went into the ash can for the duration. It is because of this conceptual discard, with its resultant wartime success in the promotion of social engineering, that I have presumed at this time to bring into the open a conflict that many, perhaps most of us, have secretly felt. Must we now resume the tattered stencils that we so recently abandoned with such good effect?

There are various indicators of improvement in theoretical outlook. I have in mind the new and vital conception of the ego that has come into psychotherapy;[25] the discovery and application of psychological principles involved in bringing the worker into a participant relation with his job;[26] the discovery and application of procedures leading to successful administration.[27] We discern an accelerated movement toward the development of such theories as can have their acid test here and now, not a thousand years hence. These theories neither strain the credulity nor stretch an inappropriate model beyond its logical breaking point.

We happily find more emphasis than before on the structuring activities of the person, on the importance of centrally initiated motive patterns, on cognitive dynamisms—including ideology, schemata of meaning and frames of reference. We find the contemporaneity of motives stressed, as well as the important functions of self-esteem and ego-involvement. Though symbols are still confused with signals, we are beginning, through content-analysis and interviewing, to study symbols both in their own right and as the basic ingredients of all complex conduct, including all morally relevant thought and behavior. We have learned, through improved polls and other methods of inquiry, to ascertain the direction of social purpose as it resides in individual minds. From such knowledge it should be possible to fashion a domestic and international social policy that will be sufficiently realistic to succeed.

All these and many more signs indicate the growing dependence of modern theories upon a model that is none the less scientific for being humane. As this design for personality and social psychology gradually becomes better tempered to our subject matter, we shall cease borrowing false notes—whether squeaks, squeals or squalls. We shall read the score of human personality more accurately for the benefit of the world audience that waits to listen.

REFERENCES

1. "Today we are faced with the preëminent fact that, if civilization is to survive, we must cultivate the science of human relationships—the ability

of all peoples, of all kinds, to live together and work together, in the same world, at peace."

2. E. G. Boring, "Mind and mechanism," *Amer. J. Psychol.*, 1946, 54:173-92.

3. See Chapter 12 of the present volume.

4. E. R. Hilgard and D. G. Marquis, *Conditioning and learning*, New York: Appleton-Century, 1940.

5. *Ibid.*, p. 101.

6. *Ibid.*, p. 88.

7. G. W. Allport, "Effect: a secondary principle of learning," *Psychol. Rev.*, 1946, 54:335-47.

8. See Chapter 9 of the present volume.

9. E. C. Tolman, "A stimulus-expectancy need-cathexis psychology," *Science*, 1945, 101:160-66.

10. It is instructive to read the perorations of two presidential addresses by psychologists, one preferring the machine model, the other the rat model. Though good-humored and witty, both authors candidly acknowledge their own escapist motives. To paraphrase Carlson's quip concerning Cannon's theory of emotions: the authors seem to entertain their models because the models entertain them.

"I believe that robotic thinking helps precision of psychological thought, and will continue to help it until psychophysiology is so far advanced that an image is nothing other than a neural event, and object constancy is obviously just something that happens in the brain. That time is still a long way off, and in the interval I choose to sit cozily with my robot, squeezing his hand and feeling a thrill—a scientist's thrill—when he squeezes mine back again." (E. G. Boring, *op. cit.*, p. 192).

"And, as a final peroration, let it be noted that rats live in cages; they do not go on binges the night before one has planned an experiment; they do not kill each other off in war; they do not invent engines of destruction, and if they did, they would not be so dumb about controlling such engines; they do not go in for either class conflicts or race conflicts; they avoid politics, economics and papers on psychology. They are marvelous, pure and delightful. And, as soon as I possibly can, I am going to climb back again out on that good old philogenetic limb and sit there, this time right side up and unashamed, wiggling my whiskers at all the dumb, yet at the same time far too complicated, specimens of *homo sapiens*, whom I shall see strutting and fighting and messing things up, down there on the ground below me" (E. C. Tolman, *op. cit.*, p. 166).

11. J. Huxley, *Man stands alone*, New York and London: Harper, 1941.

12. I. D. Suttie, *The origins of love and hate*, London: Kegan Paul, 1935.

13. An excellent example is Bertocci's analysis of man's sense of moral obligation (P. Bertocci, "A reinterpretation of moral obligation," *Phil. Phenomenol. Res.*, 1945, 6:270-83). He shows that, when we study the *ought-consciousness* phenomenologically, we discover how entirely different it is from the *must-consciousness*. This discovery leads to a justifiable suspicion that, whatever conscience may be, it does not derive merely from fear of punishment or from social coercion. Too hastily and heedlessly have psychologists accepted Freud's identification of the superego with threat of parental punishment.

14. McDougall specifically objected to the concept of intention on the

grounds that conscious intention merely obscures the instinctive motive at work (W. McDougall, *Outline of psychology*, New York: Scribner, 1923, pp. 121 f.). He had in mind the indubitable fact that men's verbal reports of their intentions may be rationalizations. But in my use of the term I do not confine intention to reportable purpose. Sometimes the essential direction of an intention is understood well enough by the subject, sometimes not. If the term, as I propose, is taken to mean *both* the understood and the non-understood direction of an act, I maintain that it can serve as a proper designation for "ultimate motives" and not merely for proximate or rationalized motives.

To my mind, it is unnecessary to have recourse to a doctrine of underlying needs or instincts. McDougall, for example, allowed far too little for the ever changing panorama of man's intentions, which, as they evolve from an original genetic equipment, undergo complete change of form and functional significance (G. W. Allport, "Motivation in personality: reply to Mr. Bertocci," *Psychol. Rev.,* 1940, 47:533-54).

15. See Chapter 9 of the present volume.

16. C. L. Hull, "Goal attraction and directing ideas conceived as habit phenomena," *Psychol. Rev.,* 1931, 38:487-506.

17. P. Lecky, *Self-consistency: a theory of personality,* New York: The Island Press, 1945, p. 122 f.

18. E. L. Thorndike, *Animal intelligence,* New York: Macmillan, 1911, p. 119.

19. R. M. Yerkes, *Chimpanzees: a laboratory colony,* New Haven: Yale University Press, 1943, p. 189.

20. E. Cassirer, *An essay on man,* New Haven: Yale University Press, 1945, p. 30.

21. Even in human beings we occasionally encounter a sharp break between symbols and signs. Some of Goldstein's aphasic patients, for example, seem capable of responding to signs but not to symbols, as in the case of the man who could understand the word-signs "drink it" when a glass full of water was presented to him, but was unable to go through the symbolic motions of drinking it if the glass was empty (K. Goldstein, *Human nature in the light of psychopathology,* Cambridge: Harvard University Press, 1940, p. 44).

Without symbols we could not make believe, dissimulate or lie; we could not form plans for our future or hold in mind those schemata that make possible consistency in moral conduct.

22. E. Cassirer, *op. cit.,* p. 25.

23. C. Morris, *Signs, language and behavior,* New York: Prentice-Hall, 1946, p. 198.

24. *Ibid.,* p. 23.

25. See Chapter 9 of the present volume.

26. See Chapter 12 of the present volume.

27. A. H. Leighton, *The governing of men,* Princeton: Princeton University Press, 1945.

PART II: *Motivation and structure in personality*

CHAPTER 5

The ego in contemporary psychology

This essay argues that the concept of self—that is, of ego—must be given a prominent position in psychological theory. It deplores the fact that, following the publication of William James's *Principles of psychology,* the self for a time suffered a virtual eclipse.

Since the first publication of this essay in the *Psychological Review* (1943), the concept has in fact been reintroduced at a rapid rate. There is much agreement concerning need for it, but less agreement concerning its precise place in personality theory. The analysis offered in the present chapter is developed more fully in my book *Becoming: basic considerations for a psychology of personality* (1955).

The essay was the presidential address at the fourteenth annual meeting of the Eastern Psychological Association at Hunter College in April 1943.

Introduction

One of the oddest events in the history of modern psychology is the manner in which the ego—or self—became sidetracked and lost to view. I say it is odd, because the existence of one's own self is the one fact of which every mortal person—every psychologist included—is perfectly convinced. An onlooker might say, "Psychologists are funny fellows. They have before them, at the heart of their science, a fact of perfect certainty, the one warrant for the being of all other things, and yet they pay no attention to it. Why don't they begin with their own egos, or with our egos—with something we all know about? If they did so, we might understand them better. What is more, they might understand us better."

Back in the 1880s, of course, it was good form for James, Royce, Dewey and their contemporaries to speak freely of the ego, the self or even the soul. The soul, to be sure, was giving way under Wundt's onslaughts, and everyone was finding it exhilarating to shake off the alleged theological domination and to emerge unfettered and positivistic into the era of the New Psychology. They forgot that their predecessors had endorsed the soul, not because of their theological leanings, but because associationism did not recognize or explain to their satisfaction the *coherence, unity* and *purposiveness* that they thought prevailed in mental life. Granted that the "soul" also failed to explain these properties, it at least called attention to their existence.

After the expulsion of the soul, these unifying properties of mental life were occasionally referred to under the designation of *self*. For a time, thanks to James, Calkins, Prince, and the French psychopathologists, self was a reasonably popular concept. But gradually it too fell into disuse.

The total eclipse of soul and the partial eclipse of self were due in part, as I have just said, to the rise of positivism in psychology. Positivism, we all know, is a scientific program for moral rearmament, whose imperatives include absolute monism, absolute objectivity and absolute reductionism—in short, absolute chastity. From this ascetic point of view, subjective certainties are suspect, selves seem a bit indecent and any hint of metaphysics (that is, of nonpositivistic metaphysics) savors of laxness. As Gardner Murphy has pointed out, there was no prestige to be gained from a psychology of the self.[1]

But for all its sumptuary control, positivism had one undisputed merit: it engendered a wholesome dislike for question-begging explanations. Much of the older psychology, it showed, suffered from a tendency to labor over words as if words were the essence of things. Thanks to positivism, faculty psychology, resting as it did on verbal realism, became discredited, and dialectics fell into disrepute. Much of self-psychology, we must now admit, dwelt on the unenlightening plane of dialectics. Its statements were often redundant or circular: in the manner of Gertrude Stein, it sometimes asserted that a self is a self is a self. Not being, by nature, especially lyrical, psychologists failed to see any deeper significance in this exalted formula. Quite understandably, they refused to admit such a stammering self to the gray citadel of their laboratories.

But when a concept becomes taboo, it is probable that the taboo will irradiate to cover a whole range of problems associated with the concept. Something of this sort seems to have happened. It is not only the soul and the self that suffered ostracism. Along with them went a vast array of problems having to do with the coherence and unity of mental life; with pride, ambition and status; with values, ideals and outlook on the future. The eclipse, of course, has not been total, but it has been considerable.

As if to compensate for the neglect of these interests within the field of psychology proper, psychoanalysis rose upon the horizon, emitting a spectacular, if sporadic, light. Small wonder that the world at large turned to psychoanalysis for guidance in dynamic psychology. There was precious little other guidance to be had. I am inclined to believe that history will declare that psychoanalysis marked an interregnum in psychology—between the time when it lost its soul, shortly after the Franco-Prussian War, and the time when it found it again, shortly after World War II.

Until psychoanalysis becomes finally fused into a broader and more adequate psychology, it may take pride in having preserved and advanced the study of certain functions of the self that positivistic psychology had consigned to oblivion. It may take credit, too, for preserving one term, more or less cognate with *self*, from the dark taboo of which I have spoken. *Ego* has featured prominently in psychoanalytic literature from its beginning. This term I am now appropriating to signify the recentering that is taking place in psychological theory.

But it is not from psychoanalysis alone that we draw our threads. The position of the ego in contemporary psychology is determined by certain other historical trends as well.

Main Conceptions of the Ego

Among the different conceptions of the ego found in psychological literature, the following are certainly the most important:

The ego as knower. The nominative form of the word *ego* implies that some subject is busily engaged, as Brentano would say, in "intending" his relations to the universe. The problem of the knower, or "Pure Ego," has been of little interest to psychologists since James gave it his lengthy *coup de grâce* in the *Principles.* It is enough, says James in effect, to admit that knowing goes on. A separate knowing-ego is not a necessary assumption. For phenomenologists[2] and personalists,[3] of course, the problem of the subject-object relationship remains uppermost. But, for the most part, since the time of Brentano and James, psychologists have passed the problem by.[4] For our purposes, we need only record this first usage and note its relative rarity.

The ego as object of knowledge. Some investigators have set themselves the problem of the nature of our experience of the self.[5] This approach, limited as it is to the deliverances of introspection, has not been particularly rewarding. It yields relatively unenlightening localizations for the ego, which is felt to lie "between the eyes" or to consist of "motions in the head" or to be situated "between right and left," "between up and down," "between behind and before." Following this line of investigation, Horowitz came upon such a diversity of results (reports locating the ego in the head, heart, chest, face, brain, genitals) that he concludes: "The localization of the self as it is reported in the literature quoted, in the responses on our questionnaire, in informal discussion, in the investigation of children, is not the basic phenomenon one might hope for to ease an analysis of the structure of the self and personality." [6]

There seem to be only two facts upon which there is general agreement: (1) Infants, all writers concur, do not recognize themselves as individuals; they behave in what Piaget calls an "undifferentiated absolute" composed of self and environment. Only gradually and with difficulty does a segregated ego evolve. (2) The ego of which we are aware is variable in its dimensions. Sometimes it includes less than the body and sometimes more. In a semi-doze we lose all sense of our egos, though we may be conscious enough of impersonal items. Our feet, perhaps, are suddenly perceived as strange objects not belonging to us. In pathological conditions, remarkable experiences of depersonalization take place.[7] Conversely, we sometimes think of a tool we are using as part of our extended ego-system, and at times we regard our children, our lodge or our ancestors as an intimate part of our extended selves. It is agreed that, in this manner, the ego-systems of which we are aware contract and expand in a most variable fashion.[8]

The ego as primitive selfishness. A century ago Max Stirner wrote *Der Einzige und Sein Eigenthum,*[9] a volume in which he developed the thesis that man is by nature unalterably egoistic. In 1918 the French biologist Felix Le Dantec handled the same theme more brilliantly in his *L'egoïsme: seule base de toute société.*[10] Unquenchable egoism is the foundation of the social edifice, says Le Dantec, and hypocrisy is its keystone. Psychologists are partial to such hardheaded realism and have themselves gone far in unveiling the hypocrisy in man's nature. Projections, rationalizations, defense mechanisms have been exposed for what they are—the whitewashing of ego-centric motivation. During this century psychologists have joined with historians, biographers and novelists in the fashionable sport of debunking human motives.

The ego as dominance-drive. Related to this view of primitive egoism, we find many investigations that deal with dominance feelings, with ascendance, with pecking orders, with euphoria. From this point of approach, the ego is that portion of the personality that demands status and recognition. The negative states of anxiety, insecurity, defensiveness, resistance are just as truly indicators that, whenever the ego is debased, there arise impulses for its defense and restoration to status.

Ego as a passive organization of mental processes. Psychoanalysis, we all know, has contributed much to the interpretation of human nature in terms of egoism. Its whole theory of motivation is based upon the assumption of hedonistic self-interest. But in psychoanalysis, egoism, oddly enough, is ascribed not to the ego but to the urges arising from the id. For Freud the ego proper is a passive percipient, devoid of dynamic power, "a coherent organization of mental processes" that is aware of the warring forces of the id, superego and external environment.[11] The ego, having no dynamic power, tries as well as it can to conciliate and to steer the warring forces; but when it fails, as it often does, it breaks out in anxiety. The ego is born of restraint of the instinctual impulses, and it continually needs strengthening. But even when, through the analytic process, it is strengthened, it is still essentially nothing more than a passive victim-spectator of the drama of conflict.

Dissatisfied with Freud's denial of dynamic power to the ego, later psychoanalytic writers, French and Hendrick among them,[12] have ascribed more *momentum* to the ego. It is the agent that plans, that strives to master as well as to conciliate the conflicts. One analyst, Heinz Hartmann, departing considerably from Freud, holds that "adaptation to reality—which includes mastery of it—proceeds to a large extent from the ego and in particular from that part of the ego which is free from conflict; and it is directed by the organized structure of ego-functions (such as intelligence, perception, etc.) which exist in their own right and have an independent effect upon the solution of conflicts."[13] To such writers the ego-ideal is no longer, as it was with Freud, a passive reflection of the superego, which in turn is conceived as a mere legacy of the parent. The ego through its ideals reaches into the future, becomes an executive, a planner, a fighter.

Ego as a "fighter for ends." We are brought, then, by some of the more modern psychoanalysts to a position not unlike that of McDougall, or of James in his more teleological moments. For McDougall self-regard was the master and controlling sentiment, in whose interest all other sentiments function.[14] The phrase "fighter for ends" I borrow from James,[15] who at times was intensely dynamic and personalistic in his conception of the self.

The purposive view of the ego may be linked to Koffka's postulate that there is ever active "a force which propels the ego upwards."[16] The same position is represented in those dynamic psychologies that recognize the subservience of the biological drives to one central drive of ego-satisfaction. One of the most forceful expressions of this point of view is to be found in Goldstein's *Human nature in the light of psychopathology*.[17]

The ego as a behavioral system. In spite of his postulation of "a force which propels the ego upwards," Koffka's position is characteristically somewhat less dynamic than that just described. The ego, he says, is only one segregated system within an homogeneous field. Much behavior occurs with no reference to the ego. Not all perception, not all action, not all emotion and not all consciousness are related to an ego-system. The ego varies widely in its boundaries from time to time and, under certain circumstances, acts as a system that determines the course of events, as does any other dynamic system according to the theory of Gestalt. But, much of the time, behavior is free from the influence of an ego-system.

More influential because of its experimental fruitfulness is Lewin's treatment of the subject.[18] Although he seldom uses the term *ego*, he too allows for a central subsystem within the person. Not all behavior is ego-linked, but many kinds of experimentally obtained results can be accounted for only by reference to the special types of tension that exist whenever the ego is "engaged." The shifting aspiration level is, most obviously, a phenomenon of ego-tensions. Satiation, substitution, encapsulation, resistance, irreality and power-field are among the Lewinian concepts whose characteristics represent various properties of ego-tensions.[19]

It is clear that Lewin, no less than Koffka, wishes to avoid thinking of the ego as a single entity and prefers to regard it as the variable set of forces that are aroused whenever the person enters into some novel and perhaps dangerous relation to his environment.

Ego as the subjective organization of culture. In recent years, as everyone knows, there has been a drawing together of psychology, psychoanalysis and social anthropology. The resulting commensalism has produced a new conception of the ego. The picture of the selfish and unsocialized ego bequeathed us by Stirner and Le Dantec has been broadened. Sherif, for example, points out that, although the ego is a "genetic psychological formation," it is acquired by the child under the ceaseless impact of influence by parents, teachers and associates, with the result that the ego "is chiefly made up of social values." [20] Since the process of segregating the ego in childhood is achieved largely by giving the child a name, a status, a code of behavior, a social sense of guilt and social standards for making his judgments, Sherif concludes that the ego is nothing but the social part of man.[21] This author's position is extreme, for if the ego is nothing but "the social in man," one wonders what to call all the antisocial impulses and the solitary strivings that are normally called *egoistic?*

Cantril's view is similar to, but less extreme than, Sherif's. Cantril admits that "a person's ego and, consequently, the way in which he regards himself, are by no means always entirely bound by the surrounding culture." [22] But what an individual regards as himself is, undeniably, in large part socially determined. When his nation's flag is torn down, *he* is insulted; when disparaging remarks are made of his parents, *he* is involved; when his political candidate loses a contest, *he* has been defeated.

By stressing the cultural content of the ego, these authors in effect eradicate the artificial Freudian distinction between ego and superego. They also rescue the ego from the antisocial solipsism of Stirner and Le Dantec and make of it a socialized agent ready to enter as an integrated unit into the complex relations of social life.

From this historical glance I have omitted many writers who have made their contribution to the literature of the ego. Nevertheless, I believe I have mentioned the chief ways in which, up to now, the ego has been conceived—that is, as knower, as object of knowledge, as primordial selfishness, as dominator, as a passive organizer and rationalizer, as a fighter for ends, as one segregated behavioral system among others and as a subjective patterning of cultural values.

The question immediately arises as to whether these eight uses of the term *ego* have anything in common, or whether, as is often the case, a single term is allowed to obscure entirely different problems. Is the ego as knower the same ego that seeks status? Is the I that is known also a fighter for ends? Has the ego-system proposed by Koffka any kinship with Freud's ego, who attempts through insight to reclaim the id?

These are questions that cannot yet be answered. We cannot say whether these eight conceptions reflect irreconcilable theories, or shade imperceptibly into one another, or are all ultimately to be subordinated under one inclusive theory of the ego.

In favor of the last possibility, I should like to point to recent experimental studies that, if I mistake not, lend support to several of these conceptions simultaneously. *The experiments result in one common finding—namely, that ego-involvement, or its absence, makes a critical difference in human behavior.* When a person reacts in a neutral, impersonal, routine atmosphere, his behavior is one thing. When he is behaving personally, perhaps excitedly, seriously committed to a task, he behaves quite differently. In the first condition

his ego is not engaged; in the second condition it is. And it is my belief that, in most of the experiments I shall report, one finds that
the ego is acting in several, if not all, of the eight capacities I have
listed. In other words, *ego-involvement* is, as the phrase implies, a
condition of total participation of the self—as knower, as organizer,
as observer, as status seeker and as socialized being. But now for the
experimental evidence.

Experimental Evidence

Generality and specificity. A few years ago I found myself involved in a controversy in the field of personality. Certain experimenters claimed that their findings demonstrated a situational
specificity in human conduct. For example, a child honest in one
situation would not be found honest in another,[23] a person confident
of one judgment would not be confident of another.[24] Whole books
were written in defense of specificity.[25] Other investigators, by
other methods, found a person honest in one situation to be honest
in another,[26] a person confident in one judgment to be confident
in another;[27] and whole books were written in defense of generality.[28]
It was a pleasant battle while it lasted. An arbitrator arose, a peace-
maker by temperament—Gardner Murphy was his name—and he
proposed a compromise. "Honesty," he suggested, "is either a general
characteristic or a set of specific habits, depending on your interest
and your emphasis."[29] Murphy was right, but it was not until recently that the deciding interest and critical emphasis became clear,
at least to me. For my own belated insight I am indebted to an
experiment by Klein and Schoenfeld.[30]

These investigators gave to a group of subjects a series of mental tests under two experimental conditions. In the first, the atmosphere was neutral, dull, *non-ego-involved.* The workers were merely
laboratory subjects going through routine motions. After each of the
six tests, they were required to rate the degree of confidence they
felt in the accuracy of their performances. For each individual, there
was little consistency in these certainty ratings.

After an interval of time, a second, equivalent set of tests was
administered. This time the atmosphere was markedly changed. The
subjects were placed under greater strain; they were told to try hard,
since the results of these "intelligence" tests would be entered on
their college records. For this set of tests, the confidence ratings were
markedly consistent. A student who felt assured in one test felt
assured in the other five; a student who lacked confidence in one of

his performances generally lacked confidence in the other performances. The authors conclude that confidence is a personality trait *when the ego is involved*, but that it is specific to each situation when the subject has no deep interest at stake.

This experiment supplies the hypothesis needed to settle a long-standing controversy: when there is ego-involvement, there are general traits; when there is no ego-involvement, there are no general traits.

From an entirely different source comes evidence to the same effect. In connection with its polling investigations, the Office of Public Opinion Research has found that *intensity* of feeling goes with *consistency* of opinion.[31] For example, in the pre-Pearl Harbor era it was found that those who felt most intensely in favor of aid to Britain were, by and large, those who endorsed all sorts and varieties of interventionist propositions. On the other hand, those who were lukewarm in their support of aid to Britain were far more inconsistent and specific in their answers. Sometimes they gave interventionist, and sometimes isolationist, replies. The measure obtained between the intensity scale and the generality of the attitude was a coefficient of correlation of +.63.

Judgment. Eli Marks worked on judgments of skin color among Negroes. He found them, in part, a function of the objective scale but also, in part, a function of an egocentric scale. A Negro of medium coloration is likely to be judged dark by a Negro of lighter complexion and to be judged light by a Negro of darker complexion.[32] For decades psychophysicists have dealt with judgments of hue as a function of wave length, but Marks makes clear that judgments of hue may be also a function of one's sense of social status. Wave length is perceived by the sensitized retina, but it is perceived no less by the sensitized ego.

In the field of simple predictive judgment, it was found in the public opinion polls of 1940 that, of the people who were strong Willkie supporters, 71 per cent predicted that he would win the election; of those who were weak Willkie supporters, only 47 per cent made this prediction.[33] Assuming, as we must, that intensity of an attitude indicates ego-involvement, we find here a clear quantitative demonstration that a 24 per cent difference in the number of predictions exists when the ego-regions of the personality are engaged. Admittedly, the ego's wish is only one factor in predictive judgments; but if conditions are right, it can become the crucial factor.

Polling research has uncovered yet another important fact con-

cerning judgment. If you ask respondents to tell you to your face
what they think about the British, or about some minority group in
this country, or even about their own educational level, you obtain
one set of results; but if you ask them to write their answers to the
same questions privately and deposit them in a padlocked ballot box,
on the average your results will be significantly different.[34] Now
this difference between open and secret expressions of opinion seems
to exist only when the answers might jeopardize the respondent's sense
of status or affect his prestige in the interviewer's eyes. The discrepancy is great enough to warrant the use of secret balloting whenever questions are of a type that might expose the person to humiliation.

Judgments concerning one's self are remarkably interesting
things to study. We know, for example, how inaccurate people are
in rating their own economic status. Nearly all prefer to overlook
the objective evidence and to identify themselves with the great
middle class.[35] We know something about the distortions that result
when people report their own traits. Frenkel-Brunswik found the
self-protective devices so powerful that her subjects would omit,
justify or completely reverse the facts in their accounts of their own
deficiencies.[36] Although it is trite to point out what all psychologists
know so well, that lack of objectivity is the rule when our egos are
involved, it is not trite to remark that very little work has been done
on the extent and nature of the distortion, or on the curious and
momentous question why some personalities attain objectivity even
in the face of extreme ego-involvement. Insight, it would seem,
grows more and more difficult to achieve as the inner regions of the
personality are approached. And yet some individuals accomplish
remarkable feats of self-objectification. Why do they succeed and
others fail?

Memory. Thanks to Bartlett we know how cultural schemata
alter our memory traces.[37] Here, of course, is an example of the
silent influence of an ethnocentric frame. But within any given
culture, striking memory-efforts can be traced to egocentric frames
as well.

Edwards has demonstrated that, if memory material fails to fit
comfortably into an ego-involved frame, it contorts itself until it
does so. Selecting three groups of students, each with a different
attitude toward the New Deal (favorable, neutral or opposed) he
first read them a ten-minute passage concerning the relations of the
New Deal to communism. The subjects knew they were to be tested
for the accuracy of their retention.

"Immediately after the reading, a multiple choice recognition test consisting of 46 items was given to the subjects. Half or 23 of the items on the test were answered in the passage in a manner favorable to the New Deal, the other 23 were answered in a manner unfavorable. The items on the test offered opportunities for rationalization of one's answer, if the correct answer was opposed to one's attitude. The subjects were re-tested after an interval of 21 days.

"Analysis of variance of the data showed that rationalization was directly associated with the degree of conflict between the correct answer and the attitudinal frames of reference of our subjects. In general the results show—as do many other studies—that it is almost impossible to expect objectivity and accuracy in perception, learning, remembering, thinking, etc., when ego-involved frames of reference are stimulated." [38]

Here one might cite also the memory experiments of Zillig, which show how members of the male sex recall fewer aphorisms favorable to women than to men.[39] Or the Watson and Hartmann study concerning the distortions that occur in memory for theological arguments, depending upon the subject's previous commitment to atheism or to theism.[40] Or Wallen's ingenious demonstration that, after an interval of time, subjects recall ratings of their own personalities in a manner that makes them compatible with their own preconceived opinions of themselves.[41]

Levine and Murphy demonstrated that pro-Communist sympathizers memorize pro-Communist textual material more easily than they do anti-Communist textual material.[42] What is more, they forget the antipathetic text more rapidly and more completely than the sympathetic text. In anti-Communists the effects are exactly reversed. It was a brilliant stroke for these authors to demonstrate in one experiment that both learning and forgetting are functions of the political identifications of the ego.

Frame of reference. Some of the studies I have mentioned have been conducted in relation to what their authors have called a "frame of reference." Now, a frame of reference seems to signify *any spatial-temporal or cultural orientation that relates many of an individual's attitudes, habits and judgments to one another and that influences the formation of new judgments, attitudes and habits.* A general orientation favorable to the New Deal will, according to Edwards, determine our specific remembrance of items from speeches concerning the New Deal.[43] A general orientation regarding various other subjects, Sells has shown, will affect our logical reasoning in all matters pertaining to them.[44]

It is important to note that not all frames are ego-involved. If I locate Ninth Avenue or East Twelfth Street readily, it is because I have a geographic frame in mind for New York City. In my case this spatial orientation is not at all ego-involved. The point I am making is that research on the problem of frames of reference is not necessarily research on the problem of ego-involvement. Many cultural frames having to do with language, etiquette or dress determine our perceptions, our memory, our conduct, but their influence is not felt as personally relevant. Margaret Mead has expressed her anthropological astonishment at the odd custom Americans have of appearing at her lectures with clothes on; but to most of us this quaint folkway causes no ego-concern, at least as long as it is operative.

But an interesting discovery came to light in World War II. Certain cultural frames, which had previously been indifferent, suddenly became acutely personal. Probably no one in Alsace felt concerned about the bilingual frame of reference until the Nazis decreed that only German should be spoken and that only Germanized names and inscriptions should appear on the tombstones. Bilinguality had always been taken for granted; but when this familiar, habitual frame was suppressed and placed under attack, it became of central importance, and people reacted as to a personal insult. Many of us have discovered that hitherto indifferent frames of reference, such as the constitutional guarantees we enjoy, previously taken for granted, have suddenly become ego-involved and, once in jeopardy, are defended as if they were parts of our physical bodies. Suppose we were forbidden to speak the English language. How enraged we would become! What had always been a mere ethnocentric frame would immediately become ego-involved.

Ethnocentric and egocentric frames both affect our conduct, and under certain conditions the ethnocentric frame is experienced also as an egocentric frame. But I think it is a mistake to confuse the concept of the ego with that of the socius (or cultural portion of our personalities) as Sherif has done. Under normal social conditions, only a relatively small portion of our culture is ego-involved.

Learning. The longest and most difficult chapter in psychology, no one will deny, is the chapter on learning. The 1942 Yearbook of the National Society for the Study of Education is devoted entirely to this subject. One searches its 463 pages in vain for any mention of the ego, and almost in vain for any recognition of the importance of *interest*. True, one finds occasional remarks to the effect that "the teacher who neglects the simple but powerful word of praise does so at her pedagogical peril," [45] but the potential significance of such remarks for learning theory seems lost to view.

⌜Clinical, educational and industrial psychologists know that the first rule of all applied psychology is that every child and every adult needs some experience of success and social approval.⌟ John E. Anderson advises the teacher to go far out of her way if necessary to find an area in which these feelings can be engendered. He adds: "Success in one area may more than compensate for failure in many areas; some accomplishment furnishes an integrating center about which the personality may be integrated." [46]

Note especially Anderson's statement that "success in one area may more than compensate for failure in many areas." Only in terms of ego-psychology can we account for such fluid compensation. Mental health and happiness, it seems, do not depend upon the satisfaction of any specific drive; they depend, rather, upon the *person* finding *some* area of success *somewhere*. The ego must be satisfied—not the hunger drive, nor the sex drive, nor the maternal drive, however temporarily insistent these segmental tensions may be.

Most theories of learning lean heavily upon the assumption of multiple drives. A segmental tension exists; the organism behaves; the tension is relieved; and the response is set. In this sequence it is often assumed that all drives are equally potent for learning. The satisfaction of any drive, through the principle of reward or confirming reaction, is held to bring about an equal degree of learning. If this is so, how can we account for the fact that praise is found almost uniformly to be the leading incentive in school, in factory and in ordinary life? If we are to hold to the theory of multiple drives at all, we must at least admit that the ego-drive (or pride, or desire for approval—call it what we will) takes precedence over all other drives.

Not only does human learning proceed best when the incentive of praise and recognition is used, but the individual's *capacity* for learning actually seems to expand under this condition. Every psychometrist knows that if he is to obtain a valid IQ, the subject must be encouraged. Terman's instructions on this point are well known: "Nothing contributes more to a satisfactory *rapport* than praise of the child's efforts. . . . In general, the poorer the response, the better satisfied one should appear to be with it. . . . Exclamations like fine! splendid! etc., should be used lavishly." [47]

In other words, to maximize the child's intelligence we must maximize his ego. For psychological theory this is really a momentous fact. Intelligence is the ego's tool for solving its own problems. It is manifestly unfair to estimate intelligence on the basis of performance in which the individual himself has no interest. For this reason, through the device of praise, the subject must be encouraged to make the test-items into ego-involved problems, which he can attack with maximally motivated effort. Intelligence is the individual's capacity to solve problems of importance to himself.

One unfavorable condition for learning must be admitted lest we oversimplify the issue. Too intense an ego-involvement may be disruptive. Its normal integrative value may be actually undetermined when eagerness or self-consciousness reach a degree of intensity that leads to embarrassment or over-anxiousness. No one learns or performs well if his autonomic nervous system is in a turmoil. We need a rule that will help us determine the optimum degree of ego-involvement required for enhancing efficiency of learning and performance.[48]

One word about the law of effect. Its principal shortcoming, I think, stems from the assumption that rewarded *responses* tend to recur. Many experiments, in fact, show that rewarded responses do not blindly recur whenever an appropriate stimulus returns. Hoppe points out that people normally do not strive again for a goal successfully achieved.[49] What they do is to raise their aspirations to a point where they clearly risk failure. A student who makes an A record in a course in college shows no tendency to repeat that course. He prefers to take new risks in the same general area. And an experiment by Rosenzweig indicates that it is definitely infantile to choose to repeat successful acts.[50] For example, a puzzle once solved, even if accompanied by a burst of elation, no longer attracts the mature individual. He wants new worlds to conquer. Reward may bring merely satiation and boredom.

The fallacy, I repeat, lies in our speaking of rewarding a *response.* The law of effect would be truer if it held simply that a *person*, being rewarded, employs his past successes in whatever way he thinks is likely to bring him satisfaction in the *future.* Israeli has shown that, except for certain psychopaths, people are much more interested in their futures than in their pasts.[51] Since this is so, an individual's past performances often mean little or nothing to him. Only if the ego would be served thereby does he engage in a repetition of the successful act. More often he chooses to vary and refine his behavior so that he may feel that he himself is growing toward new successes in the future.

The relation between success and repetition, I suspect, is much closer in the case of non-ego-involved behavior than in the case of ego-involved behavior. Over and over again I use the same motor combinations in typewriting, in driving my car, in dealing with tradesmen. They are reasonably successful acts; why should I change them? But I do not repeat successful research work; I do not repeat a gratifying conversation with a friend; nor do I restate the same goal in an aspiration-level experiment. Ego-involved tasks often demand changing goals and new responses. Rewarded behavior, it would seem, becomes stereotyped only in lower animals, or in human activities of such a routine nature that they fail to engage the ego.

To summarize this brief discussion: It would seem that, in order to employ the law of effect with human learning, we must view it as secondary to the principle of ego-involvement. The law of effect, like cue reduction, conditioning, bond-formation and most other popular principles of learning, has been worked out for the most part on animal subjects or on human beings deprived, for the duration of the experiment, of their egos. The principles may be good ones, but when the ego is engaged they operate in a contingent fashion. Learning theory of the future, let us hope, will not remain so peripheral to the ego.

Motivation. You may be thinking, "But, we've always known that one must be motivated in order to secure a response. Are you talking about anything more than the importance of motivation?" Yes. I am saying that there are two forms of motivation, one ego-involved and one not, and I am attempting by repeated citations from experiments to show the differences that exist between them.

Take, for example, the work of Huntley and Wolff on judgments based upon records of expressive behavior.[52] These investigators, working independently, instructed their subjects to make judgments concerning the personalities of many people from their handwritings, from their recorded voices, from photographs of their hands and from their style of storytelling. The subjects were motivated in a routine manner, as is any laboratory subject. Suddenly, in the midst of the series, they were confronted with samples of their own expressive behavior, which had been recorded without their knowledge. In the large majority of cases the subjects did not consciously recognize their own records and continued innocently with their characterizations. But something had happened. The characterizations began to take a different form. Even though a judge was wholly unaware that a certain expression was his own, he generally gave it a much more favorable rating than he gave similar expressive records taken from other subjects. Occasionally he gave it a vehemently unfavorable rating. Practically never did he give it an indifferent rating. Other people's records might arouse no affect, but not his. Whenever a subject became half-conscious, as it were, that a record might possibly be his, his judgments were still more intensely partisan; but, when he fully recognized his own record, his social sense of modesty prevailed, and his judgments returned to the noncommital level.

In these experiments we have a particularly neat demonstration of the fact that ego-involved systems may operate in a wholly silent manner, affecting judgments in a most extreme way without the subject knowing the reason. The experiments also prove that the limen of ego-involvement is lower than the limen for self-recognition, an interesting finding, which warns us once more that conscious report and introspection will never be a sufficient method for exploring the operations of the ego-system. But the important point for our present purpose is to note that routine motivation to perform a task is one thing and ego-charged motivation is quite another. Routine motives yield one set of results, ego-motives a different set.

When is motivation ego-involved, and when is it not? A partial answer seems to lie in the degree of frustration involved. As we have already noted, many customary frames of reference are not felt to be personally relevant and do not behave like egocentric frames, until their continuance is threatened. Many drives, too, run their course without engaging the ego unless they are interfered with. But serious frustration may instigate the clamor, the jealousy, the possessiveness often characteristic of ego-involvement. Yet frustration by no means always produces this effect, especially if one has compensated for drive-frustration by success in other realms. And, to complicate the situation further, we cannot say that ego-involvement is absent when there is no frustration. Many smooth-running instances of goal-seeking behavior are obviously ego-involved. A mother feels just as closely identified with her child when it is in good health as when her maternal care meets with frustration. A businessman is as much absorbed in his enterprise in times of prosperity as in times of adversity. Let us say, then, that frustration of goal-seeking behavior or any kind of threat to the individual is very likely to engage the ego-system, but that normally this ego-system is made up of the ordinary values that spell out the significance of life to the individual.

The level of aspiration. The history of ten years' research on this Lewinian problem is too intricate to trace here, but, unless I am mistaken, every investigation has directly or indirectly confirmed Hoppe's initial claim that the subject behaves in such a manner as to maintain his self-esteem at the highest possible level.[53] Of course, many investigators have not used the conception of the ego at all. Yet, whatever results are found, all seem to point to the essential inescapability of Hoppe's original hypothesis. Frank, for example, found that subjects in whom "self competition, and consciousness of social pressure" were present had D-scores three to seven times as large as did subjects who had no such sense of personal involvement in the situation. (D-scores, of course, indicate the discrepancy between performance and the goal that the individual wishes or expects to achieve.) Frank also found that subjects who are ego-involved do not change their estimates with every little variation in their performance. They try and try again before trimming their aspirations to fit their capacities. Subjects not ego-involved, on the other hand, quickly yield to the immediate realities of the situation and lower their aspiration level.[54] We know too that competitiveness, surely a symptom of ego-involvement, usually produces a rise and greater consistency in the aspiration level.[55] But we cannot say that competitiveness always has this effect, because subjects who dread competition will lower their level of aspiration consistently in order to avoid the risk of humiliation.[56]

In short, it seems always to be the ego-demand of the individual subject that determines the behavior of the aspiration level. Some subjects are adventurous, some cautious; their egos demand different types of satisfaction, and it is this fact that is repeatedly reflected in the results of the experiments. It is worth pointing out that historically the aspiration level may well be regarded as the door by which the ego re-entered the cloisters of academic psychology.

Industrial psychology. Most of us, I suppose, have been impressed by the demonstrations of Roethlisberger and Dickson,[57] Watson[58] and others that employees in industry are not "economic men" so much as they are "ego men." What they want, above all else, is credit for work done, interesting tasks, appreciation, approval and congenial relations with their employers and fellow workers. These satisfactions they want even more than high wages or job security. The employer's estimate of the worker's wants correlates just about zero with the worker's own report of his wants.[59] The employer thinks that wages and security are the dominant desires, whereas in reality the ego-satisfactions are primary. What a different outlook there would be on our economic life if we took firm hold on the issues of status and self-respect in industry and replanned our industrial society in a manner that would rescue the worker's ego from oblivion.

The Nature of the Ego

In the experiments I have cited, and in many others of analogous nature, it turns out that one group of subjects (those who are personally aroused and committed to a task) behave in ways quite unlike other subjects (who are not so committed). In some instances there are measurable quantitative differences as great as 50 or 60 per cent, sometimes much more. In other instances there are qualitative changes that elude measurement. Thus we are here confronted with some parameter that makes a vast difference in our experimental results.

We have seen that under conditions of ego-involvement the whole personality manifests greater consistency in behavior; it reveals not specificity in conduct but generality and congruence. In the field of judgment, we have seen how ego-involvement results in significant distortions of the ordinary psychophysical scales. In memory, we find that ego-involved retention is characteristically superior (though at times repressions also may be more likely to occur, and rationalizations may creep into memory). In intelligence, we note that ego-involvement is indispensable if we would obtain optimum performance. In learning theory, reforms seem indicated to make room for the demonstrable influence of the ego upon the acquisition of skill and knowledge. In motivation, the craving for recognition, status and personal appreciation turns out to be supreme, so much so that our conceptions of procedure and policy in industrial relations, in education and in psychotherapy are profoundly affected. And these are only a few of the operational criteria by which we may demonstrate the existence of the ego.

Its admittance to good standing in contemporary psychology has been advocated by several psychologists besides myself. Koffka, Lewin and the psychoanalysts have done so, as has Murray, who makes a distinction between "peripheralist" psychology and "centralist" psychology.[60] The thesis set forth in Rogers' book *Counseling and psychotherapy*[61] seems to me especially clear evidence that the ego is coming into its own. Rogers, in effect, asks counselors to sit back and, with little more than an occasionally well-placed *m-hm*, to encourage the patient himself to restructure and re-plan his life. The patient's ego takes command. It's about time it should.

Although we have given an adequate operational demonstration of the ego, we have not yet faced the difficult problem of definition.

Earlier we saw that eight conceptions seem to prevail. But whenever we encounter ego-involvement, the ego in *several* of its historical senses seems to be active. Furthermore, these historical conceptions seem to have much in common.

For one thing, it seems clear that all of the conceptions are less embracing than "personality." All writers seem agreed that the ego is only one portion, one region—or, as the Freudians say, one "institution"—of the personality. Many skills, habits and memories are components of personality, but seldom if ever become ego-involved. Writers seem also agreed that the ego is nonexistent in early childhood, evolving gradually as the child comes to mark himself off from his environment and from other human beings. They seem to agree in viewing the ego as the portion of the personality that is in proximate relation to the external world: it senses the threats, the opportunities and the survival significance of both outer and inner events. It is that portion of the personality, so to speak, that meets the world head-on. It is the contact-region of the personality. For that reason it is also the conflict-region. Yet it is coextensive neither with consciousness nor with unconsciousness; for much that we are conscious of is unimportant to our egos, and many unconscious stimuli silently but effectively engage them.

There is also agreement that the subjective sense of the ego varies greatly from time to time, now contracting to include less than the body, now expanding to include more. Its content keeps changing; at one moment the ego seems preoccupied with one activity and soon thereafter with a wholly different activity. This shifting scene, however, does not mean that there is no stable and recurring structure. On the contrary, if you know a person well enough, you find that you are able to predict with marked success what items will and what items will not be linked to his ego. By many writers the ego is represented as a layered structure. Certainly there are *degrees* of ego-involvement: a person may be moderately partisan or intensely partisan.

There seems to be one other property of the ego that is less often discussed—namely, its customary preoccupation with the future. Israeli, it will be remembered, reports that among his subjects over 90 per cent expressed themselves more interested in their futures than in their pasts.[62] This finding is worth stressing, for, as a rule, psychologists are more interested in a person's past than in his future. In other words, the psychologist and his subject customarily face in different directions, and that is unfortunate.

The admittance of the ego to good standing in psychology does not mean a reimportation of the *deus ex machina* of pre-Wundtian psychology. It does mean, however, a recognition of the fact that our predecessors, who regarded psychology as the science of the soul, were not wrong in setting the problems of unity and personal relevance before us. What they called the soul we may now, with good conscience, call the ego. In so doing, no clocks need to be set backward. Dialectics has already given way to experiment, to the clinic and to still newer methods for studying the common man in his normal social setting.

But, disregarding the problems of method, which are beyond the scope of this essay, we may safely predict that ego-psychology in the twentieth century will flourish increasingly. For only with its aid can psychologists reconcile the human nature that they study and the human nature that they serve.

REFERENCES

1. G. Murphy, "Psychology and the post-war world," *Psychol. Rev.*, 1942, 49:298-318.

2. M. Beth, "Zur Psychologie des Ich," *Arch. f. d. Ges. Psychol.*, 1933, 88:323-76; T. K. Oesterreich, *Phenomenologie des Ich in ihren Grundproblemen*, Leipzig: J. A. Barth, 1910.

3. For example, J. S. Moore, "The problem of the self," *Phil. Rev.*, 1933, 42:487-99.

4. Private correspondence with Koffka concerning his own usage of the term brought out the interesting fact that, in writing his chapters on the ego, he had never thought of ego in the role of the knower (K. Koffka, *Principles of Gestalt psychology*, New York: Harcourt, Brace, 1935). "To be quite frank, I never put this question to myself." He adds, "That my solution will be similar to Brentano's I doubt. At the moment it seems to me that it will be found in the theory of Ego subsystems, more particularly in the relation of the Self-system to other Ego-systems."

5. E. W. Amen, "An experimental study of the self in psychology," *Psychol. Monogr.*, 1926, Vol. 35, No. 165; E. L. Horowitz, "Spatial localization of the self," *J. Soc. Psychol.*, 1935, 6:379-87; H. Lundholm, "Reflections upon the nature of the psychological self," *Psychol. Rev.*, 1940, 47:110-26.

6. E. L. Horowitz, *op. cit.*, p. 386.

7. H. Delgado, "Psicologia y psicopatologia de la conscientia del yo," *An. Inst. Psicol.*, University of Buenos Aires, 1938, 2:135-76; P. Federn, "Narzissmus im Ichfuge," *Int. Z. f. Psychoanal.*, 1927, 13:420-38.

8. H. Lundholm, *op. cit.*

9. M. Stirner, *The ego and his own* (trans. by S. T. Byington), London: A. C. Fifield, 1912.

10. F. Le Dantec, *L'egoïsme, seule base de toute société*, Paris: Flammarion, 1916.

11. S. Freud, *The ego and the id* (trans. by J. Rivière), London: Hogarth Press, 1927.

12. R. M. French, "Some psychoanalytic applications of the psychological field concept," *Psychoanal. Quart.*, 1942, 11:17-32; I. Hendrick, "Instinct and the ego during infancy," *Psychoanal. Quart.*, 1942, 11:33-58.

13. H. Hartmann, "Ich-psychologie und Anpassungsproblem," *Int. J. Psychoanal.*, 1940, 21:214.

14. W. McDougall, *The energies of men*, New York: Scribner, 1933, p. 383.

15. W. James, *Principles of psychology*, New York: Holt, 1890, I, 141.

16. K. Koffka, *op. cit.*, p. 670.

17. "On the basis of our discussion I believe we are in no way forced to assume the existence of special drives. . . . They are special reactions in special situations, and represent the various forms by which the organism as a whole expresses itself. . . . The traditional view assumes various drives which come into the foreground under certain conditions. We assume only one drive, the drive of self-actualization, but are compelled to concede that under certain conditions the tendency to actualize one potentiality is so strong that the organism is governed by it" (K. Goldstein, *Human nature in the light of psychopathology*, Cambridge: Harvard University Press, 1940, pp. 144 f.).

18. K. Lewin, *Principles of topological psychology*, New York: McGraw-Hill, 1936, p. 181.

19. A particularly suggestive contribution of Lewin pertains to the difference between nationalities in terms of the relative ease with which the ego becomes "engaged." Thus the American is less defensive, less touchy, less reticent than the German, because the barriers of the German's ego lie nearer the "surface." He protects himself against familiarity and intrusion, whereas the American leads a much more "public" life and protects only the "core" of his personal life from public gaze (K. Lewin, "Some social-psychological differences between the United States and Germany," *Char. & Pers.*, 1936, 4:265-93).

20. M. Sherif, *The psychology of social norms*, New York: Harper, 1936, p. 179.

21. *Ibid.*, p. 186.

22. H. Cantril, *The psychology of social movements*, New York: Wiley, 1941, p. 44.

23. H. Hartshorne and M. May, *Studies in deceit*, New York: Macmillan, 1928.

24. W. C. Trow, "The psychology of confidence," *Arch. Psychol.*, 1923, No. 67.

25. P. M. Symonds, *The nature of conduct*, New York: Macmillan, 1928.

26. D. W. MacKinnon, "Violation of prohibitions," in H. A. Murray (ed.), *Explorations in personality*, New York: Oxford University Press, 1938, pp. 491-501.

27. D. M. Johnson, "Confidence and speed in two-category judgment," *Arch. Psychol.*, 1939, No. 241.

28. G. W. Allport, *Personality: a psychological interpretation*, New York: Holt, 1937.

29. G. Murphy and G. Jensen, *Approaches to personality*, New York: Coward-McCann, 1932, p. 385.

30. G. S. Klein and N. Schoenfeld, "The influence of ego-involvement on confidence," *J. Abnorm. Soc. Psychol.*, 1941, 36:249-58.

31. H. Cantril, *Gauging public opinion*, Princeton: Princeton University Press, 1943, Chap. 3.

32. E. Marks, "Skin color judgments of Negro college students," *J. Abnorm. Soc. Psychol.*, 1943, 38:370-76.

33. H. Cantril, *Gauging public opinion, op. cit.*

34. *Ibid.*, Chap. 5.

35. *Ibid.*

36. E. Frenkel-Brunswik, "Mechanisms of self-deception," *J. Soc. Psychol.*, 1939, 10:409-20.

37. F. C. Bartlett, *Remembering: a study in experimental and social psychology*, Cambridge, England: Cambridge University Press, 1932.

38. A. L. Edwards, "Rationalization in recognition as a result of a political frame of reference," *J. Abnorm. Soc. Psychol.*, 1941, 36:234.

39. M. Zillig, "Einstellung und Aussage," *Z. f. Psychol.*, 1928, 106:58-106.

40. W. S. Watson and G. W. Hartmann, "Rigidity of a basic attitudinal frame," *J. Abnorm. Soc. Psychol.*, 1939, 34:314-36.

41. R. Wallen, "Ego-involvement as a determinant of selective forgetting," *J. Abnorm. Soc. Psychol.*, 1942, 37:20-39.

42. J. M. Levine and G. Murphy, "The learning and forgetting of controversial material," *J. Abnorm. Soc. Psychol.*, 1943, 38:507-17.

43. A. L. Edwards, "Political frames of reference as a factor influencing recognition," *J. Abnorm. Soc. Psychol.*, 1941, 36:34-50.

44. S. B. Sells, "The atmosphere effect: an experimental study of reasoning," *Arch. Psychol.*, 1936, No. 200.

45. National Society for the Study of Education, *The psychology of learning*, Forty-first Yearbook, Part 2, Bloomington: Publ. School Pub. Co., 1942, p. 118.

46. *Ibid.*, p. 349.

47. L. M. Terman, *The measurement of intelligence*, Boston: Houghton Mifflin, 1916, p. 125.

48. One formulation of the needed rule is suggested by French: "So long as the tension does not exceed the available energy of the integrative mechanisms, so long will the integrative capacity of the goal-directed striving increase with increasing tension. But as soon as the tension of the need begins to exceed the available energy of the integrating mechanism, the effect of increasing tension will be the opposite" (R. M. French, "Goal, mechanisms and integrative field," *Psychosom. Med.*, 1941, 3:245).

49. F. Hoppe, "Erfolg und Misserfolg," *Psychol. Forsch.*, 1930, 14:1-62.

50. S. Rosenzweig, "Preferences in the repetition of successful and unsuccessful activities as a function of age and personality," *J. Genet. Psychol.*, 1933, 42:423-41.

51. N. Israeli, "The social psychology of time," *J. Abnorm. Soc. Psychol.*, 1932, 27:209-13.

52. C. W. Huntley, "Judgments of self based upon records of expressive behavior," *J. Abnorm. Soc. Psychol.*, 1940, 35:398-427; W. Wolff, "Selbstbeurteilung und Fremdbeurteilung im wissentlichen und unwissentlichen Versuch," *Psychol. Forsch.*, 1932, 16:251-329.

53. F. Hoppe, *op. cit.*

54. J. D. Frank, "Some psychological determinants of the level of aspiration," *Amer. J. Psychol.*, 1935, 47:285-93.

55. M. G. Preston and J. A. Bayton, "Differential effect of a social variable upon three levels of aspiration," *J. Exp. Psychol.*, 1941, 29:351-69.

56. J. D. Frank, "Individual differences in certain aspects of the level of aspiration," *op. cit.*

57. F. J. Roethlisberger and W. J. Dickson, *Management and the worker*, Cambridge: Harvard University Press, 1939.

58. G. Watson, "Work satisfaction," in G. W. Hartmann (ed.), *Industrial conflict: a psychological interpretation*, New York: Cordon Press, 1939, Chap. 6.

59. *Ibid.*, p. 119.

60. H. A. Murray, *Explorations in personality*, New York: Oxford University Press, 1938.

61. C. R. Rogers, *Counseling and psychotherapy*, Boston: Houghton Mifflin, 1942.

62. N. Israeli, *op. cit.*

59. Ibid., p. 120.

62. N. Frankl, op. cit.

The trend in motivational theory

What methods shall we use to assess a person's motives? The answer, of course, depends on what theory of motivation we hold.

This essay argues—in agreement with modern "ego-psychology"—that conscious values and intentions are important, far more important than Freudian and other irrationalist theories of motivation would allow. It holds that the best way to discover what a person is trying to do is to *ask* him (with, of course, due precautions), though the more sly "projective" methods also have their uses. The essay calls for a systematic use of both indirect and direct methods, all in accordance with a balanced theory of motivation.

Originally the essay appeared in *The American Journal of Orthopsychiatry* (1953).

Motivational theory today seems to be turning a corner in the road of scientific progress. In attempting to characterize this change in direction I wish to pay special attention to the problem of psychodiagnostic methods, for the successes and failures of these methods can teach us much about psychodynamic theory.

Let us start by asking why projective methods are so popular in both diagnostic practice and research. The answer, I think, is to be found in the history of motivational theory during the past century. All of the major influences have pressed in a single direction. Schopenhauer, with his doctrine of the primacy of the blind will, had little respect for the rationalizations invented by the individual's intellect to account for his conduct. Motives, he was sure, could not be taken at their face value. Darwin followed with his similar anti-intellectual emphasis on primordial struggle. McDougall refined the Darwinian stress on instinct, retaining in his horme the flavor of Schopenhauer's will, Darwin's struggle for survival, Bergson's *élan* and Freud's libido. All these writers were irrationalists—confident that underlying genotypes in motivation should be sought, rather than the surface phenotypes. All of them were reacting against the naïve intellectualism of their predecessors and against the rationalizations offered by self-justifying mortals when called on to account for their conduct. Among these irrationalists who have dominated Western psychology for the past century, Freud, of course, has been the leading figure. He, like the others, perceived that the mainsprings of conduct may be hidden from the searchlight of consciousness.

In addition to irrationalism, modern dynamic psychology has developed another earmark: geneticism. The original instincts laid down in our nature are regarded as decisive; or if not, then the experiences of early childhood are held to be crucial. At this point, the leading non-dynamic school of thought—stimulus-response psychology—joins forces with geneticism. Stimulus-response theorists agree with instinct psychologists and psychoanalysts in viewing adult motives as conditioned, reinforced, sublimated or otherwise elaborated editions of instincts or drives, or of an id whose structure, Freud said, "never changes."

Not one of these dominating theories of motivation allows for an essential transformation of motives in the course of life. McDougall explicitly denied the possibility, asserting that our motivational structure is laid down once and for all in our equipment of instincts. New objects may become attached to an instinct through learning, but the motive power is always the same. Freud's position was essentially identical: the concepts of sublimation and of shifting object cathexis chiefly accounted for whatever apparent alterations occur. Stimulus-response psychology is likewise geared to the assumption of remote control operating out of the past. We respond only to objects that have been associated with primary drives in the past, and we do so only in proportion to the degree that our responses have been rewarded or gratified in the past. From the stimulus-response point of view, the individual can hardly be said to be *trying* to do anything at all. He is simply *responding* with a complex array of habits that somehow were rewarded year before last. The prevailing dictum that motivation is always a matter of "tension reduction" or of "seeking equilibrium" is consistent with this point of view but scarcely consistent, I think, with all the known facts.

This prevailing atmosphere of theory has engendered a kind of contempt for the "psychic surface" of life. The individual's conscious report is rejected as untrustworthy, and the contemporary thrust of his motives is disregarded in favor of a backward tracing of his conduct to earlier formative stages. The individual loses his right to be believed. And while he is busy leading his life in the present with a forward thrust into the future, most psychologists have become busy tracing it backward into the past.

It is now easy to understand why the special methods invented by Jung (fifty years ago), Rorschach (forty years ago) and Murray (thirty years ago) were seized upon with enthusiasm by psychodiagnosticians. At no point do these methods ask the subject what his interests are, what he wants to do or what he is trying to do. Nor do the methods ask directly concerning the subject's relation to his parents or to authority figures. They infer this relationship entirely by assumed identifications. So popular is this indirect, undercover approach to motivation that many clinicians and many university centers spend far more time on this type of diagnostic method than on any other.

Occasionally, however, a client may cause the projective tester consternation by intruding his unwanted conscious report. The story is told of a patient who remarked that a Rorschach card made him think of sexual relations. The clinician, thinking to tap a buried complex, asked him why. "Oh, because," said the patient, "I think of sexual relations all the time, anyway." The clinician scarcely needed a Rorschach card to find out this motivational fact.

Still, it is probably true that most psychologists prefer to assess a person's needs and conflicts by going the long way around. The argument, of course, is that everyone, even a neurotic, will accommodate himself fairly well to the demands placed upon him by reality. Only in an unstructured projective situation will he reveal his anxieties and unmasked needs. "Projective tests," writes Stagner, "are more useful than reality situations for diagnostic purposes." [1] To my mind, this uncompromising statement seems to mark the culmination of a century-long era of irrationalism, and therefore of distrust. Has the subject no right to be believed?

Fortunately, the extensive use of projective methods at the present time is yielding results that enable us to place this technique in proper perspective and to correct the one-sided theory of motivation upon which their popularity rests.

Let us consider first the wartime research conducted with thirty-six conscientious objectors who lived for six months on a semistarvation diet.[2] Their diet was so rigorously meager that on the average they lost one quarter of their initial body weight in the course of the six months. The food need was agonizingly great, their incessant hunger most poignant. Unless occupied with laboratory or other tasks, they found themselves thinking of food almost constantly. Typical daydreaming is reported by one subject as follows: "Today we'll have Menu No. 1. Gee, that's the smallest menu, it seems. How shall I fix the potatoes? If I use my spoon to eat them, I'll be able to add more water. . . . If I eat a little faster, the food would stay warm longer—and I like it warm. But then it's gone so quickly."

Now, the curious thing is that, while these men were clearly obsessed by their food drive and all their energy seemed directed toward its fulfillment, on projective tests the need failed to appear. The investigators report that, among the tests used (free word association, first letters test, analysis of dreams, Rorschach and Rosenzweig's P-F Study), only one gave a limited evidence of the preoccupation with food—the free association test.

Here is a finding of grave significance. *The most urgent, the most absorbing motive in life failed completely to reveal itself by indirect methods.* It was, however, entirely accessible to conscious report. Part of the explanation may be that the subjects turned in relief to laboratory tasks to forget for a while their obsessive motive. They responded to the projective tests with heaven knows what available, habitual associational material. The failure of night dreams to reveal a significant amount of wish fulfillment is somewhat more perplexing. It can scarcely be ascribed to a defensive mental set. But both types of result suggest a possible law: unless a motive is repressed, it is unlikely to affect distinctly the perception of, and responses to, a projective test. It is too early to tell whether this is a valid generalization, but it is a hypothesis well worth testing.

Other studies on hunger seem to yield supporting evidence.[3] Their trend suggests that, on projective tests, the number of explicit food associations actually declines in longer periods of fasting, apparently because the motive itself gradually becomes completely conscious and is not repressed. It is true that instrumental associations (references to ways of obtaining food) continue to appear in the subject's word-responses as the state of hunger grows. This finding, however, is quite consistent with the hypothesis, since, while hunger is fully conscious, the subject in the experimental situation is prevented from seeking satisfaction and thus is still repressing his instrumental action-tendencies.

Another revealing line of evidence comes from the research of J. W. Getzels.[4] This investigator utilized two forms of a sentence completion test—one couched in the first person and one in the third. His pairs are of the following type:

When they asked Frank to be in charge he. . . .
When they asked me to be in charge I. . . .

When Joe meets a person for the first time he usually. . . .
When I meet a person for the first time I usually. . . .

In the experiment, of course, the items were randomized. In all there were twenty diagnostic items of each type. The subjects were sixty-five veterans, twenty-five diagnosed as well adjusted; forty were psychoneurotic cases discharged from service with disability involving personality disorder.

It turned out that, to a highly significant degree, the well-adjusted men gave *identical* responses to the first- and to the third-person completions. If we assume that the third-person sentence is a "projective method," then the results obtained by this method for well-adjusted subjects squared almost perfectly with the results obtained from the direct, first-person questioning. The psychoneurotics, on the other hand, to a highly significant degree varied their responses. They said one thing when queried directly (for example, "When they asked me to be in charge I agreed") and another on the projective item ("When they asked John to be in charge he was afraid"). The first-person completion is so direct that in the psychoneurotic it invokes the mask of defense and elicits a merely conventionally correct response.

Thus the direct responses of the psychoneurotic cannot be taken at their face value. The defenses are high; the true motives are hidden and are betrayed only by a projective technique. The normal subjects, on the other hand, tell you by the direct method precisely what they tell you by the projective method. They are all of a piece. You may therefore take their motivational statements at their face value, for, even if you probe, you will not find anything substantially different.

This research adds weight to the tentative judgment we formed in the case of the starving subjects. It is not the well-integrated subject, aware of his motivations, who reveals himself in projective testing. It is, rather, the neurotic personality, whose façade belies the repressed fears and hostilities within. Such a subject is caught off guard by projective devices; but the well-adjusted subject gives no significantly different response.

There is, however, one difference between the two researches. The starving subjects actually *avoided* any betrayal of their dominant motive in the projective tests. The well-adjusted veterans, on the other hand, gave essentially the *same* type of response in both direct and projective testing. It may be that the dissimilar nature of the tests used in the two situations accounts for this difference in results. But this detailed difference need not detain us here. What seems to be important is the implication of these researches that *a psycho-*

diagnostician should never employ projective methods in the study of motivation without at the same time employing direct methods. If he does not use direct methods, he will never be able to distinguish a well-integrated personality from one that is not. Nor will he be able to tell whether there are strong conscious streams of motivation that are entirely evading the projective situation (as in the case of the starving subjects).

The trend of evidence seems to indicate that a normal, well-adjusted individual with strong goal-directedness may, on projective tests, do one of two things—either give material identical with that of conscious report, in which case the projective method is not needed, or give no evidence whatever of his dominant motives. Only when the projective responses reveal emotionally laden material that is contradictory to conscious report, or to other results of direct assessment, do we find special value in projective testing. And we shall never know whether or not a neurotic situation prevails unless we use *both* diagnostic approaches and compare the yield.

Consider for a moment the diagnosis of anxiety. Using various responses on the Rorschach and TAT cards, the clinician might infer a high level of anxiety. Now, this finding taken by itself tells us little. The subject may be the sort of person who is enormously effective in life because he harnesses his anxiety to performance. He may know perfectly well that he is a harried, worried, bedeviled over-achiever. Anxiety is an asset in his life, and he has enough insight to know the fact. In this case the yield by projective methods is matched by the yield from direct methods. The projective technique was not really needed, but it does no harm to use it. Again, as in our starvation cases, we might find that projective protocols reveal no anxiety, while in actuality we are dealing with a person who is as harried, worried and bedeviled as our first subject. The explanation may be, quite simply, that he effectively controls his jitters and that his large measure of control enables him to tackle the projective tests with some mental set unrelated to his anxious nature. But we may also find—and here is where projective methods have their uses— that an apparently bland and calm individual, denying all anxiety, reveals profound disturbance and fear in projective performances. It is this type of dissociated nature that projective tests help to diagnose; yet they cannot do so unless direct methods also are employed.

In speaking so frequently of direct methods, I have referred chiefly to conscious report. To ask a man his motives, however, is not the only type of direct method that we may employ. It is, however, a good one—especially to start with.

When we set out to study a person's motives, we are seeking to find out what that person is trying to do in this life—including, of course, what he is trying to avoid and what he is trying to be. I see no reason why we should not start our investigation by asking him to tell us the answers as he sees them. If the questions in this form seem too abstract, they can be recast. Particularly revealing are people's answers to the question, "What do you want to be doing five years from now?" Similar direct questions can be framed to elicit anxieties, loyalties and hostilities. Most people, I suspect, can tell what they are trying to do in this life with a high degree of validity, certainly not less on the average than the prevailing validity of projective instruments. Yet some clinicians disdain to ask direct questions.

But by direct methods I mean also to include standard pencil-and-paper measures, such as the Strong Interest Inventory and the Allport-Vernon-Lindzey Study of Values. It often happens that the yield on such instruments is not what would come from the subject's conscious report. The subject may not have known, for example, that compared with most people his pattern of values is, say, markedly theoretical and aesthetic, or far below average in economic and re-ligious interest. Yet the final score on the Study of Values is itself merely a summation of a series of separate conscious choices that he has made in forty-five hypothetical situations. While his verbal re-port on the pattern as a whole may be faulty, this pattern not only squares with all his separate choices but is known on the average to have good external validity. People with certain patterns of interests as measured by the test do in fact make characteristic vocational choices and do in their daily behavior act in ways that are demon-strably consistent with the test results.

To sum up: Direct methods include the kind of report that is elicited in careful interviewing, whether it be the simple psychiatric variety, or the sort employed in vocational or personal counseling, or in non-directive interviewing. Autobiographic methods, when em-ployed at their face value, are likewise direct. So too are the results of any kind of testing where the final scores represent a sum or pattern of a series of conscious choices on the part of the subject.[5]

The currently fashionable term *psychodynamics* is often equated explicitly with psychoanalytic theory. Projective techniques are considered psychodynamic because they are thought to tap the deepest layers of structure and functioning. We have already indicated reasons for doubting the sufficiency of this assumption. Many of the most dynamic motives are more accurately tapped by direct methods. At the very least, the discoveries by projective techniques cannot be properly interpreted unless they are compared with discoveries yielded by direct methods.

Devotees of psychodynamics often say that no discoveries are of value unless the unconscious is explored. This dictum we find in the valuable book by Kardiner and Ovesey, *The Mark of oppression*,[6] dealing with the seriously disordered and conflictful motivational systems of Negroes in a Northern city. Unless I am greatly mistaken, however, the authors discover little or nothing about their cases through psychoanalytic probes that is not evident in the manifest situation. The conscious handicaps of a Negro in our society, the economic misery, the deteriorated family situations, the bitterness and despair constitute a painful psychodynamic situation in individual lives that in most instances receives no further illumination when depth analysis is employed.

Most of the psychodynamic evidence given by Kardiner and Ovesey concerning their cases is, in fact, drawn from straightforward autobiographical report. Their use of this method is acceptable and their findings highly instructive. But their theory seems to me out of line with both the method actually used and the findings obtained. Psychodynamics is not necessarily a hidden dynamics.

This point is well made by the psychiatrist J. C. Whitehorn[7] who holds that psychodynamics is a general science of motivation. Into its broad principles one may fit the specific contributions and insights of psychoanalysis, but psychoanalysis itself is by no means the sum and substance of psychodynamics. Whitehorn insists that the proper approach to psychotic patients, especially to those suffering from schizophrenic or depressive disorder, is through such channels of their normal interest systems as remain open. It is not the region of their disorder that requires primary attention, but those psychodynamic systems that still represent sturdy and healthy adaptations to reality. In Whitehorn's words, the therapist should seek "to activate and utilize the resources of the patient and to help him thereby to work out a more satisfying way of life with a less circumscribed emphasis upon these special issues." [8]

Sometimes we hear it said that psychoanalytic theory does not do justice to psychoanalytic practice. What is meant is that, in the course of therapy, an analyst will devote much of his time to a direct discussion with his patient of his manifest interests and values. The analyst will listen respectfully, accept, counsel and advise concerning these important and *not* buried psychodynamic systems. In many instances, as in the cases presented by Kardiner and Ovesey, the motives and conflicts are taken at their face value. Thus the method of psychoanalysis as employed is not fully sustained by the theory that is affirmed.

Nothing that I have said denies the existence of infantile systems, troublesome repressions or neurotic formations. Nor does it deny the possibility of self-deception, rationalization and ego-defense. My point is merely that methods and theories dealing with these aberrant conditions should be set in a broad conception of psychodynamics. The patient should be assumed insightful until he is proved otherwise. If you asked a hundred people who go to the icebox for a snack why they did so, probably all would answer, "Because I was hungry." In ninety-nine of these cases we may—no matter how deeply we explore—discover that this simple, conscious report is the whole truth. In the hundredth case, however, our probing shows that we are dealing with a compulsive overeater, with an obese seeker after infantile security, who, unlike the majority of cases, does not know what he is trying to do. It is peace and comfort he is seeking— perhaps his mother's bosom—and not the left-over roast. In this case, and in a minority of all cases, we cannot take the evidence of his overt behavior, nor his account of it, at their face value.

Freud was a specialist in precisely those motives that cannot be taken at their face value. To him, motivation resided in the id. The conscious, accessible region of personality that carries on direct transactions with the world—that is, the ego—he regarded as devoid of dynamic power.

It is a misfortune that Freud died before he had remedied this one-sidedness in his theory. Even his most faithful followers tell us now that he left his ego-psychology incomplete. In recent years many of them have labored to redress the balance. Without doubt the principal current in psychoanalytic theory today is moving in the direction of a more dynamic ego. This trend in theory is apparent in the work of Anna Freud, Hartmann, French, Horney, Fromm, Kris and many others. In a communication to the American Psychoanalytic Association, Kris points out that the attempt to restrict interpretations of motivation to the id aspect only "represents the older procedure." Modern concern with the ego does not confine itself to an analysis of defense mechanisms alone. Rather, it gives more respect to what he calls the "psychic surface." Present psychoanalytic techniques, he tells us, tend to link "surface" with "depth." [9] In a similar vein Rapaport has argued that a measure of true autonomy must now be ascribed to the ego.[10]

To illustrate the point at issue, we might take any psychogenic interest of maturity—say, the religious sentiment. Freud's handling of the matter is well known. To him religion is essentially a neurosis in the individual, a formula for personal escape. The father image lies at the root of the matter. One cannot therefore take the religious sentiment, when it exists in a personality, at its face value. A more balanced view of the matter would seem to be this: *sometimes* one cannot take this sentiment at its face value, and *sometimes* one can. Only a careful study of the individual will tell. In a person in whom the religious factor serves an obviously egocentric purpose—talismanic, bigoted, self-justificatory—we can infer that it is a neurotic, or at least immature, formation in the personality. Its infantile and escapist character is not recognized by the subject. On the other hand, in a person who has gradually evolved a guiding philosophy of life where the religious sentiment exerts a generally normative force upon behavior and confers intelligibility to life as a whole, we infer that this particular ego-formation is a dominant motive and that it must be accepted at its face value. It is a master motive and an ego-ideal whose shape and substance are essentially what appear in consciousness.[11]

Let us consider a final example. It is well known that most boys around the age of four to seven identify with their fathers. They imitate them in many ways. Among other things, they may express vocational aspirations for daddy's job. Many boys, when grown, do in fact follow their fathers' footsteps.

Take politics. Father and son have been politicians in many families: the Tafts, Lodges, Kennedys, La Follettes and Roosevelts, to mention only a few. When the son is at a mature age, say fifty or sixty, what is his motivation? Is he working through his early father identification, or is he not? Taken at its face value, the interest of the son in politics now seems to be absorbing and self-contained, a prominent factor in his own ego-structure. In short, it seems to be a mature and normal motive. But the strict geneticist would say: "No, he is now a politician because of a father fixation." Does the geneticist mean that an early father identification started him in a political direction of interest? If so, the answer is yes, of course. All motives have their origin somewhere. Or does he mean, "This early fixation now, today, sustains the son's political conduct"? If so, the answer is normally no. The political interest is now a prominent part of the ego-structure, and the ego is the healthy man's source of energy. To be sure, there may be cases where a person mature in years is still trying to curry Father's favor, to step into his shoes, to displace him with the mother. A clinical study of a second-generation politician may conceivably show that his behavior is compulsively father-identical. If so, his daily conduct is in all probability so compulsive, so ungeared to realistic situational needs, so excessive that the diagnosis can be suspected by any skilled clinical observer. But such instances are relatively rare.

To sum up: We need in our motivational theory to make a sharper distinction between infantilisms and motivation that is strictly contemporary and at age.

I am fully aware of my heterodoxy in suggesting that there is, in a restricted sense, a discontinuity between normal and abnormal motivation, and that we need a theory that will recognize this fact. Discontinuities are distinctly unpopular in psychological science. One theory of abnormality tells us that we are merely pleased to regard the extremes on our linear continuum as abnormal. Some culture theorists insist that abnormality is a relative concept, shifting from culture to culture and from one historical period to another. Likewise, there are many borderline cases which even the most experienced clinician could not with confidence classify as normal or as abnormal. Finally —and most important—one can, by scratching deeply enough, find *some* infantilism in the motivation of many normal people.

Granted all these familiar arguments, there is still a world of difference, if not between normal and abnormal people, then between the healthy and unhealthy mechanisms involved in the development of motivation. What we call integrative action of the nervous system is basically a wholesome mechanism that keeps motivation up to date. It tends to bring about both an internal consistency and a reality testing among the elements entering into motivational patterning. Effective suppression is another healthy mechanism, harmless to the individual and making possible the arrangement of motives in an orderly hierarchy.[12] With the aid of effective suppression, the individual ceases to act out infantile dramas. Insight, a clear self-image and the little-understood factor of homeostasis may be mentioned among the balancing mechanisms.

As Getzel's experiment shows, direct and projective performances in healthy people are all of a piece. A further test of normality—unfortunately, one psychologists have not yet developed—may lie in the harmony of expressive behavior (facial expression, gestures, hand-

writing) with the individual's fundamental motivational structure.
There is evidence that discoordination between conscious motives and
expressive movement is an ominous sign.[13] This lead for research
should be followed through.

In unhealthy motivation, unbalancing mechanisms have the upper hand. There is always some species of dissociation at work.
The individual represses ineffectively; repressed motives erupt in
autistic gestures, in tantrums, in nightmares, in compulsions, perhaps
in paranoid thinking. Above all, self-knowledge is lacking in large
regions of the life. But normally the balancing mechanisms have the
upper hand. Sometimes, in certain badly disordered lives, the unbalancing mechanisms take over. Occasionally we find them operating in a segmental way in lives that are otherwise healthy. When
the clash in mechanisms is marked, diagnosis is aided by the use of
projective techniques. But, when there is essential harmony within
the personality system, projective methods will teach us little or
nothing about the course of motivation.

From what has been said, it is clear that a satisfactory conception
of psychodynamics will have the following characteristics: (1) It will
never employ projective methods or depth analysis without allowing
for a full diagnosis of motives by direct methods as well. (2) It will
assume that, in a healthy personality, the great bulk of motivation
can be taken at its face value. (3) It will assume that normal motivation of this order has a present and future significance for the individual, which is by no means adequately represented by a study of
his past life. In other words, it will allow that the present psychodynamics of a life may in large part be functionally autonomous, even
though continuous with early motivational formations.[14] (4) It will,
at the same time, retain the epochal insights of Freud and others to
the effect that infantile fixations sometimes occur and that we do
well to check on conscious report and to supplement direct methods
by indirect.

Before such an adequate conceptualization can be achieved, one
current dogma in motivational theory must be re-examined. I refer
to the oft-encountered statement that all motives aim at "the reduction of tensions." This doctrine—found in instinctivism, psychoanalysis and stimulus-response psychology—operates to keep us on a
primitive level of theorizing.

We cannot, of course, deny that basic drives seem to seek "reduction of tension." Oxygen need, hunger, thirst and elimination are
clear examples. But these drives are not a trustworthy model for all

normal adult motivation. Goldstein remarks that patients who seek only tension reduction are clearly pathological. They are preoccupied with segmental irritations from which they seek relief. There is nothing creative about their interests. They cannot take suffering or delay or frustration as a mere incident in their pursuit of values. Normal people, by contrast, are dominated by their "preferred patterns" of self-actualization. Their psychogenic interests are modes of sustaining and directing tension rather than escaping it.[15]

We should, I think, agree that tension reduction is not an adequate statement of the functioning of mature psychogenic motives. At the time of his inauguration as president of Harvard, James Bryant Conant remarked that he was undertaking his duties "with a heavy heart but gladly." He knew he would reduce no tensions by committing himself to the new job. Tensions would mount and mount and, at many times, become almost unbearable. While he would, in the course of his daily work, dispatch many tasks and feel relief, the over-all commitment—his total investment of energy—would never result in any equilibrium. Psychogenic interests are of this order: they lead us to complicate and strain our lives indefinitely. "Striving for equilibrium," "tension reduction" and "death wish" seem trivial and erroneous representations of normal adult motivation.

The postwar years, as I have said, brought a wholesome turn in theorizing. Few authorities on war neuroses, for example, wrote in terms of tension reduction; they spoke, rather, of "firm ego structure" or "weak ego structure." Grinker and Spiegel say, "As the ego becomes stronger the therapist demands increasing independence and activity from the patient."[16] After successful therapy, these and other writers sometimes remark, "The ego now seems in full control." In such expressions as these—and one encounters them with increasing frequency—we meet post-Freudian ego psychology again. True, the flavor of these theoretical statements varies. Sometimes they still seem close to the conception of the ego as rationalizer, rider and steersman. But often, as in the statements just quoted, they go far beyond. They imply that the ego is not only normally able to avoid malignant repression, chronicity and rigidity, but is also a differentiated dynamism —a fusion of healthy psychogenic motives that can be taken at their face value.

There is no need to take fright at the conception of an "active ego." As I see the matter, the term *ego* does not refer to a homunculus, but is merely a shorthand expression for what Goldstein calls "preferred patterns." The term means that normally healthy personalities have various systems of psychogenic motives. They are not limitless in number; indeed, in a well-integrated adult they may be adequately indicated on the fingers of two hands, perhaps one. What a person is trying to do persistently, recurrently, as a function of his own internal nature, is often surprisingly well focused and well patterned. Whether these leading motives are called desires, interests, values, traits or sentiments does not greatly matter. What is important is that motivational theory—in guiding diagnosis, therapy and research—should take these structures fully into account.

REFERENCES

1. R. Stagner, "Homeostasis as a unifying concept in personality theory," *Psychol. Rev.,* 1951, 58:5-17.

2. J. Brozek, H. Guetzkow, M. V. Baldwin and R. Cranston, "A quantitative study of perception and association in experimental semi-starvation," *J. Pers.,* 1951, 19:245-64.

3. R. Levine, I. Chein and G. Murphy, "The relation of the intensity of a need to the amount of perceptual distortion: a preliminary report," *J. Psychol.,* 1942, 13:283-93; R. N. Sanford, "The effect of abstinence from food upon imaginal processes," *J. Psychol.,* 1936, 2:129-36.

4. J. W. Getzels, "The assessment of personality and prejudice by the methods of paired direct and projective questionnaires," unpublished thesis, Harvard College Library, Cambridge, 1951.

5. For the purposes of the present argument, this simplified discussion of direct and indirect techniques is adequate. Psychodiagnosis requires, however, a much more discriminating classification of the methods currently employed and of the "levels" of organization that each normally taps. An excellent beginning is Rosenzweig's proposal that three classes of methods be distinguished, each adapted in principle to tapping three levels of behavior (S. Rosenzweig, "Levels of behavior in psychodiagnosis with special reference to the picture-frustration study," *Amer. J. Orthopsychiat.,* 1950, 20:63-72). What he calls *subjective* methods require the subject to take himself as a direct object of observation (questionnaires, autobiographies). *Objective* methods require the observer to report on overt conduct. *Projective* methods require both subject and observer to "look the other way" and to base the diagnosis on the subject's reaction to apparently "ego-neutral" material. Broadly speaking, Rosenzweig's subjective and objective procedures correspond to what I here call direct methods, and projective procedures to indirect methods.

Especially noteworthy is Rosenzweig's statement that the significance of projective methods, such as his own P-F Study, cannot be determined unless the subject's projective responses are examined in the light of his subjective and objective responses.

6. A. Kardiner and L. Ovesey, *The mark of oppression,* New York: Norton, 1951.

7. J. C. Whitehorn, "Psychodynamic considerations in the treatment of psychotic patients," *Univ. West. Ontario Med. J.,* 1950, 20:27-41.

8. *Ibid.,* p. 40.

9. E. Kris, "Ego psychology and interpretation in psychoanalytic therapy," *Psa. Quart.,* 1951, 20:15-30.

10. D. Rapaport, "The autonomy of the ego," *Bull. Menninger Clin.*, 1951, 15:113-23.

11. G. W. Allport, *The individual and his religion*, New York: Macmillan, 1950.

12. L. Belmont and H. G. Birch, "Re-individualizing the repression hypothesis," *J. Abnorm. Soc. Psychol.*, 1951, 46:226-35, D. V. McGranahan, "A critical and experimental study of repression," *J. Abnorm. Soc. Psychol.*, 1940, 35:212-25.

13. G. W. Allport and P. E. Vernon, *Studies in expressive movement*, New York: Macmillan, 1933.

14. G. W. Allport, *The nature of personality: selected papers*, Cambridge: Addison-Wesley, 1950, especially pp. 76-113.

15. K. Goldstein, *Human nature in the light of psychopathology*, Cambridge: Harvard University Press, 1940.

16. R. R. Grinker and J. P. Spiegel, *War neuroses*, Philadelphia: Blakiston, 1945, p. 94.

CHAPTER 7

What units shall we employ?

Turning from the problem of motives to the problem of structure, we ask: what are the building blocks that comprise the edifice of a given personality?

The leading historical answers to this question include such proposed units as traits, sentiments, attitudes, schemata, factors and syndromes of temperament. While each of these has certain advantages, the best solution seems to lie in identifying the unique dynamic *trends* peculiar to the structure of each individual life.

This essay was orginally part of a symposium held at Syracuse University and published under the title *Assessment of human motives* (1958).

Man's nature, like all of nature, seems to be composed of relatively stable structures. The success of psychological science, therefore, as of any science, depends in large part upon its ability to identify the major structures, substructures and microstructures (elements) of which its assigned portion of the cosmos is composed.

Early Inadequate Units

From the fourth century B.C. to the seventeenth century A.D., the life sciences—indeed, all the sciences—were badly frozen because they had chosen unproductive units of analysis: the Empedoclean elements of earth, air, fire and water. These units and these alone are the "root of things"—so said Hippocrates and Galen; so said all the sages of the Middle Ages and the Renaissance, including both Christian and Islamic scholars.[1] Personality theory, such as it was, was written entirely in terms of the four temperaments arising, men said, from the humoral distillations of the four cosmic elements: black bile (*melancholic*), yellow bile (*sanguine*), blood (*choleric*) and phlegm (*phlegmatic*). "Quatuor humores in nostro corpore regnant," sang the thirteenth-century medical poem. This rigidity of analysis endured at least until the time of Harvey, whose discovery of the circulation of the blood in 1628 cast doubt upon the whole humoral doctrine.[2]

Freed at last from this incubus, psychology perversely entered a second ice age by adopting the conception of *faculties*—units scarcely more productive than the humors. The faculties set forth by the Thomists, by Christian Wolff, by the Scottish school and by the phrenologists have a certain common-sense appeal, but they do not satisfy modern theorists.

Under the influence of Darwin, personality theorists traded faculties for *instincts*. The ensuing era, lasting approximately sixty years, cannot be called an ice age, for it brought with it McDougall's elegant and consistent defense of instincts and their derivatives, the sentiments. More than anyone else, McDougall fixed our attention upon the possible existence of uniform motivational units. Freud reinforced the search, though, unlike McDougall, he himself offered no clear taxonomic scheme. During this era innumerable instincts were discovered, postulated, invented. In 1924, Bernard reported that more than 14,000 different instincts had been proposed and that no agreement was yet in sight.[3]

Sensing disaster in this direction, psychologists started fishing in fresher waters. The doctrine of *drives* (a limited form of instinct) continued to hold the behaviorist fort, and to some extent still does, but most psychologists nowadays seem to agree with Hebb[4] that to equate motivational structure with simple drives or biological needs is a wholly inadequate procedure.

Difficulties and Complexities of Contemporary Search

I mention these fragments of history in the hope that they will give perspective to our contemporary search. It is clear that we have not yet solved the problem of the units of man's nature, though the problem was posed twenty-three centuries ago. It is equally clear that psychology lags far behind chemistry, which has its periodic table of elements; behind physics, with its verifiable, if elusive, quanta; and even far behind biology, with its cell. Psychology does not yet know what its "cell" may be. It is partly for this reason that skeptics question psychology's right to be called a science. Its investigators have not yet reached agreement on what units of analysis to employ.

Some of the trouble lies in the fact that psychology could make little use of a "cell," even if it discovered one. (It has given up the "reflex arc," which for a time seemed to serve the purpose.) Psychology's peculiar problem lies in the existence of many different levels of organization, whose number and nature are as yet unascertained. Units of structure may be smaller or larger, depending on our interests. If we happen to be concerned with an elementary behavioral problem, such as the alternate extension and flexion of the leg, we may adopt *spinal innervation* as our unit. If we wish to classify forms of motor activity, *walking* seems a more acceptable unit. Should we be interested in interpersonal behavior, we can conceivably establish a measurable habit of *walking away from people* (thus approaching Karen Horney's conception). If our concern is with the generalized dispositions of personality, we may consider some such unit as a *trait of withdrawal*. Fine-grained or coarse-grained—units of both orders have their place. Ultimately, of course, our hope is to be able to reduce molar units to molecular and, conversely, to compound molecular units into molar.

But we are far from this goal. Even at the coarser levels of analysis, we are not in agreement on the kinds of units we seek. Shall they be habits or habit systems; needs or sentiments; vectors, factors, trends or traits? Shall they be drives or dimensions; *Anschauungen* or attitudes; regions, syndromes, personal constructs or ergs? All have been proposed and empirically defended.

The most hopeful note in the confused situation is that for the past thirty years there has been boundless zeal for both measurement and theory. By now the measured aspects of personality cannot fall far short of the 14,000 instinctive units reported by Bernard. When psychologists face up to this orgy of units, let us hope they will not fall into the state of collapse that terminated the earlier search for instincts. There seems to be no immediate danger, for one reads in the *American Psychologist*: "A Ford Foundation grant of $238,400 will enable a research team of the University of Minnesota to conduct a five year study aimed at developing a more adequate system of descriptive, diagnostic, and dynamic categories. . . . The team will work toward developing terms or systems of terms maximally descriptive of personality." [5]

I should like to discuss this bewildering topic, not because I have a secret solution for a two-thousand-year-old problem or because I am so clairvoyant that I can previse the final Minnesota results, but because I believe that our present research lacks perspective on its own efforts, and I should like to achieve a balanced view of the efforts of assessors to date. Toward the end of this essay, I shall venture one somewhat radical proposal for a shift of direction in our research.

Central Propositions for a New Approach

First, a few central propositions on which I hope we can all agree. It seems clear that the units we seek in personality and in

motivation are relatively complex structures, not molecular. They lie
in the upper reaches of what Hull called the habit hierarchy, and not
at the level of specific habits. We do not seek cells or even cell
assemblies; we do not seek reflexes, hedons, traces or quanta of en-
docrine discharge, or the gating processes of the nervous system. Ultimately, of course, we should like to translate complex structures into
microelements and discover their neurohumoral counterparts. But at
present, and for some time to come, we must be satisfied to search out
the generalized units that define relatively broad forms of organization.

The second proposition may admit of equally rapid agreement.
Methodologists tell us than we can never observe a motive, or a trait,
or any similar unit directly. We agree. They tell us that any unit we
discover is only a "hypothetical construct" or an "intervening variable." Here, too, they are right, though for my part I vote for "hypothetical construct," which, in the usage proposed by Mac-
Corquodale and Meehl,[6] implies that the units we seek, though invisible, are factually existing. Methodologists tell us, furthermore,
that we must have sound and repeatable operations for establishing
the units we fix upon; we may not bring them into being by merely
naming them, as did the addicts of instinct a generation or two ago.
Again we agree. In fact, we do well to accept all the cautions and
safeguards of modern methodology, save only that excess of zeal
which holds all units to be fictional, existing only in the manipulations of the investigator.

A third proposition will detain us longer, for it has to do with
the greatest stumbling block of all in our search for objectively existing structures. I refer to the unquestioned variability of a person's
behavior from situation to situation. Motivational units discovered
under laboratory conditions often seem to evaporate when the subject
moves from the laboratory to his office, to his home, to his golf club.
Indeed, his behavior in these familiar settings may often seem contradictory. Situational variability has led many social scientists to the
conviction that any search for a consistent personality with specifiable
motives and traits is doomed to failure.

Recently I attended a conference of psychologists working on the
problem of the "perception of persons."[7] At this conference one
heard much about perception but little about persons, the object of
perception. The reason, I think, is that the participants were keenly
aware of the chameleon-like changes that mark a person as he moves
from situation to situation. They much preferred to study the percep-
tion-of-a-person-in-a-situation and thus evade the question of what the

person is really like. Not only does the individual vary his behavior, but our perception of him is heavily affected by our subjective sets, by our degree of liking for him and by his degree of similarity to ourselves. The perceiver himself may, therefore, be the principal source of variance; the situation in which the object-person acts may be the second source of variance; and the fixed traits and motives of the object-person may be only a minor factor.

The hope for an accurate assessment of motives and traits is thus badly bedeviled by the person's variability and the perceiver's bias. It is also badly bedeviled by the uncertainty of criteria. When are we to know that our assessment is accurate and veridical? Not by comparing our assessment with ratings by others, who may be subject to both common and idiosyncratic errors. Not by the self-report of the subject, who is capable of self-deception. Not by prediction of future behavior, which will depend to a considerable extent on the situation that evokes this behavior. Not by other tests and measurement, for these too are fallible.

Situational Variables

All these objections are sound, and their combined force is today leading many investigators away from the assessment of motives and persons. One tempting escape is found in the concept of *role*. Emanuel Brown, to use one example, is no longer viewed as a single person: he is a colligation of roles. As a teacher he meets certain expectancies; as a father, others; still others as a citizen and as a Rotarian. In one of his enthusiastic moments, William James took the same way out. "A man," he says, "has as many selves as there are distinct groups of persons about whose opinion he cares." [8]

The extreme version of this situational doctrine is found in Coutu's book *Emergent Human Nature*, where the author argues that the search for traits of personality and their assessment is chimerical; that the most we can say of any person is that in a given situation he has a specific tendency to respond in a certain limited way. The only acceptable unit, therefore, according to Coutu, is the "tinsit" or "tendency-in-a-situation." [9]

Unless we can successfully refute the extreme forms of role theory and tinsit theory, and James's statement about the social self, our work should cease here and now. What is the use of assessing motivation or personality if behavior is as dependent on the situation as these theories assert? Let us see what may be said on the other side.

In the first place, some of our assessment methods have built into them a safeguard against situational variability. They explicitly vary the situation. Thus a person's disposition to be ascendant, or his aesthetic value, or his neurotic tendency is tested by a wide range of items depicting a great variety of situations commonly experienced. While some studies show that a trait measured in this way does vary, say, from the academic to the business situation, or from the athletic to the purely social, it is more common to find that the person carries with him, by and large, his typical level of anxiety, a typical amount of aesthetic interest and of ascendance, a typical aspiration level and a fairly constant degree of prejudice.

In the second place, it is obviously not true that a man has as many social selves as there are groups whose opinion he prizes. A man who is deferential, ambitious or compulsive in the office is not likely to shed these characteristics at home or on the golf course. Their intensity may vary, and their mode of expression may alter, but true Jekyll and Hyde cases are exceedingly rare. So far as roles are concerned, is it not a fact that characteristic styles run through a person's conduct even when he is playing diverse roles? Is it not also true that a person *seeks* the roles that are most congenial to his personality, avoiding others that cramp his style or put an undue strain upon his internal motivational structure?

That some persons are forced into roles they do not like we must admit, just as we must admit that a range of variation marks anyone's behavior according to the circumstances in which he finds himself. But though these factors greatly complicate our search for structures, they need not discourage us. There is too much consistency, too much dependability, too much sameness in a person's behavior to warrant the surrender of our task.

There are two steps we can take to meet this problem. We can continue to seek methods of assessment that cross over many situational boundaries. Pencil-and-paper techniques can do so more easily than experimental techniques, since the former can ask the subject about his behavior in many daily contexts. But if a technique is limited to a given experimental situation (as is the Rorschach, for example), we can at least insist that our diagnosis be confirmed by additional evidence drawn from ancillary techniques.

Elsewhere I have deplored our reliance on too limited a battery.[10] Projective tests, for example, need the supplement of direct methods, for otherwise we may obtain a picture of certain latent tendencies without ever knowing whether these are separated from or integrated with conscious interests and self-knowledge. It makes a world of difference whether anxiety, or homosexuality, or aggression is a repressed tendency or whether it is fully accepted and known. Projective devices alone would never answer this question.

Besides using multiple or wider devices to enlarge the coverage of situations, we may often need frankly to admit the limited range covered by our assessment. We can say, for example, that this college student in a series of tests at college displays such and such characteristics. Just what he will do at home or in business we cannot be sure. In another case, we might say that this patient, manifestly disturbed, shows such-and-such propensities, but that owing to his condition no wider generalization is allowable at this time.

Situationism, in short, is a serious obstacle to overcome. Diagnosticians should be more aware of the problem and strive for broader coverage in their instruments; at the same time, they should safeguard their statements about motivation by making clear the conditions covered by the battery.

But let us not join the camp of skeptics who say that an individual's personality is "a mere construct tied together with a name" —that there is nothing outer and objectively structured to be assessed. No scientist, I think, could survive for long if he heeded this siren song of doubt, for it leads to shipwreck. An astronomer spots a star. Like any good realist, he assumes that it has properties, elements and structure—all of which it is his scientific duty to search out and to study. When a botanist dissects a plant, he does not assume that he is dissecting a construct tied together by a name. It is a plant; and its structure and its functioning interest him. Similarly, the psychologist of personality wants to come as close as he can to the veridical structure of the person he studies; and he does so in spite of the extensive and troublesome situational variability, and in spite of his own errors of observation and measurement, which he tries constantly to reduce.

A theoretical task for the future is to relate the intra-individual structure to the recurrent situational patterns, which in themselves may be regarded as complex social or cultural structures. In the terms of F. H. Allport, we have to deal both with *trend structures* in the personality and with *tangential collective structures*. Between them exists some degree of *interstructurance*. Analytical research, such as that carried out by Tannenbaum and Allport,[11] should help us determine the differentials of energy in the individual's pattern of behavior that may be ascribed to internal-trend structures, on the one hand, and to tangential collective structures, on the other.

Units of Motivation and Units of Personality

We move now nearer to the heart of our subject. What is the relation between units of motivation and units of personality? I would suggest that all units of motivation are at the same time units of personality, but that not all units of personality are simultaneously units of motivation. Only a few writers have made this distinction systematically. Murray does so when he distinguishes motivational needs, or *vectors*, from the styles or manners of fulfilling needs represented by actones and verbones.[12] Similarly, McClelland distinguishes motives from traits and from schemata.[13] Traits he limits to recurrent patterns of expressive or stylistic behavior; schemata, to additional orientations, cognitive and symbolic habits, and frames of reference. To him motives alone are the dynamic or casual forces, and these he finds satisfactorily designated by the term *needs*.

We will all agree that some characteristics of personality are of a highly dynamic order, while some are of an instrumental or stylistic order. There is, for example, a distinct difference between a hate-filled complex or a driving ambition, on the one hand, and a style of urbanity or a hesitating manner, on the other. In Lewin's terms, certain regions are capable of greater tension than others. And some regions (the stylistic) are called into play only to guide the individual in the execution of more central motives. Thus a young man who is hungry for friendships goes out in the evening on a quest, but conducts himself according to his own peculiar style of timidity or confidence, reticence or garrulity. His need for affiliation and his style of seeking it are both characteristics of personality, the one being more dynamic (more motivational) than the other.

At the same time, we are not all in agreement about what constitutes a motivational unit. If we were to follow Murray, McClelland or Freud, we would put on the one side only the inferred forces called needs, instinctual energies or id impulses. On the other side we would put the schemata, traits, cathexes and features of ego-structure. The implication here is that there are raw, primary, urge-like forces that alone constitute units of motivation. It is chiefly these, of course, that the projective tests seek to assess.

But, for my part, I cannot believe that motivational units are as abstract as this procedure implies. Let me illustrate my misgiving by reference to a certain man's interests. He is, let us say, profoundly interested in politics. This simple statement tells you a great deal about his motivational structure. Is it helpful, for purposes of assessment, to dissipate this integral structure in some such analysis as follows? He has an aggressive drive, a need for externalization and a modicum of father fixation—all of which are cathected on politics; he has certain cultural schemata that he has learned, and has a habit of reading the political news in the morning paper, together with a history of reinforcement so far as civic participation is concerned. Or, to make the point simpler, shall we say that his need for aggression (which some might hold to be the ultimate motivational unit in his case) is somehow arbitrarily cathected by politics? Or shall we say—I think more accurately—that his aggression and his interest are now all of a piece? His passion for politics is one true structural fact, no matter what his past behavior history may have been. You will recognize that I am here enlisting the principle of functional autonomy.

There is no need to debate this issue now. I want merely to point out that ultimate motivational units are not limited to the unconscious urges, ergs, needs or instinctual energies favored by certain forms of psychodynamic theory; nor are they accessible solely through projective techniques, even though these are certainly legitimate tools to use in a total battery of assessment methods.

Classes of Units in Current Assessment Research

Let us ask now what classes of units we find in current assessment research. No single investigator deals with them all, for each specializes in his own pet dimensions. Our question is what picture emerges if we try to catch a glimpse of all the investigators at work at once.

The preference of many investigators for multivariate scales makes difficulty at the outset for our attempt at orderly classification. A generation ago we were content with one test for ascendance-submission, a wholly separate test for extroversion-introversion, and so on. While such single scales are still with us, our hunger for omnibus instruments has grown. Take the field of neuroticism. At first (in 1917) we had the Woodworth Personal Data Sheet, which measured one and only one alleged unit: a neurotic disposition. The Cornell Index developed by Weider in 1945 still yielded a general score for the selection or rejection of armed services personnel, but at the same time differentiated various types of neurotic maladjustment. More widely used today is the MMPI [Minnesota Multiphasic Personality Inventory], with its 550 items subdivided into 26 unitary tendencies. Most of these relate to pathological trends, but one cannot say that the units sought are conceptually uniform.

Our multiphasic instruments, our many-faceted inventories, our multiple-factor devices and our miscellaneous profiles make it hard to sort out the types of units involved. The current vogue is to assess everything all at once; but in the process, the possibility of theoretical analysis seems to suffer. I wonder whether this desire is not caused in part by the fact that the Rorschach Test at first claimed to measure "the total personality." Such an intoxicating possibility led us to give up our earlier slingshot scales and adopt the shotgun inventory.

In spite of the shotgun's scatter, let us try to classify the units sought in personality assessment. Without claiming any finality for my listing, I call attention to ten classes of units that seem to me to be widely studied today:

INTELLECTUAL CAPACITIES. This area is so large in its own right that we ordinarily segregate it from both motivation and personality assessment. I mention it here only because a complete assessment could not possibly leave it out of account. Someday, I hope, we may be able to relate intellectual functioning more intimately than we now do to motivational and personal functioning.

SYNDROMES OF TEMPERAMENT. In this group we note recent progress; one thinks of the work of Sheldon, Thurstone, Cattell, Guilford and others. Thanks to their efforts, we can now assess such units as general activity, sense of well-being, restraint, emotional stability, lability and somatotonia. One could wish for a stricter limitation of the concept of temperament than some of these investigators employ, but they deal constructively with units representing the prevailing "emotional weather" in which personalities develop.

UNCONSCIOUS MOTIVES. Without doubt the greatest interest of clinical psychologists is in units of this general class. Sometimes they are called needs (though no one insists that all needs are unconscious); often they involve dimensions with a Freudian flavor, such as anxiety, aggression, oral or anal trends and Oedipal fixation. Freudian theory holds that such deep and buried motives are somehow more real and basic than units tapped by other methods. This contention, as I have already indicated, can never be proved unless both direct methods and projective methods are used for the same variables with the same personalities.

SOCIAL ATTITUDES. Here are units of quite a different order. While they have been evolved chiefly in social psychology, they are part and parcel of any complete clinical assessment program. We want to know how our subject views the church or how he regards Russia. We want to know his liberal or conservative tendencies and his score on scales for authoritarianism, ethnocentrism, dogmatism and traditional family ideology. These last-mentioned units illustrate the inevitable arbitrariness of our classification, for, while they deal with social attitudes, they pretend to disclose deeper aspects of character structure and thus overlap with our other categories.

IDEATIONAL SCHEMATA. Growing out of the study of social attitudes, we find today considerable concern with generalized thought-forms. One may cite Klein's efforts to discover general styles, or *Anschauungen*, which cut through both motivational and cognitive functions; or Kelly's proposal to study the constructs a person employs in viewing the world around him. Witkin and others establish the syndromes of "field dependence" and "field independence." [14] Though Witkin's diagnostic method is anchored in perceptual measurement, he finds that the "field dependent" person is characterized also by anxiety, fear of his impulses, poor impulse control and a general lack of awareness of his own inner life.

INTERESTS AND VALUES. In contrast to unconscious motivational units, we find many dimensions that deal with structured motives rather than with their presumed underlying dynamics. Here we would cite measures of interest in art, farming or salesmanship; or the six Spranger units, as measured by the Allport-Vernon-Lindzey *Study of Values*. Perhaps here, too, we would locate the summary measure of masculinity-femininity, based on a potpourri of conscious choices.

EXPRESSIVE TRAITS. A number of units seem to fall halfway between motivational and stylistic dimensions. For want of a better term, we may call them *expressive*. Among these we may include dominance tendencies, extroversion, persistence and empathy, as well as sociability, self-control, criticalness, accessibility and meticulous, or "just so," trends.

STYLISTIC TRAITS. This group receives least attention, probably because psychologists regard stylistic traits as lying on the surface of personality. One might include here politeness, talkativeness, consistency, hesitancy and other measurable manners of behaving. Ultimately we may expect that these stylistic characteristics will be related to deeper structural units, but they are also measurable in their own right.

PATHOLOGICAL TRENDS. Many investigators prefer to analyze motivation and personality in familiar clinical terms. Hysteric, manic, neurotic and schizoid dispositions are the sort of units we find employed in the assessments of both normal and abnormal personalities. We have spoken of the evolution of these measures from the Woodworth PD Sheet to the MMPI. One could mention as equally illustrative of this group the Humm-Wadsworth Test and other derivations from the Kraepelin and Kretschmer classifications.

FACTORIAL CLUSTERS. As yet I have not referred to factors. Factorial units in part belong in the classes we have already considered. Clearly, Thurstone's "primary mental abilities" are properly classified under intellectual capacities. Most of the factors proposed by Guilford and Zimmerman can be located under temperament syndromes or under expressive traits. Most of Cattell's factors can be similarly sorted. At the same time, many of the factors that result from summarizing mathematically the data from many tests used with many people often defy conceptual analysis in any of the preceding classes. Thus Guilford and Zimmerman report an "unidentified" factor, called C_2, which represents some baffling blend of impulsiveness, absentmindedness, emotional fluctuation, nervousness, loneliness, ease of emotional expression and feelings of guilt.[15] When units of this sort appear—and it happens not infrequently—one wonders what to say about them. To me they resemble sausage meat that has failed to pass the pure food and health inspection.

I am not saying that factorial analysis does not have its place in the search for units. It seems to me that when factor analysts start with a conceptually defined field, such as extroversion and introversion, they often succeed in improving for us the clarity and accessibility of dimensions. In other words, factors are better when they follow theory than when they create it.

Factors are simply a summary principle of classification of many measures used with (usually) many people. This property does not suddenly endow them with new power. They are not, as some enthusiasts hold, "the cause of all human conduct," nor are they "source" traits as opposed to "surface" traits, nor are they the "influence" underlying all behavior. They are neither more nor less motivational than other units. Usually they are nothing more than empirically derived descriptions of the average man.

In this respect, factors do not differ markedly from the other types of units we have described. All of them presume to offer scalable dimensions—that is to say, they are common units in respect to which all personalities can be compared. None of them corresponds to the cleavages that exist in any single personality, unless the single personal structure happens to be like that of the empirically derived average man. Still, scalable dimensions are useful dimensions, and I hope that work will continue until we reach firmer agreement concerning their number and nature.

I cannot claim that the thousands of dimensions proposed to guide our analysis of motivation and personality can all be neatly included in this tenfold scheme; but it may be helpful to our thinking.

As yet investigators have reached little or no agreement; they are not yet able to say, "These are the most useful units to employ." For the guidance of elementary students, Woodworth and Marquis, basing their classification on Cattell,[16] ventured a "List of the most clearly established primary traits": "Easy-going, intelligent, emotionally stable, dominant, placid, sensitive, trained and cultured, conscientious, adventurous, vigorous, hypersensitive, friendly." [17] But professional psychologists are not yet ready to fix upon this or any other "primary" list.

A word should be said about the intercorrelation of traits. Factor analysis in its earlier years hoped to eliminate this troublesome phenomenon by seeking factors orthogonal to one another, but even factor analysts now admit that this goal is impracticable. A certain tendency to coexist must be expected among human qualities. Of course, if correlations are very high (as they would certainly be between scales for "dominance" and "ascendance," for example, or for "depression" and "melancholy"), it would be foolish to retain separate scales for synonymous or nearly synonymous traits.

One of the most insistent intercorrelations that occur indicates a general soundness, or strength, or dependability of character structure, or the opposite syndrome. Vernon shows how this pattern—he calls it "dependability"—emerges in factorial studies.[18] The Grant Study at Harvard, working intensively with normal young men, was forced to adopt a general over-all measure of "soundness." [19] In general, it does not seem that a "halo" effect deriving from the bias of raters can account for this finding.

When such persistent intercorrelations occur between any clusters of traits, what shall we call them: types? syndromes? far-reaching dimensions? My own preference would be for *syndrome*, since the term clearly indicates coexistence among conceptually distinct variables. The term *type*, I fear, would lead us into trouble, since the term has many additional meanings.

Individual Structural Pattern

Now let us turn finally to a somewhat alarming possibility. What shall we do if the cleavages in any single life do not correspond to the empirical cleavages derived from studies of the average man? Can it be that our unending search for common units, now multiplying year by year, is a kind of nomothetic fantasy? Can it be that the structural organization of Joseph Doakes's personality is unique?

If such a possibility seems too traumatic to face, let us ask the question in a milder way. Suppose we leave our common units unmolested and apply them as seems helpful in our assessment work; what shall we do when a given case seems to be completely by-passed by the common dimensions? A. L. Baldwin, for example, discussing four nursery school children, writes that the group analysis gave reasonably accurate interpretations of the behavior of three of the four children, but the fourth was not described adequately in terms of the group factors. "Even in cases where group factors were approximately accurate, some aspects of the individual's personality were not revealed." [20]

Perhaps what we need is fewer units than we now use, but units more relevant to individual structural patterns.

To gain some preliminary insight into this matter I tried a simple pilot exercise with ninety-three students. I asked them to "think of some one individual of your own sex whom you know well," then to "describe him or her by writing in each space provided, a word, phrase, or a sentence that expresses fairly well what seems to you to be some essential characteristic of this person." The page provided eight spaces, and the students were told to "use as many spaces as you need." The term "essential characteristic" was defined as "any trait, quality, tendency, interest, etc. that you regard as of major importance to a description of the person you select."

After the student had finished with the first page, he received a second page that added two additional blank spaces for further characteristics. The question was then asked, "Do you feel the need for more than ten essential characteristics? If so, about how many more do you think you would need?" A further question asked, "Do you feel that some of the characteristics you have named are duplicates (that is, more or less synonymous), so that really fewer would have sufficed? If so, about how many in all would have been sufficient?"

Faulty though this method may be, the results are not without interest. Only 10 per cent of the subjects felt that they needed more than ten essential characteristics, and for the most part these subjects were vague regarding the total number that would be required: two said they needed an additional ten, one needed fifty, others did not know.

Ninety per cent of the students, however, found the exercise meaningful and the total of ten spaces provided fully adequate. On the average, they indicated that 7.2 essential characteristics would cover their needs, the range being from 3 to 10.

One might object that the method employed had the effect of suggesting a rather small number of essential characteristics. Perhaps this is so, though I shall in a moment cite independent supporting evidence for the proposition that a relatively small number of structural units covers the major aspects of personality.

From my point of view, the weakness of the experiment lies chiefly in the somewhat sketchy definition of "essential characteristic." Many students, though not all, were content with common trait names, such as *friendly, loyal, intelligent, dependable*. I should not expect such terms ordinarily to do justice to the peculiar coherent structure of friendliness, loyalty, intelligence or dependability that mark the life in question. Here we are confronted with the universal problem in all idiographic research: adjectives cut slices *across* people rather than *within* people. It requires more deftness with language than most of us possess to put together a phrase or sentence that will pinpoint *individual* structure. It is precisely here that the gifts of the novelist and biographer exceed those of the psychologist.

Turning for a moment to the field of biography, we find confirmation of our point in Ralph Barton Perry's definitive volumes on *The thought and character of William James*.[21] Summing up his exhaustive study of this complex and fascinating figure, Perry concludes that, in order to understand him, one must deal with eight leading "traits" or "ingredients." He first lists four "morbid" or "pathological" traits—tendencies that taken by themselves would have proved to be severe handicaps. These are hypochondria, preoccupation with "exceptional mental states," marked oscillations of mood and repugnance to the processes of exact thought. Blended with, and redeeming, these morbid trends are four "benign" traits: sensibility, vivacity, humanity and sociability. While, like the students in our exercise, Perry uses common trait names, he proceeds immediately to define them in such a way that the peculiar Jamesian flavor of each ingredient is brought to light. Clinical psychologists need some of the biographer's skill in particularizing terms. Standing alone, such terms are only hollow universals.

It seems to me that George Kelly in his *Psychology of personal constructs* is approaching the same goal from a different direction.[22] He holds that the important thing about any person is the major way in which he construes his life-experiences, including his social contacts. Hence, in order to understand a person, we should adopt what Kelly calls the "credulous approach." Through interviewing or by studying self-characterizations, perhaps with the aid of the Role Construct Repertory (REP) Test, we arrive at our diagnosis. The method yields constructs that are unique to the individual, as well as constructs he has in common with others. Further, it leads to the discovery of the unique pattern of relations among the several constructs of a given person. Speaking of widely used scaling and factoring procedures, Kelly observes that, while such methods provide a quick and sure exploitation of common constructs (applicable to all people), they prevent us from discovering new and unique constructs and fall into the additional error of assuming that the greatest commonality defines the greatest truth.

In a personal communication, Professor Kelly tells me that he is not yet prepared to say how many major constructs the average individual uses, but that sometimes an individual's responses to REP "can be condensed into one or two major dimensions with two or three rows left over as specific constructs." It is true that people with an intellectual bent often seem to produce a variety of constructs, but their large vocabulary does not entirely obscure the relative simplicity of their patterns. Kelly speaks likewise of a useful therapeutic rule of thumb: "The patient may change the topic in the middle of an interview but he rarely changes the theme." Themes are persistent and recurring. While each person may have certain specific and concrete constructs that apply to limited and special areas of experience, Kelly concludes that the clinician does not ordinarily identify more than "four of five major construct dimensions." We hope that work with the REP Test and with other quantitative clinical instruments will continue until we find a firm answer to our question.

A similar promising lead lies in the techniques of "personal cluster analysis" set forth by Alfred Baldwin.[23] Analyzing an extensive written correspondence from an elderly woman, he discovers only four or five major ideational and value-laden themes.

Another related proposal was put forward some years ago by F. H. Allport, who suggested measuring the consistency of an individual's acts in relation to his own principal life purposes or "teleonomic trends."[24] The investigator could, from previous acquaintance, hypothesize the principal themes or trends—or "constructs," or "clusters"—he expects to find in a given life. He could then by observation—with due checks for reliability—order the daily acts of the individual to these hypothesized dimensions. If we use this method systematically, we might well find, as do Perry, Kelly and Baldwin, that a handful of major structures covers the life surprisingly well, even though specific and unrelated minor trends may likewise appear.

The proverbial visitor from Mars would, I think, find it incomprehensible that so little sustained work has been done in this promising direction of individuality. He would say to the earth-bound psychologist: "Human nature on your planet is infinitely diverse. No two people are alike. While you give lip service to this proposition, you immediately discard it. What is more, people's internal structural organization—individual by individual—may be far simpler and more accessible than you think. Why not take the cleavages nature offers you and follow them through? Even granted that uniformities run through nature at its lower levels of organization (the chemical elements composing the body are identical), at the higher levels of organization where the psychologist works, the units you seek are not uniform at all. A baby, once started on the road of life, will fashion—out of his unique inheritance and special environment —nodes of accretion, foci of learning and directions of growth that become increasingly individual as the years roll along. And won't you have a good laugh at yourself when you discover this elementary fact? Then, perhaps, you'll look for your units where you ought to look for them—in each developing life."

I venture to hope we shall heed the admonition of the visitor from Mars. That we have not done so is due, of course, to the prevailing conviction that science cannot deal with individual cases at all, except as they exemplify general laws or display uniform structures. The philosophers of the Middle Ages felt the same way, their dogma being *scientia non est individuorum*. But isn't the definition of science at best an arbitrary matter—at worst, an idol of the den?

Summary

In the interest of perspective, let me summarize my principal points. The search for the units that comprise motivation and compose personality is very ancient. Not until the past generation or two has appreciable progress been made. During recent years, however, we have followed a bewildering array of approaches, many of them fresh and imaginative, and resulting in more measured aspects than anyone can conveniently compute. Broadly speaking, these uncounted thousands of nomothetic units fall into ten classes: intellectual capacities, syndromes of temperament, unconscious motives, social attitudes, ideational schemata, interests and values, expressive traits, stylistic traits, pathological trends and factorial clusters not readily classifiable in the other nine categories. Some investigators, of course, propose units that combine two or more of these classes. While I suspect there may be some overenthusiasm for certain categories (the overzealous use of projective tests for tapping unconscious motives, for example, and the over-addiction to factorial units), I would not discourage research in any of these directions.

We must accept the fact that up to now relatively little agreement has been achieved. It seems that each assessor has his own pet units and uses a pet battery of diagnostic devices. But it is too early to despair. Instead of discouragement, I hope that our present disagreement will lead to continuous and wholesome experimentation. Essential to continued progress is a firm belief in the "outer reality" of personal and motivational systems. The fact that the units we seek are invisible should not deter us. Nor should we yield to the destructive skepticism of certain extreme methodologists, who hold that the whole search is chimerical. Finally, while we must admit the variabilities of the structures we seek, which are caused by changing situations without and continual growth and change within, we should take this fact into our design and theory, and not surrender our belief that reasonably stable personal and motivational structures exist.

Such, in brief, is the present state of affairs with nomothetic assessment, as I see it. But I have argued, in addition, that we will do well to turn to the fresher possibilities that lie in improved idiographic analysis. Nor should we be deterred by preconceived ideas about what science can and cannot with propriety do. The conquerors of Mt. Everest did not allow themselves to be blocked by the sacred cows they encountered in the streets of Darjeeling. Nor should we. But perhaps the goal ahead is not so formidable as Mt. Everest. It may turn out to be only as high and as wide and as human as the personality of John Citizen, who is, after all, our old and familiar friend.

REFERENCES

1. See C. Sherrington, *Man on his nature,* 2nd ed., New York: Doubleday Anchor, 1953, Chap. 1.

2. See G. W. Allport, *Personality: a psychological interpretation,* New York: Holt, 1937, Chap. 3.

3. L. L. Bernard, *Instinct: a study in social psychology,* New York: Holt, 1924, p. 220.

4. D. O. Hebb, *The organization of behavior,* New York: Wiley, 1949.

5. *Amer. Psychol.*, 1957, 12:51.

6. K. MacCorquodale and P. E. Meehl, "On a distinction between hypothetical constructs and intervening variables," *Psychol. Rev.*, 1948, 55:95-107.

7. See R. Tagiuri and L. Petrullo (eds.), *Person perception and interpersonal behavior*, Palo Alto: Stanford University Press, 1958.

8. W. James, *Psychology: briefer course*, New York: Holt, 1910, p. 179.

9. W. Coutu, *Emergent human nature*, New York: Knopf, 1949.

10. See Chapter 6 of the present volume.

11. A. S. Tannenbaum and F. H. Allport, "Personality structure and group structure: an interpretative study of their relationship through an event-structure hypothesis," *J. Abnorm. Soc. Psychol.*, 1956, 53:272-80.

12. H. A. Murray, et al., *Explorations in personality*, New York: Oxford University Press, 1938.

13. D. C. McClelland, *Personality*, New York: Dryden, 1951. See also his "Personality: an integrative view," in J. L. McCary (ed.), *Psychology of personality*, New York: Logos, 1956.

14. H. A. Witkin, H. B. Lewis, M. Hertzman, K. Machover, P. Meissner and S. Wapner, *Personality through perception*, New York: Harper, 1954.

15. J. P. Guilford and W. S. Zimmerman, "Fourteen dimensions of temperament," *Psychol. Monogr.*, 1956, No. 417.

16. R. B. Cattell, *Description and measurement of personality*, Yonkers, N.Y.: World Book, 1946.

17. R. S. Woodworth and D. G. Marquis, *Psychology*, New York: Holt, 1947.

18. P. E. Vernon, *Personality tests and assessments*, London: Methuen, 1953.

19. C. W. Heath, *What people are*, Cambridge: Harvard University Press, 1945.

20. A. L. Baldwin, "The study of individual personality by means of the intraindividual correlation," *J. Pers.*, 1946, 14:168.

21. R. B. Perry, *The thought and character of William James*, Boston: Little, Brown, 1936, Vol. II, Chaps. 90-91.

22. G. A. Kelly, *The psychology of personal constructs*, New York: Norton, 1955, I, 34.

23. A. L. Baldwin, "Personal structure analysis: a statistical method for investigating the single personality," *J. Abnorm. Soc. Psychol.*, 1942, 37:163-83.

24. F. H. Allport, "Teleonomic description in the study of personality," *Char. & Pers.*, 1937, 6:202-14.

CHAPTER 8

What is a trait of personality?

This is an early essay. It is included because it represents probably the first attempt to formulate what has come to be called "trait theory." The issues it raises are still basic to the psychology of personality.

Traits, though they may be called by various names, seem to be the "hypothetical constructs"—that is, the inescapable assumptions—in every theory that seeks to depict high-level integration of personality.

The essay was read at the Ninth International Congress of Psychology, held in New Haven in 1929, and published in the *Journal of Abnormal and Social Psychology* (1931). Later developments of trait theory will be found in *Personality: a psychological interpretation* (1937), as well as in various chapters of the present volume.

At the heart of all investigation of personality lies the puzzling problem of the nature of the unit or element that is the carrier of the distinctive behavior of a man. *Reflexes* and *habits* are too specific in reference and connote constancy rather than consistency in behavior. *Attitudes* are ill-defined and, as employed by various writers, refer to determining tendencies that range in inclusiveness from the *Aufgabe* to the *Weltanschauung*. *Dispositions* and *tendencies* are even less definitive. But *traits*, although appropriated by all manner of writers for all manner of purposes, may still be salvaged, I think, and may be limited in their reference to a certain definite conception of a generalized response-unit in which resides the distinctive quality of behavior that reflects personality. Foes as well as friends of the doctrine of traits will gain from a more consistent use of the term.

The doctrine itself has never been explicitly stated. It is my purpose, with the aid of eight criteria, to define *trait* and to state the logic and some of the evidence for the admission of this concept to good standing in psychology.

1. *A trait has more than nominal existence.* A trait may be said to have the same kind of existence that a habit of a complex order has. Habits of a complex, or higher, order have long been accepted as household facts in psychology. There is no reason to believe that the mechanism that produces such a habit (integration, *Gestaltung*

or whatever it may be) stops short of producing the more generalized habits which are here called traits of personality.

2. *A trait is more generalized than a habit.* Within a personality there are, of course, many independent habits; but there is also so much integration, organization and coherence among habits that we have no choice but to recognize great systems of interdependent habits. If the habit of brushing one's teeth can be shown, statistically or genetically, to be unrelated to the habit of dominating a tradesman, there can be no question of a common trait involving both these habits; but, if the habit of dominating a tradesman can be shown, statistically or genetically, to be related to the habit of bluffing one's way past guards, there is the presumption that a common trait of personality exists that includes these two habits. Traits may conceivably embrace anywhere from two habits to a legion of habits. In this way, there may be said to be both major, widely extensified traits and minor, less generalized traits in the same personality.

3. *A trait is dynamic, or at least determinative.* The stimulus is not the crucial determinant in behavior that expresses personality; the trait itself is decisive. Once formed, a trait seems to have the capacity of directing responses to stimuli into characteristic channels. This emphasis upon the dynamic nature of traits, ascribing to them a capacity for guiding the specific response, is variously recognized by many writers. The principle is nothing more than that which has been subscribed to in various connections by Woodworth, Prince, Sherrington, Coghill, Kurt Lewin, Troland, Lloyd Morgan, Thurstone, Bentley, Stern and others.

From this general point of view, traits might be called "derived drives" or "derived motives." Whatever they are called, they may be regarded as playing a motivating role in each act, thus endowing the separate adjustments of the individual to specific stimuli with that *adverbial* quality that is the very essence of personality.

Some psychologists may balk at the doctrine of the absorption of driving power into the integrated mechanism of traits. If so, it is equally possible, without violence to the other criteria of this essay, to accept the view that a trait is a generalized neural set, which is activated ecphorically or redintegratively. But it seems to me that this second doctrine is only slightly less dynamic than the first. The difference is simply one between trait considered as a drive aroused through the operation of a specific stimulus, and trait conceived as powerfully directive when an effective stimulus arouses the organism to action.

4. The existence of a trait may be established empirically or statistically. In order to know that a person has a habit, it is necessary to have evidence of repeated reactions of a constant type. Similarly, in order to know that an individual has a trait, it is necessary to have evidence of repeated reactions that, though not necessarily constant in type, seem none the less to be consistently a function of the same underlying determinant. If this evidence is gathered casually by mere observation of the subject or through the reading of a case-history or biography, it may be called empirical evidence.

More exactly, of course, the existence of a trait may be established with the aid of statistical techniques that determine the degree of coherence among the separate responses. Although this employment of statistical aid is highly desirable, it is not necessary to wait for such evidence before speaking of traits, any more than it would be necessary to refrain from speaking of the habit of biting finger-nails until the exact frequency of the occurrence is known. Statistical methods are at present better suited to intellective than to conative functions, and it is with the latter that we are chiefly concerned in our studies of personality.

5. Traits are only relatively independent of each other. The investigator desires, of course, to discover what the fundamental traits of personality are—that is to say, what broad trends in behavior do exist independently of one another. Actually, with the test methods and correlational procedures in use, completely independent variation is seldom found. In one study, expansion correlated with extroversion to the extent of +.39; ascendance with conservatism, +.22; humor with insight, +.83; and so on. This overlap may be due to several factors, the most obvious being the tendency of the organism to react in an integrated fashion: when concrete acts are observed or tested, they reflect not only the trait under examination but also, and simultaneously, other traits. Several traits may thus converge into a final common path. It seems safe, therefore, to predict that traits can never be completely isolated for study, since they never show more than a relative independence of one another.

In the instance just cited, it is doubtful whether humor and insight (provided their close relationship is verified in subsequent studies) represent distinct traits. In the future, it may be possible to agree upon a certain magnitude of correlation, below which it will be acceptable to speak of separate traits, and above which only one trait will be recognized. If only one trait is indicated, it will presumably represent a broadly generalized disposition. For example, if humor and insight cannot be established as independent traits, it will be necessary to recognize a more inclusive trait and name it, perhaps, "sense of proportion."

6. *A trait of personality, psychologically considered, is not the same as moral quality.* A trait of personality may or may not coincide with some well-defined, conventional social concept. Extroversion, ascendance, social participation and insight are free from preconceived moral significance, largely because each is a word newly coined or adapted to fit a psychological discovery. It would be ideal if we could, in this way, find our traits first and then name them. But honesty, loyalty, neatness and tact, though encrusted with social significance, *may* likewise represent true traits of personality. The danger is that, in devising scales for their measurement, we may be bound by the conventional meanings and thus be led away from the precise integration as it exists in a given individual. Where possible, it would be well for us to find our traits first and then seek devaluated terms with which to characterize our discoveries.

7. *Acts, and even habits, that are inconsistent with a trait are not proof of the nonexistence of the trait.* The objection most often considered fatal to the doctrine of traits has been illustrated as follows: "An individual may be habitually neat with respect to his person and characteristically slovenly in his handwriting or the care of his desk."

In the first place, this observation fails to state that there are cases frequently met where a constant level of neatness is maintained in all of a person's acts, giving unmistakable empirical evidence that the trait of neatness is, in some people at least, thoroughly and permanently integrated. Not everyone will show the same degree of integration in respect to a given trait. What is a major trait in one personality may be a minor trait, or even nonexistent, in another personality.

In the second place, there may be opposed integrations—that is, contradictory traits—in a single personality. The same individual may have traits *both* of neatness *and* of carelessness, of ascendance *and* of submission, although these will frequently be of unequal strength.

In the third place, there are in every personality instances of acts that are unrelated to existent traits, the product of the stimulus and the attitude of the moment. Even the characteristically neat person may become careless when he is hurrying to catch a train. But to say that not all of a person's acts reflect some higher integration is not to say that no such higher integrations exist.

8. *A trait may be viewed either in the light of the personality that contains it or in the light of its distribution in the population at large.* Each trait has both its unique and its universal aspect. In its unique aspect, the trait takes its significance entirely from the role it plays in the personality as a whole. In its universal aspect, the trait is arbitrarily isolated for study, and a comparison is made between individuals in respect to it. From this second point of view, traits merely extend the familiar field of the psychology of individual differences.

Geneticism *versus* ego-structure

This essay brings together trait theory and motivation theory. It argues that acquired traits may become the primary motivational units in a life. The ego, thus constituted, develops a "go" of its own.

The essay (here condensed) appeared in a symposium published in the *British Journal of Psychology* (1946). It is in part a reply to Cyril Burt, who in the same *Journal* had criticized my position and defended instincts as the permanent motivational units in human personality.

Broadly speaking, British psychologists have been more partial than American psychologists to doctrines of instinct. And so, in a sense, this essay is an argumentative epistle to colleagues across the sea.

There are two ways of looking at motivation. *Geneticism* stresses the importance either of what is "given" in human nature or of early learned formations. Instinct theory, orthodox Freudianism, stimulus-response psychology are all of this type. For several decades this psychological orientation has prevailed.

The alternative view, defended in this essay, calls for emphasis on *ego-structure*.

Geneticism regards a man's motives, say, at the age of fifty, as elaborated, conditioned, sublimated or otherwise modified editions of a primary material. This material may be labeled instincts, or drives, or id (whose structure, Freud says, "never changes"). Geneticism says, in effect, that the passionate devotion of a pianist to his instrument is an elaboration of his original grasp reflex—plus, perhaps, a continuing, instinctive need for mastery.

Granted that there is a continuous evolution of manual dexterity from the digital grasp to fluent technique, one may well doubt that the energy sustaining the present musical passion has any relation to the aboriginal energy of the grasp or to the clamor of the infant for self-assertion. The subforms of the present pattern formerly served one function in the life; but the contemporary disciplined passion for music serves a wholly different function. *Historical continuity does not mean functional continuity*.

It is encouraging to note that the anachronistic fallacy in motivation theory is not now as dominant as it used to be. The past has begun to lose its appeal to many theorists and the present correspondingly to gain. Gestalt psychology illustrates the trend. To advocate "insight" and "belongingness" is to advocate current, and even momentary, dynamisms. The discovery of the motivational character of persistence in interrupted tasks, and of other closure-activities, has led to an emphasis upon the immediate situation. The field-theory of Lewin, with its topological representation, makes it almost impossible to include genetic factors in the representation of field forces. Again, a rebirth of introspective studies brought in the "feel" of motives as parts of the self. Koffka began to speak of the ego as a region of the personality having to do with states of tension and self-reference, which are so characteristic of motivated behavior.[1] Virtually nothing in the writings of Köhler, Koffka, Lewin and others of the Gestalt persuasion suggests that what we do today is a necessary product of unchanging id, eternal instincts or early conditioning. Belongingness, the field, the ego and closure are the characteristic motivational concepts.

Furthermore, a shift has definitely occurred in psychoanalysis. Currently, psychoanalysts are inclined to ascribe much more *momentum* to the ego than did Freud. I have commented elsewhere on this development.[2] Here I will only illustrate it by a quotation from Heinz Hartmann: ". . . Adaptation to reality—which includes mastery of it—proceeds to a large extent from the ego and in particular from that part of the ego which is free from conflict; and it is directed by the organised structure of ego-functions (such as intelligence, perception, etc.) which exist in their own right and have an independent effect upon the solution of conflicts."[3]

Outside psychoanalytic circles, the powerful therapeutic movement called non-directive therapy is gaining ground with a distinctly anti-genetic platform. The patient is allowed to re-structure and re-plan his life with as little or as much reference to past motives and influences as he himself feels to be relevant. It turns out that he, unlike the geneticist, is normally interested more in the future than in the past. Indeed, if we pause to think about it, any personal problem has an *effective* relation only to one's future, since it is in the future that all problems must be solved. The ego, in taking command, projects itself forward into the future and recasts its motives largely in terms of intentions and plans.

Ego-structure

Few writers on war neuroses or morale have been able to avoid using the concept of the ego. Writings dealing with theory, like those dealing with therapy, have reintroduced the very term that long ago fell into disuse. Over and over we have read of the "firm ego-structure" and the "weak ego-structure." The former, it is often said, resists fear, whether immediate or repressed; the latter succumbs to the traumatic conditions of battle.[4] Prisoners best able to resist the tortures of a concentration camp are those who have firm purposes and strong political convictions.[5]

One may ask, "Did not Freud acknowledge ego-strength in the ability of a patient to hold his impulses in check and to steer a safe course between the tyrannies of the id, the superego and the harsh environment?" He did, but he also claimed that the ego has no energy of its own. It is passive; it is the mere rider on the horse.

War studies show indisputably, I think, that, far from being a passive agent, the ego is a dynamic process of great positive power. What but a motivational structure of immense momentum could handle the fatigue, fear, anger, apathies, disgust and conflicts aroused by wartime conditions? Morale ascribed to ego-strength is not passive; it is a matter of powerful, dominant interests, capable of promoting activity so vital that lesser, segmental, impulsive activities are inhibited effectively and without serious repression.

A few passages from one of the books on psychiatric combat casualties indicate that the primary purpose of treatment is to restore normal ego-strength (that is, normal and current interests and motives) in order to offset the ravages of segmental and impulsive fears and conflicts. "As the ego becomes stronger, the therapist demands increasing independence and activity from the patient."[6]

A soldier—or civilian—is abnormal if he cannot proceed according to the lights of his ordinary, daily motivation. Horribly shocked, he becomes fearful, uncontrollably hostile or apathetic. In any case, he finds that he cannot absorb and handle the traumatic conditions. The provocation is great: "It is difficult to describe the intensity of these hostile feelings before which the ego recoils and withdraws."[7] Yet, normally, even these incredibly severe strains are handled adequately by an ego that is so firmly attached to its present projects that it refuses to regress or to split. And, even when the break comes, the physician knows there is a *norm* for each person to which he must be helped to return. After treatment, the physician writes with gratification: "The ego now seemed in full control."[8]

It is an interesting discovery that, unless the ego resumes control soon, there is special danger of malignant repression, chronicity and rigidity. In terms of theory, this finding seems to mean that the ordinary pattern of interests that comprise morale normally balances the life but that, if denied dominance for too long a time, it may yield permanently to regressive mechanisms. Hence, it was up to the war psychiatrist to "put pressure on the ego" to make it assume control as soon as possible.[9]

Is this ego-structure, which is emphasised so much during wartime, a mere matter of instincts, or of early training, or of constitutional make-up? That it may be historically conditioned by these factors no one can deny, but is it historic in essence? We have no data to show, for example, whether an optimum degree of security in early life correlates with ego-strength. We do know that wartime writers have emphasized, rather, the role of group-identification and of ideological conviction. Both make for resistance to combat neurosis. Both reflect the high importance of *contemporary* loyalty. The man who wants *now* to stand with his outfit, to support his commander, to win a victory for democracy, is the man who stands the strain. Even if it turns out that this man was also characteristically breast fed, secure within the family, father-identified or mesomorphic, the psychiatrist finds that ordinarily he cannot appeal to, or employ, these factors. He invokes only the most recent, adult, motivational structure. Childhood security may or may not be a factor in resistance to breakdowns (I suspect the correlation is low), but ideological strength and loyalty are factors of proven importance. "If the soldier could feel that the pain, the sacrifices, and death were dedicated to a larger purpose with which he was identified, his capacity to ward off anxiety would thereby increase." [10]

Functional Autonomy

Functional autonomy is merely a shorthand phrase designed to call attention to some of the considerations I have just reviewed. It marks a shift of emphasis in the theory of motivation from geneticism in its various forms to the present "go" of interests that contemporaneously initiate and sustain behavior.

It is not necessary for me to repeat the lines of evidence I have adduced.[11] They include such diverse considerations as the high correlation between skills and interests; conative perseveration, or the haunting urgency with which tasks accepted by the individual are held in mind until completed; and the obvious dynamism of sentiments which are so individual in character that they bear no ascertainable resemblance to underlying instincts. Patriotism, stamp collecting, religion are themselves the needs of a given person—often his *ultimate* needs.

In my earlier exposition, however, there was one defect, which I have tried subsequently to remedy.[12] My picture of derived motives led some readers to accuse me of allowing for a complete anarchy among motives. A motive (I seemed to be saying) might evolve, severing itself from its root-forms, and lead a wholly independent existence, devoid not only of historical ties but also of relationship to anything else in the personality. Such a loose conception is, of course, untenable. Though motives may often be (and, I argue, usually are) independent of their origins, they are obviously not independent of the contemporary ego-structure in which they are now embedded.

Let us take an example. During World War II, a fairly large number of illiterates turned up in the American draft. The men, Negro and white, were sent to special training centers where, with the aid of ingenious methods of instruction, most of them acquired within eight weeks a degree of literacy equal to that of four years of schooling.[13] They were highly motivated to learn, the chief incentives being to correspond by post with the folks at home; to avoid the shame of using an X in place of a signature when others were watching (as in signing the payroll); and to do what was expected of them. When these men left the special training unit, and especially after they were discharged from the army and returned home, these three incentives were completely eliminated. Yet many of the men, perhaps most, had acquired an interest in reading. The interest was a product of the three motives; but, since all three became demonstrably inactive, its subsequent existence must have been autonomous of these origins. The interest in reading, we conclude, brought them *new* sources of satisfaction. It played a revised role in the economy of their lives. Not only is the ego-structure somehow served by this new skill and interest; the skill and interest are now a *part* of the ego-structure itself. Literate interests now help to *constitute* the personality.

To say that some instinct must be sustaining the new literate interests is to invoke a remote abstraction. Even McDougall, I suspect, would grant that the interest in this case is merely an aspect of the generalized sentiment of self-regard. If so, his statement of the matter would be close to my assertion that the new interest now finds itself part of the essential economy of the ego. With the sentiment of self-regard, the doctrine of functional autonomy has much in common. The chief difference is that the latter sees no necessity for invoking the energies of underlying, hypothetical instincts. An ego-structure (sentiment of self-regard) is quite sufficient to keep an individual on the move. It seems to me unnecessary to seek its dynamics, as McDougall does, in the twin and abstract propensities of self-assertion and submission.[14]

Mr. Burt's Criticisms

Cyril Burt, who has criticized the theory of functional autonomy on several counts, is no doubt still unpersuaded. I hope, however, that he may find my relating of functional autonomy to ego-structure somewhat more to his liking than the earlier version of the theory he has criticized. In any case, his objections are all closely reasoned and well taken.

First: Mr. Burt starts with the evolutionary argument. "When the ape evolved into man, what freak of innumerable mutations obliterated all traces of the instinctive mechanisms, handed down throughout the ages through all our mammalian ancestors? Surely the 'higher brain centres' have been merely 'superposed' upon the lower, not suddenly inserted into their place."[15]

Phylogenetic continuity, I grant, may not be denied. The appetites of men and animals are much alike and rest on identifiable mechanisms that are closely similar. Yet these drives and these mechanisms comprise only a fraction of the vast motivational structure of human beings. Do we not know that the "superposed" higher brain centers in many ways regulate and dominate the lower? Since this is so, we have a right to expect a shift in emphasis and dominance of mechanisms, as well as phylogenetic continuity.

Second: he argues that drives are, after all, instincts and that once this is admitted, the argument is surrendered to the instinctivist. Here a serious misunderstanding exists.

Drives are primarily viscerogenic states of excess or deficit stimulation—what Woodworth calls conditions of "tissue change." Besides the obvious pressures that arise in body cavities, blood stream and autonomic organs, we may include among drives the irritation of proprioceptors and sensitivity (with a customarily adient response) to external stimulation. This equipment and the attendant initial responses, let us concede, are innate, unlearned, universal. They account for the "absolutely dependable motives" that Klineberg finds to be the possession of every individual in every culture. What is more, their physiological foundations are clearly identifiable.[16]

If instincts are defined in this way, then, of course, instincts exist. But the doctrine of instinct generally smacks more of the pull and less of the push. It stresses the innateness of the *purpose;* and most lists of instincts exceed by far the range of physiologically grounded drives or "absolutely dependable motives" that can be universally established.

Though drives are instinctive, they don't carry us far with our theory of motivation. They account well enough for the maintenance of physiological equilibrium and for initial and vague contacts with the environment. They furnish a fairly adequate picture of *infant* motivation, but a poor picture of adult motivation. Lust and the "activity drive," even hunger and elimination, are so regulated by acquired habits and sentiments that they do not for long operate as simon-pure drives but soon take their place as dynamisms in the ego-structure. The drive-force becomes fused with, and modified by, psychogenic accretions. Tastes often become inseparable from the drives.

Mr. Burt dislikes this view. He fears, to take the example of hunger, that we should "have to abandon any notion that there might be a biological purpose in eating, because there must be as many purposes in eating as there are types of objects to eat." [17] But I see no real difficulty here. We can take the purpose of eating at its face value and acknowledge that hunger and other "absolutely dependable" drives have a uniform significance for all creatures, without denying the obvious fact that differing tastes, modes and manners do affect the operation of the drive and form (from the individual's point of view) a highly integral part of the total motive.

To admit drives in the sense here defined is not to open the door to such alleged instincts as acquisitiveness, gregariousness, appeal, parental behavior, submission or self-assertion. These concepts are not in the least comparable with drives, but are abstractions from learned human behavior and ascribed without evidence to the primordial horme.

Third: my critic wonders, naturally enough, why some acquired patterns of activity and interest become autonomous and others not. Since he doubts that a satisfactory answer is forthcoming, he suggests that any adult interest is, after all, secretly fed by the springs of some instinct or other. He believes that the concept of "instinctive reinforcement" is more helpful to the teacher or therapist than the theory of "functional autonomy," for in the former case one invokes deeper dynamisms and escapes the perils of rationalization.[18]

In attempting to answer the question why some acquired motivational patterns become autonomous and others do not, I shall have to invoke the concept of ego-structure. To take an example, one individual finds that the cause of the labor movement, let us say, becomes his passion. Everything connected with the rights of the workingman takes on an urgency. Another individual, with perhaps similar upbringing, remains cool and indifferent to the issue. My first comment on this puzzling problem is that *all* theories of motivation fail to provide a full solution. Instinctive reinforcement applied to the riddle is certainly vague. Even assuming that in one case a bit of the parental instinct is inolved and in the other case not, the question of *why* this selectivity exists between two individuals remains unanswered. The conditioned reflex theory likewise finds no solution, at least so far as the *present* absorbing role of the interest in the personality is concerned. Freud might invoke in the case of the labor enthusiast a hypothetical reaction-formation—say, a repressed hatred of the father—but he would have difficulty in either proving his point or changing the man's interest when this alleged reinforcement is uncovered.

From the point of view of functional autonomy, I would approach the problem by saying that this mature interest, like all others, is now a part of the individual's style of life; it *is* his present ego-structure. It brings satisfactions, not to this or that instinct, but to his total blended system of current sentiments, aspirations and intentions. It is not a channeling of the parental instinct, nor is it sublimated aggression (at least, not necessarily). It is *he*. There are, of course, genetic reasons why he evolved this particular zeal; but now the ego-structure, in its present economy, consists of a blending of this powerful motive with many others not sharply separated from it. Taken together they comprise the congruent pattern of the current ego-structure in which all dynamism resides.

Fourth: Mr. Burt worries lest, by taking motives at their face value, I open the door to all the misleading rationalizations of which every skilled psychologist is properly wary. Yes, there may be such a danger. We cannot always believe an individual's account of his own motives, for people have differing degrees of insight into their own ego-structures. What is more, in many cases there *are* infantile reasons for a current intense or obsessive interest. Undoubtedly *some* labor fanatics are merely expressing a neurosis. But without careful diagnosis we cannot tell, and there is certainly no reason to assume that *every* current interest is merely a mask for hidden instincts or early repressions.

I am inclined to believe that Mr. Burt will agree with me on this point, for he too seems impatient with the archaisms of psychoanalysis and with the everlasting recounting of stories of early life to the exclusion of a current, cross-sectional analysis of motives.[19]

Mr. Burt, I believe, is on solid ground when he says that, in individuals who have partly regressed or never risen above infantile level, one may look for the dominance of repressed innate tendencies. Whatever these genetic tendencies are, it is chiefly in neurotic or infantile personalities that they hold sway.[20] Normal people are not prisoners of the past. I would applaud Mr. Burt's concluding statement in the symposium, "Is the Doctrine of Instincts Dead?": "In studying the more normal adult the assessment of acquired interests, motives, and ideals may be far more important; here indeed, lies a field of research which, as is generally conceded, has been sadly neglected hitherto." [21]

Fifth: Mr. Burt wonders why habits-on-the-make should show so much functional autonomy, and why habits already formed recede in motivational force. He would think that the opposite condition ought to prevail.[22] My answer is that in learning a habit (driving a car, for example) the individual is distinctly *ego-involved*. He has accepted the task, and its accomplishment is important to his self-esteem. While this condition lasts, there is a peculiar urgency about acquiring the skill. When the skill is once acquired, it is relegated to the level of instrumentality and is called upon in the service of some more ego-involved motive.

Finally: Mr. Burt's sharpest shafts, like those of other critics, are reserved for my contention that an unavoidable corollary of the doctrine of functional autonomy is the resulting uniqueness of mature patterns of motives. Since this is a question of some moment, I shall devote the following section to it.

The Uniqueness of Personality

Mr. Maberly has presented persuasively the clinical point of view. He stressed the importance of evaluating any bit of behavior in the light of the individual's total motivational pattern as it exists at any given moment. Anyone who deals with personality in the concrete is likely to agree cordially with Mr. Maberly's emphasis. Mr. Burt apparently agrees with it, for he too writes of the need for obtaining a synoptic view of the individual with the aid of "imaginative insight." Yet, at the same time, Mr. Burt seems to land himself in something of a contradiction, for he affirms that it is the bounden duty of the scientist to occupy himself with *universals*, even in dealing with personality.

Let us look first at Mr. Burt's definition of personality, which I find to be excellent. For him, personality is the "entire system of relatively permanent tendencies, both physical and mental, that are distinctive of a given individual, and determine his characteristic adjustments to his material and social surroundings." [23]

Words like *distinctive* and *characteristic* should make Mr. Burt very chary of exalting universals to the extent that he does. He would have us study also the ego-sentiment, including the ego-ideal—which, he admits, is a qualitative matter and can best be "stated primarily in words." But all this evidence of Mr. Burt's sensitivity to the never-repeated patterns of personality does not quite fit with his scientific conscience, as expressed in his plans for the assessment of personality. He wants to find a small number of independent factors similar to "key-elements in chemistry." He favors the factorial approach. I doubt that he can easily reconcile this methodological preference with his own definition of personality.

Mr. Burt presents the dilemma, and his preference, in the following analogy: "Every man's face is absolutely unique; yet should we argue that the 'common' features—the eyes, the nose, the mouth—are not 'true' features at all? We may agree that a list of facial measurements would be no substitute for a photographic reproduction of an individual face in all its concrete completeness. But equally a set of portraits, however life-like, could not by themselves suffice for scientific purposes." [24]

It is true that every man has a nose, two eyes, a mouth and a chin, and that these are common and measurable features. It is also true that no method of measuring emotional expression of the face has been evolved, let alone the permanent configuration or set that *is* the person's face.

Yet, Mr. Burt insists, "psychology, as a science, deals with universals, not with particulars." I am tempted to reply—tartly, perhaps, but also justly—that as long as psychology deals only with universals and not with particulars, it won't deal with much, least of all human personality. His definition of psychology as science is far more rigid and narrow than his definition of personality. The consequence can only be that psychology as science is frankly and woefully inadequate to deal with personality, its natural subject matter. I wonder whether Mr. Burt really wants to accept this conclusion, to which he has inevitably committed himself.

Psychology, it seems to me, must be equipped to deal with the *whole* of personality, defined as Mr. Burt has defined it. What is "distinctive," what is "characteristic" must be included. The doctrine of functional autonomy helps to express the uniqueness of motives that confer distinctiveness to a person's characteristic adjustments.

Our difficulty here lies in the cultish conception of science, which bedevils most of us simply because of the incalculable prestige of those disciplines that have dealt so successfully with *inanimate* nature. If we no longer rivet our attention to their methods—so well adapted to their subject matter, but not to ours—and if we ask what the *aims* of science are, the dilemma can be resolved. Science aims to achieve powers of understanding, prediction and control above the level of unaided common sense. From this point of view it becomes apparent that only by taking adequate account of the individual's total pattern of life can we achieve the *aims* of science. Knowledge of general laws —including, let me repeat, the law of functional autonomy—quantitative assessments and correlational procedures are all helpful; but with this conceptual (nomothetic) knowledge must be blended a shrewd diagnosis of trends within an individual, an ability to transcend the isolated common variables obtained from current measuring devices and to estimate the ego-structure of the individual. Unless such idiographic (particular) knowledge is fused with nomothetic (universal) knowledge, we shall not achieve the *aims* of science, however closely we imitate the methods of the natural and mathematical sciences.[25]

Mr. Burt has earlier given a conspectus of methods and principles involved in assessing personality. The test-situations he has employed in his own original investigations are lifelike and situational. He believes that the proper manner of treating the data obtained is by correlational techniques. He advocates the use of variables that have been established by previous correlational studies, such as: a general factor of emotionality; certain bipolar dimensions, including introversion, cheerfulness, social responsiveness and their opposites; special factors or needs resembling McDougall's catalogue of instincts; and a measure of integration or consistency in the individual's life. He would then add (in order to repair the ravages of analysis) a "synoptic character sketch," which "calls quite as much for the imaginative insight of the artist as for the tabulated measurement of the scientist." [26]

I deplore his sharp separation of the "insights of the artist" and the "measurements of the scientist." Cannot a psychology of personality in the future do a better job of understanding, prediction and control by fusing these two modes of knowledge? Mr. Burt comes close to doing so himself in his matching studies. He demonstrates, as other studies have done, that the more information derived from many sources goes into a sketch, the more easily is it matched with a criterion. It is not, however, the mere array of psychometric scores that males matching successful; it is, rather, the *patterning* of the variables that turns the trick.[27] In short, successful scientific prediction requires knowledge of the essential relations that comprise the unique ego-structure of the individual.

But how, concretely, shall we overcome the opposition between "science" and "art," and bring them into a single psychological discipline? Though the question cannot be answered fully for many, many years, I offer one illustration. Mr. Burt seeks a few "key-qualities." He thinks their discovery will enhance our powers of predicting an individual's behavior. So do I. But the key-qualities we seek must, I submit, be *personal,* not universal. Each life seems to have a limited number of themes, a handful of ascertainable values and directions—true key-qualities. In finding them, there is an opportunity for analysis and even quantification (on a strictly intra-individual level); it is not merely by "imaginative insight" that we make our study of unique and individual traits. Life-history techniques, matching, personal structure analysis (that is, the search for personal but not universal factors) and other methods are already available; others will be invented.

Exclusive reliance on factorial dimensions is not acceptable, for two reasons. *First:* the resulting factors are completely limited by the specific kinds of tests that happened to be thrown into the matrix. One cannot draw out more than one puts in. *Second:* the resulting factors are a peculiar hash of the personalities of all participants and do not necessarily represent the living ego-structure of any single participant.

In making these criticisms, I am not repudiating the use of nomothetic factors, nor of test-scales, ratings and dimensions. More of my own research and writing has been devoted to this type of approach to personality than to any other. The resulting "common traits," I find, have utility for *comparative* purposes, for approximations to the modes of adjustment that similarly constituted individuals in similarly constituted societies can be expected to acquire, and for the training of the young psychologists in respect to a common language and in the use of analytical procedures. What I argue is that, as psychologists, we must include many other procedures in our store of tools. We must acknowledge the roughness and inadequacy of our universal dimensions. Thereby shall we enhance our own ability to understand, predict and control. By learning to handle the individuality of motives and the uniqueness of personality, we shall become better scientists, not worse.

Summary

Various forms of geneticism have long dominated theories of personality. There has been an overemphasis on constitutionalism, instincts, an unchanging id and childhood habits. But, especially under the impact of the war, a desirable shift of emphasis to the contemporary motivational structure of the ego has now occurred. One theory, in line with this modern trend of emphasis, is the doctrine of functional autonomy, which holds that, while the transformation of motives from infancy onward is gradual, it is none the less genuine. Just as we learn new skills, so also we learn new motives.

A consequence of this view, disturbing to those who define science rigidly as the study of universals, is that the motivational structure of adult lives is essentially unique. Egos have infinite variety. Methods are now developing that will enable psychology to catch up with and deal more adequately with this unassailable fact. The bifurcation of scientific and clinical psychology is false and undesirable, as is an oversharp distinction between the methods of science and the methods of art.

Since Mr. Burt's views on personality are well known, I have stated my own in comparison with his. As I see it, in many respects our views are substantially identical. My definition of personality agrees with his. Together we repudiate the theory that "concatenated reflexes" constitute personality. We both wish to study the total person, and we both regard the rubrics of abnormal psychology as inadequate to the task. We agree that goal-striving is the essence of personality and that assessment is practicable and desirable. In other respects we likewise see eye to eye.

There are two chief differences. *First:* in my opinion, personality is a post-instinctive phenomenon, and reliance upon McDougallian instincts leads us into an anachronistic conception of adult motivation. Though viscerogenic drives exist throughout life (usually in an overlaid fashion), the postulation of other instincts not only seems unnecessary but fits badly with the known facts concerning the contemporaneity and individuality of the ego-structure.

Second: it seems to me improbable that a small number of uniform factors like "key-elements in chemistry" will account for the infinite variety of normal adult motivational patterns. I see more hope in the endeavor to find unique key factors (central traits) that animate an individual life. Common (that is, comparable) traits, whether called factors, dimensions or what not, have a certain utility; but they are at best rough approximations of what goes on in a given life and must be used guardedly.

Mr. Burt holds that the "scientific" study of personality demands the use of common variables exclusively. I argue that it is possible, by broadening our theory and our procedures, to avoid the sharp bifurcation of scientific and clinical psychology. Though less developed at the present time, idiographic methods of study are basically more important—and are no less "scientific"—than nomothetic methods.

REFERENCES

1. K. Koffka, *Principles of Gestalt psychology*, New York: Harcourt, Brace, 1935.

2. See Chapter 5 of the present volume.

3. H. Hartmann, "Ich-psychologie und Anpassungsproblem," *Int. J. Psycho-Anal.*, 1940, 21:214-16.

4. J. Dollard, *Fear in battle*, New Haven: Institute of Human Relations, 1943.

5. B. Bettelheim, "Individual and mass behaviour in extreme situations," *J. Abnorm. Soc. Psychol.*, 1943, 38:417-52.

6. R. R. Grinker and J. P. Spiegel, *War neuroses*, Philadelphia: Blakiston, 1945, p. 94.

7. *Ibid.*, p. 96.

8. *Ibid.*, p. 105.

9. *Ibid.*, p. 113.

10. *Ibid.*, p. 119.

11. Especially in *Personality: a psychological interpretation*, New York: Holt, 1937, Chap. 7. See also my "Motivation in personality: reply to Mr. Bertocci," *Psychol. Rev.*, 1940, 47:533-54; and Chapter 12 of the present volume.

12. "Motivation in personality: reply to Mr. Bertocci," *op. cit.*

13. P. Witty, "New evidence on the learning ability of the Negro," *J. Abnorm. Soc. Psychol.*, 1945, 40:401-4.

14. W. McDougall, *Outline of psychology*, New York: Scribner, 1923, p. 428.

15. C. Burt, *Brit. J. Educ. Psychol.*, 1943, 13:3.

16. O. Klineberg, *Social psychology*, 1940, pp. 160 f.

17. C. Burt, *op. cit.*, p. 5.

18. *Ibid.*, p. 10.

19. *Ibid.*, p. 11.

20. *Ibid.*, p. 14.

21. *Ibid.*, p. 14.

22. *Ibid.*, p. 11.

23. C. Burt, *Brit. J. Educ. Psychol.*, 1945, 15:107. In all essential features this definition is identical with my own; see G. W. Allport, *Personality: a psychological interpretation*, *op. cit.*, p. 48.

24. C. Burt, *Brit. J. Educ. Psychol.*, 1943, 13:7.

25. The point stated here so briefly I have argued more fully in the following publications: *The use of personal documents in psychological science*, New York: Social Science Research Council, 1942, Bull. 49. "The psychologist's frame of reference," *Psychol. Bull.*, 1940, 37:1-28; "Personalistic psychology as science: a reply," *Psychol. Rev.*, 1946, Vol. 54.

26. C. Burt, *Brit. J. Educ. Psychol.*, 1945, 15:110 f.

27. Cf. N. Polansky, "How shall a life-history be written?" *Char. & Pers.*, 1941, 9:188-207.

PART III: *Normative problems in personality*

Review preface page v

CHAPTER 10

Personality: normal and abnormal

It is sometimes said that science is "value-free," that it makes no assumptions regarding good or evil. Science produces technology (including the H-bomb) and lets others worry about the ethics involved.

Whether any science can be entirely value-free is a question. One thing at least is certain: psychologists, by the nature of their profession, are persistently haunted by problems of value. Especially in the fields of therapy, guidance and consultation, a psychologist cannot escape them.

The four following chapters wrestle with common normative dilemmas confronting psychologists. In sequence, the essays attempt to answer the following questions:

What is a normal, sound, healthy personality?

By what guiding principle shall we try to resolve conflicting desires in the person and in society?

What are the requirements for a fully mature democratic personality?

Under what psychological conditions can love be maximized, hate minimized?

The present chapter is an address delivered at the Fifth Inter-American Congress of Psychology at Mexico City in December 1957. It first appeared in *The Sociological Review* (1958).

The word *norm* means "an authoritative standard," and correspondingly *normal* means abiding by such a standard. It follows that a normal personality is one whose conduct conforms to an authoritative standard, and an abnormal personality is one whose conduct does not do so.

But having said this much, we immediately discover that there are two entirely different kinds of standards that may be applied to divide the normal from the abnormal: one statistical, the other ethical. The former pertains to the average or usual, and the latter to the desirable or valuable.

These two standards are not only different but, in many ways, stand in flat contradiction to each other. It is, for example, *usual* for people to have some noxious trends in their natures, some pathology of tissues or organs, some evidences of nervousness and some self-defeating habits; but, though usual or average, such trends are not healthy. Or again, society's authoritative standard for a wholesome sex life is, if we are to accept the Kinsey Report, achieved by only a minority of American males. Here too the usual is not the desirable; what is normal in one sense is not normal in the other sense. And certainly no system of ethics in the civilized world holds up as a model for its children the ideal of becoming a merely average man. It is not the actualities, but rather the potentialities, of human nature that somehow provide us with a standard for a sound and healthy personality. *A NORM*

Fifty years ago this double meaning of *norm* and *normal* did not trouble psychology so much as it does today. In those days psychology was deeply involved in discovering average norms for every conceivable type of mental function. Means, modes and sigmas were in the saddle, and differential psychology was riding high. Intoxicated with the new-found beauty of the normal distribution curve, psychologists were content to declare its slender tails as the one and only sensible measure of abnormality. Departures from the mean were abnormal and for this reason slightly unsavory.

In this era there grew up the concept of "mental adjustment," and this concept held sway well into the decade of the '20s. While not all psychologists equated adjustment with average behavior, this implication was pretty generally present. It was, for example, frequently pointed out that an animal who does not adjust to the norm for his species usually dies. It was not yet pointed out that a human being who does so adjust is a bore and a mediocrity.

Now times have changed. Our concern for the improvement of average human behavior is deep, for we now seriously doubt that the merely mediocre man can survive. As social anomie spreads, as society itself becomes more and more sick, we doubt that the mediocre man will escape mental disease and delinquency, or that he will keep himself out of the clutch of dictators or succeed in preventing atomic warfare. The normal distribution curve, we see, holds out no hope of salvation. We need citizens who are in a more positive sense normal, healthy and sound. And the world needs them more urgently than it ever did before.

It is for this reason, I think, that psychologists are now seeking a fresh definition of what is normal and what is abnormal. They are asking questions concerning the *valuable,* the *right* and the *good* as they have never asked them before.

At the same time, psychologists know that, in seeking for a criterion of normality in this new sense, they are trespassing on the traditional domain of moral philosophy. They also know that, by and

large, philosophers have failed to establish authoritative standards for
what constitutes the sound life—the life that educators, parents and
therapists should seek to mold. And so psychologists for the most
part wish to pursue the search in a fresh way and, if they can, avoid
the traditional traps of axiology. Let me briefly describe some recent
empirical attempts to define normality and afterward attempt to
evaluate the state of our efforts to date.

Naturalistic Derivations of "Normality"

Two proposals have recently been published that merit serious
attention. Both are by social scientists, one a psychologist in the
United States, the other a sociologist in England. Their aim is to
derive a concept of normality (in the value sense) from the condition of man (in the naturalistic sense). Both seek their ethical imperatives from biology and psychology, not from value-theory directly.
In short, they boldly seek the *ought*—the goal to which teachers,
counselors and therapists should strive—from the *is* of human nature.
Many philosophers tell us that this is an impossible undertaking.
But, before we pass judgment, let us see what success they have had.

E. J. Shoben asks: what are the principal psychological differences between man and lower animals? [1] While he does not claim
that his answer is complete, he centers upon two distinctively human
qualities, and he makes the extra-psychological assumption that man
should maximize those attributes that are distinctively human. The
first quality is man's capacity for the use of propositional language *A*
(symbolization). From this particular superiority over animals,
Shoben derives several specific guidelines for normality. With the
aid of symbolic language, for example, man can delay his gratifica- *1.*
tions, holding in mind a distant goal, a remote reward, an objective
to be reached perhaps only at the end of one's life, or perhaps never.
With the aid of symbolic language, he can imagine a future for him- *2.*
self that is far better than the present. He can also develop an in- *3.*
tricate system of social concepts that leads him to all manner of
possible relations with other human beings, far exceeding the rigid
symbiotic rituals of, say, the social insects.

A second distinctive human quality is related to the prolonged
childhood in the human species. Dependence, basic trust, sympathy *B.*
and altruism are absolutely essential to human survival, in a sense
and to a degree not true for lower animals.

Bringing together these two distinctive qualities, Shoben derives

A + B.

his conception of normality. He calls it "a model of integrative adjustment." It follows, he says, that a sense of *personal responsibility* marks the normal man, for responsibility is a distinctive capacity derived from holding in mind a symbolic image of the future, delaying gratification and being able to strive in accordance with one's conceptions of the best principles of conduct for oneself. Similarly, *social responsibility* is normal; for all these symbolic capacities can interact with the unique factor of trust or altruism. Closely related is the criterion of *democratic social interest,* which derives from both symbolization and trust. Similarly, the *possession of ideals* and the necessity for *self-control* follow from the same naturalistic analysis. Shoben points out that a *sense of guilt* is an inevitable consequence of man's failure to live according to the distinctive human pattern, and so in our concept of normality we must include both guilt and devices for expiation.

Every psychologist who wishes to make minimum assumptions and to keep close to empirical evidence, and who inclines toward the naturalism of biological science, will appreciate and admire Shoben's efforts. Yet I imagine our philosopher friends will arise to confound us with some uncomfortable questions. Is it not a distinctively human capacity, they will ask, for a possessive mother to keep her child permanently tied to her apron strings? Does any lower animal engage in this destructive behavior? Likewise, is it not distinctively human to develop fierce in-group loyalties that lead to prejudice, contempt and war? Is it not possible that the burden of symbolization, social responsibility and guilt may lead a person to depression and suicide? Suicide, along with all the other destructive patterns I have mentioned, is distinctively human. A philosopher who raises these questions would conclude, "No, you cannot derive the *ought* from the *is* of human nature. What is distinctively human is not necessarily distinctively good."

Let us look at a second attempt to achieve a naturalistic criterion of normality. In a recent book entitled *Towards a measure of man,* Paul Halmos prefers to start with the question, "What are the minimum conditions for survival?" [2] When we know these minimum conditions, we can declare that any situations falling below this level will lead to abnormality, and tend toward death and destruction. He calls this criterion the *abnorm* and believes that we can define it, even if we cannot define normality, because people in general agree more readily on what is bad for man than on what is good for him. They

QUESTIONS

agree on the bad because all mortals are subject to the basic imperative of survival.

The need for survival he breaks down into the *need for growth*
and the *need for social cohesion*. These two principles are the universal conditions of all life, not merely of human life. Growth means
autonomy and the process of individuation. Cohesion is the basic
fact of social interdependence; it involves, at least for human beings,
initial trust, heteronomy, mating and the founding of family.

Halmos believes that, by taking an inventory of conditions
deleterious to growth and cohesion, we may establish the *abnorm*.
As a start he mentions, first and foremost, disorders of child training.
"Continued or repeated interruption of physical proximity between
mother and child," he says, or "emotional rejection" of the child by
the mother, is a condition that harms survival of the individual and
the group. In his own terms, this first criterion of abnormality lies
in a "rupture in the transmutation of cohesion into love." Most of
what is abnormal he traces to failures in the principle of cohesion, so
that the child becomes excessively demanding and compulsive. Here
we note the similarity to such contemporary thinkers as Bowlby, Erikson and Maslow.

Halmos continues his inventory of the abnorm by accepting syndromes that psychiatrists agree upon. For instance, it is abnormal
(inimical to survival) if repetition of conduct occurs irrespective of
the situation and unmodified by its consequences; it is abnormal if
one's accomplishments constantly fall short of one's potentialities; it
is abnormal if one's psychosexual frustrations prevent both growth
and cohesion.

It is well to point out that the basic functions of growth and
cohesion postulated by Halmos occur time and time again in psychological writing. Bergson, Jung and Angyal are among the writers
who agree that normality requires a balance between individuation
and socialization, between autonomy and heteronomy. There seems
to be considerable consensus in this matter. Let me quote from
Werner Wolff, one of the founders of this Society whose recent death
has brought sorrow to us all:

"When an individual identifies himself to an extreme degree
with a group, the effect is that he loses his value. On the other hand,
a complete inability to identify has the effects that the environment
loses its value for the individual. In both extreme cases the dynamic
relationship between individual and environment is distorted. An
individual behaving in such a way is called 'neurotic.' In a normal

group each member preserves his individuality but accepts his role as participator also." [3]

While there is much agreement that the normal personality must strike a serviceable balance between growth as an individual and cohesion with society, we do not yet have a clear criterion for determining when these factors are in serviceable balance and when they are not. Philosophers, I fear, would shake their heads at Halmos. They would ask, "How do you know that survival is a good thing?" And, "Why should all people enjoy equal rights to the benefits of growth and cohesion?" And, "How are we to define the optimum balance between cohesion and growth within the single personality?"

Halmos himself worries especially about the relation between abnormality and creativity. It was Nietzsche who declared, "I say unto you: a man must have chaos yet within him to be able to give birth to a dancing star." Have not many meritorious works of music, literature and even of science drawn their inspiration not from balance but from some kind of psychic chaos? Here, I think, Halmos gives the right answer. He says in effect that creativity and normality are not identical values. On the whole, the normal person will be creative; but if valuable creations come likewise from people who are slipping away from the norm of survival, this fact can only be accepted and valued on the scale of creativity, not properly on the scale of normality.

Imbalance and Growth

In this day of existentialism, I sense that psychologists are becoming less and less content with the concept of adjustment and, correspondingly, with the concepts of "tension reduction," "restoration of equilibrium" and "homeostasis." We wonder if a man who enjoys these beatific conditions is truly human. Growth, we know, is due not to homeostasis but to a kind of "transistasis." And cohesion is a matter of keeping our human relationships moving, not in mere stationary equilibrium. Stability cannot be a criterion of normality, for stability brings evolution to a standstill, negating both growth and cohesion. Freud once wrote to Fliess that he finds "moderate misery necessary for intensive work."

A research inspired by Carl Rogers is interesting in this connection. One series of patients manifested before treatment a zero correlation between their self-image and their ideal self-image. Following treatment the correlation was +.34—not high, but approaching the coefficient of +.58 that marked a healthy, untreated group.

Apparently this magnitude of correlation is a measure of the satisfaction or dissatisfaction that normal people have with their own personalities.[4] A zero correlation between self and ideal-self is too low for normality; it leads to such anguish that the sufferer seeks therapy. At the same time, normal people are by no means perfectly adjusted to themselves. There is always a wholesome gap between self and ideal-self, between present existence and aspiration. On the other hand, too high a satisfaction indicates pathology. The highest coefficient obtained, +.90, was from an individual clearly pathological. Perfect correlations we might expect only from smug psychotics, particularly paranoid schizophrenics.

And so, whatever our definition of normality turns out to be, it must allow for serviceable imbalances within personality, and between person and society.

Approaches to Soundness

The work of Barron illustrates an approach dear to the psychologist's heart. He lets others establish the criterion of normality—or, as he calls it, *soundness*—and then proceeds to find out what "sound" men are like. Teachers of graduate students in the University of California nominated a large number of men whom they considered sound, and some of the opposite trend. From testing and experimenting with these men, whose identities were unknown to the investigators, certain significant differences appeared.[5] For one thing, the sounder men had more realistic perceptions; they were not thrown off by distortions or by surrounding context in the sensory field. Further, on check lists they stood high on such traits as integrated pursuit of goals, persistence, adaptability and good nature. On the Minnesota Multiphasic Personality Inventory they were high in equanimity, self-confidence, objectivity and virility. Their self-insight was superior, as was their physical health. Finally, they came from homes where there was little or no affective rupture—a finding that confirms Halmos' predictions.

Most authors do not have the benefit of professorial consensus on soundness. They simply set forth in a didactic manner the attributes of normality, or health, or soundness, or maturity, or productivity, as they see them. Innumerable descriptive lists result. Perhaps the simplest of these is Freud's: he says the healthy person will be able to "love" and to "work." One of the most elaborate is Maslow's schedule of qualities, which includes, among others: an efficient perception of reality, philosophical humor, spontaneity, detachment and an acceptance of self and others. Such lists are not altogether arbitrary, since their authors base them either on a wide clinical experience, as did Freud, or on a deliberate analysis of case materials, as did Maslow.[6]

So many lists of this type are now available that a new kind of approach is possible—namely, the combining of these insightful inventories. From time to time I have assigned this task to my students, and while all manner of groupings and re-groupings result, there are recurrent themes that appear in nearly all inventories. If I were to attempt the assignment myself, I should probably start with my own list of three criteria, published twenty years ago, but I would now expand it.[7]

The three criteria I originally listed were:

Ego-extension—the capacity to take an interest in more than one's body and one's material possessions. The criterion covers, I think, the attributes that Fromm ascribes to the productive man.

Self-objectification, which includes the ability to relate the feeling tone of the present experience to that of a past experience, provided the latter does in fact determine the quality of the former. Self-objectification also includes humor, which tells us that our total horizon of life is too wide to be compressed into our present rigidities.

Unifying philosophy of life, which may or may not be religious, but in any event has to be a frame of meaning and of responsibility into which life's major activities fit.

To this inventory I now would add:

The capacity for a warm, profound relating of one's self to others, which may, if one likes, be called "extroversion of the libido" or *Gemeinschaftsgefühl*.

The possession of realistic skills, abilities and perceptions with which to cope with the practical problems of life.

A compassionate regard for all living creatures, which includes respect for individual persons and a disposition to participate in common activities that will improve the human lot.

I am aware that psychoanalysts are partial to the criterion of "ego-strength": a normal person has a strong ego, an abnormal person a weak ego. But I find this phrase ill defined and suggest that my somewhat more detailed criteria succeed better in specifying what we mean by ego-strength.

The weakness of all inventories, including my own, is that the philosopher's persistent questions are still unanswered. How does the psychologist know that these qualities comprise normality, that they are good and that all people should have them? Before I attempt to give a partial answer to our irritating philosopher friend, let me call attention to one additional psychological approach.

Continuity of Symptom and Discontinuity of Process

in abn and n cases   *stages V development*

I refer to a fresh analysis of the problem of continuity-discontinuity. Is abnormality merely an exaggerated normal condition? Is there an unbroken continuity between health and disease? Certainly Freud thought so. He evolved his system primarily as a theory of neurosis, but he and his followers came to regard his formulations as a universally valid science of psychology. Whether one is normal or abnormal depends on the degree to which one can manage his relationships successfully. Furthermore, the earlier enthusiasm of psychologists for the normal distribution curve helped to entrench the theory of continuity. The strongest empirical evidence in favor of this view is the occurrence of borderline cases. Descriptively there is certainly a continuum: we encounter mild neurotics, borderline schizophrenics, hypomanics and personalities that are paranoid, cycloid, epileptoid. If scales and tests are employed, there are no gaps; scores are continuously distributed.

But—and let me insist on this point—this continuum pertains only to symptoms, to appearances. The *processes*, or mechanisms, underlying these appearances are not continuous. There is, for example, a polar difference between confronting the world and its problems (which is an intrinsically wholesome thing to do) and escaping and withdrawing from the world (which is an intrinsically unwholesome thing to do). Extreme withdrawal and escape constitute psychosis. But, you may ask, do not we all do some escaping? Yes, we do; and what is more, escapism may not only provide recreation but also have a certain constructive utility, as it has in mild daydreaming. The process of escape can be harmless, however, only if the *dominant* process is confrontation. Left to itself, escapism spells disaster. In the psychotic, this process has the upper hand; in the normal person, confrontation has the upper hand.

Following this line of reasoning we can list other processes that intrinsically generate abnormality, and those that generate normality. The first list deals with catabolic functions. I would mention:

Escape or withdrawal (including fantasy)
Repression or dissociation
Other "ego-defenses," including rationalization, reaction formation, projection and displacement

      Impulsivity (uncontrolled)
      Restriction of thinking to concrete level
      Fixation of personality at a juvenile level
      All forms of rigidification

The list is not complete, but the processes in question are intrinsically catabolic. They are as much so as are the disease mechanisms responsible for diabetes, tuberculosis, hyperthyroidism or cancer. A person suffering only a small dose of these mechanisms may appear to be normal, but only if the *anabolic mechanisms* predominate. Among the latter I would list: *intrinsically normal*

      Confrontation (or, if you prefer, reality testing)
      Availability of knowledge to consciousness
      Self-insight, with its attendant humor
      Integrative action of the nervous system
      Ability to think abstractly
      Continuous individuation (without arrested or fixated development)
      Functional autonomy of motives
      Frustration tolerance

I realize that what I have called processes, or mechanisms, are not in all cases logically parallel. But they serve to make my point—that normality depends on the dominance of one set of principles, abnormality upon the dominance of another. The fact that all normal people are occasionally afflicted with catabolic processes does not alter the point. The normal life is marked by a preponderance of the anabolic functions, the abnormal by a preponderance of the catabolic.

Conclusion

And now, is it possible to gather together all these divergent threads and to reach some position tenable for psychology today? Let us try to do so.

First, I think, we should make a deep obeisance in the direction of moral philosophy and gracefully concede that psychology by itself cannot solve the problem of normality. No psychologist has succeeded in telling us why man ought to seek good health rather than ill, or why normality should be our goal for all men, and not just for some. Nor can psychologists account for the fact that meritorious creativity may be of value even if the creator himself is by all tests an abnormal person. These and a variety of other conundrums lie beyond the competence of psychology to solve. That moral philosophers have not agreed among themselves upon solutions is also true, but we gladly grant them freedom and encouragement to continue their efforts.

At the same time, the lines of research and analysis I have here reviewed are vitally related to the philosopher's quest. After all, it is the psychologists who deal directly with personalities in the clinic and laboratories, in schools and industry. It is they who gather the facts concerning normality and abnormality, and try to weave them into their own normative speculations. A fact and a moral imperative are more closely interlocked than traditional writers on ethics may think. Among the facts that psychology can offer are the following:

Investigations have told us much concerning the nature of human needs and motives, both conscious and unconscious. A grouping of these needs into the broad categories of growth and cohesion is helpful. Much is known concerning the pathologies that result from frustration and imbalance of these needs. It would be absurd for moral philosophers to write imperatives in total disregard of this evidence.

We know much about childhood conditions that predispose toward delinquency, prejudice and mental disorder. A moralist might do well to cast his imperatives in terms of standards for child training. I can suggest, for example, that the abstract imperative *respect for persons* should be tested and formulated from the point of view of child training.

By virtue of comparative work on men and animals, we know much about the motives common to both—but also, as Shoben has shown, about the qualities that are distinctively human. Let the philosophers give due weight to this work.

While I have not yet mentioned the matter, psychology, in co-operation with cultural anthropology, has a fairly clear picture today of the role of culture in defining and producing abnormality. We know the incidence of psychosis and neurosis in various populations; we know what conditions are labeled abnormal in some cultures but regarded as normal in others. We also know, with some accuracy, those conditions that are considered abnormal in all cultures. These facts are highly relevant to the deliberations of the moral philosopher.

Following the lead of Halmos, we may say that biologists, psychologists and sociologists know much about the conditions of individual and group survival. While these facts in themselves do not tell us why we *should* survive, they provide specifications for the philosopher who thinks he can answer this riddle.

Still more important, I think, is the empirical work on consensus that is now available. We have noted Barron's method of determining the attributes of men judged to be "sound" as distinguished from those of men judged to be "unsound." While the philosopher is not likely to accept the vote of university professors as an adequate definition of soundness, he might do well to heed opinions other than his own.

Another type of consensus is obtained from the inventories prepared by insightful writers. These authors have tried, according to their best ability, to summarize as they see them the requirements of normality (or health, or maturity). They do so on the grounds of extensive experience. As we survey these inventories, we are struck both by their verbal differences and by an underlying congruence of meaning that no one has yet succeeded fully in articulating. Here again, the philosopher may balk at accepting consensus; yet he would do well to check his own private reasoning against the conclusions of others no less competent—and probably more clinically experienced —than he.

He would also do well, I think, to explore the goals of psychotherapy as stated or implied in leading therapeutic systems. If he were to comb the writings of behavioristic therapists, for example, he might reasonably conclude that *efficiency* (the ability to cope with problems) is their principal goal. Those who advocate non-directive therapy clearly prize the goal of *growth*. The desideratum for Goldstein, Maslow and Jung is *self-actualization;* for Fromm, *productivity;* for Frankl and the logotherapists, *meaningfulness* and *responsibility*. Each therapist seems to have in mind a preponderant emphasis, which, in terms of value theory, constitutes for him a definition of the good way of life and of health for the personality. While the emphases differ and the labels vary, there seems to be a confluence of these criteria. Taken together, they remind us of the tributaries to a vast river system, none the less unified for all its variety of source and shape. This confluence is a factor that no moralist can afford to overlook.

Finally, the distinction between the anabolic and catabolic processes in the formation of personality represents a fact of importance. Instead of judging merely the end-product of action, the moralist might do well to focus his attention upon the processes by which various ends are achieved. Conceivably the moral law could be written in terms of strengthening anabolic functions in oneself and in others, while fighting against catabolic functions.

It is true that the preferred method of moral philosophy is to work "from the top down." Apriorism and reason are the legitimate tools of philosophy. Up to now, this method has yielded a wide array of moral imperatives, including the following: So act that the maxim of thy action can become a universal law. Be a respecter of persons. Seek to reduce your desires. Harmonize your interests with the interests of others. Thou art nothing; thy folk is everything. And thou shalt love the Lord thy God with all thy heart, and with all thy soul, and with all thy mind . . . and thy neighbor as thyself.

We have no wish to impede this approach from above, for we dare not block the intuitive and rational springs of ethical theory. But—and this is my point of chief insistence—each of these moral imperatives, and all others that have been or will be devised, can and should be tested and specified with reference to the various forms of psychological analysis that I have here reviewed. By submitting each imperative to psychological scrutiny, we can tell whether men are likely to comprehend the principle offered; whether and in what sense it is within their capacity to follow it; and what the long-run consequences are likely to be. We will also learn whether there is agreement among men in general, and among therapists and other meliorists, that the imperative is indeed good.

One final word. My discussion of the problem of normality and abnormality has, in a sense, yielded only a niggardly solution. I have said, in effect, that the criterion we seek has not yet been discovered, nor is it likely to be discovered by psychologists working alone, nor by philosophers working alone. The cooperation of both is needed. Fortunately, psychologists are now beginning to ask philosophical questions, and philosophers are beginning to ask psychological questions. Working together, they may ultimately formulate the problem aright—and conceivably solve it.

In the meantime, the work I have reviewed in this essay represents a high level of sophistication, far higher than that which prevailed a short generation ago. Psychologists who, in their teaching and counseling, follow the lines now laid down will not go far wrong in guiding personalities toward normality.

REFERENCES

1. E. J. Shoben, Jr., "Toward a concept of the normal personality," *Amer. Psychologist*, 1957, 12:183-89.

2. P. Halmos, *Towards a measure of man: the frontiers of normal adjustment*, London: Routledge & Kegan Paul, 1957.

3. W. Wolff, *The threshold of the abnormal*, New York: Hermitage House, 1950, pp. 131 f.

4. Cited by C. Hall and G. Lindzey, *Theories of personality*, New York: John Wiley, 1957, pp. 492-96.

5. F. Barron, *Personal soundness in university graduate students* (Publications of Personnel Assessment Research, No. 1), Berkeley: California University Press, 1954.

6. A. H. Maslow, *Motivation and personality*, New York: Harper, 1954, Chap. 12.

7. G. W. Allport, *Personality: a psychological interpretation*, New York: Holt, 1937, Chap. 8.

CHAPTER II

Circles of interest and the resolution
of conflict

Under the leadership of Pitirim A. Sorokin, a group of scientists held a symposium at the Massachusetts Institute of Technology in the fall of 1957. Their essays dealt with the relationship between various sciences and the realm of values.

The following essay was prepared for this occasion and makes a brief reference to others in the symposium.

Modern psychological research supports the principle of "maximum inclusion of interests," which is the subject of this essay. The principle has been championed by many philosophers from antiquity to the present day; and investigations conducted in industry, in the classroom, in therapy—in all settings where conflict is studied—give empirical support to this central ethical imperative.

The essay was first published in *New knowledge in human values,* edited by Abraham H. Maslow, under the title "Normative compatibility in the light of social science" (1959).

Several distinguished scientists have made the point that, although moral values cannot be derived from natural data or from science, they can in some sense be validated (confirmed or disconfirmed) by the activity of science. This point has been made by both natural scientists and social scientists. I find myself in full agreement.

Likewise, I agree with Maslow when he says that the validating capacity of social science is still somewhat feeble. Its data and methods are coarse and imprecise. One critic complained that "social science is nothing but journalism without a date line." However that may be, I offer this essay in support of the proposition that modern social science, for all its imperfections, can now aid us in selecting from among the moral imperatives prescribed by various philosophers as guides to social policy. It can do so by helping us test broad types of ethical theory in the light of our modern knowledge of human nature and human collectivities.

By way of illustration, and without offering detailed evidence at this time, let me mention some of the broad types of ethical theory that seem to fare badly when they are exposed to social-scientific analysis:

Theories of renunciation or asceticism, to give one example, make the error of assuming that men seek a life that is one-sided rather than one that is full and abundant. According to this view, morality is largely a matter of repression or negation—a denial of much or most of man's endowment for growth. We cannot, of course, deny that this path of life, with its implied beatific vision, may be well suited for a few; but it is doomed to failure if it is prescribed for the masses of mankind.

Authoritarian morality, of which we have seen much in our day, defines goodness merely in terms of obedience. The adult, with all his potentialities for growth, is kept at the childhood level. While it is easy for many people to adopt the authoritarian code in order to "escape from freedom," the result, we know, is stultification, tyranny and war—and thus the destruction of virtually all values.

Legalistic theories prescribe morality in terms of "thou shalts" or "thou shalt nots." The psychological error here is that the letter of the law, being inflexible, does not guide men in the novel and changing encounters of daily life.

Utopian theories are inept, not because they counsel perfection—all morality does that—but because they plot no pathway from today's quandaries to the ultimate beatitude they depict.

Utilitarian ethics—in fact every version of *hedonism*—fixes men's minds on a will-o'-the-wisp. Happiness can never be a tangible goal; it can only be a by-product of otherwise motivated activity. We may add that, in the mid-nineteenth century, ethical hedonism (*laissez faire*) was given an explicit trial in the social policies of Britain and America, where it succeeded in creating moral dilemmas, not in solving them. Its failure was experimentally demonstrated, much as the failure of authoritarian morality has been demonstrated in our own day.

With these negative examples before us, we may ask: what type of ethical theory does social science find most congruent with recent researches on human nature and on human aggregates?

Before answering this question, let us remind ourselves that all theories of moral conduct have one primary purpose: they set before us some appropriate formula for handling conflict—conflict between warring interests in one individual, or conflict among individuals. In testing rival ethical theories, therefore, it is necessary to know a good deal about the interests of men—about the motives that are likely to come into conflict within the individual or between persons or groups of persons.

Desires Versus Demands

While our present interest is in validatable moral theory, not in motivation, let me refer to one relevant finding concerning motivation, which comes from industrial research. Summarizing a number of studies of motivation and morale in industry, Likert concludes that workers have, in effect, two primary sets of interests. They want *ego-recognition*—a broad motivational category that includes credit for work done, economic security, praise and many other means of building self-esteem. But they also, and no less urgently, want *affiliation with the group*—a dimension that includes pleasant relations with the foreman, a sense of participation in teamwork and, above all, the satisfaction of conducting themselves in terms of the values and normative expectations prevailing within the group of co-workers.[1]

The point is important. In industry, and probably in any form of human association, men wish to preserve their self-esteem—their self-love—and simultaneously wish to have warm, affiliative relations with their fellows. No one seems initially to want to hate. Hatred grows up as a consequence of blocked self-esteem and blocked affection.

It has been further discovered that high production, high morale and successful relations can be achieved only when formulae are discovered that permit the adequate expression of these two sets of interests on the part of all participants. The movement called human relations in industry teaches this lesson over and over again —in terms of labor-management councils, group decision, the retraining of foremen and basic changes in managerial philosophy.[2] In former days industry ran almost entirely on the basis of punishment—or, we may say, subtraction. Workers were asked to give up their identity, their pride, their social impulses during the hours they were earning a living. Today, the saying is, "The whole man goes to work." Realizing this fact, certain industries now have counselors on personal and family problems. Through improved communication the individual is given a means of participating in his own destiny. His private life and his work life are integrated; the interests of management and employees come together to a greater degree than formerly. I am not saying that utopia is achieved in industry, but only that experimentation has already gone far enough to demonstrate the validity of ethical theory that advocates the resolution of conflict through the harmonious integration of interests.

This approach to morality does not aim at the reconciling of conflicting *demands*. Demands are usually nothing more than ways and means prematurely conceived to be the only channels for the realization of desires. All theories of the enlargement of interests stress the distinction between demands and desires—that is to say, between instrumental and intrinsic values—and insist that the moral individual himself must at every step distinguish between his demands and his desires. E. B. Holt calls the process *discrimination;* Ralph Barton Perry calls it *reflection*.[3]

To illustrate the distinction; let us borrow a classic incident from Mary Follett.[4] It seems that, in a certain part of Vermont, dairy farmers who lived up the hill from the railway station and those who lived down the hill from the station both claimed the right to unload their milk supply first at the platform. Their demands were irreconcilable, and for a long time a feud prevailed. Finally they perceived their error. Their root-desire was not, as they thought, to unload first. This was a demand. The underlying desire of each faction was that it not be kept waiting. Profiting from this discriminative insight, they joined forces on a Saturday afternoon and lengthened the railway platform. Thereafter they were both able to unload "first."

Although the illustration may seem a bit pat, it does contain the paradigm for moral action: Two or more conflicting sets of apparent purposes collide. They are analyzed reflectively and so purged of preconceived ways and means. The root-desires themselves are then brought to fulfillment through the invention of a larger framework, which renders them compatible. In Weisskopf's term, a *union upward* is achieved.

The Principle of Enlargement of Interests

Wartime research is filled with examples of our principle. Let me cite one study, drawn from Stouffer's investigation of the American soldier.[5] Men in combat, we should expect, would show the maximum of destructive, self-preserving motivation. A number of them were asked, "When the going was tough, how much were you helped by thoughts of hatred for the enemy?" Roughly a third said such thoughts "helped a lot." But when they were asked, "When the going was tough, how much did it help you to think that you couldn't let the other men down?" approximately two-thirds said that it "helped a lot." Thus the affiliative motive, even under extreme stress, seems to hold twice as many men to their task as does the motive of hate. The point to note is that an enlargement of interest systems to include one's comrades is, even in the time of physical combat, a natural bent of man.

Successful psychotherapy offers a basic illustration of the principle. The most elementary formula for encouraging a patient is to assure him that "lots of people suffer from your difficulty." Most patients brighten when they know that they are not alone in their misery. Such assurance does not, of course, solve the patient's problem, but even this imaginative integration of interests proves helpful. True neuroses, we know, are best defined as stubborn self-centeredness. No therapist can cure a phobia, obsession, prejudice or hostility by subtraction. He can assist the patient to achieve a value-system and outlook that will blanket or absorb the troublesome factor.

The successful resolution of *social conflict* proceeds always along the same lines. Take the issue of desegregation, a problem of the first magnitude not only in this country but in the world at large. On the social level, it is a matter of bringing resistant provincial interests in line with more inclusive national and world values. On the personal level, it is a problem of enlarging the outlook of individuals who live now according to an exclusionist formula that secures for them self-esteem at the expense of dark-skinned people. At present, these individuals are willing to form no inclusive unit with the federal majority in this country or with the world majority; nor will they form inclusive units with the Negro minority in their midst. They are not able even to resolve the moral dilemma in their own breasts. In all directions the principle of inclusion fails.

At the moment this particular problem is most acute in the United States and in South Africa. Although I have not the space to diagnose the situation in detail, let me say briefly that, so far as South Africa is concerned, the chief blunder of the Nationalist Party government, morally and politically, lies in its failure to consult with the Bantu peoples concerning their own destiny. The master group *tells* the servant group, who outnumber the masters three to one, that they have nothing to contribute to the life of the multiracial society except manual labor. Thus cultural pride, love of homeland and all other normal human aspirations and abilities of the Bantus are excluded from the existing matrix of values. The policy of *apartheid* extends to housing, transportation, schools, public assemblies, recreation and politics, so that there is no legal opportunity to become acquainted. And, needless to say, the precondition of all normative compatibility is communication.

Both South Africa and the United States are exciting test cases for social science at the present time, the one following officially a policy of *excluding* interests, the other an official policy of *inclusion*. The world is watching the outcome.

We could pile up evidence from areas of conflict I have not yet touched upon—from family, classroom, neighborhood, municipality and deliberative assemblies. But I shall limit myself to one question that cuts across all these areas: how far is it possible for people, especially for children, to learn the moral principle of discrimination and inclusion?

The Process of Enlargement in Childhood

A study by Piaget and his associates is enlightening.[6] These investigators find that children around six and seven years of age, living in the city of Geneva, are unable to think of themselves as *both* Genevese and Swiss. Given a crayon and asked to draw two circles, one for Geneva and one for Switzerland, they ordinarily draw the circles side by side. They insist that if they are Genevese, they cannot simultaneously be Swiss. As for foreign lands, the children suffer from even greater cognitive impoverishment. Concerning Italy they know only that their father visited Italy, or that an aunt comes from there. Even loyalty to the homeland does not yet exist. The child's affective reactions are wholly egocentric: "I like Lausanne because I ate chocolate there." "I like Bern because my uncle lives there." In Piaget's term, these children have not yet commenced the process of "decentering" from the unit of self to any larger social unit.

Ages eight and nine are transitional. Although the child draws a circle for Geneva properly inside the circle for Switzerland, he still has difficulty translating spatial enclosure into terms of social enclosure. He may say, for example, "I'm Swiss now, so I can't be Genevese any longer." True, the concept of the homeland is gradually growing, but in a self-centered way. The child says, "I like Switzerland because I was born there." As for foreign lands, he knows of their existence but commonly views them with scorn. The French are dirty; the Americans want war; and people living in other lands all wish, of course, that they were Swiss. The child at this age has taken bits of conversation from his home and school and fitted them to this own affective self-centeredness.

Only at the ages of ten and eleven do we find that decentering has made appreciable progress. Egocentricity begins to give way to the principles of reciprocity and inclusion. The child of ten or eleven understands his dual membership, in a smaller and a larger political unit. He also gives fewer personal reasons for his affective attachment to his homeland. Switzerland now becomes the land of the Red Cross; it is the country without war. Further, the child understands that members of other countries are as attached to their own lands as he is to his; this is the principle of *reciprocity*. But cognitive reciprocity does not necessarily mean that the child is capable of seeing good in all the peoples he knows about. He may still despise them. Whether the child outgrows his affective provincialism along with his cognitive provincialism seems to depend largely on the attitudes he learns from his parents.

Now, this study teaches us certain lessons. For one thing, it shows that maturation and time are needed to achieve a decentering from the unit of self to a progressively larger social unit. Further, this process may be arrested at any stage along the way, especially in its affective aspects. It is significant that Piaget gives no evidence that his children, at least up to fourteen years of age, discern the possibility of membership in any supranational grouping. Decentering has not reached the point where the child feels himself as belonging to the European region or to the United Nations; certainly none mentions his membership in the inclusive collective of mankind. Even if, in later years, such a cognitive enlargement takes place, the chances are that the corresponding affective enlargement will be lacking. We may then say that adults in all nations are still incompletely decentered. Cognitively they may stumble at the threshold of supranational chambers, but affectively they fail to enter.

Resolving International Conflicts

A study conducted in Belgium by de Bie shows how few adults are concerned with identification across national boundaries. Even those of a higher level of education have little sense of international relationships. Membership in any unit larger than the nation simply is not a psychological reality. Let international problems be handled by our leaders, they say.[7] But most, though not all, leaders themselves lack affective, or even cognitive, decentering beyond the sphere of purely national interests.

In its *Tensions and technology* series, UNESCO has recently published a volume entitled *The nature of conflict,* surveying much relevant research. In summing up the results, R. C. Angell concludes that interacting nations will enjoy peace only when they become parts of a social system that embraces them.[8] It is not necessary to destroy national loyalties, only to include them. In Angell's words, "The social system which is painfully coming to birth will grow out of national states, but their structures will not be annihilated in the process." J. C. Flugel has made the same point: "We must probably agree that intra-group behavior is on the whole far more moral than inter-group behavior; and in so far as the latter is moral it is often because the groups in question are for certain purposes themselves members of a larger group, so that it can at bottom be reduced to behavior of the intra-group variety." [9]

Such conclusions are based on a considerable amount of historical and contemporary research. This research, broadly speaking, indicates the relative futility of the moral creeds and strategies that are hortatory, authoritarian, hedonistic, legalistic or utopian. To abolish war, some of these theories have said: *Let us give up our prejudices, our malice and our fear. Let us remove barriers to trade, to communications and travel. Let nations surrender land, money, aspirations, armaments, pride and sovereignty.* Though it is necessary that some of these subtractions take place, they will not do so if the approach is negative. Each and every local interest, deplored by us as making for international discord, serves a legitimate purpose so long as no social system exists to transcend nationhood. To state the case psychologically, individuals who favor the conditions making for war do so because they have no embracing circle of loyalties or expectations that would render these present conditions maladaptive to their purposes. Conflicts of value are never solved by the process of direct collision or defeat, nor by the double-edged subtraction that comes through compromise, but only through a process of inclusion and decentering.

Although the subtractive, authoritarian, legalistic and utopian moralities still prevail, we view with hope certain signs of progress. The United Nations, of course, is organized for the express purpose of resolving conflict through the enlargement of interest systems. True, its major activities seem for the present to be hopelessly blocked by a centering on national interests. There are even signs of regress in the present violent upsurge of national, religious and linguistic provincialism. So we must count our gains humbly: evidences of regional grouping and of increased student and personnel exchanges (though evaluative studies of this policy seem to show somewhat less gain than we might hope).[10] We note progress against illiteracy—progress that eventually may establish a firmer ground for communication. International meetings of scientists and other scholars are all to the good; so, too, the Olympic games. But perhaps our firmest gain is the widening circle of enlightenment and discussion that our common problems have evoked.

Returning to Piaget's research for a moment, we can surely say of the average adult that cognitively and affectively he is potentially capable of considerable decentering. The average man has no difficulty at all thinking of himself as a member at one and the same time of his family, neighborhood, town, state and nation. Along the way he manages to include his church, lodge and friendship circles. The principle is thus established that larger loyalties do not clash so long as they allow for the maximum possible inclusion of smaller loyalties. Trouble, to be sure, arises when values conflict at the same level: a bigamist cannot comfortably apportion his loyalty between two wives, nor can a traitor serve two countries. But it is clearly within the capacity of men to continue the decentering process illustrated by Piaget's children and to go well beyond them. Empirically we can point, as Sorokin and Maslow have done, to individuals who have already realized this capacity.[11] Unfortunately, they are still relatively few in number.

Nothing that I have said is intended to detract from the positive values of rivalry, or of pride in one's kin and kind. Rival scientists struggle vigorously to prove their respective theories against their opponents, but they do so within the frame of loyalty to science as a whole. What is good in free enterprise comes from competition regulated by common loyalty to the rules of the game. One's pride in one's way of life is not incompatible with an attitude of "let both grow together until the harvest." To critics who reply that conflict is the essence of existence—that "to live is to struggle; to survive is to conquer"—we reply that we aim not to eliminate struggle but to establish it within a framework that will actually lead to survival in a fully human sense, not to extermination in a strictly literal sense.

Preparing the Individual

The root of the matter, of course, lies in the posture of the individual's mentality. Psychologists today like to speak of "cognitive style." Now, the style of mind that welcomes rivalry within the constraints of potential inclusion is marked by a kind of *tentativeness*.

It does not insist upon the absolute validity of its equations; it prefers a way of life without prescribing it for all; it possesses humor; it maintains its loyalties within an expanding and yet discriminating frame. Its judgments are tentative, its religion heuristic, its ultimate sentiment compassion. There are people with this outlook; and it is they who, in this period of rapid social change, give the world such stability as it possesses. Our problem is to increase their numbers.

On this particular problem I shall say only one thing at this time. The cognitive style I have defined is the precise opposite of the prejudiced style of life. The past decade or so has produced hundreds of studies of the sources and correlates of prejudice.[12] If the prejudiced style of life can be learned—and certainly it is not innate—then surely the tentative style (in Gandhi's term, the *equiminded* outlook) can also be acquired. There is no simple formula for teaching it, but the books lie open for those who can adapt current research to educational policy for the home, school and church. In the home there is much to be said for the method of the family conference wherein all the members, from the oldest to the articulate youngest, can seek a rational, inclusive plan for the fulfillment of their interests. In schools, I suggest that we discard if necessary up to 10 per cent of the present content and replace it with suitably chosen instruction and experience in the principle of integration of interests. The lesson should include classroom and playground activities, as well as studies in neighborhood, national and international experiments in inclusion. In my opinion, our knowledge to date warrants this deliberate change in educational policies.

Final Word

But, of course, our knowledge, solid as some of it is, has many deficiencies. Let me conclude by stating explicitly four implications of my remarks for a possible research program:

First: at the level of the individual person, we need to know much more about the frame of mind that I have called tentative or equiminded, for to me it seems to be the very essence of altruism. Research by Sorokin and by Maslow has given us valuable insights, but much more of the same order is needed.

Second: a problem of joint concern to psychology, anthropology and philosophy confronts us. The moral guideline we have laid down requires discrimination between root-desires and demands, between intrinsic values and instrumentals. It seems probable that the root-desires (not the demands) of men in all countries are very similar and therefore not incompatible. Hence, I advocate cross-cultural investigations that will compare men's motives in many lands, but always with a view to distinguishing their root-desires from their demands.

Third: how can we develop symbols of inclusion that will assist children, and citizens, and statesmen to look beyond the confines of egocentricity? Without images it is impossible to form attitudes. Our symbols today are overwhelmingly local and nationalistic. We continue to view our membership circles, as did Piaget's children, as lying side by side, not as concentric. We have few symbols of inclusion; but even if effective supranational symbols existed, they would have no magic property. Men's choices can be only among sequences they have known, and so our problem of training involves also the giving of experience, especially in childhood, that will enlarge the cognitive style and turn the mind automatically toward the integrative mode of handling conflict.

Finally: continued philosophical research is needed concerning the principle of enlargement of interests. The harmonious realization of abilities, interests and purposes is, of course, a familiar theme in philosophies as diverse as those of Plato, Spinoza, Kant, Dewey and Perry—to name but a few. What philosophy must now do, with the aid of social science, is to specify which inclusive sets of interest can best be achieved by which available techniques—in industry, in education and in statecraft. Philosophy has the further critical task of refining the principle and examining instances where it may not fully apply. I am aware that not all conflicts are easily brought under our formula. Yet the philosophical task, I am convinced, is one of refinement, not of refutation, for the principle of maximal inclusion has the overwhelming testimony of social science in its support.

REFERENCES

1. R. Likert, *Motivational dimensions in administration,* Ann Arbor: University of Michigan Press, 1951.
2. The story is told in F. Roethlisberger and W. J. Dickson, *Management and the worker,* Cambridge: Harvard University Press, 1939; and in S. D. Hoslett, *Human factors in management,* New York: Harper, 1946.
3. E. B. Holt, *The Freudian wish and its place in ethics,* New York: Holt, 1915; R. B. Perry, *Realms of value: a critique of human civilization,* Cambridge: Harvard University Press, 1954, Chap. 6.
4. See M. P. Follett, *Creative experience,* New York: Longmans, Green, 1924; and *The new state,* New York: Longmans, Green, 1920.
5. S. A. Stouffer *et al.,* *The American soldier,* Princeton: Princeton University Press, 1949, II, 178.

6. J. Piaget and A. Weil, "The development in children of the idea of the homeland and of relations with other countries," *Int. Soc. Sci. Bull.,* 1951, 3:561-78.

7. P. de Bie, "Certain psychological aspects of Benelux," *Int. Soc. Sci. Bull.,* 1951, 3:540-52.

8. R. C. Angell, "Discovering paths to peace," in *The nature of conflict,* New York: UNESCO, 1957, Chap. 4.

9. J. C. Flugel, "Some neglected aspects of world integration," in T. H. Pear (ed.), *Psychological factors of peace and war,* Hutchinson & Co., 1950, Chap. 6.

10. *J. Soc. Issues,* 1956, Vol. 12, No. 1; *Ann. Amer. Acad. Pol. Soc. Sci.,* 1954, Vol. 295.

11. P. A. Sorokin, *Altruistic love: a study of American good neighbors and Christian saints,* Boston: Beacon, 1950; A. H. Maslow, *Motivation and personality,* New York: Harper, 1954. See also P. A. Sorokin (ed.), *Forms and techniques of altruistic and spiritual growth,* Boston: Beacon, 1954.

12. G. W. Allport, *The nature of prejudice,* Cambridge: Addison-Wesley, 1954.

CHAPTER 12

The psychology of participation

American psychology bears the stamp of American democracy. Its assumptions, its directions of research, its applications are consonant with the American creed. We cannot escape this value frame, nor do we wish to do so. On the contrary, it is a valid concern of psychology to identify those qualities of a citizen which prepare him to play his role in a participant democracy.

This essay is the chairman's address to the Society for the Psychological Study of Social Issues, delivered at Columbia University in September 1944 and published in the *Psychological Review* (1945). It bears an Author's Note:

"Were it customary for the Chairman to dedicate his address, I should offer my remarks in honor of John Dewey. He more than any other scholar, past or present, has set forth as a psychological problem the common man's need to participate in his own destiny."

John Dewey has shown that psychological theories are profoundly affected by the political and social climate prevailing in any given time and place. For example, an aristocracy produces no psychology of individual differences, for the individual is unimportant unless he happens to belong to the higher classes.[1] Dualistic psychology flourishes best when one group holds a monopoly of social power and wishes to do the thinking and planning, while others remain the docile, unthinking instruments of execution.[2] And apologists for the status quo are the ones who most readily declare human nature to be unalterable.

"The ultimate refuge of the stand-patter in every field," he declares, ". . . has been the notion of an alleged fixed structure of mind."[3] It was no accident that psychological hedonism flourished as a justification for nineteenth-century *laissez faire*; or that reflexology, blended with dialectical materialism, dominated Russian psychology after 1917. All of us watched with dismay the abrupt perversion of German psychological science after 1933.[4] With such evidence before us, can we doubt that American psychology too bears its own peculiar stamp of political and social dependency?

It is not my purpose to determine whether social and economic determinism has been decisive in the history of psychology, or whether the facts about human nature must be true regardless of any politico-ethical frame that we may hold. Dewey boldly declares that democracy and sound psychology are forever coextensive, that it is impossible to have one without the other. He would frankly banish all psychological postulates that are not democratically oriented.[5] Alluring as this whole problem is, let us limit our consideration to one distinctive, culturally conditioned feature of American psychology.

A Motorized Psychology

The genius of American psychology lies in its stress upon action—or, in slightly dated terminology, upon the motor phase of the reflex arc. Of all the schools of psychological thought we might name, only behaviorism, in both its muscle-twitch and its operational versions, is primarily American. Functionalism is American (rather than German or British) chiefly in its motor emphasis. Capacity psychology and mental testing in America deal primarily with accomplishment, activity and performance. The individual differences that are said to be a typical American interest have to do chiefly with measurable operations. We seldom record, for example, an individual's unique and subjective pattern of thought-life.

Of the many potential lines of development laid down in James's *Principles* over fifty years ago, the threads that were picked up were the radical motor elements. In the hands of Holt, Washburn and Langfeld, they led to a *motor theory of consciousness;* in the hands of Dewey, to a psychology of *conduct, adjustment* and *habit.* James himself established *pragmatism,* a doctrine that invites attention almost exclusively to the motor consequences of mental life. When James waxed ethical, as he frequently did, his moral advice was generally: "If you really care about something, you should *do* something about it." Even Josiah Royce, whose thought is often said to be the opposite of James's, agreed (like a good American) with his emphasis on *action.* Loyalty, said Royce, "is complete only in motor terms, never in merely sentimental terms. It is useless to call my feelings loyal unless my muscles somehow express this loyalty. . . . Nobody can be effectively loyal unless he is highly trained on the motor side." [6]

Returning on every ship from Europe, in the first decades of this century, were fresh young American *Doktoranden.* Their intellectual luggage was filled with European theories and concepts. But when unpacked at our motor-minded laboratories, these importations looked alien and were promptly subjected to a strenuous course in Americanization. *Feelings of innervation,* for example, were promptly dubbed outlandish. *Innervation* would do; feelings were *de trop. Ideo-motor* theory arrived and, though given a hospitable welcome by James, made little headway. *Ideas,* as the sovereign source of movement, smacked too much of the divine rights of Herbart. When *ideas* were offered to American psychologists, they commonly replied, "Keep them: stimulus and response will do quite nicely, thank you." *Empathy* arrived in a portmanteau packed in Munich. It was embedded in a whole self-psychology and in an epistemology of *Wissen von fremden Ichen.* Everything went into the ash can, save only a greatly oversimplified version of what Lipps originally intended. *Motor mimicry* was all we wanted. What would we be doing with a "mental act that held a guarantee of the objectivity of our knowledge"?

Importations in the psychology of thought were so roughly handled that they scarcely survived at all. What was *unanschaulich* in Würzburg became *anschaulich* at Cornell. To think without images seemed mildly treasonable; but to think *with* them gradually became unpatriotic. Better to think with our larynx, hands and viscera—or better still, in recent years, with our action currents. To explain volition in Würzburg, an impalpable decision factor, a *Bewusstheit,* was needed. But it all became so much simpler in Berkeley —a mere matter of rat vibrissae quivering with VTE at a choice point in a maze.

Other transformations were equally drastic. Of the countless dimensions for the study of personality proposed by Stern, the IQ alone was picked up. Wertheimer died perplexed by the selective attention Americans were paying to the visible, tangible portions of his work.[7] The entire *Geisteswissenschaft* is known in this country chiefly through an absurd little pencil-and-paper test leading to the inevitable profile. Small wonder that Spranger exclaimed, "Die grösste Gefahr Deutschland's ist die Amerikanisierung." [8]

One might think that phenomenology, since it derives from *Akt* psychology, might take hold in this country. But *mental* acts are not popular; it is *motor* acts that count. Or one might suppose that Americans would take to *intentionality,* a concept dealing with the orientation of the subject toward an object from which one might predict his future action. But such a concept is still too subjective; it is hard for us to even understand what it means. *Attitude* we will admit—if it can be operationally defined—but intentionality is just too Central European.

In short, we Americans have motorized psychology. Our theories of human nature transform meditative functions into active functions. The process clearly reflects the demand of our culture that inner life issue quickly and visibly into tangible success—that closures be reached both overtly and swiftly.

Do I seem to deplore the one-sidedness of our approach? I do not mean to. Quite the contrary: it is our way of going at things. Our preference for action, for objectivity, has carried us to new levels of attainment and will carry us still further. In the future, European models will be followed even less than formerly. What we produce must be indigenous within our culture and must harmonize with our active orientation. Especially in social psychology, I think, our derivations from Europe are virtually at an end. What may have been valid in Wundt, Durkheim, Le Bon, Tarde and Pareto will find better expression in the fresher, behavioral approach of America.

It will do so, that is, if our psychology of social action expands to give fuller play to the activities of the total organism than has been customary in the past. Even though subjective categories do not appeal, we need to find better ways of linking our psychology of action to the central regions of personality. Up to now, little progress has been made in this direction.

Motor Activity and Higher Mental Processes

True, American psychologists have to their credit the discovery that motor activity plays a pivotal role in higher mental functions. Take, as an example, *learning*: we have repeatedly insisted that learning is not passive absorption but an active response. In the classic experiment by Gates, learning scores jumped 100 per cent when four-fifths of the subject's time was devoted to recitation rather than to passive reading.[9] Haggard and Rose, reviewing many learning studies, including those that have to do with the simple conditioning of reflexes, report that in all cases learning seems to be facilitated if the subject himself overtly takes part, perhaps by turning the switch that rings the conditioning bell, or by drawing a line to accompany the apparent movement of the autokinetic phenomenon, or even by clenching his fist while memorizing nonsense syllables. These authors generalize these studies under a *Law of Active Participation*: ". . . When an individual assumes an active role in a learning situation (a) he tends to acquire the response-to-be-learned more rapidly, and (b) these response-patterns tend to be more stably formed, than when he remains passive."[10]

How to permit such helpful motor activity in a classroom where fifty pupils are busy learning is a large-sized pedagogical problem. "The chief source of the 'problem of discipline' in schools," says Dewey, "is that the teacher has often to spend a larger part of the time in suppressing the bodily activities" of the children.[11] The situation is wholly abnormal: the teacher tries to divorce bodily activity from the perception of meaning, yet the perception of meaning is incomplete without full manipulation and adequate bodily movement.

Memory for material learned in school and college is notoriously poor, so poor that educators are forced to console themselves with the wistful adage that education is "what you have left when you have forgotten all you learned in school." Perhaps a few studious attitudes, a few analytical habits are left; but should content disappear from the mind as rapidly as it does? We know that content acquired through personal manipulation does not seem to evaporate so rapidly. I recently asked 250 college students to write down three vivid memories of their schoolwork in the eighth grade. Afterward I had them indicate whether the memories involved their own active participation in the events recorded. Were they reciting, producing, talking, playing, arguing; or were they passively listening, watching, not overtly involved? Three-quarters of the memories were for situations in which the subject himself was actively participating, even though the percentage of time actually spent in participation in the average eighth grade room must be small.

We may mention also the problem of voluntary control. Although America has contributed little enough to the psychology of volition, what it has contributed is typical—namely, the finding of Bair[12] and others that a large amount of excessive, and apparently futile, motor involvement is necessary before one can gain control voluntarily over a limited muscular segment of the body. We know that a considerable overflow of effort is needed before fine skills can be differentiated, and before the individual can develop any satisfactory degree of self-determination.

In the realm of modern therapy, self-propelled activity plays an increasing part as the "Rogers technique" becomes more and more widely applied.[13] Analogously, the Kenny treatment for infantile paralysis requires the patient to take more and more responsibility and to be more and more active. Otherwise, it is discovered, the suggestions given by the therapeutist will not accomplish their purpose.[14] Angyal refers to the universal experience of psychiatrists that healthy ideas can be easily conveyed to the patient on the intellectual level without the slightest benefit accruing. The difficulty is to induce a state in which the idea "permeates the personality and influences the behavior." [15] In World War II we learned the importance of reconditioning at the front—that is, of allowing the patient himself quickly to work out his *own* relations with the terrifying environment that shocked him.

Facing the problem of re-education in postwar Germany, Lewin pointed to the impossibility of ideological conversion until the requisite experience is available: "To understand what is being talked about, the individual has to have a basis in experience." No amount of verbal defining will convey the meaning of such concepts as "his Majesty's loyal opposition" or "fair play." To most Germans, loyalty is identified with obedience; the only alternative to blind obedience is lawless individualism and *laissez faire.*[16]

One of the chief problems confronting military government is to keep the inhabitants of liberated countries active in shaping their own destiny.[17] Handouts beget apathy, and apathy prevents an interest in one's own future. How much better it was for Parisians to retake their own city than for the Allies to have done all the work, handing over the finished product. In his excellent book *Mental hygiene,* Klein expresses the point: "Without action there is no shift from the wish to the deed. There is motive, but no purpose. There is yearning without striving; hence the potential self-improvement dies stillborn." [18]

Activity Versus Participation

Facts of this sort prove to us that people must be active in order to learn, and to store up efficient memories, to build voluntary control and to be cured when they are ill or restored when they are faint. But implied in much American work is the proposition that one activity is as good as any other activity. It is *random* movement, according to much of our learning theory, that brings the organism to an eventual solution. And, according to one experimentalist, "If the body muscles are tense, the brain reacts much more quickly and intensely, if they are relaxed, it may react weakly or not at all." [19] The implication seems to be that tenseness of any kind makes for mental alertness. Activity as such is approved.

Random movement theories of learning, muscular tension theories of efficiency, speed theories of intelligence and motor theories of consciousness do not make a distinction that seems to me vital—

namely, the distinction between mere *activity* and true, personal *participation*.

Before we examine this distinction as it affects psychological theory and practice, I should like to point out that the selfsame distinction occurs in the economic and social life of the common man. Take, for example, Citizen Sam, who moves and has his being in the great activity wheel of New York City. He spends his hours of unconsciousness somewhere in the badlands of the Bronx. He wakens to grab the morning's milk left at the door by an agent of a vast dairy and distributing system, whose corporate maneuvers, so vital to his health, never consciously concern him. After paying hasty respects to his landlady, he dashes into the transportation system, whose mechanical and civic mysteries he does not comprehend. At the factory he becomes a cog for the day in a set of systems far beyond his ken. To him, as to everybody else, the company he works for is an abstraction. He plays an unwitting part in the "creation of surpluses"; and, though he doesn't know it, his furious activity at his machine is regulated by the "law of supply and demand," "the availability of raw materials" and "the prevailing interest rates." Unknown to himself, he is headed next week for the "surplus labor market." A union official collects his dues; just why, Sam doesn't know. At noontime that corporate monstrosity, Horn and Hardart, swallows him up, much as he swallows one of its automatic pies. After more activity in the afternoon, he seeks out a standardized daydream produced in Hollywood to rest his tense but *not* efficient mind.

Sam has been active all day, immensely active, playing a part in dozens of impersonal cycles of behavior. He has brushed against scores of corporate personalities, but has entered into intimate relations with no single human being. The people he has met are idler-gears like himself, meshed into systems of transmission and far too distracted to examine any one of the cycles in which they are engaged. Throughout the day Sam is on the go, implicated in this task and that —but does he, in a psychological sense, *participate* in what he is doing? Although constantly *task-involved*, is he ever really *ego-involved*?

This problem is familiar to all of us, and one of the most significant developments of the past two decades is its entrance into both industrial and social psychology. The way the problem has been formulated by industrial psychologists is roughly this: the individual's desire for personal status is apparently insatiable. Whether we say that he longs for prestige, self-respect, autonomy or self-regard, a dynamic factor of this order is apparently the strongest of his drives. Perhaps it is an elementary organismic principle, as Angyal [20] and Goldstein [21] would have it; perhaps it is, rather, a distillation of more primitive biological drives, with social competitiveness somehow added to the brew. For our purposes, the distinction does not matter.

The industrial psychologist has discovered that when the work-situation in which the individual finds himself realistically engages the status-seeking motive—when the individual is busily engaged in using his talents, understanding his work and having pleasant social relations with foreman and fellow-worker—then he is, as the saying goes, "identified" with his job. He likes his work; he is absorbed in it; he is productive. In McGregor's term, he is industrially *active*. That is to say, he is participant. [22]

When, on the other hand, the situation is such that the status-motive has no chance of gearing itself into the external cycles of events, when the individual goes through motions that he does not find meaningful, when he does not really participate—then come rebellion against authority, complaints, griping, gossip, rumor, scapegoating and disaffection of all sorts. The job satisfaction is low. In McGregor's term, under such circumstances the individual is not active; he is industrially *reactive*.

In the armed forces, in federal employment, in school systems, the same principle holds. Ordinarily, those at the top find that they have sufficient comprehension, sufficient responsibility and sufficient personal status. They are not the ones who gripe and gossip. It is the lower-downs who indulge in tendency-wit against the brass hats, complain, go AWOL, become inert or gang up against a scapegoat. In actual combat, all the energies, training and personal responsibility of which a soldier is capable are called upon; egos are engaged for all they are worth. Men are then active; they have no time to be reactive—nor have they reason to be.

Accepting this analysis as correct, the problem before us is whether the immense amount of reactivity shown in business offices and factories, in federal bureaus and in schools, can be reduced, as it is when men at the front are using all their talents and are participating to the full in life-and-death combat.

We are learning some of the conditions in which reactivity does decline. Friendly, unaffected social relations are the most indispensable condition. Patronizing handouts and wage-incentive systems alone do not succeed. Opportunities for consultation on personal problems are, somewhat surprisingly, found to be important;

and group decision, open discussion and the retraining of leaders in accordance with democratic standards yield remarkable results. One of Lewin's discoveries in this connection is especially revealing: people who dislike a certain food are resistant to pressure put upon them in the form of persuasion and request; but when the individual himself as a member of a group votes, after discussion, to alter his food-habits, his eagerness to reach this goal is independent of his personal like or dislike.[23] In other words, a person ceases to be reactive and contrary in respect to a desirable course of conduct only when he himself has had a hand in declaring that course of conduct to be desirable.

Such findings add up to the simple proposition that people must have a hand in saving themselves; they cannot and will not be saved from the outside.

In insisting that participation depends upon ego-involvement, it would be a mistake to assume that we are dealing with a wholly self-centered and parasitic ego which demands unlimited status and power for the individual himself.[24] Often, indeed, the ego is clamorous, jealous, possessive and cantankerous. But this is true chiefly when it is forced to be *reactive* against constant threats and deprivations. We all know of "power-people" who cannot, as we say, "submerge their egos." The trouble comes, I suspect, not because their egos are unsubmerged, but because they are still reactive toward some outer or inner features of the situation that are causing conflicts and insecurity. Reactive egos tend to perceive their neighbors and associates as threats rather than as collaborators.

But, for the most part, people who are participant in cooperative activity are just as much satisfied when a teammate solves a common problem as when they themselves solve it.[25] *Your* tensions can be relieved by *my* work, and my tensions by your work, provided we are co-participants. Whatever our egos were like originally, they are now, for the most part, socially regenerate. Selfish gratifications give way to cooperative satisfaction when the ego-boundaries are enlarged.

A revealing study by Leighton conducted at a Japanese relocation center during World War II makes this point clear.[26] When the Japanese were asked to pick cotton at nearby ranches to help save the crop, very few responded. The reason was that they were expected to donate all wages above $16.00 a month to a community trust fund, to be used for the common good. There was as yet insufficient community feeling; the over-all trust fund seemed too big, too distant, too uncertain. All that happened was endless argument for and against the trust fund, while the cotton stood in the fields. At this point, the schools asked to be allowed to go picking and to use the money for school improvements. This request was granted, and soon church groups, recreational societies and other community units showed themselves eager to go on the same basis. The project was a success.

What we learn from this study is that self-interest may not extend to include an object so remote and impersonal as a community trust fund, but may readily embrace school improvements and church and recreational centers. For most people there is plenty of ego-relevance to be found in teamwork, provided the composition of the team and its identity of interest are clearly understood. Thus Americans will endorse international cooperation in time of peace (and not only in time of war), provided they continue to see its relevance to their own extended egos, and provided they feel that in some way they themselves are participating in the decisions and activities entailed.

Nearly everyone will bear testimony to the superior satisfaction that comes from successful teamwork as contrasted to solitary achievement. Membership in a group that has successfully braved dangers and surmounted obstacles is a membership that is ego-involved, and the egos in question are not parasitic but socialized.

An important by-product of participation, as I am using the term, is the reduction of stereotypes. Sam's mind, we can be sure, is a clutter of false stereotypes concerning the dairy company, the transportation system, the abstract corporation for which he works and the economic laws and federal regulations that determine much of his routine, to say nothing of the tabloid conceptions begotten in Hollywood and by advertisers. If he really participated in his employment, his notions of "the Company," of surpluses and of labor unions would become realistic.

Participant Democracy

Even in a presidential election, only about three in every five eligible voters go to the polls. In a primary, the ratio is more likely to be one in every four. Yet voting is the irreducible minimum of participation in political democracy. People who do not vote at least once in four years are effectively nonparticipant; those who vote only in a presidential election—that is to say, at least a third of all voters —are scarcely better off. If we wished to complicate matters, we might ask whether those who go to the polls are really participating with the deeper layers of personality or whether their voting is, so to speak, a peripheral activity instigated perhaps by fanfare or by local bosses. It would not be hard to prove that participation in political affairs, as well as in industrial, educational and religious life, is rare. In this respect, most people resemble Citizen Sam.

Two social psychologists have concerned themselves deeply with this problem. They see that increasingly, since the days of the industrial revolution, individuals have found themselves in the grip of immense forces whose workings they have no power to comprehend, much less to influence. One of the writers, John Dewey, states the problem this way: "The ramification of the issues before the public is so wide and intricate, the technical matters involved are so specialized, the details are so many and so shifting, that the public cannot for any length of time identify and hold itself. It is not that there is no public, no large body of persons having a common interest in the consequences of social transactions. There is too much public, a public too diffused and scattered and too intricate in composition." [27]

Dewey spent many years seeking remedies for this situation. Chiefly he laid emphasis upon the need for face-to-face association, for evolving democratic methods within school and neighborhood so that citizens may obtain in their nerves and muscles the basic experience of relating their activities in matters of common concern. Some political writers, such as Mary P. Follett,[28] have held that the solution lies in reconstituting political groups on a small enough scale so that each citizen can meet face-to-face with other members of a geographical or occupational group, electing representatives who will in turn deal face-to-face with other representatives. Though the town may no longer be the best unit for operation, the spirit of the town meeting is thus to a degree recaptured. "Democracy," says Dewey, "must begin at home and its home is the neighborly community." [29]

Central to Dewey's solution also is freedom of publicity. To obstruct or restrict publicity is to limit and distort public opinion. The control of broadcasting and of the press by big advertisers is an initial source of distortion. Other groups need freer ventilation for their views in order to reduce rigidity, hostility and reactivity.

The second social psychologist, F. H. Allport, states the problem rather differently. He asks how an individual enmeshed within innumerable cycles of activity, all imposed upon him from without, can retain his integrity as a person. Like Sam, he finds himself a cog in countless corporate machines. State, county and federal governmental systems affect him, as do economic cycles, the impersonal systems known as private enterprise, conscription in wartime and social security. So, too, do city transportation, milk production and delivery, consumption, housing and banking. But he does not affect them. How can he?

F. H. Allport points to an inherent contradiction that seems to lie in Dewey's position.[30] The latter hopes that the individual will participate in every public that his own interests create in common with others. That is to say, Sam should join with others who are affected by the same municipal, banking, transportation, feeding and housing cycles. Together they should work out common problems. But Sam would be a member of hundreds of segmental types of public; and in dashing from one "common interest" meeting to another, he would not find his interests as an individual truly fulfilled. He would still be a puppet of many systems. As complexities increase under modern conditions, total inclusion of the personality in specialized publics becomes increasingly difficult to achieve.

Like Dewey, F. H. Allport has given various suggestions for the solution of the problem, but chiefly his emphasis has been upon the creation of a scientific spirit in the common man, encouraging him to call into question the corporate fictions and the sanctity of the economic cycles that, unthinkingly, he takes for granted. By questioning the transcendental reality commonly ascribed to nationhood, to "consumer competition" and to institutional fictions, and by substituting direct experience with the materials affecting his life, the individual can eventually work out a measure of integrity and wholeness within himself.[31]

Both Dewey and F. H. Allport seem to agree that the only alternative to a keener analysis of the behavioral environment and more active participation in reshaping it is to give way progressively to outer authority, uniformity, discipline and dependence upon the leader. This battlefield exists here and now within each of us. The answer to growing complexity in the social sphere is either renewed efforts at participation by each one of us, or else a progressive decline of inert and unquestioning masses, submitting to government by an elite that will have little regard for the ultimate interest of the common man.

Drawing together the threads of this problem, we are confronted with the following facts:

First: since the industrial revolution, there has been increasing difficulty on the part of the ordinary citizen in comprehending and affecting the forces that control his destiny.

Second: potentially the individual is a member of many, many publics, defined as groups of people having a common interest—as, for example, voters, motorists, veterans, employers, consumers or coreligionists.

Third: no public includes all of an individual's interests.

To these facts, we add our earlier conclusions:

Fourth: activity alone is not participation. Most of our fellow citizens spin as cogs in many systems without engaging their own egos even in those activities of most vital concern to them.

Fifth: when the ego is not effectively engaged, the individual becomes reactive. He lives a life of ugly protest, finding outlets in complaints, in strikes and above all in scapegoating. In this condition he is ripe prey for a demagogue whose whole purpose is to focus and exploit the aggressive outbursts of nonparticipating egos.

Toward a Solution

It is risky indeed to suggest in a few words the solution of such an immense social problem. Certainly it will require the combined efforts of educators, statesmen and scientists to rescue the common man from his predicament. But, from our preceding discussion, one line of thought stands out as particularly helpful.

Is it not true that all of us find coercive demands upon our motor systems imposed by the corporate cycles in which we move, generally *without* serious frustration resulting? Speaking for myself, only the outer layers of my personality are engaged in my capacity as automobile owner, insurance holder, Blue Cross member, consumer of clothing and patron of the local transit system. Perhaps I should be more interested in these cycles; but one must choose, and other things are more important to me. In this age of specialization, all of us are willing to delegate expert functions to experts. We simply cannot be bothered about the innumerable technical aspects of living that are not our specialty. In matters of broad political or ethical policy-making, the story is different; we cannot so easily avoid responsibility. Political reforms making possible good schools, recreation and health are presumably the concern of all people. National policy in securing a lasting peace is a matter of great moment for each one of us. But even among these broad social and political issues I find some that excite me more than others.

Thus I cannot share Dewey's dismay at our failure to create innumerable self-conscious publics wherever there are common interests. These publics need operate only on the broadest policy-forming level, and a relatively few members of a group can often serve adequately as representatives of others who are like-minded. I do not mean that a few public-spirited citizens should do all the work. There should be wider distribution of responsibility. But talents differ, and what warms one ego chills another.

Assuming that the major fields of activity open to all normal people are the economic, the educational, the recreational, the political, the religious and the domestic, we might assert that a healthy ego should find true participation in all of them. Or, allowing one blind spot to the bachelor, the constitutional hater of sports or of politics and the agnostic, there is still need for a balanced diet of participation in, say, five fields.

Against some such norm we might test our present situation. Do we find Citizen Sam truly participating in some *one* political undertaking? In some *one* of his economic contacts—preferably, of course, in his job, where he spends most of his time? Is he really involved in *some* religious, educational and recreational pursuits, and in family affairs? If we find that he is not actively involved in all these areas of participation, we may grant him a blind spot or two. But unless he is in some areas ego-engaged and participant, his life is crippled and his existence a blemish on democracy.

In brief, it is neither possible nor desirable that all of our activities and contacts in our complex social order should penetrate beneath the surface of our personalities. But unless we try deliberately and persistently to affect our destinies at certain points, especially where broad political policies are concerned and in some of the other representative areas of our life, we are not democratic personalities. We then have no balance or wholeness, and society undergoes proportionate stultification.

New Directions for Social Psychology

Returning to our starting point, my contention is that the earlier emphasis of American psychology on motor activity as such is now changing into an emphasis upon ego-involved participation. As time goes on, it will mark increasingly the essential differences that exist between movement initiated at the surface level and that initiated at the deeper levels of personality.[32] To do so will not be to abandon our dependence on the social climate in which we work. Quite the contrary: at last the genius of American psychology will be brought into line with the century of the common man.[33]

What, concretely, are the roles that psychologists will play in this process? Several can already be fairly well defined:

To those who serve in some consulting or guidance capacity, Citizen Sam will come as a client. He will have this symptom or that —perhaps resentment, depression, bewilderment or apathy. Among college students, one study suggests that 20 per cent are apathetic, complaining that they have no values whatever to live by. It calls for great therapeutic skill to lead such clients to commit themselves unreservedly to something. I have suggested that a balanced personality needs deep-rooted participation in all or most of the six spheres of value: political, economic, recreational, religious, educational and domestic. But commitments cannot be too comprehensive. It is not politics or economics as a whole that evokes participation, but merely some one limited and well-defined issue in the total sphere. The democratic personality needs to influence *some* but not all of the factors that influence him in representative fields of his activity.

The consultant may go one step further. Sam should not only feel that he is a citizen participating at crucial points in common activities; he should be oriented as well, toward the inner crises such as will occur in middle age, when his vitality recedes and his furious activity can no longer be sustained, when he faces old age and death itself. Sam, if I may put it this way, needs to find that metaphors and images are ultimately more important than motor gyrations. The consulting psychologist has responsibility for encouraging subjective richness in personality. For, in the broader sense, participation extends beyond the days when active citizenship is possible. The ego needs to be wholesomely attached to life, even after efficiency of action declines.

Industrial psychologists and group workers have already found a rewarding line of work in educating management, foremen and employees about the conditions that increase efficiency through participation in the job. The same type of effort is also yielding returns in other directions, especially in recreational and educational enterprises.

As teachers, both in college and in adult centers, we have a job to do in encouraging the participation of the public in the progress of science itself. The layman now finds it impossible to keep pace with science. Dazed by the benefits of television, auto, airplane and vitamins, all of which regulate his life, he stands on the side lines and cheers as the procession of science goes by. He has little real contact with the material from which his life is fashioned. Exhibitions, demonstrations and simplified experiments will help him understand.[34] But the layman needs even more: he needs to know how to *control* the applications of science. While bestowing upon him many blessings, science has also given its bounty to tyrants and to the self-appointed elite, with the result of fabulous fortunes for the few, slums and squalor for the many, violent wars and suffering beyond endurance. The common man has not chosen these consequences. He was never consulted, was never participant in guiding the applications of science.

Half a century ago, psychologists characteristically ascribed to the personality certain governing agencies: the will, the soul, the self, the moral sentiments or some other ruling faculty. Subsequent emphasis upon the motor processes, especially in America, resulted in a kind of entropy for personality. Being deprived of its self-policing functions, personality seemed to dissolve into endless cycles of motor activity controlled by stimulus or by habit. Like a taxicab, its successive excursions had little relation to one another. Then, gradually, some principles of self-regulation returned to psychology, a bit timidly and not too clearly, under the guise of *integration, vigilance* and *homeostasis.*

Ego-functions, too, were introduced, to provide for a recentering of personality with an increase in its stability. Ego-functions, as I have shown elsewhere, are of many kinds, and the ego is susceptible of many definitions.[35] Perhaps the most important distinction concerns *reactive* ego-functions, which are resistant, contrary and clamorous, as opposed to *active* ego-functions, which find full expression in participant activity. When participating, the individual discovers that his occupational manipulations grow meaningful; his community contacts are understood and appreciated. He becomes interested in shaping many of the events that control his life.

Participation, as opposed to peripheral motor activity, sinks a shaft into the inner subjective regions of the personality. It taps central values. Thus, in studying participation, the psychologist has an approach to the complete person.

Random movement, derived from the sensori-motor layer of the personality, has too long been our paradigm for the behavior of man. It fails to draw the essential distinction between aimless activity and participation. The concept of random movement denies dignity to human nature; the concept of participation confers dignity. As American psychology increasingly studies the conditions of participation it will elevate its conception of human nature, an event, we can be sure, that will at last gratify the man in the street.

In focusing upon problems of participation social psychology will also be advancing democracy, for, as Dewey has shown, the task of obtaining from the common man participation in matters affecting his own destiny is the central problem of democracy.

REFERENCES

1. J. Dewey, *Psychology as philosophic method*, Berkeley: University Press, 1899.

2. J. Dewey, *Human nature and conduct*, New York: Holt, 1922, p. 72.

3. J. Dewey, "The need for social psychology," *Psychol. Rev.*, 1917, 24:273.

4. F. Wyatt and H. L. Teuber, "German psychology under the Nazi system—1933-1940," *Psychol. Rev.*, 1944, 51:229-47.

5. G. W. Allport, "Dewey's individual and social psychology," in P. A. Schilpp (ed.), *The philosophy of John Dewey*, Evanston: Northwestern University Press, 1939, Chap. 9, especially pp. 281, 283, 290.

6. J. Royce, *Race questions, provincialism, and other American problems*, New York: Macmillan, 1908, pp. 239, 241.

7. W. Köhler, "Max Wertheimer: 1880-1943," *Psychol. Rev.*, 1944, 51:143-46.

8. Cf. E. Spranger, *Kultur und Erziehung*, Leipzig: Quelle & Meyer, 1923, p. 199.

9. A. I. Gates, "Recitation as a factor in memorizing," *Arch. Psychol.*, 1917, Vol. 6, No. 40.

10. E. A. Haggard and R. J. Rose, "Some effects of mental set and active participation in the conditioning of the autokinetic phenomenon," *J. Exp. Psychol.*, 1944, 34:56.

11. J. Dewey, *Democracy and education*, New York: Macmillan, 1919, p. 165.

12. J. H. Bair, "Development of voluntary control," *Psychol. Rev.*, 1901, 8:474-510.

13. C. R. Rogers, *Counseling and psychotherapy*, Boston: Houghton Mifflin, 1942.

14. C. Bohnengel, "An evaluation of psycho-biologic factors in the re-education phase of the Kenny treatment for infantile paralysis," *Psychosom. Med.*, 1944, 6:82-87.

15. A. Angyal, *Foundations for a science of personality*, New York: Commonwealth Fund, 1941, p. 326.

16. K. Lewin, "The special case of Germany," *Publ. Opin. Quart.*, 1943, 7:555-66.

17. G. W. Allport, "Restoring morale in occupied territory," *Publ. Opin. Quart.*, 1943, 7:606-17.

18. D. B. Klein, *Mental hygiene*, New York: Holt, 1944, p. 319.

19. A. G. Bills, *The psychology of efficiency*, New York: Harper, 1943, p. 23.

20. A. Angyal, *op. cit.*

21. K. Goldstein, *Human nature in the light of psychopathology,* Cambridge: Harvard University Press, 1940.

22. D. McGregor, "Conditions of effective leadership in the industrial organization," *J. Consult. Psychol.,* 1944, 8:55-63.

23. K. Lewin, "The dynamics of group action," *Educ. Leadership,* 1944, 1:195-200.

24. H. D. Spoerl, "Toward a knowledge of the soul," *The New Phil.,* 1944, 47:71-81.

25. H. B. Lewis, "An experimental study of the role of the ego in work. I. The role of the ego in coöperative work," *J. Exp. Psychol.,* 1944, 34:113-26

26. A. H. Leighton, *et al.,* "The psychiatric approach in problems of community management," *Amer. J. Psychiat.* 1943, 100:328-33.

27. J. Dewey, *The public and its problems,* New York: Holt, 1927, p. 137.

28. M. P. Follett, *Creative experience,* New York: Longmans, Green, 1924.

29. J. Dewey, *The public and its problems,* op. cit., p. 213.

30. F. H. Allport, *Institutional behavior,* Chapel Hill: University Press, 1933, Chap. 5.

31. F. H. Allport, "The scientific spirit and the common man," *Proc. Conf. on Sci. Spirit & Dem. Faith,* New York: 2 West 64th St., 1944.

32. See Chapter 5 of the present volume.

33. C. J. Friedrich, "The role and the position of the common man," *Amer. J. Sociol.,* 1944, 69:421-29.

34. F. H. Allport, "The scientific spirit and the common man," *op. cit.*

35. See Chapter 5 of the present volume.

CHAPTER 13

A basic psychology of love and hate

The human hunger to give and to receive love is insatiable. No one ever feels that he can love or be loved enough. Yet this root fact of human nature is seldom acknowledged or studied by psychologists.

The present essay attempts to explain the curious neglect. It examines the evidence and proposes a theory to advance our understanding of affiliative motives and of their pathological distortion into hate.

Originally an address at the Conference on Educational Problems of Special Culture Groups, held at Teachers College, Columbia University, in September 1949, the essay was printed in its present form in *Explorations in altruistic love and behavior,* edited by Pitirim A. Sorokin (1950).

> *While it is inevitable that self-love should be positive and active in every man, it is not inevitable, and it is very far from necessary, that it should be sovereign with him.*
> —Theophilus Parsons

A persistent defect of modern psychology is its failure to make a serious study of the affiliative desires and capacities of human beings. If I am not mistaken, only two sustained theories concerning their nature have been developed. Both seem to me somewhat abortive. One is the approach of those writers who postulate a *gregarious instinct.* This pallid conception turned out to give us little more than a name and, at the hands of McDougall and Trotter, led nowhere in particular except into a curious kind of British chauvinism. The other approach is that of Freud, who, with an oddly limited perspective, contrived to reduce affiliative motives to sexuality—a blunder that even the ancient Greeks, with their distinction between *eros* and *agape,* knew enough to avoid.

The "Flight from Tenderness"

Why psychologists, by and large, have side-stepped the problems of human attachment is an interesting question. Ian Suttie speaks of it as their "flight from tenderness." He believes that, in repudiating theology, modern mental science overreacted and deliberately blinded itself to the tender relationships in life so strongly

199

emphasized by Christianity.[1] Somehow it feels more tough-minded to study discord. The scientist fears that, if he looks at affiliative sentiments, he may seem sentimental; if he talks about love, he may seem emotional; and if he studies personal attachments, he may appear personal. Better leave the whole matter to poets, saints or theologians.

Besides overreacting against theology, the psychologist has, of course, a well-grounded suspicion of hypocrisy and of rationalization. Protestations of friendliness, he knows, do not always signify friendliness; they are often a mask for more basic conditions of bitterness and hate. His fear of appearing pious is not altogether a matter of yielding to a currently fashionable scientific taboo. He knows the error that lies in rationalized accounts of human motivation.

But there is yet another reason, still more fundamental, for this flight from tenderness. Desires for affiliation are—as I shall try to show—the inescapable groundwork of human life. As such they are quite naturally overlooked, for normally we do not perceive groundwork at all; we notice only the superimposed figures. The white page of the book I am reading fails to interest me; it is merely the necessary ground for the black type that I perceive. And is it not always the waterspout, rather than the otherwise calm surface of the sea, that rivets our attention? Alfred North Whitehead has pointed out that we do not even have words with which to describe what is always with us; we tend to take the ubiquities of our lives for granted and never feel the need to discuss them. It is for this reason, I think, that we pay so little attention to the prior state of concord that alone confers meaning on discord. Even the expressions of the human face illustrate the principle I am discussing: the emotion of love brings a wholly relaxed, "neutral" set to the musculature of the face. By contrast, anger, jealousy and hate are well-figured expressions. In the human face, as in life itself, it is far easier to identify and to fix for study the manifestations of intolerance and hate than the manifestations of love and tolerance: these are taken for granted.

In their theories of motivation, psychologists have been misled by this figure-ground relationship. They see antagonism as more salient and exciting than good will—and, of course, it is. Hostile emotions are warlike emotions, stimulating to the possessor and visible to the observer. Frustration and aggression interest the psychologist, but not friendship and trust. Yet it is unescapably true that hostility derives its very existence from the prior groundwork of affiliative desire with which it so sharply contrasts. Unless one first loves, one cannot hate. For hatred is an emotion of protest, directed always toward real or imagined obstructions that prevent one from reaching objectives that are positively valued—that is, loved.

The Trend in Research Findings

Although psychologists are backward in their conceptualizations of the affiliative needs of mankind, they have recently shed considerable empirical light on the nature of these needs. Modern techniques of research in the study of human relations are being profitably employed in many different kinds of groups—in the classroom, in the community, in industry. It is pleasing to watch the results of research converge. A common thread seems to run through every set of findings; before long, we may hope, this thread will lead to unifying theory.

In industrial research, investigations have been particularly fruitful. They have made it clear that management has been guilty in the past of disastrous blunders in its relations with employees. For one thing, management formerly assumed that men could be best motivated by fear and punishment. If employees came late to work, fines were levied; if they spoiled material or disobeyed rules, they paid more fines. Afraid of losing their jobs, they toed the line at the command of foremen who, more likely than not, were saturated with an authoritarian view of their own status. The policy worked so badly that industries began to give rewards and to make concessions. But these inducements had the flavor of patronage and raised the workers' expectations, rather than their morale. Psychologically, the blunder was that the rewards did not grow directly out of the workers' own activity, but were arbitrary in character, being conferred by the employer rather than generated by the work process. Rest periods, bonuses and badges are extrinsic to the work situation. Industry then tried to improve matters through time and motion studies; but such "efficiency management" does not touch the human problem. Finally, in despair, industry often multiplied its efficiency and personnel departments until the plant developed a Goliath of bureaucracy—all to no avail. Industrial relations were not improved.

Then came the modern period of research. It did not take long to discover the source of the trouble. Workers, it turns out, like jobs that are free from condescension and overclose supervision, give free play to their talents, give credit for work done, allow them to participate in decisions affecting themselves, bring together small teams of congenial co-workers and permit personal growth and advancement.

Whether investigations are conducted in factories, in business offices, in schools, in camps or in the armed forces—the same pattern of findings always emerges. People want to remain integrated human beings in a work situation, as well as at home. It is the whole individual who goes to school, to work or to war. He desires congenial, informal relations with his fellows and wants to participate in his own destiny. And he will not for long tolerate patronage.

The common thread that emerges seems to have two interwoven strands. People in any form of human association wish to preserve their self-esteem—their self-love, if you wish—and simultaneously to have warm, affiliative relations with their fellows. No one seems initially to want to hate. But hatred, none the less, grows up in many lives as a consequence of blocked self-esteem and blocked affiliation.

I dip again into research. Stouffer's extended study of the motivation of soldiers in combat in World War II revealed that the affiliative motive, even under extreme stress, seems to hold twice as many men to their task as does the motive of hate. The only reported form of help that exceeded the desire not to let other men down was religious. Fully three-quarters of the soldiers reported that prayer "helped a lot"—and prayer obviously reflects some deep affiliative (certainly not a destructive) desire.[2]

For the moment, these few examples drawn from modern research may serve our purposes.[3] They indicate that men are basically eager for friendly and affiliative relations with others, provided these relations preserve their own sense of integrity and self-esteem. Thus a double finding must be taken into account in our theorizing: people want close, warm, loving relationships with their fellows—but, at the same time, they are exceedingly sensitive to slights to their *amour-propre*. Indignity to one's self-esteem quickly generates hatred.

Here, then, is our dilemma: neither our economic nor our political life is arranged to accommodate this dual pattern of need. Except in limited ways, chiefly within the family, opportunities are not provided for the expression of the craving for love—to give and to receive. Nor is the maintenance of self-respect a serious concern of our economic and political institutions. Since the affiliative needs are so badly met, we must not be surprised to find reactivity, hostility and anxiety as the most common by-products of our social relationships. Though people want love above all else, prejudice and hostility take command of their lives. One study establishes the fact that group prejudice is an appreciable factor in the mental life of perhaps four-fifths of the American population.[4] Yet the affiliative need remains somehow basic.

Such being our quandary, it behooves us to study far more closely than we have in the past the place of love and hate in human personality, and to pay particular attention to the swift and easy manner in which hostility comes so readily to take over the management of a life.

The Nature of Love and Hate

Up to now, it is the philosophers who have formulated our major theories of love and hate. We think first, of course, of Empedocles, the pre-Socratic, who tells us that love and hate are cosmic forces—the only cosmic forces that exist. They act upon the material elements of the earth, from which they fashion harmonious and inharmonious creations. From the time of Empedocles onward, we find the history of philosophy haunted by the dialectic of love and hate. Always hate has been regarded as a less desirable emotion than love, as a disruptive and dangerous emotion unless mastered. When the Christian religion came along, it gave absolute sanction to love and absolute dissanction to hate. Perhaps it was the very severity of this sanction that led science, as Suttie suggests, to avoid the subject.

Though many philosophers have emphasized equally, as did Empedocles, the forces of love and of hate in the process of life, there is a distinct tendency among many of them to regard hatred and its attendant aggressions as somehow more fundamental. The influential Hobbes did so. To him, mortals are by their very nature impelled to seek honor, precedence, glory. We are driven above all else by "a perpetual and restless desire of power after power that ceaseth only in death." This "state of nature" leads all men to aggress against each other, to condemn their fellows and to find them offensive. Hate, aversion and suspicion are far more easily engendered than are love and loyalty, for are not man's two fundamental passions vainglory and fear? To be sure, laws, customs and religion may keep an uncertain and uneasy control over us by invoking fear; but against this restraint our vainglory presses hard. Since, according to Hobbes, everyone wishes others to value him as highly as he does himself, a cycle of fierce competition is inaugurated. Men are truly equal in one respect: they are all highly satisfied with themselves.

A more modern writer, the French biologist Felix Le Dantec, goes still further: he declares egoism to be the only keystone in our social edifice. He who professes fondness for his fellows is a hypocrite. Machiavelli, La Rochefoucauld, Schopenhauer and Nietzsche all see irrevocable egoism in human nature. For them, only one form of love ultimately exists—self-love. If this basic assumption is sound, the outlook for improving human relations is dim. Rationalize our self-love as we will, we remain frauds. Human relations cannot be improved; they can only be prettified.

Now, nothing could be more important than to know whether this view of human nature is right or wrong. Some moralists, of course, have declared it wrong. Hume, for example, poured his scorn on the principle "that all benevolence is mere hypocrisy, friendship a cheat, public spirit a farce, fidelity a snare." To Hume there is a basic sociality in man that engenders a capacity for genuine sympathy and benevolence. Shaftesbury, Adam Smith and Kropotkin agree. But it gains us little to cite venerable authorities pro and con. What is more important is that nowadays we have become wholesomely critical of our own motives. We do not wish to prate of love if self-love is at the root of our behavior, or if sympathy is merely a mask for aggression. For this grace of self-criticism we have largely Freud to thank.

But Freud's picture of human motivation, though not so simple as Hobbes's, is basically similar: all of us have a primal instinct making for death and destruction. Aggressive urges are therefore as natural as the outpouring of hot lava from a volcano. Paralleling this destructive urge are the life instincts, whose representative is the sexual drive. Taken by itself, this drive may be regarded as constructive and binding in social relationships. In fact, the best we can hope for is that a child's sex life will so develop that the libidinal striving will somehow neutralize the destructive forces in his life.

But, alas, the two instincts (destruction and sex) often fuse. Aggression is intimately bound up with each stage of developing sexuality and, in Freudian theory, seems necessary in order that the sex impulses reach their aim. The fusion is so marked that all our benign human relations, including good leadership, good will, religion and our virtues generally, can be viewed best as mere "sublimations"—mere incidents, mere by-products—of sex and aggression. There is little indication in Freud, just as there is little in Hobbes, that the affiliative desire may be basic in the constitution of human nature.

Yet is it not obvious that, from the very moment of its inception, the business of life calls for adherence, for mutuality? *In utero* the mode of life is symbiotic: the associative relationship reigns supreme, and there is no evidence whatever of destructive instincts. After birth the affiliative attachment of the child to its environment still remains dominant—in nursing, playing, resting. The social smile early sym-

bolizes his contentment with people. Toward his entire environment
he is positive, approaching nearly every type of stimulus, every type
of person. From no human being does he by instinct withdraw. His
life is marked by eager adience. To be sure, in the process of relating
himself positively to his environment, the child may do damage and
may unwittingly violate the rights of others. A two-year-old is, in
one sense of the word, very destructive. But his depredations are
psychologically irrelevant to what he is trying to do. From his point
of view, he is greedily ingesting his environment, eagerly affiliating
with it—nothing more.

When negative emotions of fear and anger arise, they owe their
whole existence to the interruption of this zeal for approach. Affiliative tendencies, when threatened or frustrated, give way to alarm
and defense. Suttie puts the matter picturesquely: "Earth hath no
hate *but* love to hatred turned, and hell no fury but a baby
scorned." [5]

So obvious is the priority of affiliative groundwork that one must
perform contortions in order to give equal footing to the alleged aggressive instincts. Some psychoanalysts achieve the feat by assuming
that eating, perhaps the most conspicuous of an infant's activities, is
a destructive act—"oral aggression," it is called. Our primordial
ancestors, writes one Freudian, "were cannibals." "We all enter life
with the instinctive impulse to devour not only food, but also all
frustrating objects. Before the infantile individual acquires the capacity to love, it is governed by a primitive hate relationship to its
environment." [6] This statement precisely reverses the order of love
and hate in ontogenetic development. Furthermore, it inverts the
meaning of the act of feeding. When I devour roast beef, it is not
from hate but from love. Acts of incorporation into myself are, from
my point of view, affiliative.

The truest statement that can be made of a normal person is
that he never feels that he can love or be loved enough. He always
wants more love in his life. One reason why religion is an almost
universal attachment of mankind is that religion maintains the basic
love relationship of the individual with some embracing principle.
The major religions represent not only a free, indestructible attachment to one's Creator, but likewise the unattained ideal of the brotherhood of man. When we imagine a perfect state of being, we invariably imagine the unconditional triumph of love.

But the desire for love, when rejected or threatened, turns to
anxious fear. No one can remain indifferent if the bid he is making
for affiliation is rebuffed. A recent study of delinquent boys shows

that in virtually every case of incorrigible delinquency there was gross emotional inadequacy in the home. The boys were rejected by their parents or had parents incapable of providing affectional security. Their bid for affiliation was blocked; and, only half-aware of their misery, they turned as a means of defense to antisocial acts.[7] During the war a thirteen-year-old boy, rejected at home, "spat on the American flag and announced that the other boys were fools to believe in our government, that he was for Hitler and Nazism, and intended to become a traitor. 'I hate all Americans,' he added."[8] Children deprived of secure affection often rant against "dirty niggers," "Jew bastards" and other minority groups.

Misanthropy—I think we may now generalize—is always a matter of frustrated affiliative desire and the attendant humiliation to self-esteem. What is so fascinating psychologically is the displacement that frequently occurs in the resulting hatred. Few of the children in the research I have cited are aware of the source of their distress. Their hatred and aggression are fixed on irrelevant objects. That the process of displacement is subtle, a California research study on anti-Semitism abundantly shows. College girls high in prejudice, it was found, ordinarily profess complete love and respect for their parents—more so than do tolerant girls. But deeper study shows that their lives are marked by much buried hostility toward their parents. In spite of appearances, they do not have a free affiliative relation in the home; and, surprising as it may seem, their anti-Semitism reflects this situation.[9]

A study among war veterans has a similar result. In this investigation, a significant relation was discovered between the recollection of love and affection enjoyed in childhood and the present tolerance for minority groups. Veterans who reported that their parents were lacking in affection toward them were found far more often among the intolerant.[10] Granted that retrospective reports of affection in childhood are not fully reliable, this stricture does not affect the proposition before us. The very fact that the men in this study *reported* basic love disturbance shows that somehow in them a bitter wound existed, and this wound had a demonstrable relation to their later intolerance.

It is necessary here to add the caution that not all hatred is displaced. Conceivably, members of a minority group may be genuinely frustrating agents and may be hated or despised directly for the obstructions they create. Not all victims of prejudice are lily-white in their innocence; but, if we look closely at the process, we find that in almost every case they attract additional displaced animosity for which they are not conceivably to blame.

Hatred is a normal enough response whenever intensely held, positive values are threatened or destroyed. The threatened values may be self-love, or the desire to be loved, or altruistic love. The point is, as Suttie said, "There is no hatred but love to hatred turned." It is an error, therefore, to regard the numerous hostile sentiments of men as merely the outpouring of aggressive instincts. Since hate is a contingent phenomenon, it is, theoretically at least, avoidable. Actually, in proportion as man's affiliative needs are met, aggression and hostility disappear. To know this fact is the first requirement for improving human relations.

Are Love and Hate Instincts?

Since hatred is a contingent phenomenon, it is not proper to argue, as the Freudians do, that it stems from an instinct of aggression or of destruction. To be sure, hostility is a normal—seemingly almost a reflex—capacity of men when severe frustration blocks the affiliative trend in their behavior. But a capacity, though native, is not itself a drive in the sense that it must find an outlet for its energy.

But how do matters stand with what I have called the affiliative desires? I realize that I may seem to imply that here, at last, is the root instinct of life. If hate exists only when affiliation is threatened, must we not therefore assume that the affiliative need itself is primordial instinct? Psychological literature has many references to this possibility—to the instinct of gregariousness, to the parental instinct, to the "wish" for response, to the "need" for affiliation.

While I would agree to endorse a postulation of this order if it seems logically necessary, I feel compelled to point to the essential emptiness of all instinct formulae. An "instinct of love" could mean nothing more than that the nature of human life seems to require strong personal attachments. Regarding the nature of this need in the individual case, it says nothing. Nor does it allow for the myriad transformations that a person's attachments undergo, including the subtle interplay of self-love and socialized love. The really important questions concerning love—and concerning hate—are postinstinctive questions. It is always our contemporary attitudes, our present loyalties and aversions, that rule our behavior; not, as Freud and others maintain, unchangeable instinctual forces.[11] I do not believe that we can view the myriad forms of attachment and repulsion in the ever growing personality as merely so many channels of outlet for the permanent instincts of sex and aggression, or of gregariousness and love, or of anything else.

Motivation—it seems obvious to me—is always a contemporary process directed toward the future, comprising attitudes, beliefs and forms of adjustment that, in the individual's mind, bind him successfully to his world. There is a concrete character in motivation to which instinct doctrines cannot do justice. Starting fairly early in our lives, we are propelled, I maintain, not by instincts but by *interests*.

In the earliest months of life, a child develops systems of positive attachments. He loves his own mother, not someone else's. His initial, undifferentiated adience is quickly polarized by objects. He develops attachments to groups of which he is a member: his family, his church, his ethnic group—and later his lodge, his office and his own offspring. The love and loyalty are concrete. They are fashioned into sentiments, and these sentiments are learned. To say that a person's positive attachments are nothing but an adventitious channeling of an instinct is simply not helpful. It is the sentiments that are the ongoing, postinstinctive motives of the developing personality.

Hatred too is concrete. When a Negro child makes friendly advances to a white child and suffers a rebuff, and the humiliation turns into hate, shall we say that the instinct of aggression has become channelized? Or shall we say that a very particular attitude of resentment is built up, which becomes dynamic in its own right because the child must thereafter adjust to this new phase of his experience? The hatred did not exist until it was learned. Always the growing child learns specific sets of ideas concerning specific sets of people and builds his sentiments accordingly. It is these sentiments (not instincts) that thereafter guide his behavior. And these postinstinctive units in personality are basic to the understanding of human relations, for they alone specify the course that the individual will take.

Let me repeat that, if we wish, we can speak of an affiliative need or instinct and in this way universalize the phenomena we are discussing. It seems to me, however, a somewhat hollow procedure; for, in so doing, we are likely to overlook the fact that each person's life history is unique and that his motives are not strictly commensurable with those of other individuals. It is always the focalized forms of affiliation that concern us in dealing with concrete human beings.

How these postinstinctive units are developed is, of course, the riddle of learning—a subject we cannot here explore. We know that attitudes take shape partly under the pressure of conformity and imitation. We know that parents are the chief influences, but that educators likewise do their part, for good and for ill. We know that displacement and generalization loom large in the process. We know, too, that a curious projectivity marks all hostile attitudes: the person we dislike is almost always regarded as wholly to blame. It seldom occurs to us that the basis for our hate may lie wholly within ourselves, that we may be merely scapegoating the individual we dislike. No person ever asks to be cured of his prejudice. Hate behaves like jaundice: the sufferer overlooks the state of his own liver; it is the world *out there* that appears maliciously yellow.

Some hostility, as I remarked earlier, can be logically justified when the hated individual or group has deliberately obstructed our path. But it seems to be one of the hardest tasks in the world to persuade an individual to sift his hostile attitudes and to separate correctly the causes that lie *out there* from the causes that lie *in here*.

In the view of motivation that I am here proposing, the important thing is the person's systematized design for living. This design—not his hypothetical instincts—is the dynamic force in his life. Whenever an adjustment confronts him, he will make it with his *present* equipment—with his current prejudices, attitudes and sentiments. It is to the credit of most neo-Freudians that they see this point: they recognize that the ego is not a servant of the id, as Freud declared. Rather, one's *present* philosophy of life may hold the key to one's conduct. One person views the world as a jungle, where men are basically evil and dangerous; another views it as a friendly place inhabited by potentially congenial fellow beings. Each acts according to his own present belief.

This postinstinctive view of motivation has two great merits. First, it assures us that improvement in human relations is possible. We are not doomed by our inherent nature to do something—pro or con—with our "instinctual" aggression; we don't have to worry about it. Our behavior results from the sentiments and prejudices we have learned. But improved education can make for better learning, and suitable therapy can make for relearning.

The second merit is that we can now grapple fruitfully with the hardest problem of all: how the affiliative needs of an individual can be reconciled with his self-love and self-esteem.

Self-Love and Altruism

The issue may be formulated as follows: *how far have the indi-vidual's affiliative desires become extended?* Does his picture of his own security and personal integrity include only a few or many affiliative relations? Does he say, as did E. M. Forster's Englishman in India, "We must exclude someone from our gathering, or we shall be left with nothing"? How many we invite to our gathering is purely a matter of our past learning. We may fashion a tiny island of security embracing a small affiliated circle, or a larger island where our self-esteem is identical with the interests of an extended circle. Some individuals are so well socialized that they feel actually stronger when they reach further in their attachments, when they invite more and more people to their gathering.

If I read the course of ontogenetic development aright, the sequence of stages is approximately as follows: There is, first of all, the symbiotic phase that I have described. After this period of dependence and security with the mother, the child enters vigorously into affiliative relations with his environment. His curiosity and friendly interest know no bounds. Such frustrations as he suffers are but ripples in the onrushing tide. Around the age of two or three, when restrictions increase, frustrations grow more severe and help to intensify the growing sense of selfhood that marks the child off more sharply from his social and physical environment. Though he normally continues for many years to have warm and positive emotional identification with his parents, he learns also to be clamorous for his rights and quick to resent slights to his *amour-propre*. Self-love becomes a prominent factor in his life—perhaps the most prominent. But, often, the welfare of others is likewise an authentic concern.

It is at this point, however, that life histories markedly diverge. Some children never seem to lose the egocentricity of their early orientation; life revolves entirely around their own interests as conceived by themselves. In other children, the introceptive, enlarging process takes hold. Just how it comes about that some youths remain essentially infantile in their self-love, while others merge their developing ego-awareness with interests that reach far beyond their own hedonistic demands, is something we do not yet know. For our purposes it may be enough to note that individuals come to have different ranges of values—all emerging from an initial affiliative thrust at the start of life, then deflected by early egotism, but finally crystallized in narrow or in broad sentiments of greater or lesser degrees of socialization.

Hobbes was certainly not entirely wrong. Vainglory, pride and insatiate self-love are found in most mortals, even where a broadly socialized structure of values exists. This fact appears in all the relevant researches I have cited. People want congenial associations, but of the sort that maintain their own self-esteem. Very few individuals are saintly enough or humble enough to maintain friendly regard for individuals who offend their self-love. At the same time, myriad patterns develop, and myriad combinations of self-love and altruism. A really mature person has a wide range of socialized interests; and his altruistic sentiments, whatever they may be, are no less genuine components of his nature than are his narrower patches of pride and egotism.

Although loving regard is seldom able to survive when self-esteem is wounded, sometimes it does; and our theory must cover this fact. Forgiveness, though surely less common than resentment, may follow upon an offense to one's ego, and the preceding love may continue unabated. A serene and highly developed personality may forgive even when forgiveness is not sought. It is possible, likewise, for some personalities to distinguish sharply between *deed* and *doer,* to hate the evil while holding the perpetrator in true esteem. It is generally true that these charitable virtues stem only from an essentially religious philosophy of life, developed to a high degree and now functionally autonomous within the personality. In these cases of extreme affiliativeness, we are dealing with an extension of the ego to a very marked degree. The autonomy of the sentiment thus developed represents a genuine transformation of the proud, clamorous ego so characteristic of personality in its early juvenile years. But saints are rare among us.

The Economy of Hate

Why is it that, in our society today, relatively few people seem able to enlarge their scope of affiliation to include the larger gathering? The prejudiced or exclusionist style of life appears to predominate.

The answer to this question seems to have something to do with the principle of least effort. There is a marked short-run economy in holding a negative view of other people. If I can reject foreigners as a category, I shan't have to bother with them, except to keep them out of my country. If I can then ticket all Negroes as constituting an inferior and objectionable race, I conveniently dispose of a tenth of my fellow citizens. If I can put the Catholics into another category and reject them kit and caboodle, my life is still further simplified. To pare down again, I slice off the Jews, the Democrats and the members of labor unions. As for experts, professors and reformers, they are easily exiled along with all the other "communists." Soon there isn't much left for me to worry about except my own group on Suburban Heights—and I can proceed at leisure to destroy them one by one through gossip. I shall probably do so, depending on the extent of emotional deprivation in my own life.

That this easy, exclusionist style of life is exceedingly common is shown not only by recent studies in the *extent* of prejudice but also by the strikingly high correlation that exists among various *forms* of prejudice. A person who is anti-Negro is usually anti-Semitic, antilabor, antiforeigner. Conversely, if a person's self-esteem and his esteem for others have blended, he is likely to be friendly with members of all groups.

Perhaps the biggest obstacle to the improvement of human relations is the amazing ease with which the human mind creates categories. To categorize human groups is a simple, socially sanctioned way of sorting one's emotions and integrating one's behavior. The process is especially clear-cut in wartime. To make a fair-minded statement about the enemy in time of conflict is regarded as treason, or at least as weakness; and to criticize one's own side is taboo. We are expected to divide our sentiments sharply between institutional friend and institutional foe. To the out-group we ascribe all vices, all evil intentions, all atrocities; to the in-group belong all virtues. By this simple device the in-group flourishes, and our lives are economically arranged.

In peacetime the process is more subtle; but even here we tend to view those who are not in our orbit as ominously outside. An interesting lesson can be found in the word *rival*. In Latin, *rivales* meant two neighboring communities on the two banks of a common stream. Even in Shakespeare's English, rival meant companion.[12] But to us it means opponent, one whom we contend against. Unless a person is clearly *for* me I come to regard him as a competitor. People who live on two sides of a stream (or an ocean) might be friends—but more often they are rivals.

The categorizing effect is seen in the responses of American troops in World War II when they were asked about their attitudes toward foreign populations. Interestingly enough, almost all questions that referred to members of other groups *as individuals* fetched a friendly enough response. Thus, the soldiers on the whole liked the German people, Englishmen, and civilians "back home." But when categorical questions were asked about Germany or Britain as a country, or about Negroes, Jews or labor groups "back home," negative prejudice was apparent. For example, although the attitude toward English civilians was usually friendly, the categorical cleavage between national groups appeared in answers to the question, "Do you think England is doing her share in helping win the war?" The same question was asked about the United States. Seventy-eight per cent of the American troops said that the United States was doing *more* than its share; only 5 per cent said that England was doing so.[13]

So easy and socially approved is this black-white arrangement of groups in our thinking that one is tempted to ask, "Why challenge it?" The answer is that, in a shrunken world, such categorizing is a peril. Contacts between *ins* and *outs* are becoming more frequent; and whenever conflicts occur—in strikes, in riots or in war—they are too deadly to tolerate. Further, our democratic ethic tells us that the exclusionist philosophy of life is somehow subpersonal; it is less than mankind is capable of.

We have not yet learned how to control or to change the exclusionist philosophy of life, but progress is certainly being made in understanding its essential nature. I have already referred to the investigations at the University of California that show a definite connection between disturbance in a child's affiliative relationships with his parents and bigotry in his outlook upon minority groups.

The youthful (and older) authoritarian personality is one that feels insecure and threatened; as a result, it creates safe little islands of self-esteem. Mental hierarchies are formed, with most groups standing below one's own. Human relationships are regarded chiefly in terms of power, not of love. Institutional securities are prized. Patriotism is important, as are the church, the sorority, and any other established in-group. Much that happens outside this circle seems alien and menacing. Any sort of ambiguity or indefiniteness is troublesome—and democracy is replete with indefinite situations. The exclusionist personality wants his categories fixed and clear; he believes "there is only one right way to do a thing"; his mind is rigid. He will not extend his circle of affiliation. As a result he is suspicious, provincial, hostile.[14]

Of course we cannot say that personalities fall neatly into two groups: the bigoted and the tolerant, or the democratic and the authoritarian. No one, least of all the average American, has a wholly consistent pattern of affiliation and hostility. A foreign student in this country recently remarked, "When it comes to minorities, you Americans talk like heaven and feel like hell. I wonder, when the time comes, whether you will act more as you talk or more as you feel." And what a tangle of conflicts the white Westerner is! Often he is fair-minded and compassionate, following political, ethical and religious codes that are unexcelled in their universalistic ideals of respect for the person. On the other hand, he is often smug, self-righteous and insufferably patronizing in his dealing with the majority of the inhabitants of the earth, who happen to have skins of different pigmentation and older, if less technical, civilizations.

The Outlook

What are the chances for widening the scope of affiliative sentiments within our preferred political structure, democracy? I find two contrasting views. E. M. Forster wrote in 1938: "Two cheers for democracy—one because it admits variety, and two, because it permits criticism. Two cheers are quite enough; there is no occasion to give three. Only Love, the Beloved Republic, deserves that." Precisely the opposite view is found in the concluding sentence in the 1950 research report *The authoritarian personality*: "If fear and destructiveness are the major emotional sources of fascism, *eros* belongs mainly to democracy."

Overlooking the too narrow implications of the term *eros*, it seems self-evident that the chances for human beings to broaden their affiliative relations are better under democracy than elsewhere. Yet Forster, too, is right in saying that, though democracy allows diversity and criticism, it has not yet found methods for releasing the potential of love in human relations. History does not indicate that it will ever do so unaided. Even organized religion today would seem to require technical assistance.

To me, the most hopeful sign lies in the developments within modern social science. Research in personality and in human relations is teaching us much concerning the nature of affiliation and hostility. Though theory lags, there is hope that serviceable inductive generalizations, properly tested against philosophy and the wisdom of the ages, will soon emerge. In fact, I venture even now to list principles that seem to me already fairly established:

It is the nature of human life to crave affiliation and love, provided such attachments are not inimical to one's sense of personal security and self-esteem. Love that entails forgiveness likewise exists, but is more rare.

When the bid for affiliation is rebuffed or self-esteem is wounded, ordinarily a secondary hostility develops. This hostility is often displaced upon irrelevant "enemies."

The operations of both affiliative and hostile motives are properly regarded, not as manifestations of instincts, but as expressions of the learned sentiment structure of the individual.

Each person, through circumstance and training, develops an exclusionist, an inclusionist or a mixed style of life that guides his own human relations.

There is a short-run economy in the exclusionist style of life—that is, in a sentiment structure narrowly built around a limited conception of self-interest and a small "safety island" of affiliation. Yet a person who experiences his own integrity only in opposition to other people, who feels secure only by undermining the security of others, can scarcely be said to have a significant purpose or integrity of his own.

There is no inherent limitation in the nature of man or in the nature of learning that requires self-esteem to be secured only through the exclusionist style of life. Personal integrity is entirely compatible with a wide circle of affiliation.

Finally, to implement these principles in action, we must maximize situations in which the individual (child or adult) can participate fully and on terms of equal status in projects of joint concern to him and his associates. By so doing, we shall realize affiliation, safeguard self-esteem and reduce hostility. Whenever this formula is applied, it goes far in improving human relations in home, school, factory and nation—and between sets of "rivals" who live on the two banks of the stream of life.

REFERENCES

1. I. Suttie, *The origins of love and hate*, London: 1935.
2. S. A. Stouffer *et al.*, *The American soldier: I, combat and its aftermath*, Princeton: Princeton University Press, 1949, p. 174; see also Chapter 11.

3. For additional evidence along the same lines see Chapter 12 of the present volume; K. Lewin, *Resolving social conflicts*, New York: 1948; and F. J. Roethlisberger and W. J. Dickson, *Management and the worker*, Cambridge: Harvard University Press, 1939.

4. G. W. Allport and B. M. Kramer, "Some roots of prejudice," *J. Soc. Psychol.*, 1946, 22:9-29.

5. I. Suttie, *op. cit.*, p. 23.

6. E. Simmel, *Anti-Semitism, a social disease*, New York: 1946, p. 41.

7. E. Powers and H. Witmer, *An experiment in the prevention of delinquency*, New York: Columbia University Press, 1950.

8. S. K. Escalona, "Overt sympathy with the enemy in maladjusted children," *Amer. J. Orthopsychiat.*, 1946, 16:333-40.

9. T. W. Adorno, E. Frenkel-Brunswik, D. J. Levinson and R. N. Sanford, *The authoritarian personality*, New York: Harper, 1950.

10. B. Bettelheim and M. Janowitz, *Dynamics of prejudice*, New York: 1950.

11. See G. W. Allport, *Personality: a psychological interpretation*, New York: Holt, 1937, Chap. 7.

12. Well, good-night.
        If you do meet Horatio and Marcellus,
        The rivals of my watch, bid them make haste.
                                                    Hamlet, Act I, Scene I

13. S. A. Stouffer *et al.*, *op. cit.*, II, 627.

14. H. W. Adorno *et al.*, *op. cit.*, *passim*.

PART IV: *Group tensions*

CHAPTER 14

Prejudice in modern perspective

During the past two decades we have learned much about the causes of human prejudice, about its nature and evil consequences. In these twenty years, more research, more writing and more objective analysis have occurred than in all previous centuries taken together.

The creed of brotherhood is ancient; it has long been present in all the great religions of the world. But the pathway to this high goal has only recently become a concern of social and psychological science. The three following essays deal with selected aspects of the problem. The issues receive fuller consideration in *The nature of prejudice* (1954).

The first essay deals with racial tensions. In two lands—South Africa and the United States—the conflict is especially acute. There are important differences between these two countries, but the underlying causes and manifestations of their prejudice are the same. What we learn in one land has considerable applicability to the other.

An invitation to give the twelfth annual Alfred Hoernlé Memorial Lecture in Durban, South Africa, in July 1956 provided the occasion for this essay. The South African Institute of Race Relations sponsored the lecture and published it in pamphlet form at its Johannesburg headquarters in 1956.

Between 1913 and 1920, R. F. Alfred Hoernlé lectured in philosophy at Harvard University, adding strength and luster to a department already famous for its scholars and teachers. I had the privilege of studying with him the thought of Descartes and Spinoza and the philosophic mood of the Enlightenment. As is the case with all great teachers, he influenced his students not only by what he said but even more by what he was. We knew him to be a truly international personage. Our student gossip mistakenly identified his birthplace as England, as Germany, as France, as Belgium, as South Africa. One of our number suggested that he might have come from Tristan da Cunha. But to our minds he was also an authentic Bostonian, so well did he fit into our special corner of New England.

For many decades I have admired him as a cosmopolitan scholar who offered us a compassionate conception of man and an idealism with firm terrestrial roots. Therefore I know that you will understand my sense of pride and gratitude in being invited to pay my personal tribute to his memory in the land of his adoption.

It is in his own broad, synoptic spirit that I venture upon my assignment. My desire is to bring the perspectives of social philosophy and of social science to bear upon man's agelong struggle with the disorder of bigotry, which lies deeply embedded in his own nature. You will forgive me if, as a visitor to South Africa, I make few direct references to problems in the Union. I think you will agree with me that, by dealing with issues which transcend national boundaries, we can on this occasion more fittingly honor Alfred Hoernlé as a figure of world significance.

Prejudice and Loyalties

One sometimes hears people of unquestionable sincerity ask, "Isn't prejudice, after all, a good thing?" I have met the query both in the United States and in the Union of South Africa. Really, I suspect, the questioner is asking, "Isn't loyalty to one's own group and to one's cherished values a good thing?" To this question, the answer is, of course, emphatically yes. In a world where the cement of positive values is badly loosened, we welcome any evidence of loyalty; for loyalty, as Josiah Royce taught us, is intrinsically a virtue. From this point of view, even the spectacular rise of nationalism today is not necessarily evil; it becomes so only when it arbitrarily circumscribes the domain of loyalty. Alfred Hoernlé himself examined the sentiment of patriotism and found it altogether good, provided only that it is neither aggressive nor exclusive.[1] Like Royce, he would require of our personal attachments only one condition— that they give due respect to our neighbor's loyalties. Only one virtue stands higher than our separate and special devotions, and that is loyalty to the concept of loyalty itself.

When a man asks, "Isn't prejudice a good thing?" he is probably confusing prejudice with particular loyalties. The very ease of this confusion places upon us an obligation to define *prejudice* carefully.[2] Prejudice, I hold, is an almost universal psychological syndrome marked by two—and only two—essential features. The first is the affective disposition that makes us lean toward or away from an object. Spinoza rightly speaks of both "love prejudice" and "hate prejudice." We can be prejudiced for or against an object. This ingredient by itself does not distinguish prejudice from any liking or disliking.

The second ingredient is more crucial—the basing of love or

hate on beliefs that are wholly or partially erroneous. To take an example: belief in witchcraft, today as in the past, rests upon a wrong diagnosis of our distress. Our cows do go dry; disease does torment us; a vague *ufufunyane* affects our nerves—but the cause is not witches. In the world at large, many such false diagnoses lead us to accuse whole nations, races or cultures of evil intentions and witch-like attributes that they do not in fact possess.

The commonest form of erroneous belief is the overgeneraliza-tion which holds that *all* members of a group possess some alleged characteristic. We say that Jews as a group are dishonest; Americans as a group are materialistic; or Africans as a group are like children. These assertions, and others like them, are either demonstrable ex-aggerations or total falsehoods. Any negative attitude based on such errors entails prejudice.

I am not, of course, implying that human antagonisms are always based on an error. Some, on occasion, may be based on a true op-position of values in which prejudice plays no part. One is not prejudiced against a gangster who invades one's premises and threatens one's life; this is a realistic conflict, and antagonism is based on a correct appraisal of facts. It is still too early to attempt an esti-mate of the amount of human conflict that is realistic and the amount that is imaginary. We now know, however, that if we can lead men to correct their erroneous appraisals of human groups, they tend to abandon long-standing antagonisms. They cease to fear what is not fearful and to hate what is not hateful. No longer do they tilt at windmills. Rather, they reserve their animus for real problems and real enemies.

A crisp but satisfactory definition of prejudice is one derived from the writings of St. Thomas Aquinas: *Prejudice is thinking ill of others without sufficient warrant.* Our examples of witch-hunting, anti-Semitism and anti-Americanism fit the definition well. If you happen to prefer slang to the discourse of the angelic Thomas, I recommend as an equivalent definition: *Prejudice is being down on something you are not up on.*

So much for the term itself. The question still remains: is pre-judice an evil thing in human relationships? Might it not be argued that partisanship, even if based on error, is necessary to the achieve-ment of desirable goals? And that prejudice against prejudice is merely the currently fashionable bigotry of the liberal? I am, as you can see, committed to answer the charges that we are all creatures of prejudice, that nothing can be done about it and that, anyway, prejudice is sometimes a good thing.

Value and Disvalue

There are, I think, two modes of reasoning which lead us to the conviction that, while prejudice is a common enough pattern of mental existence, it is not inevitable—and that it is invariably an evil. The first mode of reasoning is employed by deductive theories of value; the second is more pragmatic in character and is closely meshed with the operation of social science itself.

Philosophers ordinarily employ the deductive mode. They ask, in effect: what ethical goal, if consistently followed, would prove most viable for mankind? That is to say, what goal would lead to the maximum fulfillment of men's interests, or to the greatest possible happiness for the greatest possible numbers of human beings. All ethical inquiry seeks rules that, if followed, would be fecund for the maximization of human values. The search led Kant to the conclusion that man may *never* treat another human being as a means to an end. It led Royce to affirm loyalty to loyalty as the supreme imperative. It led Hoernlé to conclude that what he called "the liberal spirit" is most conducive to safeguarding and promoting *quality* in human life. Any social order is evil, writes Hoernlé, "in which, from the nature of its internal arrangements, any group of its members is, in principle, condemned to stunted bodies and to stunted minds." [3]

Philosophic reasoning of this type leads to the conclusion that prejudice is indefensible, since it can never lead to an increase in value over a wide range of human concerns. By its very nature, it hinders loyalties, constricts man's reason and sows disvalue.

The deductive approach is manifested also in the ethical imperatives of religion. Starting with a universalistic outlook, all the great religions of the world establish rules that would make life maximally livable for mankind. To Christians, *Love thy neighbor as thyself* is perhaps the most familiar rendering of this golden rule, but every great religion has a precise equivalent. Mahatma Gandhi sought long and hard for a term in English that would represent the exact opposite of prejudice. The term he chose was *equimindedness,* a condition of spiritual generosity wherein one's own firmly held beliefs permit others to hold equally firm beliefs of a different order. A Christian equivalent is the moving injunction of Jesus to His disciples: "Let both grow together until the harvest." [4] We do not know our ultimate worth to the harvester; but we can, if we will, grow together peaceably until the day of reckoning arrives.

Unfortunately, we may not assume that all religious reasoning is of this equiminded order. While every major religion endorses the golden rule and extols the values of brotherhood, each has generated contradictory, if minor, principles whose consequences are divisive and ethnocentric. Forgetting the universalistic implications of their monotheism, certain Moslems believe that destruction of the infidel is a high duty. Christianity, through its doctrines of election, revelation and theocracy, opened the door for a special and self-serving interpretation of God's plan for His creation. The special dogmas of election and revelation invited men to set themselves at the summit of God's supposed hierarchical arrangement for the human race. Theocracy made it possible to enforce this arrangement. Until the seventeenth century, it was never doubted that the State should implement the reasoning of its theologians. In certain lands today, the tie between theology and politics is still close.

Bigotry is thus a paradoxical product of Christianity. To justify bigotry, theologians are often forced back upon certain obscurities in the Book of Genesis. The story of the tower of Babel, for example, they interpret to mean that equimindedness is not only impossible but clearly opposed to God's will. Especially interesting to psychologists is the manner in which adherence to the bigotry-inspiring portions of the Old Testament is reconciled with the clear imperatives of equimindedness in the New. A historical example is the serpentine reasoning of Menno Simons, the Anabaptist theologian of the sixteenth century, who wrestled with St. Paul's injunction: "Therefore judge nothing before the time, until the Lord come" [5]— a precept identical with Christ's command: "Let both grow together until the harvest." Menno Simons interpreted the Pauline text to mean: "None may judge unless he have the judging word on his side." [6]

Here is the trap into which every religious bigot falls. Claiming to have the "judging word" on his side, he finds that he can conveniently violate the universalistic imperatives of his religion. Accordingly, he reverses the humility of Job and says, in effect, to the Lord, "Thy ways are, after all, only the same as my ways."

No need to dwell longer on deductive answers to the question: is prejudice an evil? I have tried to indicate that all the synoptic philosophies of man and all the great religions concur in their answer: only a condition of mind that is prejudice-free can consistently augment human values. I have also sounded the warning that it is all too easy to argue from selected and partial premises to a conclusion that justifies particularistic prejudices. Bigotry, one may say, is the result of ethical reasoning wherein an ontological premise is secretly abandoned in favor of a hidden premise of self-interest.

How does social science stand in relation to this matter? First, of course, some social scientists are philosophically or religiously inclined. They accept the universalistic view and lead their scientific lives in accordance with this commitment. A few are not so universalistic; they proceed from partisan premises. One thinks of the meretricious Nazi and Communist scientists who have contrived to prove what their leaders desire them to prove. Both these groups, however different their premises, are deductive in practice.

But for the most part, I suspect, social scientists are *inductive* by temperament. They ask, "Cannot science shed light on man's quest for an adequate ethics, and help build sound standards for moral conduct?" They say, in effect, "Let's look at man's social behavior and see why so much of his conduct is self-defeating and unproductive of what he himself considers to be good."

Inductive studies show, for one thing, that many of our thought-models become set early in life and that they prove maladaptive to our adult needs. Scientific concepts such as *stereotype, rationalization, defense mechanism, cognitive rigidity* and *semantic therapy* are testimony to the new type of insight we have gained. As contributors to this enlightenment we think of such writers as Walter Lippmann, Stuart Chase, Korzybski, Freud, Moreno, Wittgenstein, Richard Thouless, Trigant Burrow and Cantril. The exposure to ourselves of our own prejudices, though only the first step toward cure, is a significant achievement.

But the work of social science does not stop with a mere challenge. It offers means for clarifying our values and for implementing them in a rational way. Until relatively recent years, for example, it was thought that the only way to conduct an industry or business was on an essentially punitive basis. Harshness and hierarchy dominated the practices of management. Workers were nameless; they were hired or fired on whim. Placements in jobs were haphazard, and praise was an unused incentive. Above all, the worker did not participate in the many decisions affecting his destiny. This dark age of industry is, of course, far from ended; but in many shops and offices we see wholesome results that come from applying social science. When workers are no longer nameless, nor punished, nor patronized, nor overlooked; when it is realized that the whole man goes to work, carrying with him his deep need for affection, his hopes, fears and troubles; when industry meshes into his life so that he feels participant in his own destiny; when his purposes are making use of his abilities; when his aspirations are socially understood and approved—then the whole productive process improves.[7]

Social science has played a significant part in bringing about this new stage in the industrial revolution. It is by no means a matter of teaching management superficial tricks for manipulating workers. On the contrary, social science demonstrates to the employer that he cannot achieve his own purposes unless he ceases to use his workers as targets for his own private anxieties and hostilities. It teaches him self-knowledge and, in this way, knowledge of others. It teaches him a new conception of human relations. In so doing, it reveals prejudices for what they are—a prime source of suffering and disvalue.

Moving to the field of race relations, think what would happen to our prejudices if we were to admit to our minds the following *findings* fairly certain scientific discoveries:

Racial membership accounts for only a negligible fraction of ① *human attributes.* For complexion, hair form and shape of shinbone —yes. For intelligence, temper, talent, outlook, virtue and worth— not at all.

There are no instinctive aversions of human races one toward ② *another.* All such aversions are built into children, and only with considerable difficulty.

In almost every case where segregation is practiced, the financial ③ *loss is enormous,* thus lowering the standards of nourishment, shelter, health, recreation and freedom for all groups concerned. Prejudice sows only economic disvalue.

Most hostility arises not from unacceptable characteristics in ④ *other people, but from our private emotional disorders* for which the hated group is not responsible.

When people live in such a way as to have equal-status contact ⑤ *with one another in the pursuit of common objectives, they ordinarily cease to perceive one another as threats* and are likely to develop a tolerance and liking for one another.

These are but a few of the almost certain scientific laws that bear on our racial relationships. A prejudiced person who can be brought to admit these laws to his mental store will find his previous creed of exclusiveness untenable.

To restate my point: The net effect of modern science is to show that prejudice can never maximize value. While it may make for short-run emotional gains for the individual, in the long run it is uneconomic, fecund for violence and for war, trivializing to human reason and stultifying to both its possessor and its victim. It is impossible to see how value—define it as you will—can be enhanced through prejudice. Social science therefore joins its answer to that of philosophy and religion: prejudice is not, never has been and never will be a good thing in human society.

This being the case, we must next inquire: what can social science contribute to the *conquest* of prejudice in modern life?

Group Differences

The most logical place to start is with the factual study of group differences. We have already observed that the distinction between realistic conflict and prejudice lies chiefly in the erroneous beliefs, especially the overgeneralizations, on which prejudice is based. To distinguish fact from falsity, we need an accurate perception of peoples and their institutions, and an understanding of their real purposes and capacities. The first duty of the social scientist is to discover what *truth* lies behind such concepts as "mind of the nation" or "ethnic character." Like the medical diagnostician, he may start by asking embarrassing questions: *Are* Armenians a bad credit risk? *Are* Jews clannish and exclusive? *Are* Africans inherently stupid and unteachable? (It so happens that the answer to these questions is almost certainly no.)

Even though our methods of research are imperfect, such scientific evidence as we have regarding these and similar allegations is far sounder than the guesswork and anecdotalism customarily employed to support prejudiced accusations. Yet the social scientist who insists upon discovering the objective facts concerning group differences runs the risk of opprobrium. Some sentimentalists prefer on a priori grounds to deny the existence of racial or national differences; bigots are certain that they know all the differences in advance. But the social scientist wards off these attacks as best he can and affirms that his first logical duty is to *find out the facts*.

We cannot here survey all the results that are coming to light.[8] Research has still far to go. But, as I read the preliminary results, there seems to be little justification for most of our racial accusations. Differences that are expected to appear fail to do so, or else they are of a trivial order.

Let us take one sample finding of a positive difference. It concerns the incidence of alcoholism among ethnic groups in the United

States. After making a comprehensive survey, one sociologist concludes: "In statistics of admissions for alcoholic disorders to various hospitals in this country the Irish have consistently had rates two to three times as high as any other ethnic group." [9] In one institution, for example, the rate of admission for the Irish is fifty times that of the Jews.[10] Here is a factual ethnic difference; yet it is pure prejudice to say, "I don't like the Irish because they drink too heavily." For even among the Irish, the rate of alcoholic psychosis is only about 25 in any group of 100,000 Irishmen. The only realistic statement of personal preference that could be made, therefore, is somewhat as follows: "Since I don't like heavy drinkers, I probably would not like approximately 1 per cent of the Irish."

What a world of difference it would make in our human relationships if we could learn to say *one per cent* instead of *all*; this *Irishman* instead of *the Irish*; and *he* or *she* instead of *they*.

Techniques for the study of national and ethnic differences are rapidly developing. Vital statistics of the sort just cited are one source of information; international public opinion polls are another. Cross-national studies using scaling techniques are entering the scene. This topic is too specialized for further discussion here, but I do wish to sound two warnings:

First: in uncovering differences in the character of peoples, we must not forget to look also for similarities—for what Kluckhohn calls "cultural universals." [11] While differences readily strike the eye, the existence of a common ground in all cultures and in all branches of the human family is a more pervasive fact. It is true that each group has some defining attribute that makes it a group. Polish people speak Polish; most Africans have dark complexions; most Moslems hold the Koran in high regard. But these valid *defining* attributes (technically called J-curve attributes) are few.[12] Our error is to assume that all other alleged attributes are also of this order, as when we say that Poles as a group are stupid, Africans are childlike and Moslems are bloodthirsty.

Second: we must not assume that even validly discovered differences justify hostility. People can differ from us without menacing us. Suppose, for example, that one group turns out to be shorter than we in stature, less educated, less humorous, more irascible, more suspicious, even less trustworthy. Are we justified in hating members of this group or in regarding them as a threat? Do not the same differences exist within our own families? Some brothers and sisters are ill-favored compared with others; but they are often loved in spite of their oddity.

While the study of group differences is rapidly expanding, we still stumble at thresholds. Unless I am mistaken, there are few studies under way in South Africa of the beliefs, capacities, aspirations and hopes of the several ethnic groups composing the Union. Assertions are rife; data are few.

Phenomenological Studies

Besides the factual appraisal of group differences, what has social science to offer? Well, for one thing it teaches us the manner in which we *perceive* other groups of people. This area of investigation is *phenomenological*. Some years ago Dr. Malherbe reported an early study of this type: In a public service examination, candidates were instructed to "underline the percentage that you think Jews constitute of the whole population of South Africa: 1 per cent, 5 . . . 10 . . . 20 . . . 25 . . . 30 . . . per cent." When tabulated, the modal estimate turned out to be 20 per cent. The true answer is just a little over 1 per cent.[13]

This neat little experiment shows how our fears and hostility tend to inflate our perceptions out of all proportion to the facts. The American public, we know—and probably also the public of South Africa—tends to overestimate the size of the Communist party in its own land.[14]

A particularly important line of phenomenological investigation concerns the effect of equal-status contact upon our perceptions. Several studies have demonstrated that equal-status contact between groups leads to mutual regard and respect. This favorable effect is greater if members are working together for common objectives and if law and custom sanction this type of contact.[15]

Examples of this research, neat in design and convincing in result, are the two large-scale studies of public housing projects conducted respectively by Deutsch and Collins, and by Wilner, Walkley and Cook.[16] In both studies, integrated and segregated occupancy patterns were investigated. (In the former study, Negroes constituted approximately 50 per cent of the integrated housing units; in the latter they constituted 10 per cent.) From both investigations the same basic findings emerged: white people living closer to Negroes felt more friendly to them; proximity brought favorable attitudes. And what for our present purpose is most important, proximity tended to change perceptions. People living in segregated units tended to see the Negroes as a dirty people, aggressive, hostile, dangerous, not to be trusted. People living in integrated units more often reported that the Negro inhabitants of the projects were much the same as white people. Unfavorable stereotyped attributes vanished on closer acquaintance. Segregation, we may now reasonably conclude, makes for mystery, stereotypy and unfriendliness.

The phenomenological approach is broader than I have yet indicated. For example, there is the well-known tendency in man to perceive a living human agent as the cause of his miseries. Belief in witchcraft, still widespread, locates the cause of one's sufferings in a malign human agency. But it is not only among primitive people that the anthropomorphizing tendency exists. We find the same disposition in our own society, although the witches we accuse are more likely to be collective than single. Is my business shaky? *They* are to blame. Is my job insecure? *They* want to take it from me. Am I worried about my immoral impulses? Well, just look at *them*. *They*, of course, are the Jews or Bantus, Catholics or men from Mars, according to the fixations of our fantasy.

Psychodynamic Research

Which brings us to psychodynamics, an area of investigation in which marked advances have been made. Psychodynamics focuses attention upon the type of person who, because of his own needs and structure of character, is prone to develop strong prejudices. Bigotry stands revealed as one of the psychological crutches adopted by people who are crippled in their encounters with life. The crippling may have occurred in childhood, or it may come from feelings of insecurity and wounded pride in adult years. In any case, prejudice exists in many lives because it fulfills a protective and even sedative function for its bearer. The first major series of researches establishing this fact was published as recently as 1950 under the title *The authoritarian personality*. This pioneer production has since been followed by many additional studies dealing with character-conditioned prejudice.[17]

To my mind, the crux of this extensive work is its demonstration that bigotry is an easy and natural style of life to adopt. Most people are buffeted by the anxieties of existence—the normal fears of death and disaster, augmented by economic insecurity, affectional deprivation and feelings of guilt. This total "existential anxiety" fuses with the irritations of daily life. The resulting complex may lead one to seek human agents to explain his distress: it is *they* who are to blame. A punitive and exclusive style of life gradually evolves. One feels secure only in the bosom of his own group. There his pride is fed by myths of superiority, and there his two fiercely possessive needs—property and sex—are focused. There he finds social support for his prejudice; religion, literature, humor, tradition and the usages of language help sustain his exclusionist mode of life.

We owe to MacCrone some of our understanding of this life-style. He demonstrates the interlocking of suspiciousness, exclusiveness and ethnic hostility in human lives, and their blending with rigid religious ideology. He also offers us a theory of "ethno-erotism," which relates this disorder to a fixation of man's capacity-for-love exclusively upon his immediate in-group.[18] In still another sense, it is wise to note the erotic complications in prejudice. To a surprising extent, sex-conflict and guilt seem to enter the process. It is comforting to think that the demon of impulse resides not in our own breasts so much as in the lascivious black man, or Italian, or Frenchman, or Jew. As Goethe says, we never feel so free from sin as when we expatiate upon the sinful deeds of others.

Since the clamorous needs of the body and the ego, and the insistent goads of fear and anxiety, dispose us to develop a prejudiced pattern of life, we need no longer wonder at the ubiquity of our problem. We marvel, rather, at the frequency with which we encounter equiminded mortals. We should be asking: how is it that so many people develop self-insight, self-criticism and a universalistic ethic to counteract the bent toward bigotry? Up to now, psychology has given less attention to the tolerant personality than to the intolerant.

Genetic Studies

Basic to the study of both types is the study of child development, including teaching at home, in school and in the culture at large. In this area, too, there is progress to report.

Children, we know, manifest no prejudice whatever in the early years of life. Such awareness of race difference as exists is for the most part neutral or friendly, though sometimes marked by puzzlement. A little boy of four was playing for the first time with a little black girl. He said to her, "You are very nice." Then screwing up his eyes with intense effort, he added, "But I can't quite see you." There was a perceptual adjustment to be made, but the simple fact of skin color was not for him a cause for dislike.

Certain styles of child training, we now know, lead more surely than others to the production of prejudice. Broadly speaking, children who feel a warmth and security in their parents—children who know that, however badly they misbehave, they are still loved—are less prone to prejudice in later years than are children who encounter at home a rejective situation, where discipline is both harsh and capricious. It is ominous for the future of a child when the discipline he receives is based on the emotional needs of the disciplinarian rather than on any consideration of the child's own needs.[19]

Sociocultural Studies

Hastily I move on to the perspectives of sociology, anthropology and economics.

We are familiar with the Marxist theory that holds all prejudice to be rooted in an exploitation. The theory holds that ruling groups devise an ideology to justify and maintain the "surplus value" accruing to dominant groups from the ill-paid labor of subordinate groups. It seeks the roots of prejudice in one and only one human passion: greed. Herein lies its one-sidedness, for we know that prejudice also draws nourishment from fear and insecurity, from feelings of inferiority and pride, from frustration and irritability, from deprivation of love and from the sheer need to conform. Yet greed surely is to be reckoned with, as are all the economic trappings of prejudice that it brings in its train.

Economics teaches us also to look to the ecological structure of a region in order to understand the immediate nature of group conflicts, and to look to the cycles of depression and prosperity for upswings and downswings in prejudice. Above all, economics confronts us with a supreme paradox of prejudice. Through greed, men seek to reap economic profit from their prejudices, but they are betrayed by these same prejudices into behaving in most uneconomic ways. Segregation and discrimination—fruits of prejudice—turn out to be economically debilitating.[20]

From sociology and anthropology we learn additional facts to correct and supplement our psychological analysis. These social sciences warn us that prejudice is not always a crutch employed by immature or crippled personalities. It may be a phenomenon of sheer conformity, barely skin-deep. But whether it is skin-deep or bone-deep, we cannot understand prejudice unless we know its social context. What strata exist in a given society? Which are traditionally regarded as high in status, and which low? Does the culture offer a ritualized target for aggression, such as formally sanctioned anti-Semitism, a dogma of white supremacy or a belief in witchcraft? Answers to these and similar questions are needed if we are to achieve adequate perspective.

Research in sociology and in anthropology has resulted in several important laws. Let me cite three:

> *In a heterogeneous society there is more group prejudice than in homogeneous societies.* South Africa, for example, which has several "perceptual points for alarm," harbors more prejudice than, say, St. Helena or Sweden, both remarkably homogeneous societies.

> *Prejudice is greater whenever there are severe barriers to communication between groups.* This law has as its reciprocal the law of contact: prejudice lessens whenever there is equal-status contact between members of groups in the pursuit of common objectives.

> *Assuming that there is germinal prejudice against a certain group, this prejudice will become stronger in proportion to the size of the group in the total population.* Only about one thousand people from India live in the United States, but there are about thirteen million Negroes. The former group is overlooked; the latter is a target for much prejudice and discrimination. If the number of Indians were to rise to the proportion obtaining in Natal, there is no doubt that fear, suspicion and dislike would rise accordingly.

Yet it would be an error to assume that the mere density of a group in the total population brings about prejudice against it. In South Africa, for example, I find myself quite overwhelmed by South Africans. I am not for this reason prejudiced against them. Populational density, I suggest, is never a causal factor, but rather a multiplier of whatever prior prejudices exist.[21]

Historical Horizons

We have not yet spoken of the perspective of history. The truth of the matter is that, without the lens of history, we fumble along in shortsighted confusion. Take, for example, that stubborn prejudice bequeathed to us from antiquity: anti-Semitism. Only history can show us how, throughout the ages, Jews have been forced to occupy a position "at the fringe of stable values" as money-lenders, entertainers and entrepreneurs; and how such marginal people are regarded by conservatives in every era as agents of threat.

Again, without a knowledge of the Civil War in the United States and the Anglo-Boer War in South Africa, and of the heartbreaks and bitterness engendered by each, it would be impossible to understand the present family quarrels in the two lands. Only with the aid of this perspective can we come to see that, in both countries, the black man is to a certain extent an innocent bystander. He is caught, through no fault of his own, between two bitter trains of memory.

Besides adding to our knowledge of specific prejudices in specific eras, history teaches us that the official morality of a nation—what we may call its stateways—has always exerted an influence of major importance. One can point to countless violations of the spirit of the Magna Charta, the Fourteenth Amendment to the Constitution of the United States and the Charter of the United Nations, but it is impossible to deny that these statements of policy have a continuing and meliorative effect upon human relationships.

Speaking for myself, I cannot yet decide which is a more important factor in the creation of bigotry: stateways or folkways—folkways being defined here to include child training and the individual's style of life. If we are dedicated to the reduction of prejudice, is it better to fight the battle on the political front or in the home, classroom and church? Fortunately, this question need not be answered in terms of either-or. Each of us may work according to his lights and his talent. There is plenty to be done at both ends.

Finally, a lesson of history which I consider the most important of all: history helps us to determine whether we are, in fact, waging a losing battle. The prejudiced style of life is so easy to develop, so natural, so ubiquitous and, in many places, so solidly supported by the social and political structure that one could easily despair. We are tempted to say that there is no solution to our dilemma; in Sartre's words, "No exit." Among white South Africans I have encountered this pessimism. Black South Africans, too, assume the impasse. One tribe has an imaginative explanation for the situation: it holds that God Himself is good, wishing the whole human race well, but that unfortunately He has a half-witted brother who constantly interferes with His plans. It is this half-witted brother who has taken charge of relationships within the human family.

But to despair is to misread the long lesson of history. Relationships within the human family have always been strained and often fratricidal. No story is more depressing than the history of the Christian Church, which for the most part has disregarded its Founder's injunction, "Let both grow together until the harvest." Yet, during the sixteenth century and even earlier, golden words were spoken in defense of religious liberty and toleration; in the nineteenth century, many of these words were realized in practice; and in the twentieth century, we begin to descry a genuine purging of the religious conscience from much of its bigotry.

Similarly, stateways, if viewed in historical perspective, reveal slow but true advance. The progress is signalized in recent years by the United Nations' Declaration of Human Rights. Especially striking is the banding of private citizens for the extension of racial sanity and the reduction of prejudice. The South African Institute of Race Relations is an example. Comparable organizations exist in the United States for the same purpose; many are international in scope.

I have already drawn special attention to one recent historical thread: the perspective on the causes and cures of prejudice disclosed by modern social science. Its discoveries have no magical power, but they do bring a cleansing spirit and new hope into the oppressive caves of human ignorance and hate. The current outpouring of research and books; the training of younger people who, in increasing numbers, are dedicating themselves to the betterment of human relationships—these are signs of progress. At long last, in every land, enlightened men and women are determined that man's intelligence shall be brought to serve the cause of man's redemption. They see more clearly than ever before that living together as a single human family is the only future mankind can have.

Thus, viewing the matter in historical perspective, we detect a new spirit in the land. Whether it will spread rapidly enough to avert disastrous clashes of nation and race we cannot yet predict. We can say only that the age-old disorder of prejudice is beginning to yield to diagnosis and treatment, much as other endemic diseases have yielded. The more we learn of its nature, the more we discover about modes of possible cure.

The road ahead looks discouraging, but it is marked with these beacons of hope. We have, therefore, abundant reason to keep faith with all humane prophets of equimindedness in the past. They labored—and so must we—to bring rationality and compassion to bear upon our common problem.

REFERENCES

1. R. F. A. Hoernlé, *Race and reason,* Johannesburg: Witwatersrand University Press, 1945, pp. xxii, xxxii.

2. Elsewhere I have considered the problem of definition in greater detail; see G. W. Allport, *The nature of prejudice,* Cambridge: Addison-Wesley, 1954, Chap. 1. Here I summarize briefly the conclusion reached.

3. R. F. A. Hoernlé, *South African native policy and the liberal spirit,* Johannesburg: Witwatersrand University Press, 1945, p. 112.

4. St. Matthew 13:30.

5. I Corinthians 4:5.

6. Menno Simons, "A foundation and plain instruction of the saving doctrine of Christ" (trans. by I. D. Rupp), *On the ban: questions and answers,* 1550, Lancaster: Elias Baar, 1863.

7. The story of this modern chapter in the industrial revolution has been told many times. A significant publication is F. J. Roethlisberger and W. J. Dickson, *Management and the worker,* Cambridge: Harvard University Press, 1939. One may also consult S. Chase, *The proper study of mankind,* rev. ed., New York: Harper, 1956; likewise, Chapter 12 of the present volume.

8. For discussions of methods, findings and theory in this area of research see G. W. Allport, *The nature of prejudice, op. cit.,* Chaps. 6, 7, 13; see also A. Inkeles and D. J. Levinson, "National character: a study of modal personality and sociocultural systems," in G. Lindzey (ed.), *Handbook of social psychology,* Cambridge: Addison-Wesley, 1954, Vol. II, Chap. 26.

9. R. F. Bales, "Cultural differences in rates of alcoholism," *Quart. J. Stud. Alcohol,* 1946, 6:484.

10. H. W. Haggard and E. M. Jellinek, *Alcohol explored,* Garden City: Doubleday, Doran, 1942, p. 252.

11. C. Kluckhohn, "Universal categories of culture," in A. L. Kroeber (ed.), *Anthropology today,* Chicago: Chicago University Press, 1953.

12. See G. W. Allport, *The nature of prejudice, op. cit.,* Chap. 6.

13. E. G. Malherbe, *Race attitudes and education,* Johannesburg: South African Institute of Race Relations, 1946. Second Annual Hoernlé Memorial Lecture.

14. S. A. Stouffer, *Communism, conformity and civil liberties,* New York: Doubleday, 1955.

15. Cf. G. W. Allport, *The nature of prejudice, op. cit.,* Chap. 16.

16. M. Deutsch and M. E. Collins, *Interracial housing,* Minneapolis: University of Minnesota Press, 1950; D. M. Wilner, R. P. Walkley and S. W. Cook, *Human relations in interracial housing,* Minneapolis: University of Minnesota Press, 1955.

17. T. W. Adorno, E. Frenkel-Brunswik, D. J. Levinson and R. N. Sanford, *The authoritarian personality,* New York: Harper, 1950. More recent summaries of the topic may be found in H. J. Eysenck, *The psychology of politics,* London: Routledge & Kegan Paul, 1954; and in G. W. Allport, *The nature of prejudice, op. cit.,* Chaps. 25-27.

18. I. D. MacCrone, "Ethnocentric ideology and ethnocentrism," *Proc. S. A. Psychol. Assoc.,* 1953, 4:21-24.

19. G. W. Allport, *The nature of prejudice, op. cit.,* Chap. 18.

20. See, for example, E. de S. Brunner, "Problems and tensions in South Africa," *Pol. Sci. Quart.,* 1955, 70:368-86.

21. The factor of density and other sociocultural principles here mentioned are discussed in greater detail in G. W. Allport, *The nature of prejudice, op. cit.,* Chap. 14.

Techniques for reducing group prejudice

Can social science help us reduce bias through a more effective use of law, of the classroom, of mass media, of individual therapy? The question is audacious, for prejudice is deeply ingrained and will not yield easily to remedial treatment. Yet in recent years a good deal has been discovered that can serve as a guideline for the reduction of prejudice.

This survey of the subject is based on the Leo. M. Franklin Memorial Lecture, delivered at Wayne University in April 1951, and published in its present form in P. A. Sorokin (ed.) *Forms and techniques of altruistic and spiritual growth* (1954).

All sorts of methods have been tried in the attempt to change ethnic attitudes for the better. Roughly they seem to fall under the following headings (although each could be extensively subdivided): legislation, formal educational methods, contact and acquaintance programs, group retraining (group dynamics), mass media, exhortation and individual therapy.

Millions of dollars are being spent annually in the attempt to reduce group conflict and prejudice by these methods. Is the money well spent? Or should some of the money and effort spent in one direction be diverted to another, more successful direction? These are entirely practical questions, but their answer cannot be found except through painstaking research devoted to the evaluation of present action programs.

Let it be said at the outset that we are today only just starting the needed evaluative research. The studies summarized in this essay are of a pioneer character, and, while they yield many valuable indications concerning the merits and limitations of action programs, they cannot yet be considered final or definitive. They do, however, blaze a trail of progress.

Can We Expect Change?

First, it is proper to ask ourselves: is it reasonable to expect any single action program to achieve an appreciable change in the prejudices that people carry with them? One estimate says that group prejudice plays an appreciable part in the lives of four-fifths of the

American adult population.[1] Can we reasonably expect to alter this ominous proportion?

Certain weighty considerations prompt us to say no. A mounting array of evidence tells us that a person's whole life economy may be erected on prejudice. The habits of categorizing, projecting and scapegoating may be too ingrained to be disturbed. To change the attitudes would require a recentering of the whole personality. There is no medicine strong enough to counteract the functional significance of prejudice in certain lives. Moreover, prejudiced attitudes receive such continual support from the social environment that isolated target-programs seem insufficient and feeble. The child, for example, cannot possibly escape the ethnic, religious and class membership of his parents—and this anchorage is so firm that a few hours of "social science studies" in school are unlikely to affect the basic structure of his attitudes. Also, the sanctions of his gang and his neighborhood are likely to hold him within the prevailing framework of prejudice, even though films or specially prepared Sunday school lessons spray him with the message of tolerance.

But there are arguments on the other side. Not only a prejudiced outlook, but all of its ingredients, are learned. What is learned can theoretically be unlearned; or at least the learning can, from the start, be prevented.

Moreover, Americans seem to have inexhaustible faith in the changeability of attitudes. The Goliath of advertising in this country is erected on this faith. And we are equally confident in the powers of education. We brush aside aristocratic slogans, such as "blood will tell," "you can't change human nature" and "instincts of the herd," and set out to slay any attitudinal dragon that we decide to eradicate. This extreme faith in environmentalism may not be justified, but the faith itself is a factor of prime importance. If everyone expects attitudes to change—through education, publicity or therapy—then, of course, they are more *likely* to do so than if no one *expects* them to change. Our gusto for change will bring it about, if anything can. The result may yet surprise us.

The Research Approach

We have reached a point where we can begin to submit this dispute to objective tests. Efforts to improve human relations are as old as the hills. What is new is the ability and the will to evaluate the success of these efforts.

True, methods for measuring change are still in their infancy, and the more we attempt to apply them, the more complexities come to light.[2] The following instance indicates some of the difficulties:

In 1950 the National Association of Colored Graduate Nurses disbanded after forty-two years of independent existence. It did so because Negro nurses were at last welcomed to membership in most local chapters of the American Nurses' Association. Here is an example of attitude change resulting in the termination of one form of segregation. But to what was it due? Did it come about through the crusading efforts of certain Negro and white nurses? Was the present trend in FEPC legislation, or the tenor of recent Supreme Court decisions, a factor? Did the good will and brotherhood propaganda of various national bodies play a part? Or was the change a result of all these and many additional pressures? Some cause or causes had an effect, but it is not easy to trace the sequence.

There are three ideal essentials for evaluation research:

First: there must be an identifiable program to be evaluated (a course of instruction, a law, a moving picture, a new type of contact between groups). This factor is called the independent variable.

Second: there must be some measurable indices of change. Attitude scales might be administered before and after the program, or interviews conducted, or indices of tension within the community computed (for example, the number of group conflicts reported to the police). Such yardsticks are known as the dependent variable.

Third: less vital but still important is the use of control groups. When the independent variable is applied, we should like to prove that the measured change is unquestionably a result of this fact. We can do so best if we have a control group of people (matched for age, intelligence and status) who are not submitted to the impact of the independent variable. If they too show an equivalent amount of change, we cannot conclude that our independent variable was effective. Some other influence, as yet unidentified, must have been reaching both groups.

The need for a control group is not often realized by investigators. In one survey of eighteen evaluations of college programs in intercultural education, it was revealed that only four had employed controls.[3] And even when used, controls are not always effective. Suppose two groups of students are being investigated—one receiving a course of instruction, the other acting as a control. If the students gossip outside of school, the lessons learned by one group may be passed along informally to the other. In such a case, the experimental group "contaminates" the control.

A problem also arises in selecting the time when the effects of a program should be evaluated. It is ordinarily easiest to do the evaluating (testing, interviewing, etc.) immediately after the close of the program. But even if we find change at this point, who knows whether it will endure? And, if no change is found, who knows whether the program may not have "sleeper effects" and first show its influence months or even years later? Perhaps the ideal plan is to measure the effects immediately and then *again* after a lapse of a year.

Enough has been said to show that the field of evaluative research has many obstacles. It is difficult to keep the independent variable uncontaminated; it is hard to devise suitable measures of change; and when the findings are in, one cannot always interpret them with confidence, for all sorts of unwanted variables have intruded themselves into the design. The hurly-burly of everyday life in a complex community is very different from the test tube in a chemical laboratory. Yet, in spite of these difficulties, there are scores of evaluative studies that pretend to tell how effective some one type of program has been with a specified population.[4]

All organizations devoted to the betterment of group relations— and there are thousands of them—can be classified as either public or private. The former include the so-called mayor's committees, governor's committees and civic unity committees, established either by the city or state executive or by legislative ordinance. Public agencies likewise include city, state and federal commissions empowered to enforce anti-discrimination laws—sometimes all relevant laws, sometimes only specific laws, such as those dealing with housing or fair employment practices. Often a public agency is simply a fact-finding body, a notable example being the President's Committee on Civil Rights, whose incisive report in 1947 became a rallying point for the forces of tolerance.

Public efforts come to a focus in legislation. I shall try, first, to summarize available evidence and opinion regarding this technique for reducing prejudice. The story is complex, and my comments will necessarily be condensed.[5]

Legislation

Laws against discrimination are of three types: *civil rights* legislation, *employment* legislation and *group libel* legislation. Against all of these is advanced one customary argument: "But you can't legislate against prejudice." Toward the close of the nineteenth century, the Supreme Court of the United States declared that it was hopeless for laws to expect to counter "racial instincts."

This argument is weak in two respects. _First,_ we know that segregation and other anti-minority laws increase prejudice against groups. Most historians agree that the legal establishment of second-class citizenship for Negroes in the South has stimulated racism, contempt and abuse. A white child who sees segregation legally enforced is very unlikely to grow up with ideas of equality and friendliness. If legislation can thus increase prejudice, why can it not _diminish_ prejudice?

Second, legislation favorable to minority groups never aims to reduce prejudice directly. Its intent is to equalize advantages and lessen discrimination. As a by-product, people gain the experience of working or studying side by side; and such equal-status contact makes indirectly for lessened prejudice. Increasing the skills of minority groups, raising their standard of living, improving their health and education—such measures may have a similar indirect effect. Further, the establishment of a legal norm for behavior creates a public conscience and a standard for expected behavior that lessens _overt_ signs of prejudice. Legislation aims at controlling, not prejudice, but only its open expression. Yet, when expression changes, thoughts, in the long run, are likely to fall into line.

When discrimination is reduced, prejudice tends to lessen. The vicious circle begins to reverse itself. The legal termination of bias in employment, housing and the armed forces has the result, evidence shows, of raising the respect one ethnic group holds for another. Experience tells us that the difficulties of integrating hitherto segregated groups are ordinarily less than anticipated. But it often takes a law or a strong executive order to start the process moving. The _principle of cumulation,_ as Myrdal calls it, holds that raising the Negro plane of living will lower prejudice on the part of the white, and that this in turn will again raise the Negro plane of living. Benign circles of this order can be established under the initial prompting of law.

To sum up: While it is true that most Americans will not obey laws of which they disapprove strongly, most of them, deep inside their consciences, do approve civil rights and anti-discrimination legislation. They often approve even while they squeal in protest. Laws in line with one's conscience are likely to be obeyed; when not obeyed, they still establish an ethical norm that holds before the individual an image of what his conduct should be. The goad of the law often breaks a vicious circle, so that a process of healing can start to occur. Forces in the individual and in the community that have nothing whatever to do with the law are thus liberated. It is not true that legislation must wait on education, at least not on complete and perfect education. For legislation itself is one root of the educational process.

Formal Educational Programs

It is not possible to report all of the available evaluative studies of educational programs. These programs range widely in type, and a number of them are omnibus, containing many varieties of teaching techniques.

Some evaluations are concerned with the impact of special and limited programs. The latter may be classified under six headings: the *informational approach*, which imparts knowledge by lectures and textbook teaching; the *vicarious experience approach*, which employs movies, drama, fiction and other devices that invite the student to identify with members of an out-group; the *community study-action approach*, which calls for field trips, area surveys and work in social agencies or community programs; *exhibitions, festivals and pageants*, which encourage a sympathetic regard for the customs of minority groups and our Old World heritage; the *small group process*, which applies many principles of group dynamics, including discussion, sociodrama and group retraining; and the *individual conference*, which allows for therapeutic interviewing and counseling.

We are not yet able to say categorically which of these six approaches brings the greatest return. While it is fairly certain that desirable effects appear in approximately two-thirds of the experiments, and ill effects very rarely, we still do not know for sure what methods are *most* successful. The trend of evidence, as Cook points out, seems to favor indirect approaches—that is, programs which do not specialize in the study of minority groups as such, or focus upon the phenomena of prejudice as such. The student seems to gain more when he loses himself in community projects, when he participates in realistic situations and develops, as William James would say, *acquaintance with* the field rather than *knowledge about* it.

The informational approach. This tentative conclusion clearly puts the informational approach on the defensive. Traditionally it has been thought that planting right ideas in the mind would engender right behavior. Many school buildings still display the Socratic motto, *Knowledge Is Virtue*. But the student's readiness to assimilate and to use knowledge, it is now pretty well agreed, depends upon his attitudes. Information seldom sticks unless mixed with attitudinal glue. Facts themselves are inhuman; only attitudes are human. Purely factual training often has one of three equally abortive results: it is soon forgotten, or it is distorted in such a way as to rationalize existing attitudes, or it is allowed to sit in one corner of the mind, isolated from the main determinants of living conduct.

This segregation of knowledge from conduct is revealed in certain investigations that have tested both beliefs and attitudes. Authoritative instruction may have the power of correcting erroneous beliefs without appreciably altering attitudes. Children may learn the facts of Negro history without learning tolerance.

Yet there is an argument to be made on the opposite side. Perhaps students may, in the short run, show no gains or twist the facts to serve their prejudices. But in the long run, accurate information is probably an ally of improved human relations. To take one example: Myrdal has pointed out that there is no longer any intellectually respectable "race" theory that can justify the position of the Negro in this country. Since people are not wholly irrational, the fact that scientific evidence fails to support the theory of racial inferiority can scarcely fail *gradually* to penetrate into the marrow of their attitudes.

The fundamental premise of intercultural education is, in effect: *no person knows his own culture who knows only his own culture.* A child who grows up to believe that the sun rises and sets on his own in-group, and who views foreigners as strange beings from the outer darkness, is a child lacking perspective on the conditions of his own life. He will never see the American way for what it is—one of many alternative patterns of living that men have invented for their needs. Without intercultural information obtained at school, a child cannot acquire this perspective, for most children come from homes and neighborhoods where they have no opportunity to learn about out-groups in an objective way. Thus, while the teaching of correct information in the school does not automatically change prejudice, it may be an indispensable condition of change.

But may not scientific and factual instruction contain information *unfavorable* to minority groups? Yes, it is conceivable that the incidence of evil traits may be higher in one group than in another. If so, this information should not be suppressed. If we are going after the truth, we must go after the whole of it—not merely after the part that is flattering to minorities. Enlightened members of minority groups favor the publication of *all* scientific and factual findings; for they are convinced that, when the whole truth is known, it will show that most of the common stereotypes and accusations are false. If a small percentage of the accusations prove to be justified, the explanation of the findings probably lies in the adverse conditions under which many minority groups live. Properly understood, this finding will improve perspective and motivate reform. For example, the fact that *some* members of persecuted groups may *sometimes* develop ego-defenses is a fact not to be suppressed but to be faced and sympathetically understood.

How shall I sum up? Information does not necessarily alter either attitude or action. Its gains, according to available research, seem slighter than those of other educational methods employed. At the same time, there is virtually no evidence that sound factual information does any harm. Perhaps its value may be long delayed, and may consist in driving wedges of doubt and discomfort into the stereotypes of the prejudiced. It seems likely, too, that the greater gains ascribed to action and project methods require sound factual instruction as underpinning. All in all, we do well to resist the irrational position that invites us to abandon entirely the traditional ideals and methods of formal education. Facts are not enough, but they still may be indispensable.

Direct versus indirect approaches. A related question arises concerning the merits of focusing attention directly upon intergroup problems. Is it well, for example, for children to discuss the "Negro problem," or is it better for them to learn facts through more incidental methods? Some people think that courses in English or geography supply a better context for intercultural studies than do courses focused directly on social issues.

There surely is no call to sharpen in the child's mind a sense of conflict. Yet we cannot be categorical about the matter. While a child may, through indirect methods, learn to take cultural pluralism for granted, he is still perplexed by visible differences in skin color, by the recurrent Jewish holidays, by religious diversity. His education is incomplete unless he understands these matters. Some degree of directness would seem to be required. And with older and more sophisticated people there may be even greater value in a direct approach, particularly with advanced students who are prepared to face issues head-on.

In an experiment devoted to three modes of teaching one-week seminars, Rabbi Kagan reports greatest gains by the direct method.[6]

To one group of Christian students he taught Old Testament literature, avoiding any mention of Christian-Jewish friction or of present-day problems. In this indirect method, he merely stressed the positive contribution of Jews to biblical history. A second group was taught the same subject, but with frequent, direct reference to the problem of prejudice, allowing catharsis and a recounting of personal experiences in the class. A third group was taught by the indirect method, but the instruction was supplemented by personal conferences covering the student's experiences and allowing catharsis. This method Kagan called *focused interview*. Before-and-after tests were administered to all students by a Christian colleague.

The author concludes that the indirect method resulted in no significant change, but that the direct method was markedly effective and the focused interview yielded positive results. On the whole he favors the direct method group. It is important to add that a few extremely anti-Semitic students in the population were unchanged by any of these methods of approach.

It seems probable that the relative success of the direct method in this research was due to the composition of the group. The students were of high school age and were selected for their interest in religious matters. Most of them were thus probably prepared to face issues frankly and to shift their attitudes in a favorable direction. The evidence, therefore, remains uncertain. Only in the future can we decide with what groups and under what circumstances direct or indirect methods are to be preferred.

The approach through vicarious experience. Some evidence indicates that films, novels and dramas may be effective if they induce sympathetic identification with minority group members. While we are not yet certain of the facts, it seems likely that strategies of realistic participation constitute too strong a threat to some people. A milder invitation to identification at the fantasy level may be a more effective first step. Perhaps in the future we shall decide that intercultural programs should *start* with fiction, drama and films, and move gradually into more realistic methods of training.

Most of the remaining methods in intercultural education call for active participation on the part of the student. He makes field trips into the neighborhoods where minorities live; he participates in festivals or community projects with them. He develops an *acquaintance with*, not merely *knowledge about*, them. Most investigators favor the participation method above all others. It is considered good for both young and old; it can be adapted to the school program and also for use with adults. Let us consider this important technique further.

Contact and Acquaintance Programs

Contact brings friendliness: this assumption lies at the basis of many so-called action programs. The assumption, however, is stated too broadly. We know that, while some kinds of contact make for mutual understanding and friendliness, the reverse is also true. Contacts are not helpful between people of unequal status or between people who equally *lack* status (poor whites and poor Negroes). Residential contacts are unhelpful if these are perceived in terms of threatening invasion.

Yet studies are accumulating to show that, under certain conditions, increased contact does make for lessened prejudice. We can state the situation in the form of a tentative law: *prejudice tends to diminish whenever members of different groups meet on terms of equal status in the pursuit of common objectives.*

The law, it will be noted, contains two propositions: the contact must be one of equal status, and the members must have objective interests in common. While it may help to place members of groups side by side on a job, the gain in tolerance is greater if these members regard themselves a part of a team. Lewin has pointed out that many committees on race or community relations do not really engage in common projects of mutual interest. They merely meet to talk about the disease. Lacking a definite objective goal, such good-will committees often experience frustration and irritation.[7]

It follows from this law that enforced segregation should be abolished. Otherwise, equal status contacts cannot take place; until they take place, cooperative projects of joint concern cannot arise. And until this condition is fulfilled, we may not expect widespread resolution of intergroup tensions. Hence the attack on segregation must continue. Gandhi, it will be remembered, called for elimination of untouchability as the *first* point in his program. Without this gain, he felt, no other improvement in Hindu life could be achieved.

A final word of caution concerning the law. It would be easy to point to apparent exceptions, but these exceptions are usually not actual test cases. For example, it may be found that boys in a mixed school are as prejudiced against Negroes as are boys in an all-white school. Apparently, equal-status contact does not have the expected result. But status is a subtle thing, and minority groups in a school system do not always enjoy true equality. Furthermore, contact alone is not enough. The contact must lead to further action in the pursuit of common ends. In many schools, this form of mutuality does not occur.

Last but not least, this law, like all social laws, can claim to hold only when other things are equal. It is quite possible that counter-currents may set the law temporarily in abeyance. For example, if economic conditions should suddenly become stringent for both Jewish and gentile doctors, and if conditions led them to perceive each other as rivals, their former cooperativeness in pursuit of common ends might cease. But the existence of counter-tides does not mean that there are no lawful currents.

Group Retraining

One of the boldest advances in modern social science is the deliberate formation of groups for the express purpose of changing the members' outlook. People band together voluntarily in programs of group dynamics because they are dissatisfied with their skill in human relations. They wish to study techniques of democratic leadership. True, they do not join the retraining group expressly to get rid of their prejudices, but they may soon learn that it is their own attitudes and biases that are blocking their effectiveness as foremen, teachers or executives.

Unlike the citizen who reads a pamphlet or listens to a sermon on Brotherhood Sunday, the individual who submits himself to a retraining program is in it up to his eyes. He may be required to act out the roles of other people—employees, students, Negro servants—and he learns through such psychodrama what it feels like to be in another's shoes. He also gains insight regarding his own motives, anxieties and projections. Sometimes the training program is supplemented by private sessions with a counselor, who helps him further along the road of self-examination. As perspective grows, a deeper understanding of the feelings and thoughts of others develops.[8]

Evaluations of this type of training have shown that the gains are greater if social support is maintained. For example, in a study designed to increase skills in community relations work, it was found that if, after training, workers return to localities where no other members of the training team live, they tend to be less effective. They become discouraged and overwhelmed by the mores. On the other hand, two or more people who have been retrained give each other the needed support and carry through their newly acquired insights and skills more effectively.[9]

Not all retraining is of this direct, self-conscious, self-critical type. It may be more objectively centered. An example is the retraining that comes to people who band together to investigate group relations in their city or region. The experience of designing the study, framing questions, conducting interviews and computing the discrimination indices (in housing, employment and education) is highly beneficial. The follow-up activities are even more so; for as people work to improve the situation, further gains in knowledge, community skills and sympathy are bound to result.[10]

Another example of outwardly centered retraining is found in connection with the technique known as *incident control*. Its purpose, as in any group retraining, is to break down inhibition and rigidity in several individuals at once, so that they may become more effective in the pursuit of common ends. In this particular case, those who submit to training wish to develop a skill for use in everyday life—skill in answering the bigoted remarks that stain our national habits of conversation. What does one say, for example, to a stranger in a public place who has let fall a venomous comment on the Jews that reaches uninvited the ears of many bystanders? Of course, there are many situations where propriety would have us keep silent; but there are other situations where silence would lend consent, and here our sense of justice prompts us to speak up. Research shows that a calm voice, marked by obvious sincerity and expressing the view that such comments are un-American, has the most favorable effect on bystanders. But it is not easy to summon the courage to speak at all, let alone to find the right words and to control one's voice. Hours of practice under supervision in a group setting are required.[11]

Some of the retraining programs discussed thus far have a marked limitation. They are designed to free the tolerant person of his inhibitions and to provide him with skills, if he wants them. But it is clear that full-scale group retraining cannot be used with people who resist both the method and its objectives. Yet, with patience and tact, groups or classes formed for other purposes may be led by easy stages into practicing the techniques of group dynamics.

Furthermore, partial use may be made of these techniques of group dynamics without going the whole way. School children, for example, can easily be led into role-playing.[12] By playing the part of a child in an out-group, the juvenile actor may begin to appreciate, through his own sensations, the suffering and defensiveness engendered by discrimination. A related technique has been employed by Axline, who reports that play therapy in a group of young children results in the amelioration of serious racial conflicts within the group.[13] Three or four children, white and colored, are put together in a play situation with dolls and miniature house furnishings. This arrangement offers opportunities for the projection of conflicts and nascent hostility. It was found that, as the play progresses, accommodation sets in and a lasting friendly adjustment between the Negro and white playmates is established.

Mass Media

There are good grounds for doubting the effectiveness of mass propaganda. People whose ears and eyes are bombarded all day with blandishments of special interests tend to develop a propaganda blindness and deafness. And what chance has a mild message of brotherhood, sandwiched in between layers of war, intrigue, hatred and crime? Furthermore, pro-tolerance propaganda is selectively perceived. Those who do not want to admit it to their sanctuaries of belief find no trouble in evading it. Usually those who admit it do not need it. But this general pessimism should not block our search for more detailed knowledge. After all, we know that advertising and films have molded our national culture to a considerable degree. May they not profitably be used in the task of remolding it?

Research, though still somewhat meager, suggests even now certain tentative laws: [14]

1. While a single program—a film, perhaps—shows only a slight effect, several related programs produce effects even greater than could be accounted for by simple summation. This principle of *pyramiding stimulation* is well understood by practical propagandists. Any publicity expert knows that a single program is not enough; there must be a campaign.

2. Propaganda must cope, however, with the law of *specificity of effect.* In the spring of 1951, a motion picture theater in Boston ran the film, *The Sound of Fury.* The picture concluded with the clearly stated moral that conflicts can be solved only through patience and understanding, not through violence. The audience, deeply moved by the dramatic story, applauded the moral. Later in the same program, a newsreel depicted Senator Taft speaking on international relations. He made the identical point—that conflict can

be solved only through patience and understanding, not through violence. The same audience hissed. What they had learned in one context did not carry over to another. Several researches confirm the conclusion; opinions may change, but the change tends to be limited to a narrow context and to generalize very little if at all.

3. Propaganda must also cope with *attitude regression*. After a period of time, opinions tend to slip back toward their original configuration—but not all the way.

4. This regression, however, is not universal. Studying both the short-run and long-run effect of indoctrination films in the army, Hovland and his associates found that, while attitude regression was common enough, in some people a reverse trend occurred.[15] *Sleeper effects* came to light. These delayed effects occur in "die-hards" who at first resist the message of the film but later accept it. The sleeper phenomenon is noted especially among well-educated people whose initial opinions are contrary to those held by most other educated people. The authors suggest that these individuals have predispositions favoring the propaganda message but must first overcome some inner resistance to it. The moral seems to be that pro-tolerance propaganda reaching people who are ambivalent in their attitudes may have long-range effects, especially among the better educated portions of the population.

5. Propaganda is more effective when there are no *deep-seated resistances*. Research shows that people who are on the fence are more likely to be affected than those who are deeply committed.

6. Propaganda is more effective when it has a *clear field*. The monopoly of propaganda that exists in totalitarian lands forces a monotonous barrage upon the defenseless citizen, and he cannot long maintain his powers of resistance. Counterpropaganda, if it is permitted, throws the individual back upon his own resources of judgment and frees him from a one-sided view of reality. In the light of this principle, it may well be argued that pro-tolerance propaganda is needed—not only for its positive effects but also as an antidote to agitators who work on the other side.

7. To be effective, propaganda should *allay anxiety*. Bettelheim and Janowitz found that propaganda striking at the roots of a person's frame of security tends to be resisted.[16] Appeals geared into existing systems of security are more effective.

8. A final principle concerns the importance of *prestigeful symbols*. A Kate Smith can sell millions of dollars in war bonds over the radio in a single day. An Eleanor Roosevelt or a Bing Crosby

have prestige for great masses of people. Their espousing of tolerance helps to win many fence-straddlers.

Exhortation

We do not know the effects of preachment, admonishment or ethical pep talks. Religious leaders have exhorted their followers for centuries to the practice of brotherly love. The cumulative effect seems slight; yet we cannot be too sure that the method is futile. Without such constant admonishment, matters might be much worse than they are.

A reasonable guess might be that exhortation helps strengthen the good intentions of those already converted. And this achievement is not to be scorned, for without religious and ethical reinforcement of their convictions, the already converted might not maintain their efforts toward the betterment of group relations. For the character-conditioned bigot, however, and for the conformist who finds his social environment too powerful, hortatory eloquence is likely to have small effect.

Individual Therapy

Theoretically, perhaps the best of all methods for changing attitudes is individual psychotherapy. The person who, in distress, seeks the aid of a psychiatrist or counselor is usually desirous of change. He is likely to be ready for a realignment of many of his basic orientations toward life. While it is safe to say that a patient never comes to a therapist for the express purpose of changing his *ethnic* attitudes, these attitudes may assume a salient role as the course of treatment progresses, and may conceivably be dissolved or re-structured along with the patient's other fixed ways of looking at life.

No conclusive study has been made of this hypothesis, although various psychoanalysts have reported their clinical experience.[17] This experience is particularly cogent, for most patients think of psychoanalysis as a "Jewish movement" and this fact alone is almost certain to stir up such anti-Semitic prejudice as may exist. The course of the treatment may be somewhat as follows: Early in the course of his analysis, the patient enters the phase known as negative transference. He blames the analyst for the suffering the therapeutic process causes, and hates him for his position of dominance and advantage, for being *pro tem* a parent-substitute. Sometimes the analyst is a Jew; even if he is not, the patient thinks of psychoanalysis as a Jewish movement. This circumstance elicits his private anti-Semitic feelings, which more likely than not explode in his outbursts against the analyst. As the treatment progresses, and as the patient gains insight into his whole pattern of values, the anti-Semitism may abate. Indeed, in principle we should expect that, whenever prejudice of any sort intersects with a neurosis, amelioration of the neurosis will result in a reduction of the prejudice.

Psychoanalysis is only one mode of treatment. Almost any prolonged interview with a person concerning his personal problems is likely to uncover all major hostilities. In talking about them, the patient often gains a new perspective. And if in the course of the treatment he discovers a more generally wholesome and constructive way of life, his prejudice may abate. For example, one student engaged in research was conducting a long interview with a woman concerning her experience with, and attitudes toward, minority groups. There was no therapeutic intention whatsoever. In the course of the interview, the woman told of her anti-Semitic feelings. Pursuing her whole past experience with Jews and with neighborhood anti-Semitism, she gradually gained greatly in self-insight. At one point she exclaimed, "The poor Jews, I guess we blame them for everything, don't we?" Unless she had fixed her attention for considerable time (about three hours) on this feature of her belief system, she would not have tracked it down to its sources and placed it in rational perspective in her life.

The frequency of transformations under therapeutic or quasi-therapeutic conditions is unknown. More research is needed. But even if individual therapy proves to be the most effective of all methods—and because of its depth and interrelatedness with all portions of the personality, it should be—the proportion of the population reached will always be small. We cannot psychoanalyze each and every bigot.

Catharsis

Experience shows that in certain situations—especially in individual therapy and in group retraining sessions—an explosion of feeling often occurs. When the subject of prejudice comes up for discussion, a person who feels his views are under attack or disapproved may need the purging that comes with such explosion.

Catharsis has a quasi-curative effect. It temporarily relieves the tension and may prepare the individual for a change of attitude. < It is easier to mend an inner tube after the air has been released. Blake's poem expresses this relation between catharsis and tension:

> I was angry with my friend;
> I told my wrath, my wrath did end.
> I was angry with my foe;
> I told it not, my wrath did grow.

Yet not every expression of hostility has a cathartic effect. Only under special circumstances does a person who "blows his top" then become willing and able to understand the other side of the argument. While he remains at all tense and aggrieved, he cannot and will not listen.

In an eastern city, a number of unpleasant instances of ethnic conflict had occurred. Aroused citizens put pressure on the local police force to introduce a course of instruction dealing with the backgrounds of group antagonism and the policemen's role in preventing and handling outbreaks. The police officers who attended this compulsory course were resentful, for the very circumstances under which it was arranged cast reflections upon their competence and fairness. This sense of injustice, together with their own prejudices against certain minority groups, created a condition of tension that made instruction difficult—almost impossible. Whenever an objective point was made concerning Negroes in the community, some police officer would be sure to respond with a story of a vicious Negro who bit him while being arrested.

Under such conditions of injured self-esteem it is unlikely that existing prejudice can be changed. No one can be taught who thinks himself under attack. The course of instruction encountered stereotypes, caustic anecdotes and expressions of hostility from the police. None of the instruction seemed to register; it provoked only a torrent of abuse, directed partly against the teacher and partly against the minority groups under discussion. Often the class would complain: "Why does everyone pick on the police?" "We've never had any trouble. Why do we need this course?" "Why don't the Jews mind their own business? If they find a dead cat in the ash can, they call it anti-Semitism." "The Negro leaders ought to control their people and not set them against the police."

The course lasted for eight hours. The first six were largely occupied with this type of catharsis. The instructor offered no counterarguments and listened as sympathetically as possible to the hostile outbursts.

Gradually, a change seemed to occur. For one thing, the class became bored with its own complaining. The attitude seemed to be, "We've had our say; now we'll listen to what you have to say on the subject." Furthermore, so many obvious overstatements had been made in anger that a certain sheepishness crept in. The man who asserted, "We've never had any trouble; there is no problem here," was soon recounting several incidents of conflict that he had encountered and, as a policeman, did not know how to handle. A man who at first railed against Jews tried in later remarks to make amends.

Catharsis, then, may occasionally be effective because one's irrational outburst shocks one's own conscience. When the immediate tensions have been released, the individual is freer to reconstruct his perception of the total situation. Even while expressing hostility, he may be developing private plans for future conduct that will be more acceptable to the community at large. Thus a given official might have been thinking, especially toward the end of the course, "Well, I certainly have blown my top. Damn it, I had a right to; it's terrible the way we're picked on. Everybody's got prejudices. But it *is* tough on the minorities in this community. I don't want any trouble in my district. I'd better look out for so and so; he's likely to make trouble, the way he hates Negroes and Jews. I guess I'll. . . ." And here he begins to construct in imagination a plan for future handling of the problem in his precinct.

It cannot be proved that such mental processes occur following catharsis, but the impression of observers of this particular course of instruction was that during the last two hours, when the antagonism had worn out, the lessons commenced to register and the gain in self-insight was appreciable.[18]

Catharsis itself is not curative. The best that can be said for it is that it prepares the way for a less tense view of the situation. Having had his say, the aggrieved person may be more ready to listen to the other point of view. If his statements have been exaggerated and unfair—as they usually are—the resulting shame mollifies his anger and induces a more balanced point of view.

It is not recommended that every program start off by inviting catharsis. To do so would create a negative atmosphere at the outset. When catharsis is needed, it will come without special invitation.

This is most likely to occur when prejudiced people feel that they themselves are under attack. When this situation prevails, no progress can be made until catharsis is allowed. With patience, skill and luck, the leader may at the right moment guide the catharsis into constructive channels.

Final Word

The improvement of human relations is a broad subject—considerably broader than the scope of this essay. Our aim has been to pass in review a large variety of recent research in the area of ethnic antagonism. From it we have learned two things: *First:* there is an immense amount of activity and interest in applying scientific methods to the discovery of effective techniques for reducing prejudice. *Second:* present indications favor certain techniques over others, and indicate to some extent the specific conditions when we would do well to select one technique and not another.

While I sincerely believe in the value of the work reviewed, I have no desire to oversimplify the problem of building altruistic character. The issue is so complex, and the need so great, that every resource must be called upon. It would be a grave error to think that we have devised a bag of tricks, which, if adroitly manipulated, will conjure up a good neighbor. But it would be an equally grave error to assume that the plodding and serious investigations here reported have nothing to contribute to the improvement of human relationships. Education and religion, mass media and legislation, child training and psychotherapy—these and all other channels of human effort must be followed if we are to produce a race of men who will seek their individual salvation, not at the expense of their fellows, but in concert with them.

REFERENCES

1. G. W. Allport and B. M. Kramer, "Some roots of prejudice," *J. Psychol.*, 1946, 22:9-39.

2. Technical discussions concerning the measurement of attitudes, of prejudice, of group tension are omitted. The reader is referred to M. Jahoda, M. Deutsch and S. W. Cook, *Research methods in social relations*, New York: 1951.

3. L. A. Cook (ed.), *College programs in intergroup relations*, Washington: American Council on Education, 1950.

4. Surveys of these evaluational studies have been reported by O. Klineberg, *Tensions affecting international understanding: a survey of research*, New York: Social Science Research Council, 1950, Bull. 62, Chap. 4; R. M.

Williams, Jr., *The reduction of intergroup tensions: a survey of research on problems of ethnic, racial, and religious group relations,* New York: Social Science Research Council, 1947, Bull. 57; A. M. Rose, *Studies in the reduction of prejudice,* Chicago: American Council on Race Relations, 1947 (mimeographed).

5. For fuller accounts of the relationship between legislation and prejudice containing evidence for the statements made in the present discussion, see: J. H. Burma, "Race relations and anti-discriminatory legislation," *Amer. J. Sociol.,* 1951, 56:416-23; W. Maslow, "The law and race relations," *Ann. Amer. Acad. Pol. Soc. Sci.,* 1946, 244:75-81; T. S. Kendler, "Contributions of the psychologist to constitutional law," *Amer. Psychologist,* 1950, 5:505-10; M. Deutscher and I. Chein, "The psychological effects of enforced segregation—a survey of social science opinion," *J. Psychol.,* 1948, 26:259-87.

6. H. E. Kagan, *Changing the attitudes of Christian toward Jew,* New York: 1952.

7. K. Lewin, "Research on minority problems," *Tech. Rev.,* 1946, 48: 163-64, 182-90.

8. An elementary exposition of "group dynamics" is given by S. Chase, *Roads to agreement,* New York: 1951, Chap. 9.

9. R. Lippitt, *Training in community relations,* New York: 1949.

10. M. H. Wormser and C. Selltiz, *How to conduct a community self-survey of civil rights,* New York: 1951.

11. A. F. Citron, I. Chein, and J. Harding, "Anti-minority remarks: a problem for action research," *J. Abnorm. Soc. Psychol.,* 1950, 45:99-126.

12. G. Shaftel and R. F. Shaftel, "Report on the use of 'practice action level' in the Stanford University project for American ideals," *Sociatry,* 1948, 2:243-53.

13. V. M. Axline, "Play therapy and race conflict in young children," *J. Abnorm. Soc. Psychol.,* 1948, 43:279-86.

14. A bibliography of research is contained in the monograph by J. T. Klapper, *The effects of mass media,* New York: Columbia University Bureau of Applied Social Research, 1950 (mimeographed).

15. C. I. Hovland *et al., Experiments on mass communication,* Princeton: 1949.

16. B. Bettelheim and M. Janowitz, "Reactions to fascist propaganda: a pilot study," *Publ. Opin. Quart.,* 1950, 14:530-60.

17. See N. W. Ackerman and M. Jahoda, *Anti-Semitism and emotional disorder,* New York: 1950; R. M. Lowenstein, *Christians and Jews: a psychoanalytic study,* New York: 1950; E. Simmel (ed.), *Anti-Semitism: a social disease,* New York: 1948.

18. This case is recounted more fully in G. W. Allport, "Catharsis and the reduction of prejudice," *J. Soc. Issues,* 1945, 1:1-8.

Religion and prejudice

We all know some religious people who are bigoted against various ethnic and religious groups. But we also know others who sincerely practice brotherhood. In both types of people, religion seems to be largely responsible—for their prejudice, or for their tolerance.

This essay first dips into the history of the Christian church and finds that, while the opposed strands of bigotry and tolerance have always been with us, in recent years the clash has grown acute.

The essay then offers a functional analysis of the two forms of religiosity. *Extrinsic* religion is a self-serving, utilitarian, self-protective form of religious outlook, which provides the believer with comfort and salvation at the expense of out-groups. *Intrinsic* religion marks the life that has interiorized the total creed of his faith without reservation, including the commandment to love one's neighbor. A person of this sort is more intent on serving his religion than on making it serve him. In many lives, both strands are found; the result is inner conflict, with prejudice and tolerance competing for the upper hand.

Originally presented as the Ratcliff Lecture at Tufts University in April 1959, the essay was first published in *The Crane Review* (1959).

Brotherhood and bigotry are intertwined in all religion. Plenty of pious people are saturated with racial, ethnic and class prejudice. At the same time, many of the most ardent advocates of racial justice are religiously motivated. Like Gandhi they labor for equimindedness within the whole human family. This is the paradox I wish to explore.

The paradox is one to haunt both the psychologist and the clergy. Within the past decade, social and psychological scientists have made great advances in understanding the dynamics of prejudice, although they tend to overlook the tie with piety. Usually they are content merely to point to the common finding that, on the average, churchgoers are more intolerant than non-churchgoers. As for the clergy, can any minister fail to spot both bigotry and anti-bigotry in his own flock? Can he fail to sympathize with the plight of the Christian clergy in Little Rock, which has been so well described by Campbell and Pettigrew in their recent book *Christians in racial crisis*? [1]

257

Let me first briefly outline the nature of the problem in historical terms, for I urgently desire to emphasize its pervasive and apparently permanent character. In the concluding sections I shall try to unravel the paradox from a psychologist's point of view and point the road to a solution.

I

In the Christian religion, and to a varying degree in other religions, there are three intrinsic sources of bigotry.

The first is the doctrine of *revelation*: truth once revealed cannot be tampered with. This doctrine has a curious consequence for successive generations of believers: it leads to a rigidity that the original Scriptures do not warrant. Take, for example, St. Paul's injunction, "Therefore judge nothing before the time, until the Lord come." [2] St. Paul seems here to be enlarging on the words of Christ: "Let both grow together until the harvest." [3] Later believers have difficulty with these permissive sentiments. How can one be tolerant of those who depart from the revealed formula for salvation? Menno Simons, the Anabaptist, worried about the matter, and his narrow solution is typical of all the centuries. He simply reinterpreted St. Paul to mean, "None may judge unless he have the judging word on his side." [4] In effect, Simons—like many men of piety—interposed his right to judge according to his own view of the revelation. Since all sects and creeds claim to have the judging word on their side, the door swings wide to bigotry. Unbelievers are sharply judged here and now.

The second intrinsic source of bigotry lies in the doctrine of *election*. Whatever theological justification the doctrine may have, the view that one's own group is chosen (and that other groups are not) leads forthwith away from brotherhood and into bigotry. It does so because it feeds one's pride and hunger for status—two important psychological roots of prejudice. Some groups have claimed to be the lost tribe of Israel; the claim enhances the status of the members and consigns all "gentile" groups to a position of inferiority. A cardinal example of election is based on certain obscurities in the Book of Genesis. Noah, it seems, cursed Ham and declared that his children should forever be "the servants of servants." Legend has it that the children of Ham are the black race. By this sleight of hand, many white people in South Africa and in our own Southern states declare that they are divinely elected to the position of permanent white supremacy.

Thus the doctrines of revelation and election provide open channels to prejudice—but do they *necessarily* have this end-result? If so, we should have to despair of many religions. The Roman Catholic Church holds firmly to the revelation that it alone is the True Church, divinely established and protected from error. The Jewish religion could not exist at all without its revelation that the Jews are God's chosen people. Does it follow that Roman Catholics and Jews and comparable bodies are destined to bigotry?

Speaking to this very point, Bishop Lesslie Newbigin of the Anglican Church writes: "We must claim absoluteness and finality for Christ and His finished work; but that very claim forbids us to claim absoluteness and finality for our understanding of it." [5] Revelation and election, being divinely ordained, are not susceptible to human interpretation. Only God knows His plan for the human race. It is not for us to judge those who do not share our understanding of this plan.

This more relaxed interpretation of revealed religion and election requires a subtle mind, one that can embrace absolutes and at the same time judge nothing "until the Lord come." It may take a long time for the masses of religious people to acquire this delicate balance. As matters stand, we can safely say that the majority of the people will continue to regard religious outsiders with condescension and even with contempt. This will be true among Jews, Catholics, Fundamentalists—and even among liberal Christians, who often hold to a special version of revelation and election akin to intellectual snobbery.

The third intrinsic source of bigotry in Christian history—*theocracy*—has lost much of its power. It is the view, prevalent for many centuries, that rulers are divinely ordained to enforce through civil and military power the currently fashionable interpretations of revelation and election. This doctrine of divine rights and divine obligation drove the Western world into centuries of persecution and bloody bigotry under the banner of Holy Zeal. It took a very long time for the West to rid itself of physical coercion as a device for enforcing the judging word. Not only the rulers themselves, but also the people—even many saintly people—felt that it was the duty of civil authority to enforce agreement with the then prevailing interpretations of election and revelation.

One thinks of St. Augustine's appeal to the emperor to crush the Pelagians, who disputed his views on the damnation of unbaptized infants. Of the persecution of the Jews by St. Ambrose, St. Gregory of Nyssa and St. John Chrysostom.[6] Of the fanaticism of Pope

Urban II, who launched the Crusades, wherein political and economic gain at the expense of the "unspeakable Turk" was sanctified in the frenzied battle cry, "Deus vult." Of Pope Sixtus IV, who, while building the Sistine Chapel, authorized Spain's sovereigns to make a ruthless inquisition. Of the thousands of Jews burned at the stake in 1485, when Tomas de Torquemada took over the management of the Inquisition. Of St. Bartholomew's Eve in 1572, when twenty to thirty thousand Huguenots were massacred.[7] Of Pope Innocent VIII, who in the fifteenth century anathematized all who refused to believe in witchcraft.[8] Of the inconclusive savagery of the wars of religion, which subsided only toward the close of the seventeenth century.

When Protestantism arrived on the scene, it behaved no better, for it was founded on the same three pillars of bigotry: revelation, election and theocracy. It is the parodox of Protestantism that, except at high moments of its history, it has not lived by its primary tenet—that the channel of revelation is personal. Although the individual is told to seek revelation, he is expected to reach the "right" answer from his communion with the Scriptures and the Holy Spirit. Death at the stake was the punishment for Servetus, who, according to Calvin, misinterpreted the promptings of the Holy Spirit. Under Protestantism, heresy remained for a long time a capital crime, though its definition shifted capriciously through the evolution of sects and through the theocratic reigns of assorted sovereigns.

Queen Elizabeth I required every Roman Catholic to attend the Church of England. During much of the eighteenth century, the saying of the Roman Mass in England was punishable by "perpetual imprisonment"; and, as late as 1825, foreigners who wished to become English citizens had to take the Sacrament of the Lord's Supper from a minister of the Anglican Church.[9] The General Court of Massachusetts decreed in 1647 that "no Jesuit or spiritual or ecclesiastical person (as they are termed), ordained by the pope of the see of Rome, shall henceforth come into Massachusetts. Any person not freeing himself of suspicion shall be jailed, then banished. If taken a second time he shall be put to death."

II

The history of bigotry is tiresome and painful to recount. But unless we have it in mind, we shall not be able to understand the nature of our present problem. The horrors are not by any means all in the past. But what is new is our comprehension of some of the psychodynamic factors that add fire and flame to theological dispute.

Anti-Catholicism in the United States, like anti-Negro prejudice, has often drawn on the appetite for sexual disclosures. Incited by stories of immorality in convents, a mob in Charlestown, Massachusetts, on August 11, 1834, burned the Ursaline Convent. One influential political party, the Know-Nothings, rose to considerable power in the mid-nineteenth century largely on the basis of such legends. Later in the century the American Protective Association flourished, sustained by anti-Catholic periodicals. Typical among such periodicals was *Watson's Magazine*, not only anti-Catholic but anti-Negro and anti-Semitic as well. Its logic is illustrated by the following typical quotation: "Heavens above! Think of a Negro priest taking the vow of chastity and then being turned loose among women who have been taught that a priest cannot sin. It is a thing to make one shudder." Similarly, the "libertine Jew" was said to have a "ravenous appetite for the forbidden fruit—a lustful eagerness enhanced by the racial novelty of the girls of the uncircumcised." [10] This combination of the sexual and the religious is receiving considerable attention in contemporary psychology.[11]

In the present century, no less than in the past, political self-interest has sparked religious persecution. We think of the Jewish pogroms of Czarist Russia and of the slaughter of Muslim by Hindu and of Hindu by Muslim only a decade ago. A kind of religious rapture intoxicated the Nazis: " 'Hitler is a new, a greater, a more powerful Jesus Christ. Our God, our Pope, is Adolph Hitler.' So rhapsodized Nazi leader Binve. And not to be outdone in ecstatic homage, Propaganda Minister Goebbels in an address at Berlin, instructed the regimented German nation: 'Our leader becomes the intermediary between his people and the throne of God. . . . Everything which our leader utters is religion in its highest sense, in its deepest sense, and in its deepest and most hidden meaning.' " [12]

Even these few examples show us why many thoughtful people today discredit religion. A college student summed up a common judgment: "Religion has tried for centuries to establish a brotherhood of man. It has had its day. . . . The problems religion tries to solve need solving, but religion has failed." A second student speaks of organized religion as "another schism in a divided world—a curse." [13]

III

The history we have reviewed up to now is one-sided. We should not forget that even in times of persecution there have been great-souled prophets who, often to their peril, spoke out against bigotry and preached the Gospel of equimindedness. Socrates did so. So too did Christ—many centuries ahead of His church.

Early in the Christian era the voices were timid and clouded. Tertullian, for example, asserted that God did not wish to be worshiped unwillingly; salvation could not be coerced but must be freely appropriated. And it was Tertullian who so brilliantly perceived the dynamics of scapegoating: "They take the Christians to be the cause of every disaster to the state, of every misfortune to the people. If the Tiber reaches the wall; if the Nile does not reach the fields; if the sky does not move, or if the earth does; if there is a famine, or if there is a plague—the cry is at once 'The Christians to the lions.'" [14] Yet it was also Tertullian whose rigid interpretations of election and revelation led him to speak so fiercely against recusants that he has been called the first Christian bigot.

Toward the end of the fifth century, Pope Gelasius I likewise opposed coercion and questioned the right of any emperor to interpret the Sacrifice of the Cross or to prescribe how its benefits shall be spread among mankind. St. Ambrose, too, opposed the emperor's right to interpret the Christian trust, but he did not hesitate to denounce the Jews. In the thirteenth century Raymond Lully dared to oppose both the Crusades and the rising Inquisition. And a century later Cardinal Cusa suggested that human transcripts of the divine will are always contaminated by the blindness of self-interest of mortal men. He proposed a parliament of religions to which even the Muslims should be invited. But such voices were feeble and sporadic.

The Reformation added its pleas, even while it took over the three pillars of bigotry. In 1554, Sebastian Castellio issued his manifesto advocating religious toleration. Christianity, he insisted, is beneficence; persecution is its antithesis, and if persecution belongs to religion, religion is a curse to mankind. At the height of witchburning, Montaigne expressed his misgivings in golden words: "After all, it is rating one's conjectures at a very high price to roast a man alive on the strength of them." Also in the sixteenth century, Schwenkfeld taught that a sense of divine immediacy should keep us from hatred: the Holy Spirit has sevenfold gifts, and we should acknowledge their diversity among men of all kinds. Irenicism, a search for peaceful unity among churches, grew on this foundation, as did modern Quakerism. But the full flower of this sixteenth-century spiritualism was slow in being achieved. As Bainton remarks, "The best things on religious liberty were said in the sixteenth century but not practiced until the nineteenth." [15]

But advocates of equimindedness were seldom wholehearted. Milton advanced the principle of religious freedom but would have denied its benefits to Catholics and atheists—a position held likewise by John Locke. Cromwell declared for freedom of conscience but denied it, for political reasons, to Catholics, Anglicans and Baptists.

But slowly there arose strong champions of the separation of church and state. Preliminary skirmishes were fought by dissenters in Holland and by Roger Williams in the New World. The decisive turning point came, of course, when James Madison wrote and Congress adopted the First Amendment to the Constitution of the United States: "Congress shall make no law respecting the establishment of religion, or prohibiting the free exercise thereof. . . ." For the first time in the history of the Western world, men canceled the claim of divine sanction for the state, and therewith the possibility of official persecution for religious deviance. This decisive step has been called by one of America's foremost jurists, David Dudley Field, "the greatest achievement ever made in the course of human progress."

The First Amendment eliminated the possibility of theocracy in America, and its repercussions were so wide that today heresy or any other form of religious deviance is seldom if ever punished as a legal crime in any country of the world. The theocratic pillar of bigotry is gone, and the other two pillars are weakening. It is this fact that helps create the current crisis, with its potential for profound change.

Only in certain markedly orthodox sects today do we find the doctrines of revelation and election explicitly used to justify anti-Negro, anti-Jewish, anti-Gentile or any other prejudice. Yet if explicit theological justification is rarer than it was, an analogous psychological process is still at work.

IV

Let us take a not uncommon form of the religious-prejudice syndrome. A certain child, let us say, is taught the usual adult complex of ideas. Christ came into the world to save all men—black, brown and white—but dreadful things will happen if any but a white man should move into the neighborhood. He is taught that his family's church is the best and that all others are inferior. He learns that the Heavenly Father grants favors when asked, but especially to a child who belongs to the elect.

Now, suppose this teaching is absorbed by a child who has deep psychological needs engendered by insecurity, inferiority of status, suspicion and distrust. He may never think explicitly of the doctrines of revelation and election; yet his background prepares him for the same type of reasoning that has marked bigotry throughout the course of history: "God is partial to me. Through prayer I can conjure His special favor. Since God is created in my image, His role is to confer security and other benefits upon me. My economy of living is one of exclusion—of barring from my presence out-groups, which threaten my comfort. My religion and my prejudice both serve my exclusionist style. They are islands of safety in a threatening world. They are custom-tailored lifejackets to be donned in frightening waters." In such a life, religion is not the cause of ethnic prejudice, nor is prejudice the cause of the religion. Both strategies are protective; both confer security, a sense of status and of encapsulation.

This syndrome appears to be exceedingly common; many investigations show that, on the average, churchgoers and professedly religious people have considerably more prejudice than do non-churchgoers and nonbelievers. Today, as in former times, countless people assume that the Almighty meant to arrange the human family in a hierarchical order, with themselves at the top. And some will still cite Holy Scripture to prove their point.

In the case we have described, it is clear that religion is not the master-motive in the life. It plays an instrumental role only. It serves and rationalizes assorted forms of self-interest. In such a life, the full creed and full teaching of religion are not adopted. The person does not serve his religion; it is subordinated to serve him. The master-motive is always self-interest. In such a life-economy, religion has extrinsic value only. And it is *extrinsic* religion, thus defined, that we find most closely associated with prejudice.

V

But now we turn to the opposite, or *intrinsic*, type of religious sentiment. It too gets an early start in life. The child's mind is, as in the other case, early tuned to the favors that God can render—a gift of skates for Christmas, or cancellation of an appointment with the dentist. It is hard at the start for any child to avoid a self-centered and family-centered view of religion. But there is an early difference: the youngster we are now describing has the benefit of basic trust and security within his home. He does not need to look on people as threats to his well-being. He does not need to use religion as a talisman. He does not become fixated on an immature level of development. At adolescence he can take the leap that Piaget calls *reciprocity,* the ability to perceive that others too have convictions and preferences (for their own religion, culture and race) that are analogous to—and, from their point of view, as reasonable as—his own.

The youth we describe is not crippled by his fears and anxieties. He has them, to be sure, but he accepts them as normal afflictions of the human race. It is a sound principle of psychology that the acceptance of one's anxieties makes for a compassionate understanding and acceptance of others.

Advancing thus into maturity, the individual does not necessarily lose his religious faith, nor even his belief in revelation and election. But dogma is tempered with humility: in keeping with biblical injunction, he withholds judgment until the day of the harvest. A religious sentiment of this sort floods the whole life with motivation and meaning. It is no longer limited to single segments of self-interest. And only in such a widened religious sentiment does the teaching of brotherhood take firm root.

I do not wish to imply that people are wholly intrinsic or wholly extrinsic in their religious outlook. Gradations occur along a continuum. Extrinsic religionists have moments when the universalism of the Christian teaching breaks through to them, causing them perhaps to doubt their own stand on such issues as Negro segregation. Intrinsic religionists too may have their lapses, as when they slip into snide and socially fashionable anti-Semitism.

Yet, in principle, the distinction is crucial. Unless we accept it, we shall fail to explain the age-old paradox that troubles us all: how does it come about that religious people tend to be more prejudiced than nonreligious people, while at the same time most of the fighters for equality and brotherhood throughout the centuries have been religiously motivated? We think of Pope Gelasius, Castellio, St. Francis, Schwenkfeld and Roger Williams; in more recent days, of Gandhi, Father Huddleston, Martin Luther King and Albert Schweitzer; and of countless active members of the American Friends Service Committee, the Catholic Interracial Councils, the Unitarian Service Committee and other religious groups too numerous to mention.

VI

The relationship between religion and prejudice hinges on the type of religion that the personal life harbors. When it is extrinsic, the tie with prejudice is close; when intrinsic, prejudice is restrained. Now that religious bodies are becoming self-critical and alert to the issue, they would do well to employ this central fact to guide their policies and plans for the future. Their problem, if I may venture to state it for them, is how to transform the prejudice-linked, extrinsic style of religion held by most of their members—whatever the religious body may be—into intrinsic religion, where the total creed of equimindedness becomes woven into the fabric of personality itself.

REFERENCES

1. E. Q. Campbell and T. F. Pettigrew, *Christians in racial crisis*, Washington: Public Affairs Press, 1959.
2. I Corinthians 4:5.
3. St. Matthew 13:30.
4. Menno Simons, "A foundation and plain instruction of the saving doctrine of Christ" (trans. by I. D. Rupp), *On the ban: questions and answers*, 1550, Lancaster: Elias Barr, 1863. And see Chapter 14, p. 223, of this volume.
5. Rt. Rev. L. Newbigin, "The quest for unity through religion," *J. Rel.*, 1955, 35:17-33.
6. The history of anti-Semitism in the Catholic church is told by M. Hay, *The foot of pride*, Boston: Beacon, 1950, reissued in 1960 as a Beacon Paperback under the title, *Europe and the Jews*. In one of the sermons of the golden-mouthed St. John Chrysostom (whom Cardinal Newman called "a sensitive heart . . . elevated, refined, transformed by a touch of heaven"), we read: "The synagogue is worse than a brothel . . . it is the den of scoundrels and the repair of wild beasts . . . a criminal assembly of Jews . . . a house worse than a drinking shop . . . a den of thieves; a house of ill fame, a dwelling of iniquity, the refuge of devils, a gulf and abyss of perdition. . . . As for me, I hate the synagogue. . . . I hate the Jews for the same reason," pp. 27 ff.
7. For convenient accounts of these and many similar episodes, see G. Meyers, *The history of bigotry in the United States*, New York: Random House, 1943. See also R. H. Bainton, *The travail of religious liberty*, Philadelphia: Westminster, 1951.
8. H. Kramer and J. Springer, *Malleus Maleficarum* (trans. by M. Summers), London: Pushkin Press, 1948, p. xx. See also A. Huxley, *The devils of Loudon*.
9. M. Freedman (ed.), *A minority in Britain*, London: Valentine, Mitchell, 1955, p. 39 f.
10. G. Meyers, *op. cit.*, pp. 252, 259 f.
11. G. W. Allport, *The nature of prejudice*, Cambridge: Addison-Wesley, 1954, Chap. 23.

12. G. Meyers, *op. cit.*, pp. 389 ff. A useful account of the mixing of political bias with Protestant bigotry is R. L. Roy, *Apostles of discord*, Boston: Beacon, 1953.

13. G. W. Allport, J. M. Gillespie, and J. Young, "The religion of the post-war college student," *J. Psychol.*, 1948, 25:3-33.

14. Tertullian, *Apology*, Chap. 40, in Migno: *Patrologia Latina*, Vol. 1, Col. 542.

15. R. H. Bainton, *op. cit.*, p. 253. Other sources regarding the growth of religious toleration are K. S. Latourette, *A history of Christianity*, New York: Harper, 1953; and W. K. Jordan, *The development of religious tolerance in England*, 4 vols., Cambridge: Harvard University Press, 1932-40.

PART V: *Perception and social programs*

Social service in perspective

A psychologists's interests often range widely. He is sometimes concerned with the way people perceive their worlds—that is to say, how they define the situation they are in. He may also be concerned with the process of communication—including rumor, public opinion and persuasion—and may want to know how these and other psychological factors can lead to improvement in the human condition. Part V deals with these topics.

My earliest years of teaching were in the Department of Social Ethics at Harvard University. This in part explains my interest in applying psychological principles and methods to the professional field of social work.

The essay was read at a conference held as part of the Bicentennial Celebration of Columbia University from June 2-5, 1954. It is reprinted here from a volume of proceedings entitled *National policies for education, health, and social services* (1955), where it appeared under the title, "The limits of social service."

A century ago both Thoreau and Emerson spoke out sharply regarding the limits of social service—of "philanthropy," as they then called it. In *Walden,* Thoreau criticized the tendency of the would-be benefactor to project his own ailments onto others. Because he himself suffers a stomach-ache he thinks that the whole world has been eating green apples. Thoreau advised the benefactor to cure himself, to grow cheerful, to abandon his melancholy projections and thus to permit the victims of his "charitable" impulses to do the same.

Emerson pointed to a different shortcoming. In *Self-Reliance* he wrote: "I tell thee, thou foolish philanthropist, that I grudge the dollar, the dime, the cent I give to such men as do not belong to me and to whom I do not belong." Where no spiritual affinity exists, charity is in vain. Emerson deplored the thousandfold impersonal relief societies devoted to distributing "alms for sots."

When we think back on the unwisdom of nineteenth-century benevolence, we applaud these thrusts of criticism. But we recognize the critics' error. Thoreau and Emerson were presuming to condemn all social service because they mistook momentary limitations for ultimate limits. They could not foresee the enlargement of horizons and improvement in practice that would come through the labors of

Octavia Hill, Arnold Toynbee, Jane Addams, Richard Cabot, Mary Richmond and many other thoughtful leaders. Nor could they predict the future influence of psychological science and psychiatry upon social service. They could not foretell the evolution of public policy as guided by Bismarck in Germany, by the Fabians and the Labor Party in Britain and by the New Deal in the United States.

We therefore take warning. It would be folly to set dogmatic and premature limits upon the sciences and arts that comprise social service. Unlike Thoreau and Emerson, we know that its methods and its philosophy are still evolving. Present faults and shortcomings surely exist, but most of them, we suspect, are removable. As such they constitute *limitations* in social service but not *limits*. In the course of our discussion we shall hit upon boundaries beyond which neither public nor private social work may proceed. But for the most part we shall be concerned with limitations that can in principle be overcome.

Evaluating Social Service

The brightest feature of the present situation is the spirit of self-objectification, self-scrutiny and self-criticism that marks contemporary social services. We are less inclined than formerly to mistake our good intentions for good results, or our own professional growth for growth in our clients. We have reached a stage of wholesome skepticism. Today the question is whether social service, in any of its philosophies and methods—public or private; family-centered, community-centered or person-centered; manipulative or interpretative; based on psychoanalytic theory, economic theory, religious theory or no theory—does in fact achieve the results we aim to achieve.

It is now thirty years since leaders of social service began to call for an evaluation of results. To some extent the impetus came from donors who rightly wondered whether society actually benefits from their financial support of social work. But chiefly, I think, the impetus for evaluation has come from ardent workers who wish to know whether their efforts are truly in the public interest or reflect merely pleasant conceits of their own. Among the early voices raised in behalf of evaluative research were those of Porter R. Lee, Dr. Haven Emerson and Dr. Richard Cabot.[1] Two of the earliest investigations were those of Miss Theis, who followed the later careers of nearly eight hundred foster children, and of the Gluecks, who traced five hundred former inmates of the Concord Reformatory.[2]

The former study made us hopeful concerning the policies and practices of child-placing agencies, while the latter thrust us into a state of despair regarding the outcome of our efforts to rehabilitate delinquents. No subsequent evaluation of penal practices has in any respect restored our hope. But when evaluative results turn out to be negative, we are not entitled to say, "Nothing can be done." Rather, we feel goaded to restate our aims, alter our approach and redouble our efforts. For example, we might decide to study the few cases of successful reformation, and re-tool our practices by them.

Deeply disturbed by this failure with adult delinquents, Dr. Richard Cabot, shortly before his death in 1938, established and subsidized the Cambridge-Somerville Youth Study, perhaps the most elaborate evaluative investigation yet attempted. The study was action research; it instituted a program of long-continued treatment of pre-delinquent children for the express purpose of discovering whether such social service could check later delinquency. Specially established action research of this type has marked advantages over the cursory evaluative investigations that are all we can expect from agencies busy with daily demands. The financial resources are more adequate; research specialists are employed; and the important condition of having a control group can be observed. The three hundred boys in treatment were matched at the outset of the study with an equal number of controls. It was thus possible to estimate accurately the amount of change that occurred as a result of treatment rather than as a result of gradual maturing in the average community setting, where schools, churches and assorted social agencies are likewise engaged in the building of character. The treatment plans were badly interrupted, however, by the coming of the war; many of the boys entered service at the age of seventeen, the very time when the most effective casework might have been done.

The results of this elaborate study, as set forth by Powers and Witmer, are not as conclusive as we might wish.[3] In general terms, the study showed that, by police standards, approximately the same number of treatment and control boys turned out to be delinquent. Thus, in a sense, even five to seven years of casework, commencing between the ages of six and ten, proved ineffective. This pessimistic generalization, however, masks certain subsidiary findings of potentially great importance. There is some evidence, for example, that treatment boys, though they tangled with the courts as often as control boys, did not continue into careers of serious and aggravated criminality. There is also evidence that those who benefited most from the program were boys who, like their parents, were genuinely fond of the counselor; were relatively free from severe neurotic or pathological traits; and seemed to need most of all guidance and example in making up for minor defects in the home. At the same time, the study found that caseworkers were rarely, if ever, able to provide full and sufficient emotional anchorage for a boy whose own parents rejected him. Social service—at least of the type we are here discussing—seems unable to compensate for wretched emotional situations in the home. This example shows that evaluative research can help us determine the limits of an agency's work and identify the types of cases that can and cannot be rehabilitated.

It also came to light in the Cambridge-Somerville Youth Study that certain types of caseworkers seemed to have greater success than others. Specifically, the warm or friendly or informal workers, who to some critics seemed actually "unprofessional" in their approach, apparently had more success than the highly trained, diagnostic-minded, theoretically oriented workers. While too few cases are involved in this comparison to justify a generalization, the finding is potentially of great significance. If substantiated, it will cause us to examine sharply some of our current presuppositions regarding the selection and training of personnel—indeed, our whole philosophy of the "professional approach."

While I have used for illustrative purposes a study in the field of delinquency prevention, I could point to numerous areas that have recently yielded to evaluative penetration. The advances have been impressive. In 1952, David G. French published his book *Measuring results in social work,* a survey that places the whole subject in excellent perspective. One merit of the book is that it sets forth a detailed proposal for an Institute for Research in Social Work, which would supply agencies and programs with expert assistance in conducting evaluative investigations. Meanwhile, an avalanche of special and limited evaluative studies have been tumbling from the press.[4]

The trend toward social evaluation reaches far beyond casework. It embraces psychotherapy, health education, recreational programs; the effects of study in foreign lands, of summer camps, of programs for the reduction of ethnic prejudice; the efficiency of information services, even of general education in our colleges; and many other socially relevant policies and practices.

In the field of social service, anecdotal proof of success has given way. We can no longer say that failure to assess our efforts is in principle a major limitation. The chief obstacles in evaluation now are scant funds and a shortage of technical skills. Evaluation is not a job for amateurs; it requires shrewd planning, inventiveness, technical training and great caution in interpreting results. But these barriers are not insurmountable. If progress in the next twenty-five years matches progress in the past, we shall soon have this important instrument well under control.

The Goals of Social Work

One cardinal requirement for successful evaluation forces us to pause and take stock. Every evaluator agrees that we cannot measure progress unless we know our objectives, and these objectives must be stated in accessible (that is, operational) terms. We are thus brought face to face with the question of the goals of social service. While the question is familiar, it is none the less true that only a tiny fraction of the mountainous literature on social service is concerned with its *raison d'être*, with its philosophical guidelines and moral objectives. Such formulations as we do encounter are often too general or too vague to help the evaluator.

It may well be that—in certain respects, at least—we face an insoluble problem. If we accept as our goal "growth in personality" (and this is a goal upon which, I suspect, most of us would agree), how can we measure progress? How long after a program of treatment shall we attempt to determine growth? And what is our *criterion* for "growth in personality" or "improvement in character" —or, for that matter, for "self-reliance," "wholesomeness," "good citizenship," "happiness" or even "normality of adjustment"?

Occasionally our stated objectives are less elusive. When we say, for example, that our goal is economic rehabilitation of a client, we can set a reasonable criterion, such as holding a job steadily for a year. We can then determine what proportion of our clients reach this criterion of success. Even more general objectives, which may appear at first like clouds of vapor to a social scientist, can be and have been reduced to accessible operations. I have in mind the criterion of "movement," deemed desirable in certain casework philosophies; Hunt and Kogan have captured this will-o'-the-wisp and, with considerable success, impounded it for reliable measurement.[5]

It remains true, however, that our deepest concerns and highest ideals are not likely to lend themselves to exact measurement. And so we are faced here with the necessity for compromise. Measurement we surely want, but not if it tempts us to state our aims and objectives in brittle or trivial terms. Where meaningful and concrete operations are statable, let us use them in our evaluative procedures; but let us not assume that our total philosophy is reducible to criteria of this order.

Social service now proceeds under a wide variety of philosophies. While we hear a good deal about the need for "a single integrative professional philosophy," such articulate axiology as exists—and there is not a great deal of it—is far from receiving unanimous endorsement. Scientific humanism, as represented by Bisno, asks social service to adhere to a philosophy of science that is empirical in outlook, pragmatic in method, relativistic respecting values and negative toward all absolutes.[6] Some form of the philosophy of self-realization is, I suspect, more widely endorsed. For example, Richard Cabot, Mary Richmond and many like-minded workers hold that the supreme test of social service is "growth in personality": [7] does the personality of clients change, and change in the right direction? ("Right direction" is determined always by reference to the unique potentialities of the individual in relation to the rights and privileges of others.) The emphasis of Roman Catholic social service is somewhat different. It advocates bringing man under the sway of reason, in order that this distinctive human faculty may assist man, who is made in the image of God, to "find his way back to God." [8]

Is such disagreement on basic philosophy a serious limitation? The matter can be argued both ways. On the one hand, it could be said that social service, lacking a single ethical direction, slips easily into adulation of techniques. It does so because science and technology are the idols of our society and, lacking an explicit conscience of its own, social service unconsciously adopts the idolatry of the day. Four hundred years ago Rabelais warned us that "science without conscience spells only the ruin of the soul." We have minimized the warning of Rabelais and have lived rather by the faith of Karl Pearson, who, in his *Grammar of science,* prophesied that the gradual spread of scientific objectivity to the common mind will cure us of all passionate prejudices and improve our human relationships. Yet up to now science has brought only slight visible improvement in this regard. Like social service, it seems to require a doctrine of man, and a firm ethics by which to test its practices.

On the other hand, it may be argued that agreement on matters of such ultimate importance is impossible to achieve and not really desirable. Final truth we cannot know; human wisdom evolves best through diversity. A rough proximate agreement is all we need, and this we have already achieved. We know that social service aims to insure the survival and smooth functioning of the group; also, that in a democracy it aims to contribute to the fullness of individual life by helping to remove limitations that impede self-reliance. Sophisticated philosophers may try, if they will, to order these proximate goals under a framework of ultimates; but the harder they press their logic of values, the greater will be the resulting disagreement. Their final formulations will be as diverse as positivism and Thomism, humanism and existentialism, quietism and socialism. Why worry about the matter, when a rough working basis is already at hand?

What shall we say about this dispute? My own inclination is to concede that agreement on ultimates is neither possible nor, at this time, desirable. Yet if we are content with only a crude working basis, we may easily be trapped by the ideology of engineering and find ourselves preoccupied with techniques and gadgets, thus embracing, without fully knowing it, a directionless and conscienceless scientism. The safeguard, I think, is to foster continuous consideration of the aims of social service and the frames of axiology into which it may fit. Students should receive nutritive doses of ethics in schools of social work and should be encouraged to debate the matter in order to develop their own views. No one is bound to accept the final philosophy of another, but a philosophy of some kind he must have. It is, I believe, a serious shortcoming of social service that it pays too little attention—in its curricula of training and in later professional years—to its goals, objectives, policies and ethical premises, and to philosophies of life under which the daily activities of social workers may be ordered.

Public and Private Service

Modern social work developed from the attempt to offset the pauperizing effects of almsgiving and indiscriminate charity. It soon became apparent that private efforts, as represented in the Charity Organization movement, were hopelessly inadequate to repair the ravages caused by the industrial revolution and by the long period of *laissez faire* that accompanied it. Action by the state became imperative; and gradually, throughout the Western world, the ideals of social insurance, social security and governmental assistance to the sick, the aged, the unemployed and the young became accepted practices.

In a democracy, having a free economy and reasonable opportunities for upward mobility, as well as respect for the dignity of the individual, the ideals and aims of governmental and private social service are essentially the same. Whatever the division of functions, both forms of service wish to reduce unnecessary suffering, preserve a basic social order and maximize the opportunities of individuals to develop their potentialities.

Unless I am mistaken, the division of function that has occurred follows essentially the arrangement predicted and approved by Sidney Webb forty years ago.[9] This author employs the metaphor of the extension ladder. Public welfare services are charged with filling the gaps that exist in the basic economic and institutional structure of society. They provide means by which individuals obtain physical care, decent housing and protection against disability and poverty in old age, even though they cannot pay for such services in a competitive market. Thus public agencies provide a standardized form of assistance to all who meet certain specifications.

It is commonly agreed that the function of private social service, on the other hand, is to help individuals make the most of the resources of society, including the benefits that the government provides. Relieved of many of the burdens of economic relief, private social service has turned more and more to the understanding and treatment of personality. The ideal of "casework above the poverty line" emerged in the First World War, when the home service rendered by the Red Cross to the families of men on military duty demonstrated that human needs are by no means always economic. As early as 1909, Richard Cabot had written that he could see no reason why social work should be done only with the poor.[10]

This ideal of professional service above the poverty line has spread so widely that today we find a large percentage of the services privately rendered paid for by the client. This trend seems to hold not only for casework and guidance services but also for recreational and group work. A decreasing proportion of the funds raised by Community Chests go into direct relief and a larger proportion into administration, organization and even research. The trend is made possible by the creation of what has come to be called the "welfare state," in which unemployment benefits, industrial safety, health services, child care and social security are recognized matters for public rather than private responsibility.

Originally Sidney Webb held that voluntary agencies are superior to public authorities in three main features: (1) invention and experimentation with new services and new methods, (2) ability to give special and individualized care to particular cases and (3) freedom to bring religious or other moral influences to bear on clients. On the whole, it has been felt that voluntary agencies maintain high standards, which act as a model and monitor for public service. Today these distinctions are less sharp than formerly. Excellent casework is now done by civil service appointees, and public officials may be as imaginative and experimental as private workers. Nearly all of our personnel in public service is trained in private schools of social work, where the ideals and methods of voluntary agencies prevail.

Whatever their functions may be, the spread of public agencies has been continually and vigorously fought by economic and political conservatives. They profess to see in it the undermining of initiative, as well as threatening dislocations caused by excessive taxation, bureaucracy and loss of freedom. A century ago, conservatives objected to the elimination of the workhouse test for relief and held firmly to the principle of "less eligibility." Unless a pauper is stigmatized, they argued, we shall all lose our sense of shame and gladly become paupers. No battle was ever lost more decisively. Conservatives have been losing ground for decades—to such an extent, in fact, that we are now obliged to ask whether there is not some validity in their position. We need not include here conservatives whose transparent motivation is the preservation of their own privilege and status.

The plain fact is that the scope of social service has expanded, and is still expanding, at a spectacular rate. Private social services now receive and spend approximately one and a half *billion* dollars a year. In one cluster of 117 cities, gifts to Community Chests more than doubled between 1941 and 1954.[11] Government expenditures have mounted at a still more rapid rate. Two and a half billion dollars is the annual outlay of states, while the federal government spends many more billions on its social services, including programs for health and welfare, veterans' benefits and social security. In all, the total annual expenditure is over thirteen billion dollars, and ever rising.[12]

The reason for this mounting outlay is not increased destitution, but, rather, a change in the public's attitude toward social responsibility. Problems that received no attention a few decades, or even a few years, ago, now are accepted as legitimate and pressing obligations of society. The conservative's alarm merits fresh attention. Are we growing reckless and extravagant in our outlay? Do individuals cease to exert themselves and weakly prefer public bounty? Are we all passengers on the gravy train?

The danger, if I may venture an opinion, does not lie in the expansion of social services, or even in the fraction of the national income invested in them. The philosophy of both public and private service, and of their interrelationships, is essentially sound. The danger is more subtle: we might phrase it in terms of the growing insistence upon "rights" and the diminishing emphasis upon "duties." Take the social worker's own mental attitude, for example. His profession sensitizes him to the injustices he encounters. He is led to demand basic rights for dependent children, for victims of desertion, for the aged, for minority ethnic groups. It is proper that he should do so. But there is a reciprocal question: in fighting for rights, are social workers—and American citizens generally—aware of the duties they in turn owe to their community and their state? We greedily scramble for our share of public benefits, but pay our taxes reluctantly, and sometimes not at all. Almost half of us do not vote. Very few participate in civic affairs. Do social workers, in dealing with clients, try to inculcate in them an awareness of their duties? Or do they merely intensify the sense of "rights," already so prominent in the American's mind? In the Japanese culture, we are told, heavy emphasis is placed upon the sense of obligation, far less on rights. In our culture the burden of emphasis is precisely reversed.

Another example: unless I am mistaken, most young people training for the profession of social service prefer to work for private agencies and shun opportunities for public service. This is true, I think, even though half the openings in social service today occur in public agencies and a large number of scholarships and other inducements are offered by public agencies, including the Veterans Administration, the National Mental Health Foundation and state welfare departments.[13] The reason for this disaffection is fairly apparent. It is felt to be somehow less pleasant to be bound by public bureaucracy than by private bureaucracy. It is disagreeable to be exposed to political control and the hazards of McCarthy-like persecutions. Yet how are we to build and maintain our public services, if we as citizens shun them? The basic philosophies of public and private agencies do not greatly differ. What we need is a more cordial and equal relationship between them, and in particular a higher sense of obligation to public service, an area that will continue to grow by leaps and bounds.

While I am deploring overemphasis upon private and proprietary conceptions of social service, let me bemoan also our national provincialism. When we view the world situation as a whole, we are forced to conclude that some of our refined distinctions and preoccupations look like fancy embroidery. We quarrel, for example, over the hairlike boundary between casework and psychotherapy, while most of the world has never heard of either. In most countries of the earth, the poor survive only with the help of the poor. The professions of social work and psychiatry are totally unknown. Voluntary service is nonexistent. Most countries have no public assistance, no social security, no community resources to which the needy can be referred. Sickness, poverty and desolate old age are so familiar that the people, submerged in despair, ignorance and apathy, are benumbed. In these countries, social service for the present can mean only the launching of some vast social change that will lift the masses to the point at which individual problems can be perceived and differential treatment become possible.

It is a limitation of American social service that, lacking world perspective, it cosily believes that the United States lives safely on an island, unaffected by the misery of other nations. Their revolt into communism and into other desperate experiments can easily cause a world conflagration that will wipe out the painful gains of social service in the United States. I suggest that those of us who are engaged in social service are living, to some extent, in a fool's paradise. It would seem to be high time for us to concern ourselves more actively with the new international ethics of mutual aid.[14]

Professionalism

A dilemma of a different order confronts us when we consider the motivation that sustains social service. Unless there are elements of love, compassion and a desire to share one's own life-benefits with others, the whole process of social service is likely to be a husk. At the same time, it is fatal if these altruistic impulses are concentrated into fitful ecstasies and allowed undisciplined expression. Nor is it enough for the social worker to engage in the immediately rewarding contacts of good casework. The needed discipline requires also a long-range focus, sustained by a social and personal philosophy tempered by patience, a sense of political strategy and all other virtues of sturdy citizenship. Discipline requires also freedom from self-deception.

I realize that in these days of strict self-scrutiny, social workers are expected to examine their own motives. They are, for example, supposed to be aware of the dangers of projection—the same pitfall Thoreau denounced when he accused philanthropists of surrounding others with the remembrance of their own cast-off griefs and despair, and mistakenly calling the process "sympathy." Most social workers today agree that their professional equipment requires, first of all, a fundamental security in themselves, and, secondly, an ability to understand that other people have different needs and ways of thought.[15]

But projection is only one form of self-deception. There is also the bias of optimism, which often leads a worker to put a too rosy complexion on his relationships with a client. Technically we speak of a "parataxic dyad" whenever a worker or his client (or both) seriously misperceives the attitude of the other respecting their relationship. In a study of delinquency prevention, Teuber and Powers discovered that, in about a third of the cases, the counselor or the boy was ignorant of the other's true attitude. A counselor, for example, might describe a boy's attitude toward him as trusting and affectionate, while the boy really believed that the counselor was a paid detective, hired to spy on bad boys. Instead of affection and trust, the boy felt fear and hostility in the relationship. In parataxis it is usually the worker who takes the rosier view of the state of rapport and overestimates the therapeutic value of his efforts. In the Teuber-Powers study, it turned out that parataxis was greater, and rapport less, in cases where the worker approached his task with rigid ideas concerning what constituted admissible and inadmissible professional practices. The dyadic relationship, in general, was much better among workers who adhered to a "friendship theory" of social service.[16]

The "friendship theory" has met strenuous objections. Its opponents argue convincingly that we do not choose clients on the same basis that we choose a friend. There are insuperable barriers of age, of contrasting educational and economic status, and of lifelong differences in habits of thought. Still worse, clients demand of the caseworker far more patience, objectivity and self-control than do friends.

Here, then, is the dilemma. The basic motives for social service can only be charity, compassion and tolerance—all of which are central ingredients in friendship. At the same time, we are rightly warned that these virtues may lead us into sentimentality and unwisdom. Only strict objectivity and a professional view of our roles will save us; yet professionalism may freeze the heart, lead to parataxis in our relationships and betray us into harmful excesses of specialism.

Specialism is a peculiar hazard in social service, medicine, the ministry or any other profession devoted to helping people in distress. Distress defies job analysis. We know how, in medicine, the decline of the general practitioner has created problems for many a sick

Social service in perspective

person whose real difficulties elude the succession of specialists he visits. In social work, the problem is growing acute. Increasing emphasis on defining "agency function" can lead to a rat-race of referrals, sometimes demoralizing to the client and hence unethical. Even if referrals themselves do not damage the client, he may find at the end of his trek that there is no rubric for his distress and therefore no agency to help him. An unmarried girl in a certain town could find no help: she was seven months pregnant, and the only appropriate agency had a rule that no applicant more than six months pregnant could be accepted. Good casework, the agency said, could not be done at this late stage of pregnancy. But is good casework an end in itself? Are we wrong in assuming that social service exists to aid mortals in distress, not to sharpen skills or gratify the professional self-image of the worker?

Another peril of excessive professionalism is overemphasis upon diagnosis. Ever since the ideal of "social diagnosis" was set before us forty years ago in Mary Richmond's epoch-making book, *What is social case work?* it has seemed self-evident that it is folly to launch into a program of treatment without knowing the nature of the problem and its roots. No one wishes to retard the development of diagnostic methods; yet we do well to keep their limits in mind.

In the first place, a worker—whether in a public or a private agency—may be so preoccupied with diagnosis that, by placing his client under a lens, he sets up a relationship that endangers his ultimate chances of helping him. Even in medicine, successful therapy may be blocked by excessive shunting of the patient from laboratory to laboratory, and the therapeutic relationship in social work is even more delicate and easily torn. A client who discovers that he is regarded as a specimen, an exercise in diagnosis and manipulation, draws back from the friendly relation that, in most cases, is the essential condition of helping him.

In the second place, it is simply not true that successful treatment invariably presupposes accurate diagnosis. Many a client, like many a medical patient, has with friendly support and encouragement mastered his trouble without enjoying the luxury of a diagnosis.

Finally, diagnoses are likely to be little more than coarse classifications. Certainly the present rubrics of psychiatry and of psychology are not final. It is not particularly helpful to decide that a certain client had unfortunate conditioning, or feels rejected, or harbors resentment against authority figures. All these diagnoses may be true, but one cannot pluck out the root causes one by one. Better to view the person himself, in all his maladaptive complexity, and the immediate environment he faces, as the "cause" of his trouble. Best work with him where he stands.

Let me repeat: I am not arguing against diagnosis, but I am pointing to the fact that excessive emphasis upon diagnosis, as one aspect of excessive professionalism, may constitute a serious limit to the effectiveness of social service.

Another dogma of social service may prove a handicap if it is carried to an extreme—the dogma that help should be offered only to those individuals and families who express a conscious need for help. Granted that the chances for effective work are greater with those who present a "growing edge" to the social worker, I question whether such initiative is a *final* measure of ability to profit from an agency's service. I have heard of an agency that rejected a dependency case because the five-year-old child in question had expressed no "felt need." Such extremes engender countermovements: we hear nowadays about "aggressive casework"—first practiced on a large scale, I believe, by the Cambridge-Somerville Youth Study—and about "reaching the unreached." Without presuming here to judge the merits of these new movements, I venture merely to point out the need for sensible balance in settling this matter of policy in social service.

My remarks on certain aspects of professionalism in social service may seem excessively critical. If so, I can only plead that my subject calls for a certain acidulousness. And if my criticism is in part justified, it points to a wholly understandable weakness. Social service is a young profession. In setting its standards and defining its policies, it is very likely to overshoot the mark, to exalt its insight into the realm of dogma—and then, perhaps, to oscillate between extreme positions. In time we can expect a better equilibrium to be achieved, but only if we recognize dogmas and excesses for what they are.

The Foundations in Psychology

Social service is what Auguste Comte called "concrete" science— that is to say, it borrows and applies theories and principles derived from the more basic "abstract" sciences. The laws and formulations of biology, sociology and psychology supply the foundations for the practices of social service, as they do for education, therapy and all other skills in human relations.

One weakness of social service lies, I think, in its faddist tendency—its tendency to borrow too heavily from some theory currently fashionable in the underlying "abstract" sciences. Early in the present century, we know there was an almost total blindness to psychological laws of motivation and learning, as well as dense disregard for psychiatric principles. It was thought that the capacity for normal living could be restored merely by observing one sociological law—that the family is the primary unit of human association, survival and adjustment. Somewhat later the biology of tonsils became an obsession; social workers stood their charges in line outside tonsillectoria, hoping for biological magic to restore a capacity for normal living. But these fevers were as nothing compared with the awesome regard for the human psyche that settled upon us during the 1920s.

At first William Healy, Ernest Southard, Richard Cabot, Adolf Meyer and Mary Jarrett pushed us gently toward the psychiatric point of view. Then, suddenly, depth psychology descended upon us! Our watchwords became "transference," "countertransference," "attitude therapy," "rebirth," "clarification" and "insight development." We were supposed to "support neurotic equilibrium" and to re-create in our client "a sense of the security and emotional dependency of the childhood period." (These quotations, incidentally, are all from the recent literature of casework.)

It would be most unbecoming for a psychologist to criticize social work for giving enthusiastic if belated recognition to the basic importance of the human psyche. I do, however, wish to point out that the enthusiasm has generally been directed toward *psychiatry* (the art of treating sick people), rather than toward *psychology* (the science of the normal mind). Psychology is a less vivid, more mundane and more time-consuming subject for study. Like psychiatry and psychoanalysis, it is fallible. Yet it offers principles of learning, motivation, social interaction, leadership, group dynamics, thought-processes, personality growth, assessment and diagnosis—principles that ought not be overlooked in favor of easier and more dramatic formulations, even though these too have great merit.

If social service follows the best thinking available in psychology and psychiatry—and I would not have it do otherwise—it will be subject to the limitations of this best thinking. Psychology, psychoanalysis and psychiatry are in a stage of rapid development. It would be unreasonable to expect social service to advance more rapidly than they. But because the change is so rapid, caution and balance are necessary in appraising dicta that may be more fashionable than true.

Let us consider one example. Freud, seconded by Rank, Bowlby and Melanie Klein—all of whom have had a marked influence upon social work—tells us that the essential foundations of character are established by the age of three. This proposition is startling. It may be true. But as yet it is unproved. A great many social workers, however, accept it as if it were gospel.

Such a fatalistic and dispiriting view leaves only a few relatively mean functions for the social worker to perform. He can, to be sure, enter the family constellation and help steer its prevailing neurosis. In a self-sacrificing mood, he might offer himself as a scapegoat and try to channel the mother's aggression from her long-suffering husband and children. At best a "limited therapy" might be undertaken with a client, provided there are vestiges of warmth and security in early childhood upon which to build. But for infants wholly deprived and therefore irretrievably warped, nothing can be done in later life except to distract them from their errant ways with such ingenuity as the worker can muster.

Within this framework of thinking, there is little merit in friendliness or in spiritual support unless there is also a suitable early soil on which to build, and unless the personality of the client can be suitably matched to the personality of the worker. But by the time depth diagnosis is accomplished, and the matching of the neurosis of the client with that of the worker is completed, all human impulses to sympathy and understanding may have evaporated.

Recent researches have, indeed, indicated the importance of early years in the formation of character. But these researches are as yet of limited scope, and do not justify a sudden and complete revising of the whole philosophy of social service. While Freudian and Rankian theories undoubtedly contain valuable truths, I venture to believe that they contain no more truth than certain opposing theories —those which maintain that personality is subject to constructive influences all through life; that it possesses inherent resources for growth and change at every period; and that no character is conclusively set at the age of three, or thirteen, or thirty.

If we knew the full truth about the foundations of human nature, we should have to include within our view the limitations that heredity sets upon our efforts. At present, psychology, psychoanalysis and social work all proceed with an environmental bias (though for psychoanalysis the environment is of little consequence after the infant years). The social worker secretly knows that nature sets ironclad limits to his labors, through constitutional defects, perverse temperament and mental inadequacy. But until we understand human genetics better than we do, we cannot say how serious these limits may be. Meanwhile, it seems sensible to continue to attack human problems with an environmental bias, remaining ready to correct our bias if and when it becomes necessary to do so.

I am sure that those who engage in social service, as well as those charged with the curricula in our schools of social work, would reply that no school of psychological thought today is followed blindly, but that the insights gained are synthesized and adapted to the realities of casework. Certainly the admirable effort spent on devising "an integrated program of professional education for social work" reflects a commendable breadth of view.[17] My fear is not directed primarily toward the unbalanced curricula of instruction, though more varied psychology, more philosophy and ethics, and more concern with public policy are certainly needed. I am worried, rather, that individual social workers, confronted by the tangled skein of a human life, might oversimplify what they learn and gravitate toward pet psychological formulas in order to "understand" the problems presented. It takes detachment, maturity and wide study of psychology not to compress a given life into an easy, and probably erroneous, formula.

In no field of human endeavor is it more essential to balance science and art. On the one hand, a client is a representative of the human species, and universal laws of health and disease, instincts and impulses, frustration and resentment, ego-defense and prejudice, reason and the irrational are likely to apply. General laws of economics, cultural expectation and taboo, family structure and the role requirements of our society are likewise relevant to each concrete case. At the same time, every individual is an idiom unto himself. His course of becoming is unlike any other. His problems and his assets are his alone; so, too, his suffering and his bid for affection.

The busy social worker is likely to let the particular be overwhelmed by the general. It is easier to conjure with the principles of psychoanalysis than to make a separate study of development and growth in each individual. It is easier to recall the general principles of criminology than to understand the particular malefactor. It is simpler to categorize in terms of neuroses and therapeutic roles than to comprehend and treat personal patterns of trouble. The balancing of general knowledge against a knowledge of the particular poses a harder problem for social service, I suspect, than for any other occupation.

This problem is directly related to the issue previously mentioned: the need for balance between the "professional" theory and the "friendship" theory of social service. Friendship is precisely that human relationship in which the particular takes precedence over the general. Yet, as we have seen, social service cannot be exclusively a relation of friendship, for the relationship from the beginning imposes certain restrictions. One member of the dyad is, by definition, older, or wiser, or stronger, or more resourceful. The other is the weaker, the suitor, suffering from adversity. Yet little can be done for the client unless some of the virtues of friendship, along with the perception of the particular and the art of individualizing, are well represented.

In short, it is the fate of social service to seek broad and accurate foundations for its policies and practices, but it should balance its dependence upon the general with a regard for the particular. Such a dexterous balance is difficult to achieve. Many of our current disputes over the "true function" of social service arise, I feel, from denying its essential and unavoidable versatility. Who can say whether the social worker is an "adjustment adviser," a "teacher," a "resource person," a "big brother" or a "psychotherapist"? If he places the need of the client first, he will be all these things at different times and under different circumstances. Only when we mistakenly place "agency function" or one-sided theories of science first do we find ourselves quarreling over the precise role or attitude that is, or is not, appropriate to social service.

Before leaving the relationship between social service and social science, I should like to protest the present one-sidedness in their communication. Why should social service do all the borrowing? Why should not the bulging files of social agencies be made to yield their buried knowledge to help build a more comprehensive psychology of motivation, of learning, of personality growth and of human relations? There are mountains of case records awaiting analysis and inductive handling. Our files are for the most part graveyards of *knowledge*. They should, rather, become treasure-troves for the development of new *principles* of human nature and of social relations.

Social Change and Public Apathy

An atomic war may force all of us who survive to forage for edible weeds and a cave to dwell in. One spasm of international madness could, at a single sweep, destroy the intricate fabric of social service and turn its fine philosophy into an absurdity. Even short of an atomic war, we rightly fear what may happen to the values of our unique democratic society as communism spreads more widely in the world. Already we see how its grim pressure is straining our historical conceptions of civil liberties, of individual rights and of mutual trust and respect. The extension of public service, which we welcome, can conceivably slide into the crude statism of Stalin or, more likely, the subtler but equally destructive statism of Hitler. Our demagogues are pushing hard. We feel ourselves on the defensive before titanic forces of social change.

The ideals and practices of social service are among the finest fruits of the orchard of democracy. Their existence depends upon maintaining the soil, the roots and the main trunks of our way of life. It is fatal blindness if social service does not realize this fact and act in accordance with it. Today the social worker who does not labor to preserve the foundations of democracy is like a squirrel nibbling fruits others have planted in an orchard now withering.

Here I am speaking from the "structural" point of view. Sociologists and historians often tell us that, as individuals, we are nearly helpless before the sweep of social change. It is the total frame in which we live that conditions our acts. Social service as we know it will survive only so long as it is maintained by political democracy and economic free enterprise—and by our subtly evolved sense of social responsibility, based on a delicate blend of protectiveness toward and autonomy for the individual person. The structural argument is harsh. It holds that this intricate framework is subject to historical changes, no matter what you and I may will to do.

The same argument also takes another form, drawing not on the inevitabilities of social change but upon the now familiar creed of natural selection. It asks whether social service is viable from the point of view of nature. Evolutionists from Herbert Spencer to Raymond Pearl have warned us that arrogant interference with nature's law can bring misery, if not actual destruction, to the human race. From their point of view, the protection and unnatural preservation of the inept fills the earth with misfits whom nature, left to herself, would promptly dispatch. Like medicine and public health, social service conspires to negate nature.

This issue has been tiresomely debated, though it has never been definitely settled. One thing only is clear: we have decided deliberately to disregard the simple logic of natural selection. We have asserted, once and for all, that nature's coarse standards are not a proper measure of man's worth or of his right to survive. In place of "rugged individualism," our society has chosen "socialized individualism." We may be wrong, but we shall have to make the best of it. As we reap the consequences in terms of high birth rates, increasing maladies of old age and overpopulation, we shall have to learn gradually to solve the problems that medicine and social service may have caused in our society.

In this matter, social service has contracted to transcend its own limits. It hopes that, by adapting to altered conditions, it can continue to work out its ideals. A cataclysm might prove fatal; but short of that, we shall endeavor to adjust to—and, when possible, guide and direct—social change. So far as the specter of natural selection is concerned, we believe that here too the strategies of intelligence will enable us to meet and master whatever dislocations may result from abandoning the jungle theory of survival in favor of higher ethical ideals.

I do not mean to imply that these commitments are conscious and deliberate on our part. Few people think about the philosophy that underlies their support of social service. The public gives generously to private philanthropy and votes decisively for an extension of state and federal benefits, yet the social worker knows that he cannot count on consistency in the public's attitude. While wanting more state and federal services, people are definitely antagonistic toward paying taxes. While wanting freedom for themselves, many people are ready to deny it to others. While wanting better opportunities for their children than they themselves enjoyed, people hold to resistant and stagnant ideologies of child training, from which neither social workers nor educators can successfully convert them. While deploring the contagion of delinquency in society, neither the public nor its legislative representatives will sanction the drastic types of reform we know to be needed. All in all, public attitudes are conservative—far more so, as a rule, than the attitudes of those who are active in social welfare. It is, therefore, a major frustration of our calling that those who are engaged in its practice will be limited, and often defeated, by public ignorance and apathy.

Self-confidence and Its Enemies

Since social service is severely restricted—by social structure on the one hand, and by public apathy on the other—it seems ungracious to blame it for feelings of inadequacy. Yet this is, I think, one of its defects, the final defect of which I wish to speak.

Social service lacks self-confidence; it lacks a firm sense of conviction in its own goals.[18] In part, our confidence is weak because we feel at a disadvantage in a society where competitiveness and aggressiveness reap conspicuous rewards, while the ideals of cooperation, to which social service is committed, represent a minority point of view. In part, our low confidence is engendered by the very atmosphere of doubt in which we live, by the same atmosphere that causes us to engage in wholesome self-scrutiny, self-evaluation and self-criticism.

But self-assessment should take into account assets as well as liabilities. Among its assets social service can reckon its recent achievement of the status of a full-fledged profession. The two major characteristics of any profession, writes Dean Ralph Tyler, are its use of technics derived from general principles and its possession of a code of ethics.[19] I have already mentioned the present alertness of social work in deriving its procedures from underlying sciences. I have, to be sure, criticized a certain one-sidedness in the derivations now popular, but the trend in general is wholesome. And social service is making good progress in the formulation of an explicit code of ethics.[20] Thus the advance to professional status, in both public welfare and private social work, is clear and gratifying.

Still, some of us, caught in the current atmosphere of doubt, tend to lack courage. We are not as certain as we once were that our efforts will succeed. Who can be? Yet the existentialists remind us that men can be half-sure without being half-hearted. Accepting our doubt, and admitting every hazard, we are still free to elect and pursue our option. Living requires that we know the worst and make the best of it. Some of us would benefit from a generous injection of this type of existentialist courage.

But we need not rest content with a philosophy of make-the-best-of-it. Deep inside, each of us knows that the spirit behind social service knows no limits. This spirit, the finest fruit of Judeo-Christian ethics, is eternally sound. How ironical it is that the scriptural word "charity," as used by St. Paul, has in our profession become a sign of opprobrium rather than of inspiration! The motive behind social work always has been, and will continue to be, *caritas*, and this motive is infinitely valid.

The root problem of social service is how to express the impulse of charity effectively with the technical skill and flexible intelligence required by complex modern conditions. The chief lesson we learn from the nineteenth century is that good intentions are not enough. Nowadays we know a great deal more about sound means of fostering growth in personality, about the basis of human motivation, about a proper relationship between public and private effort. When we reflect on our progress in theory and in practice, we have every right to reassert our faith and stiffen our courage. There are plenty of obstacles in our path and many trends that need correcting; but, barring global catastrophe, we can expect continued development in the right direction.

Social service has a greater clarity of perspective than does politics or commerce. It can therefore press for the stabilizing reforms that are needed to make life rich, meaningful and just in a system of free initiative and individual liberty. By asserting its convictions more loudly than it has, social service can make itself not only the servant but also the prophet of democracy. And today, as never before, democracy needs both servants and prophets.

Social service has limits and limitations. But it has also the saving virtue of self-criticism, and is daily growing in shrewdness and sense of strategy. Its foundations are eternally valid. The balance, therefore, is in its favor.

REFERENCES

1. Dr. Cabot's presidential address to the Fifty-eighth National Conference of Social Work in 1931 is an important historical landmark. In it he reviews the handful of evaluative studies available at that time and pleads with unmatched eloquence for a continuing program of evaluation in all social agencies. R. C. Cabot, "Treatment in social casework and the need of criteria and of tests of its success or failure," in *Proceedings of the national conference of social work,* Chicago: University of Chicago Press, 1931.

2. S. van S. Theis, *How foster children turn out,* State Charities Aid Association, 1924. S. Glueck and E. T. Glueck, *Five hundred criminal careers,* New York: Knopf, 1930. See also E. T. Glueck, *Evaluative research in social work,* New York School of Social Work, 1936.

3. E. Powers and H. Witmer, *An experiment in the prevention of delinquency* (Foreword by G. W. Allport), New York: Columbia University Press, 1951.

4. Among representative evaluative studies I would call attention to the following:

G. W. Allport, *The nature of prejudice,* Cambridge: Addison-Wesley, 1954, Chaps. 29-31.

S. Axelrad, J. Frings and E. Herzog, *A study of short term cases,* New York: Research Department, Jewish Family Service, 1951.

I. A. Berg, "Measures before and after therapy," *J. Clin. Psychol.,* 1952, 8: 46-50.

M. Blenkner, "Obstacles to evaluative research in casework," *Social Casework,* 1950, 31: 54-60, 97-105.

C. F. Cannell, F. G. Wale and S. B. Withey, "Community change: an action program in Puerto Rico," *J. Soc. Issues,* 1953, Vol. 9, No. 2.

H. S. Coffey, M. Freedman, T. Leary and A. Ossorio, "Community service and social research—group psychotherapy in a church program," *J. Soc. Issues,* 1950, Vol. 6, No. 1.

H. J. Eysenck, "The effects of psychotherapy: an evaluation," *J. Consulting Psychol.,* 1952, 16:319-24, No. 5.

S. Glueck and E. T. Glueck, *Unraveling juvenile delinquency,* New York: Commonwealth Fund, 1950.

W. Healy and A. F. Bronner, *Treatment and what happened afterward,* Boston: Judge Baker Guidance Center, 1939.

P. Hoch (ed.), *Failures in psychiatric treatment,* New York: Grune and Stratton, 1948.

J. McV. Hunt, "The problem of measuring the results of psychotherapy," *Psychol. Ser. Cen. J.,* 1949, 1:122-35, No. 4.

L. S. Kogan, "Evaluative techniques in social casework," *Soc. Ser. Rev.,* 1952, 26:305-09, No. 3.

L. S. Kubie, "Objective evaluation of psychotherapy: roundtable," *Amer. J. Orthopsychiat.,* 1949, 19:463-91.

H. H. W. Miles, E. L. Barrabee and J. E. Finesinger, "Evaluation of psychotherapy with a follow-up study of 62 cases of anxiety neurosis," *Psychosom. Med.,* 1951, 13:83-105.

R. E. Perl and A. J. Simon, "Criteria of success and failure in child guidance," *Amer. J. Orthopsychiat.,* 1942, 12:642-58.

H. A. Rashkis and D. A. Shaskan, "The effects of group psychotherapy on personality inventory scores," *Amer. J. Orthopsychiat.,* 1946, 16:345-49, No. 2.

G. J. Rich, "Preschool clinical service and follow-up in a city health department," *Amer. J. Orthopsychiat.,* 1948, 18:134-39, No. 1.

S. B. Sells, "Problems of criteria and validity in diagnosis and therapy," *J. Clin. Psychol.,* 1952, 8:23-28.

R. I. Watson, "Research design and methodology in evaluating the results of psychotherapy," *J. Clin. Psychol.,* 1952, 8:29-33.

5. J. McV. Hunt and L. S. Kogan, *Measuring results in social casework: a manual on judging movement,* New York: Family Service Association, 1950.

6. H. Bisno, *The philosophy of social work,* Washington: Public Affairs Press, 1952, p. 92.

7. R. C. Cabot, *The meaning of right and wrong,* New York: Macmillan, 1933. M. Richmond, *What is social case work?* New York: Russell Sage Foundation, 1922.

8. M. J. McCormick, *Diagnostic casework in the Thomistic pattern,* New York: Columbia University Press, 1954, pp. 13, 51.

9. S. Webb, "The extension ladder theory of the relation between voluntary philanthropy and state or municipal action," *The Survey,* 1914, 31:703-07.

10. R. C. Cabot, *Social service and the art of healing,* New York: Moffat, Yard and Co., 1909.

11. *Trends in giving,* Community Chests and Councils of America, 345 East 46th Street, New York 17, New York, Table 12.

12. R. H. Kurtz (ed.), *Social work year book, 1954,* New York: American Book-Stratford Press, 1954, p. 221.

13. See *Social work fellowships and scholarships in the United States and Canada,* Council on Social Work Education, 345 East 46th Street, New York, New York.

14. A good place to start our self-education in this regard is with the valuable reports of the Economic and Social Council of the United Nations,

such as the "Programme of concerted practical action in the social field of the United Nations and specialized agencies," Report E/CN.5/291, March 2, 1953. Also significant is the work of private international organizations, such as the International Conference of Social Work with its many branches, the International Federation of Social Workers and the International Committee of Schools of Social Work.

15. Cf. V. P. Robinson, *A changing psychology in social casework,* Chapel Hill: University of North Carolina Press, 1930, p. 180.

16. H. L. Teuber and E. Powers, "Evaluating therapy in a delinquency prevention program," in *Psychiatric Treatment,* Vol. 21, *Proc. of the Assoc. for Research in Nervous and Mental Disease,* Baltimore: Williams and Wilkins, 1953, Chap. 12.

17. Report of Annual Meeting–1952, New York, American Association of Schools of Social Work, 1 Park Avenue, New York 16, New York.

18. L. H. Towley has made this point forcefully in his address "Professional responsibility in a democracy," in *Education for social work: proceedings annual program meeting,* New York: Council on Social Work Education, 1953, pp. 10-21.

19. R. W. Tyler, "Distinctive attributes of education for the professions," *Soc. Work J.,* April 1952, p. 5.

20. "A proposed code of ethics for the social worker," *Soc. Work J.,* April 1949.

Perception, proception and public health

An exciting development in recent years is the joining of forces between the medical and the social sciences. The points of contact are numerous and the results beneficial. We are now becoming familiar with the social structure of hospitals, with the role of the family and of cultural background in cases of illness, and with the importance of the patient's attitude toward his physician and nurses. We are exploring ever more deeply his attitude toward medication and surgery, toward life and death.

This essay focuses attention on certain important points of contact between the psychology of perception and the practical work of public health practitioners. It introduces the new but, I trust, useful concept of "proception."

The Health Education Monographs first published the essay in 1958 under the title "Perception and public health." It was the second annual Dorothy B. Nyswander Lecture, delivered at the School of Public Health at Berkeley, California, in May 1958.

During the past decade, the outlook and duties of health education have changed significantly, principally in the direction of closer cooperation with psychological and social science.[1] At the beginning of that period, terror of infectious diseases was still uppermost. Since these specific scourges had specific causes, research in public health meant chiefly finding the antitoxin or antibiotic that would defeat the invading microbe. This work required little cooperation or knowledge on the part of the ordinary citizen. He was not deeply involved in sanitary engineering, water purification or rodent control. But he did develop, thanks to public health education, a "bacterio-technological perspective on illness."[2] He became vaccine conscious, as the recent rush of the public for Salk vaccine shows. Miracle cures he now understands; and his faith in them is still growing.

But where is the vaccine to prevent mental breakdowns? to lead people to early examinations for cardiac and cancer conditions? to abolish harmful practices of eating, sleeping and recreation? to control alcoholic and other addictions? to eliminate reckless automobile driving? to establish wholesome practices of child training? Health workers agree that we have now entered an era when the human factor—the whims, values and perceptions of the ordinary citizen—must be considered before further progress can be made. Future advances will require the consent and cooperation of people: the *public* part of public health will increasingly concern us.

It is not possible to review in a single essay all the exciting advances in social science that have potential value for future progress in public health. Many of these developments are already familiar, perhaps especially those concerned with opinion and communication, with leadership and group process, and with the differing ethnic and regional requirements of public health work. I shall concentrate, rather, on the less often considered question of perception and public health—in practical terms, the question: *Does the receiver hear and comprehend the health message as the health educator intends?*

The Paradox of Perception

A traveler to Naples tells the following story: Arriving at his hotel overlooking the fabulously beautiful bay, his cab driver burst forth in rapture. Although the driver had seen the lovely view a thousand times, he cried out, *"Come e bello, come e bello!"* The traveler agreed with his ecstatic driver and entered his hotel. There the innkeeper confided that he was having much trouble with a rich American oil magnate who had come to Naples to escape boredom in his retirement. This American, after glancing at the view, had merely sniffed, "Just trees and water and a city—I've seen them thousands of times." Hiring a taxi, he drove to Pompeii and returned full of wrath. "I've seen enough good houses in my lifetime," he said, "without going to look at a lot that are in ruins." The oil magnate retreated to his only solace, a concoction made of schnapps and champagne. A few weeks later he developed delirium tremens and was shipped back to the United States.

The story illustrates our first principle: *environment may be less a matter of physical surroundings than of perception.* Two men in the same geographical spot do not live in the same environment. It is for this reason that a health worker, even though he does not alter his approach in the slightest degree as he goes from house to house, may be perceived as threatening or consoling, as a friend to be welcomed or as a pest to be avoided. The worker thinks that he plays a steadfast professional role; but he doesn't. Like the Bay of Naples, he is two things to two perceivers—and ten things to ten perceivers.

But here we run into the prime paradox of perception: there *is*, after all, a Bay of Naples. The process of perceiving is subjectively swayed, but it is objectively anchored. Perception is governed by both outer and inner factors; in the language of Plato, "The light within meets the light without." What we see and hear is, therefore, both veridical and distorted, both true and false.

The fact that we perceive the world around us fairly accurately is due to the evolution of sensory and brain processes well tuned to outer reality. Eyes perceive color, line and shape with exquisite fineness; ears register accurately a wide range of air vibrations. The skin, less perfect in sensitiveness, still mediates evidence of shape and the finer gradations of temperature. The reason for this mirroring ability is undoubtedly its "functional usefulness." The organism has a better chance of survival if the sensory equipment is finally accurate. As Woodworth maintains in a recent book, the first and foremost motive in life is man's pervasive need to handle his world competently.[3] For Woodworth, the process of perception is the fundamental dynamism serving this fundamental motive.

Yet, by following the same line of reasoning, we can say the perceptual process must *depart* from true mirroring in order to be of maximum use to us. Not every tree in the forest comes into perceptual focus; only the one we are chopping. Not every object on the dinner table is perceived with clarity; only the bite we are about to put into our mouths. If you hear a babble of vague conversation, how quickly *your* name stands out if it is mentioned. Selective perception is as much a functional necessity as is veridical perception.

In coping with our world, it would not be enough to follow only "the light without." We have first to select what we shall see; in so doing, we become hypervigilant toward some cues and indifferent or actively defensive toward others. We perceive in order to cope, but coping means more than passive mirroring. It means fulfilling our needs; it means finding safety and reassurance, love and self-respect, freedom from worry, opportunities for growth—and, ultimately, a satisfying meaning for our existence. Our coping may thus be best served by disregarding some stimuli entirely, by modifying our interpretation of others and by blending incoming meanings with our past habits, our present needs and our future directions.

The point is illustrated in a recent health investigation conducted by Dr. Dorrian Apple of the Boston University School of Nursing. Her problem was to determine when people "perceive" sickness—that is to say, what configuration of experience tells a person that he, or someone else, is sick. The answer, she found, is that the symptoms must be *actively present* now; they must be *acute and well-defined;* and they must lead to an *impairment of activity.* These criteria are additive, and a really sick person will show all three conditions. Thus a man with a present fever and a head cold, unable to go to work, is perceived as sick. But a man with a vague and chronic discomfort in the chest who suffers no interruption in his daily duties is seldom seen as sick.[4] From the health worker's point of view, of course, the latter may be far more seriously ill and may need medical attention more urgently. But how shall the health worker deal with a sick person who perceives no sickness?

And when a person does perceive that he is ill, how greatly his perceptual field changes. Objects previously of interest lose their demand; the health visitor is no longer perceived as a busybody but as an angel of mercy; bodily functions loom large; minor as well as major discomforts fill the horizon. As Charles Lamb observed: "How sickness enlarges the dimensions of a man's self to himself! He is his own exclusive object. Supreme selfishness is inculcated upon him as his only duty." [5] In illness the "bacterio-technological perspective" of which we have spoken melts away. The sick person cannot take an impersonal, aseptic view of the health worker, even though he may pretend to do so. He is sensitized, as is the child, to his own fears and to signs of love and support from those who care for him. Small matters arouse aggression or querulousness, ill humor or shame. An inadvertent frown on the face of the examining doctor or health worker may be perceived as a prophecy of doom.[6] A proud adult may even view his illness as a reflection on his heredity and therefore as a disgrace to his family. Clearly the perceptual worlds of health and disease are not the same.

Percept or Procept?

Before examining the application of modern perceptual research to health education, may I invite your close attention to a current technical issue in the psychology of perception?

Up to now I have been employing the term *perception* broadly, as indeed many psychologists today do. There is good reason for this broad usage. Psychologists have always known that perception is the process of adding meaning to sensory input. It is the process that creates a stable environment out of what would otherwise be a chaos of unsorted sensory impressions. Perception is the stabilizer of our mental life. Yet, while this fact has been known, psychologists' curiosity until recently has been restricted to a few standard laboratory problems. Size and depth, localization and movement were studied on the assumption that somehow the structure of the outer world is cast in a veridical manner upon our sense organs, with a few minor exceptions known as "illusions."

Then, suddenly, less than two decades ago, psychologists grew excited by the discovery (though they should have known it all along) that perception is not simply the faithful translation of outer configurations into inner experience. Perception is profoundly influenced by two additional factors: social and cultural custom, and the personality of the perceiver. We sense what the outer world offers, yes; but we sense it through social and personal lenses. So startling was the discovery that it became known as the "new look" theory of perception (deriving its nickname from the then current fashion in women's clothes).

This theory says, in brief, that unless the external stimulus is unusually strong and compelling, what we perceive is a blend of the external message and our own subjective meanings. Innumerable experiments have by now established the fact that the words we hear or the sights we see—at least when they are not compellingly clear and well structured—are influenced by subjective conditions. Among these conditions, various investigators have identified the influence of hunger, thirst, fear and hate; of deep-lying interests and values; of traits of temperament; and of one's total character-structure and way of looking at life.[7]

The specific influence of social and cultural customs also shapes our perception of words, of time and of worth. Examples of so-called *social perception* are to be found in Benjamin Paul's book *Health, culture and community*. An American physician in a village in India, for instance, will be perceived as a powerful and revered figure if he pronounces the confident words, "The patient will recover." In Chile the same degree of confident prediction may make the physician seem arrogant and hence not to be trusted.[8] In India a cow that falls sick on the streets of a city may be perceived as an object of compassion, whereas a dying man who falls on the same street is avoided, because to touch him would bring defilement.

The enthusiasm of psychologists for these "new look" discoveries led them to use the concept of perception somewhat promiscuously. But a specialist is known by the words he uses carefully. And among the careful words for the psychologist should certainly be *perception*.

Even if used scrupulously, however, the concept of perception inevitably covers the energy from the stimulus, the receptor activity, a sensory core projected and organized through expectancy and intention, blended with subtle muscular adjustments and capped by a lightning process of categorization, made possible by bewilderingly swift associations with past experience—the whole baffling sequence occupying only a split second and resulting in a firm, well-configurated experience of objectified meaning. Even the most careful use of the term must cover all these interlocking processes.

At the same time, *perception* should not be extended to cover other so-called higher mental operations. It should not be stretched to include the judgment, reflection, evaluation or emotional response that follow rapidly on a percept; nor should it cover the trains of memory, imagination and motor performance that ensue. Strictly speaking, a percept is a quasi-sensory organization—though involving central as well as peripheral processes—located "out there." It is a complex interpretation of sensory experience, but it is not coextensive with the whole of mental life.

Suppose you ask a sample of people: *Would you agree that the world is a hazardous place and that men are basically evil and dangerous?* About half the replies are likely to be yes and about half no. Now, do those who reply affirmatively really *perceive* the world as threatening and *perceive* men as evil, or do they merely *judge* them to be so? Neither term is entirely satisfactory. To judge is to make an intellectual assertion; but a person who gives an affirmative answer probably has such a deep-seated suspicious outlook that he actually *sees* malice in people's faces, much as did H. A. Murray's children after they had played a scary game of "murder." [9] A person with such a deep suspicion might, on opening the door to a health worker, actually *see* the visitor as having a hostile face and menacing manner. At the same time, not every distrustful attitude is a perception. In his extensive analysis of research and theories of perception, F. H. Allport has shown that very often what is called a percept is, in reality, the judgment of a percept or a response to a percept.

The truth of the matter is that psychologists today are in a predicament. While the classical account of perception is not adequate, it does offer us at least two concepts directly pertinent to our problem. One of these is *apperception,* a recognition of the role of past experience and association in shaping a present percept. The other is the concept of *set,* a recognition of the incontestable fact that a person will for the most part perceive what he is at this moment "tuned" to perceive. But these concepts antedate depth psychology. They seem a trifle intellectualistic and fail to allow for the fact that perceptions may be rooted in deeper layers of personality, in what

Tolman calls our "belief-value matrix." Not long ago Postman help-fully proposed that the concept of *perceptual response disposition* (really a modern version of set) may help us account for all the clearly identifiable factors that enter into the "subjective" shaping of perception. And by distinguishing "perceptual response disposi-tions" from "mnemonic response dispositions," we can avoid con-fusing perception proper with the total process of cognition.[10]

This type of discussion is important for the psychologist who wishes to avoid terminological promiscuity and hopes for a model by which he can distinguish one cognitive process from another. But what of the health worker? He too is a behavioral scientist—or, as Dr. Griffiths has expressed it more accurately, a *practitioner* of be-havioral science.[11] As such, he needs a new concept that will by-pass the fine distinctions so important for the psychologist—a concept that will enable him to deal with the *integrated* disposition of a person to perceive, pay attention to, extract meaning from, feel, think about and respond to a situation, and to hold it in memory. It is this larger unitary process of the human organism that we seek to christen, for it is this more molar disposition with which the health worker must deal.

Borrowing from the philosopher Justus Buchler, I propose that the term we need is *proception*.[12] The term recognizes the fact that each individual carries with him his past relations to the world—his cumulated experience—and at the same time is strongly propelled into the future. Every human being has "proceptive directions," which are his potentialities for seeing, hearing, doing, thinking, making and saying. These potentialities are derived in part from his own temperament and in part from the culture and situation in which he has acquired his proceptive directions. The term designates the total process of personally relevant behavior from input to act. Unlike *percept,* the term *procept* gives full weight to cumulative habit, emotional direction and all other forms of "gating" that the complex psychophysical dispositions of the individual exert upon his behavioral sequence. It is wholly in keeping with modern research in neurophysiology to suggest that the procept "gates" (that is, opens and closes pathways to) the percept.

Why do I deal with this terminological issue in an essay on public health? I do so partly to fortify the health educator in his future encounters with psychologists. If a critical laboratory psychologist says to you, "Look, you are using the term 'perception' too broadly, and I find this a sloppy practice," the proper reply is, "Well, in the first place, many of you psychologists are equally sloppy;

but in the second place, if it pleases you better, I'll speak when appropriate of proception, rather than of perception." This sophisticated reply will probably bewilder your critic. It will surely shut him up.

But there is a still better reason for this terminological digression. The health worker of the future cannot overlook the dynamic propulsion that causes one individual to accentuate, another to reject and a third to distort a given health message. Its reception will vary according to the nationality, the class membership, the ethnic group and, above all, the personality and present situation of the client. By suggesting the concept of "proception," I hope to fix your attention upon this variable of prime importance and to allow you no escape from it. *Perception* you might be tempted to shrug off as a problem for the psychologist; *proception* is clearly the concern of both pure and applied behavioral scientists.

Proceptive Types

We must next ask whether there is such a thing as basic proceptive types. Without using this particular label, many of the "new look" researches are converging on precisely this problem. It is characteristic of these investigations that they first demonstrate some inner consistency among an individual's perceptions (considered in the narrow sense) and then discover that these ways of perceiving are linked to the person's needs, his "directive states," his character structure or his whole "cognitive style."

Thus, for example, Witkin and his collaborators describe two basic and contrasting proceptive types (admitting, of course, that many people fall between the extremes). One type they label *field-dependent*; the opposite, *field-independent*. First they study certain elementary perceptual tendencies by placing a subject in a chair that can be mechanically tilted. The chair is in a room whose walls, ceiling and floors can likewise be tilted. The subject is asked to adjust a movable rod so that it stands vertically. Field-dependent subjects tend to adjust the rod so that it remains parallel to the tilted walls of the room. Field-independent subjects are able to disregard the visual field; they take their cues from their own sensations of gravitational pressure and locate the rod closer to the true vertical.

Thus far the experiment demonstrates nothing more than individual differences in a very limited perceptual task. But studying the same subjects further, it is discovered that field-dependent persons are limited in other ways by the perceptual context. They cannot, for example, easily analyze out a particular geometrical design that lies embedded in a complex visual pattern. Field-independent people seem more able to disregard the context and discriminate the needed detail.

These perceptual styles turn out to be merely a part of a wider proceptive syndrome. The field-dependent person is usually characterized by a general passivity in dealing with the environment, a certain unfamiliarity and distrust of his own impulses and a low degree of self-esteem. The independent or analytical perceptual performer is in general more active and independent in meeting the environment; he is higher in self-esteem and shows greater control and understanding of his own impulses.[13]

Let me mention very briefly several researches which have broadly confirmed Witkin's. In a series of experiments, Klein discovered what he calls "levelers" and "sharpeners," the former behaving much like Witkin's field-dependent cases and the latter showing the more highly differentiated ability of the field-independent type.[14] Even before the advent of the "new look," Goldstein identified "concrete" and "abstract" styles of cognitive operation which have much in common with Witkin's and with Klein's.[15] Ericksen overlaps this typology with his conception of *repressers* and *intellectualizers*.[16] Barron discovered that *simplicity* and *complexity* are basic proceptive dimensions.[17] Boldest of all is the work of our late friend and neighbor, Else Frenkel-Brunswik. She has related a purely perceptual tendency (called "intolerance of ambiguity") to the deepest proceptive layers of character structure, showing that people whose emotional lives are filled with prejudice and rigidity concerning their relations with other groups must also, by and large, have definiteness and structure in what they see and hear in the outer world.[18] There seems to be a relation here to the work of Hastings, who, using Dr. Knutson's *Personal Security Scale,* found that observers low in personal security tend to locate objects—if the objects have no firm anchorage in the environment—as closer to themselves than do people with a high sense of personal security.[19] It is as though anxious people are distrustful, apprehensive and insecure in handling even simple percepts. Postman and Bruner have discovered a kind of "perceptual recklessness" among persons under stress: [20] such persons seem to jump at premature hypotheses and demand a definiteness in the outer world that it may not in fact possess.

All this varied work, I am well aware, is not yet firmly collated; and some researches, as Postman and other critics have pointed out, are imperfect in design and execution. But one cannot help feel that important knowledge is emerging, establishing beyond doubt the dependence of perception upon broad underlying proceptive directions.

Now for further applications to public health. The health worker himself is a selected, well-educated, highly specialized person. In terms of these proceptive types, he is likely to be field-independent, an intellectualizer, a sharpener, an abstract thinker. But the people with whom he deals are likely *not* to be so, especially in times of illness, anxiety and strain. When a health worker calls on the distraught mother of a sick child, for example, the mother almost certainly is not listening, in a field-independent way, for coldly rational instructions. She is listening in large measure for approval of what she is doing, for reassurance and hope. She is field-dependent: the health worker is seen as a global agent of mercy. Unless the health worker somehow puts his instructions within this context, they are very likely to be unperceived, distorted or repressed.

Every health worker knows too that some people over-react to the educator's message, even to the point of hypochondria, whereas others turn a deaf ear and repress what they hear. Workers on cancer control will surely recognize the over-vigilant and over-defensive types. Since the health worker tends to dislike both hypervigilance and defensiveness, his own proceptive directions may lead him to assume erroneously that his client is an intellectualizer like himself.

Physicians, like all other health workers, have their own proceptive tendencies to guard against. It is a known fact, for example, that, in the field of mental health, patients who most nearly approach the therapist's own syndrome of proceptive dispositions are likely to receive from him the best treatment and most sympathy.[21]

Such class-anchored procepts are of great importance. For example, it is said that the main goal of public health work is "the inculcation in each individual of a sense of responsibility for his own health." This is a pleasant, middle-class, democratic-sounding axiom; it resonates sweetly among our own proceptive dispositions. But to some people, especially among what we call the "lower classes," such a maxim may not resonate at all. They may perceive it as a slap at their cherished domestic values. To them individual responsibility is a kind of self-centeredness; what is important is to take care of one's family in times of trouble and to be taken care of by them. Self-responsibility is isolationism; it is even disloyal.

A similar misunderstanding may attend our middle-class emphasis on preventive medical, dental and child guidance work—all of which demands present sacrifice for future good. The message of preventive medicine is less meaningful to people who, from economic necessity, have to live from day to day, seizing present gratifications where they can and leaving tomorrow's evil, as the Bible admonishes, to the morrow. . . . Likewise with "cleanliness": you and I are likely to see in a dirty house an index of moral turpitude, but those who live in such a house may view our concern for cleanliness as compulsive and downright neurotic. In this case, who is to say whose perceptions are correct? [22]

Ethnic Procepts

An exciting new field of research is the proceptive study of health problems in cross-cultural perspective. Take the case of pain. One might think that such an elementary perception would have no cultural variation. And the best scientific evidence does seem to indicate that the threshold of pain is more or less the same for all human beings, regardless of nationality, sex or age.[23] Can we, then, conclude that people perceive pain in the same way? In a limited and literal sense, yes; but we can also safely assert that they do not *proce*ive it in the same way. Dr. Zborowski shows that, by and large, Italians regard pain as a physical misery to be complained about, to be relieved immediately and then to be forgotten. Jewish patients, on the other hand, often regard it as something to be complained about and also to be worried about, in terms of its significance for one's future and the future of one's family. Old-line Americans generally view it as something *not* to be complained about, but to be relieved scientifically with an optimistic expectation regarding the eventual outcome.[24]

In our own culture, then, and especially in foreign cultures, health workers must learn how to circumvent proceptive rigidities. In South Africa I found myself admiring the resourceful strategies of public health workers who, when confronted with cultural beliefs harmful to health, invented artful detours.

At one health station in Zululand, the nutritional state of expectant and nursing mothers was found to be deplorable. Milk was badly needed in their diet. The whole wealth of a Zulu homestead is in its cattle, so in most cases the needed nutrient is available. It is forbidden by taboo, however, to partake of milk from cattle belonging to another kin group; and the wife, of course, lives with her husband's kin group. Worse still is the belief that a pregnant woman who partakes of milk will bewitch the cow who gave it. Hence, of all people in the community, the married woman is most rigidly excluded from partaking of milk. The belief systems here are too deep for the health educator to challenge, but his imagination comes to the rescue. Powdered milk, because of its texture, is regarded by the tribe as a wholly different substance, hence prescriptions of powdered milk meet no resistance. Through this strategy, the health of the mothers is greatly improved.

Again, in Zululand tuberculosis is rife. It is possible with tact to persuade acutely affected cases to go to a sanitarium for treatment. But if the educational effort goes further and explains to the tribesmen that acute cases are carriers of the disease, resistance will arise. This explanation is proceived as an accusation of witchcraft, for a person who carries a disease must certainly be a witch. A father will insist on keeping his sick daughter at home, rather than accept the implication that she is an evil agent.[25]

A physician friend of mine found that Zulu mothers were giving their children an opium-laden nostrum as protection against bewitchment. Rather than counter the mothers' fixed belief in witchcraft prophylaxis, the physician persuaded them that the drug would be just as effective if it were poured into the child's bath water. He told no lie, aroused no resistance and improved the babies' health.

Such deceptions are occasionally necessary to circumvent proceptive rigidities. But there is an ethical hairline between beneficent deception and mendacious condescension; and this is a matter requiring constant moral vigilance. Kutner reports that one of the commonest complaints of surgical patients is, "They won't tell me anything" or "I want to ask them a question, but they are always too busy." And the research of Dr. Beryl Roberts concerning reasons women delay in seeking treatment for breast lesions has shocked me with evidence of indifference and intellectual patronage on the part of some physicians.[26]

Proceptive dispositions, cultural and personal, run deep, but not deepest. They are incident to the one basic desire of all mortal men: *the desire for meaning.* The health and suffering, the life and death of each individual are his own existential concern. The health worker should help, and not hinder, the person's quest for meaning in this sequence of mystery. To assume that the patient's perceptions are those of scientific medicine is certainly an error; but to assume that he neither wants nor deserves the truth is intolerable condescension. There is no solution to this ethical predicament of the health worker, except to develop sensitivity to each patient at each stage of growth, to respect him as a unique being-in-the-world and to advance his quest for meaning with all the skill at one's command.

Further Explorations

I feel I have touched only the fringes of my subject. I should like to trace an additional score of contacts between perceptual research and public health work, but shall content myself with a brief mention of two.

First: modern laboratory work on sensory deprivation has particular relevance. Until recently we have not known how important for our lives is the perceptual flood of sights, sounds, smells, touches, muscular strains and speech that engulfs us. Like fish, we live in an environmental water; and like fish, we are slow to discover this fact. Recent research has shown how profoundly disturbing it is for a subject, even a healthy college student paid twenty dollars a day for his pains, to lie in a room from which this perceptual bombardment is almost excluded. In this drastic isolation he develops a fierce hunger for perception—any kind of perception. He also develops hallucinations and loses an integrated image of himself and his body. He perceives his body as one thing, his "self" as another. Most remarkable of all, if his hunger for perception is in a small way appeased by the voice of the experimenter, he seems to develop unusual receptivity to the message. If, for example, the experimenter tries to persuade him that ghosts exist, he accepts the suggestion— and retains it even after he returns to normal life. All indications are that this planted idea has taken firm root.[27]

Obviously, this finding has a bearing upon the macabre problem of "brainwashing"; but it also has implications for the health worker. It clearly relates to the phenomenon Spitz has called "hospitalism." [28] Patients who have suffered even mild sensory deprivation through a long illness may develop unusual perceptual disturbances and suggestibility. In the same way, the apparent stupidity and deficiency in learning ability of some children and some primitive tribes may well be due to the relatively low level of perceptual bombardment from their impoverished environments.

Second—and finally: research in the critical area of child and parental guidance is of profound concern to health workers. Probably all of us are convinced that future advances in the physical and mental welfare of our nation require improvement in the attitudes and practices of parents, especially mothers. But one cannot change a mother's attitudes without realizing that she has her own proceptive biases, that she sees her child and her world in her own peculiar way.

Take the case of the young mother who applies excessive discipline too early in a child's life. She almost certainly is not intentionally cruel. Rather, she lacks the ability to proceive the child's destructive acts for what they are. Every exploring infant is destructive: he pulls off eyeglasses, spills his cup of milk and soils himself. A young mother may perceive these acts as aggressive on the part of the child and forthwith start her scolding, spanking and withdrawal of love. Some mothers proceive aggressive intent when the child is only two or three months of age and punish him accordingly. At the other extreme, there are mothers so patient or so blind that they do not undertake to socialize the child even when, a year or two later, his destructiveness does involve aggressive intent.[29] In either case, the health worker cannot expect to change the mother's socialization practices until he corrects her proceptions of her baby's behavior.

Final Word

The alert health worker, in short, has no choice: from now on, he must develop skill as an *oculist*, training himself to look *at* his spectacles and not merely *through* them—and to look both at and through the spectacles of the client with whom he deals.

He will soon discover that his habit of viewing sickness and health in a sharpened, field-independent way is not often his client's mode of perception, especially if the client is ill. He will discover that culture, social class and personality lay down stubborn proceptive dispositions that in part control what a person sees and hears, what he thinks and feels and what he does. Since, in the last analysis, every percept bears the imprint of the individual, no reliance on rules of thumb, routine curricula, or mass media can adequately guide health education. To sense and to nourish the growing edge of each individual in his present situation is the only formula for success.

There is another lesson that all of us who teach need to learn. We are habitually tempted to present to our students and clients a summary statement of our hard-won conclusions. We entrust our cryptic wisdom to a burnished lecture or a polished pamphlet, hoping thereby to bring our audience rapidly to our own level of knowledge. I try in a single essay to give the gist of my conclusions respecting proceptive processes—and I largely fail. A health worker may, at the clinic or on a doorstep, present his client with a finely wrought sonnet on sanitation or child care—but he too will largely fail. The sad truth is that no one learns by having conclusions presented to him. Learning takes place only when there is a need, a curiosity, an interest; an exploring, erring and correcting of errors; a testing and verifying—all carried through by the individual himself. In school, in college, in the clinic we cannot scamp the process.

It is hard to know how to present our invitation to learning to students or clients who, because of their own proceptive directions, have a need for safety, a need for simple and gratifying rubrics to reinforce their own prejudices; who are untrained in following evidence or logic; who are emotionally fearful and cognitively self-centered. It is usually approval they want and not fact; reassurance and not alarm; certainty and not challenge. Even those who, on the surface, appear objective and responsive often are not so; for them, too, the message is darkened, blurred and misshapen.

Discouraging as the outlook may be, it is still inescapably the moral duty of the health worker to advance the learning process, even in the most resistant cases, as best he can, so that the client may participate constructively in his own destiny and become creatively aware of factors making for sickness and for health.

The time has passed when we can impose a mere routine of sanitation, nutrition and hygiene, leading to a controlled, calculated, technically efficient life of conformity with our antiseptic cultural ideal. Such mechanical regulation leaves untouched the client's future role in managing his and his family's affairs. However important it may still be in certain respects to impose hygienic practices from the outside, our task now is increasingly to win the participation of the public in seeking sounder personal, domestic and civic values, so that the physical and spiritual welfare of our nation may increase.

REFERENCES

1. M. Derryberry, "Health education in transition," *Amer. J. Pub. Health*, 1957, 47:1357-66.

2. T. Parsons and R. Fox, Introduction to "Sociocultural approaches to medical care," *J. Soc. Issues*, 1952, 8:2.

3. R. S. Woodworth, *Dynamics of behavior*, New York: Holt, 1958.

4. D. Apple, "Definitions of illness," unpublished research from the Boston University School of Nursing.

5. C. Lamb, "The convalescent," in *The essays of Elia*, New York: Macmillan, 1905, p. 222.

6. H. D. Lederer, "How the sick view their world," *J. Soc. Issues*, 1952, 8:4-15.

7. For a recent review of the "new look" literature see N. Jenkin, "Affective processes in perception," *Psychol. Bull.*, 1957, 54:100-27.

8. B. D. Paul (ed.), *Health, culture, and community*, New York: Russell Sage Foundation, 1955, cf. pp. 112, 340.

9. H. A. Murray, "The effect of fear upon estimates of the maliciousness of other persons," *J. Soc. Psychol.*, 1933, 4:310-29.

10. For critical discussion of this issue see: F. H. Allport, *Theories of*

perception and the concept of structure, New York: Wiley, 1955; L. Postman, "Perception, motivation, and behavior," *J. Pers.,* 1953, 22:17-31; and E. C. Tolman, "A psychological model," in T. Parsons and E. A. Shils (eds.), *Toward a general theory of action,* Cambridge: Harvard University Press, 1951.

11. W. Griffiths, "Communication problems facing our profession," *Health Educ. Monogr.,* 1957, 1:27.

12. J. Buchler, *Nature and judgment,* New York: Columbia University Press, 1955.

13. H. A. Witkin *et al., Personality through perception,* New York: Harper, 1954.

14. G. S. Klein, "Personal world through perception," in R. W. Blake and G. Ramsey (eds.), *Perception: an approach to personality,* New York: Ronald Press, 1950.

15. K. Goldstein and M. Scheerer, "Abstract and concrete behavior: an experimental study with special tests," *Psychol. Monogr.,* 1941, Vol. 53, No. 239.

16. C. W. Ericksen, "The case for perceptual defense," *Psychol. Rev.,* 1954, 61:175-82.

17. F. Barron, "Complexity-simplicity as a personality dimension," *J. Abnorm. Soc. Psychol.,* 1953, 48:163-72.

18. E. Frenkel-Brunswik, "Intolerance of ambiguity as an emotional and perceptual personality variable," *J. Pers.,* 1949, 18:108-43. See also G. W. Allport, *The nature of prejudice,* Boston: Addison-Wesley, 1954, Chap. 25.

19. P. K. Hastings, "A relationship between visual perception and level of personal security," *J. Abnorm. Soc. Psychol.,* 1952, 47:552-60, No. 2. Supplement.

20. L. Postman and J. S. Bruner, "Perception under stress," *Psychol. Rev.,* 1948, 55:314-23.

21. F. C. Redlich, A. B. Hollingshead and E. Bellis, "Social class differences in attitudes toward psychiatry," *Amer. J. Orthopsychiat.,* 1955, 25:60-70.

22. For a discussion of the "belief-value matrix" in relation to social class, see O. G. Simmons, "Implications of social class for public health," *Human Organization,* 1957, 16:7-10.

23. J. D. Harley, H. G. Wolff and H. Goodell, *Pain sensations and reaction,* Baltimore: W. Wilkins Company, 1950, p. 122.

24. M. Zborowski, "Cultural components in responses to pain," *J. Soc. Issues,* 1952, 8:16-30.

25. These instances are described by J. Cassel, "A comprehensive health program among South African Zulus," in B. D. Paul, *op. cit.*

26. B. Kutner, "Surgeons and their patients: a study in social perception," in G. E. Jaco (ed.), *Patients, physicians and illness,* Glencoe, Ill.: The Free Press, 1958. See also B. J. Roberts, "A study of selected factors and their association with action for medical care," unpublished thesis, 1956, Harvard Medical School Library.

27. D. O. Hebb, "The motivating effects of exteroceptive stimulation," *Amer. Psychologist,* 1958, 13:109-13.

28. R. A. Spitz, "Hospitalism: a follow-up report," *Psychoanalytic Study of the Child,* 1946, 2:113-17.

29. R. R. Sears, E. E. Maccoby and H. Levin, *Patterns of child rearing,* Evanston, Ill.: Row, Peterson and Co., 1957, Chap. 7.

The analysis of rumor

As old as human society itself, rumor has flourished in wars and depressions, in peace and prosperity.

Why do rumors spread? What motives do they satisfy? What basic laws govern the quantity of rumor in circulation and the distortions that individual rumors undergo in transmission?

The essay was written collaboratively with Leo Postman and appeared in the *Public Opinion Quarterly* (1946-47). It is, in effect, a condensation of our book, *The psychology of rumor*, which was published in 1947 and is now out of print.

Rumor became a problem of grave national concern in the frenzied years 1942 and 1943. At that time a high official in the Office of War Information gave a reason for rumor and a recipe for its control that were partially—but only partially—correct. "Rumor," he said, "flies in the absence of news. Therefore, we must give the people the most accurate possible news, promptly and completely."

It is true that rumor thrives on lack of news. The almost total absence of fear-inspired rumors in Britain during the darkest days of the blitz was due to the people's conviction that the government was giving full and accurate news of the destruction and that they therefore knew the worst. When people are sure they know the worst, they are unlikely to darken the picture further by inventing unnecessary bogies to explain their anxieties to themselves.

At the same time, it would not be hard to prove that rumor also flies thickest when news is most plentiful. There were few rumors about our desperate losses at Pearl Harbor until the papers themselves had published an official report on the disaster. Although there were scattered rumors of Hitler's death before the papers told of the assassination attempt in the summer of 1944, there were many more immediately afterward. The deluge of peace rumors in late April and early May 1945 coincided with the open discussion of the approaching collapse of Germany in the press. Similarly, a flood of rumors swamped the country during the final hours before V-J Day: premature stories of the war's end spread faster than they could be officially denied. One of the odd episodes in the history of rumor was the fact that, within a few hours after the release of the news of President Roosevelt's sudden death on April 16, 1945, tales spread regarding the death of many other notable persons, including General Marshall, Bing Crosby and Mayor La Guardia.

If public events are not newsworthy, they are unlikely to breed rumors. But, under certain circumstances, the more prominence the press gives the news—especially momentous news—the more numerous and serious are the rumored distortions this news will undergo.

The OWI official made his error in assuming that rumor is a purely intellectual commodity, something one substitutes, *faute de mieux,* for reliable information. He overlooked the fact that, when events of great importance occur, the individual never stops at a mere acceptance of the event. His life is deeply affected, and the emotional overtones of the event breed all sorts of fantasies. He seeks explanations and imagines remote consequences.

Yet the official did state, inexactly and too simply, a part of the formula for rumor-spreading and rumor-control. Rumor travels when events have *importance* in the lives of individuals and when the news received about them is either *lacking* or *subjectively ambiguous.* The ambiguity may arise if the news is not clearly reported, or if conflicting versions of the news have reached the individual, or if he is unable to comprehend the news he receives.

The Basic Law of Rumor

These two essential conditions—importance and ambiguity—seem to be related to rumor transmission in a roughly quantitative manner. A formula for the intensity of rumor might be written as follows:

$$R \sim i \times a$$

In plain words, this formula means that the amount of rumor in circulation will vary with the importance of the subject to the individuals concerned *times* the ambiguity of the evidence pertaining to the topic at issue. The relation between importance and ambiguity is not additive but multiplicative; if either importance or ambiguity is zero, there is *no* rumor. For instance, an American citizen is not likely to spread rumors concerning the market price for camels in Afghanistan because the subject has no importance for him, ambiguous though it certainly is. He is not disposed to spread gossip concerning the doings of the people in Swaziland, because he doesn't care about them. Ambiguity alone does not launch or sustain rumor.

Nor does importance. Although an automobile accident in which I lose my leg is of calamitous significance to me, I am not susceptible to rumors concerning the extent of my injury because I *know* the facts. If I receive a legacy and know the amount involved, I am resistant to rumors that exaggerate its amount. Officers in the higher echelons of the army were less susceptible to rumor than was GI Joe, not because coming events were less important to them, but because, as a rule, the plans and strategies were better known to them. Where there is no ambiguity, there can be no rumor.

Motives in Rumor-Mongering

This principle—that rumor does not circulate unless the topic has importance for the individual who hears and spreads the story— is linked to the *motivational factor* in rumor. Sex interest accounts for much gossip and most scandal; anxiety is the power behind the macabre and threatening tales we so often hear; hope and desire underlie pipe dream rumors; hate sustains accusatory tales and slander.

It is important to note that rumor is not a simple mechanism; it serves a complex purpose. The aggressive rumor, for example, by permitting us to slap at the thing we hate, *relieves* a primary emotional urge. At the same time—literally in the same breath—it serves to *justify* us in feeling as we do about the situation, and to *explain* to ourselves and to others why we feel that way. Thus rumor rationalizes even while it relieves.

But to justify our emotional urges and render them reasonable is not the only kind of rationalization. Quite apart from the pressure of particular emotions, we continually seek to extract *meaning* from our environment. There is, so to speak, intellectual pressure along with the emotional. To find a plausible reason for a confused situation is itself a motive; and this pursuit of a "good closure" (even without the personal factor) helps account for the vitality of many rumors. We want to know the why, how and whence of the world that surrounds us. Our minds protest against chaos: from childhood we are asking *why, why?* This effort after meaning is broader than our impulsive tendency to rationalize and justify our immediate emotional state.

The result of this demand for meaning is curiosity rumors. A stranger whose business is unknown to the small town where he takes up residence will breed many legends, each designed to explain to curious minds why he has come to town. An odd-looking excavation in a city inspires fanciful explanations of its purpose. The atomic bomb, only slightly understood by the public, engenders much effort after meaning.

When a person's emotional state is reflected, unknown to himself, in his interpretation of his environment, we speak of *projection*. He is failing to employ exclusively impartial and objective evidence in his explanations of the reality surrounding him.

In dreams, everyone projects. Only after we awaken do we recognize that our private wishes, fears or revengeful desires have been responsible for what came to pass in our dream-imaginations. The child asleep dreams of finding mountains of candy; the inferior youth asleep triumphs on the athletic field; the apprehensive mother dreams of the death of her child.

Daydreams too are projective. Relaxed on a couch, our minds picture events that actualize our hopes, desires, fears. We find ourselves in fantasy successful, satisfied or sometimes defeated and ruined —all according to our temperament or the type of emotion that is, for the time being, steering the associational train of thought.

Rumor is akin to the daydream at second hand. If the story we hear gives a fancied interpretation of reality that conforms to our secret lives, we tend to believe and transmit it.

In short, in a homogeneous social medium, rumor is set in motion and continues to travel by its appeal to the strong personal interests of the individuals involved in the transmission. The powerful influence of these interests harnesses the rumor largely as a rationalizing agent, requiring it not only to express but also to explain, justify and provide meaning for the emotional interest at work. At times the relationship between the interest and the rumor is so intimate that we must assume the rumor to be simply a projection of an altogether subjective emotional condition.

The Basic Course of Distortion

It is a notable fact that the same pattern of distortion is found both in the changes an individual's perceptions and memories suffer in the course of time and in the transformations a tale undergoes as it travels from person to person. This pattern of change in both social and individual memory has three aspects: *leveling, sharpening* and *assimilation*.

As a rumor travels, it tends to grow shorter, more concise, more easily grasped and told. In successive versions, more and more of the original details are *leveled* out; fewer words are used and fewer items are mentioned. In our laboratory experiments on rumor, we found that the number of details retained in transmission declines most sharply at the beginning of a series of reproductions. The number continues to decline, but more slowly, in each successive version. The same trend is typically found in individual retention, but "social memory" accomplishes as much leveling within a few minutes as individual memory accomplishes in weeks of time.

As leveling of details proceeds, the remaining details are necessarily *sharpened*. Sharpening denotes the selective perception, retention and reporting of a few details from the originally larger context. Although sharpening, like leveling, occurs in every series of reproductions, the same items are not always emphasized. Much depends on the constitution of the group in which the tale is transmitted, for those items will be sharpened which are of particular interest to the reporters. There are, however, some determinants of sharpening which are virtually universal: unusual size, for example, and striking, attention-getting phrases.

What is it that leads to the obliteration of some details and the pointing up of others? And what accounts for the transpositions, importations and other falsifications that mark the course of rumor? The answer is to be found in the process of *assimilation*, which results from the powerful attractive force exerted by habits, interests and sentiments already existing in the listener's mind. In the telling and retelling of a story, for example, there is marked assimilation to the principal theme. Items become sharpened or leveled to fit the leading motif of the story, and they become consistent with this motif in such a way as to make the resultant story more coherent, plausible and well rounded. Assimilation often conforms to expectation: things are perceived and remembered as they *usually* are. Most important of all, assimilation expresses itself in changes and falsifications that reflect the agent's deeply rooted emotions, attitudes and prejudices.

Leveling, sharpening and assimilation, even though distinguished for purposes of analysis, are not independent mechanisms. They function simultaneously, and they reflect the singular, subjectifying process that results in the autism and falsification so characteristic of rumor.

The Fusion of Themes in Rumor

To enumerate the emotions that launch and sustain rumors is a difficult task because the motivational pattern is always complex and often runs very deep. One scheme of classification, however, based on the dominant type of motivational tension reflected in rumors, was attempted during the war.[1] The analysis of one thousand wartime stories current in 1942 indicated that nearly all seemed to express either hostility, fear or wish. To sort rumors in terms of their motivational mainsprings was probably much easier in wartime than in peacetime; but even in wartime, the hate-fear-wish trichotomy is much oversimplified. A fear rumor (concerning an enemy atrocity, for example) may be sustained by elements of sexual interest, adventure and feelings of moral superiority. The complex of motives to which a rumor is assimilated is a personal matter, and to learn why a given individual falls for a certain story would require a clinical study of that individual. Because of the diversity of motivational blends that may nourish a rumor, any psychological classification will be inevitably oversimplified and crude.

Thus we must not expect to find any one rumor correlated with only a single emotion or with only a single cognitive tendency. Assimilation does not work on a unit basis. Even an apparently simple story may serve as explanation, justification and relief for a *mixture* of feelings.

Anti-Negro Rumors

A fusion of hatred, fear, guilt and economic bewilderment is found in the curious rumors of the "Eleanor Clubs," which circulated busily in Southern states in 1943. The theme of these stories was that large numbers of Negro women, especially domestic servants, were banded together under the spiritual sponsorship of Eleanor Roosevelt for the purpose of rebellion against the existing social order. Here the most obvious fusion is that of antagonism against New Deal liberalism with traditional anti-Negro feeling. But the complex of motives goes even deeper.

There were many versions of the rumors, in which the "Eleanor Clubs" were sometimes called "Daughters of Eleanor," "Eleanor Angel Clubs," "Sisters of Eleanor" and "Royal House of Eleanor." [2] These fanciful titles represent, of course, assimilation of the rumor to the stereotype concerning the religiosity of the Negro and his supposed flair for pompous institutional names. It was widely told that the motto of these groups was "A white woman in every kitchen in a year." A typical Eleanor story ran as follows: "A white woman was away for a while; and when she returned, she found her colored maid sitting at her dresser combing her hair with her comb." Others represented the Negro servant as bathing in her employer's bathtub or entertaining her friends in the parlor. One rumor had it that when a white lady called her cook to come and prepare dinner for her guests, the cook demanded, in turn, that the mistress be at *her* home by eight o'clock Sunday morning to fix breakfast for *her* guests. One Negro maid was reported to have offered to pay a white woman to wash her clothes. Occasionally the stories hinted at coming violence, charging that the clubs were saving ice picks and butcher knives for a rebellion.

All these versions, besides reflecting anti-Roosevelt and anti-Negro feeling, show a distinct fear of *inversion of status*. The colored people are represented, not merely as nursing resentment beneath the surface, but as being on the verge of revolt. They threaten to take over, to reverse the social scale. Why? Because the white rumor-spreaders find their feelings of economic and social insecurity to some extent explained and relieved by these stories. Suffering a vague anxiety, they justify their jitters by pointing to Negro aggression and derive a melancholy consolation from alerting one another to the menace.

But we must probe still further. A rumor of inversion of status admits in a circuitous way that a relationship other than the *status quo* between the races is conceivable. And, according to the American creed, the *status quo,* being essentially unjust, should not be permanent. Every American, as Myrdal points out, believes in and aspires to something higher than the present plane of race relations.[3] At heart he agrees with Patrick Henry, the slave owner, who as long ago as 1772 wrote: "I will not, I cannot, justify it." At the same time, most whites permit themselves only a squint-eyed insight into their moral dilemma. A century and a half after Patrick Henry, the conflict still persists. Were whites to face the issue squarely, they would be torn asunder by their conflicting loyalties—to the American creed, and to their convenient belief in white supremacy.

Rather than face this pointed and irreconcilable conflict between two cherished loyalties, many white people twist and squirm and rationalize. The guilt-evasion rumor is eagerly seized upon as a means of escape. If, as the Eleanor Club stories hold, the Negro is overly aggressive, illegally plotting and vulgarly menacing, then he has no *right* to equal status. He must expect no more consideration than we give to trespassers, marauders and blackmailers. He must be kept in his place; and if there are instances of injustice, do not our patience and indulgence more than make it up to him? After all, he is only an unruly child and must be treated as such—kindly but firmly. By this devious mental maneuvering, the bigot is able to escape his feelings of guilt.

Guilt-evasion is likewise detectable in innumerable rumors detailing incidents of the Negro's criminal and disloyal tendencies. One wartime story had it that Negroes were not being drafted as rapidly as whites because authorities were afraid to let them get their hands on guns. Even humorous yarns concerning Negro stupidity, gullibility and laziness have the same functional significance; so, too, the myriad tales of Negro sexual aggression. All of these tend to allay the white man's sense of guilt; for what can we do with a black man who is disloyal, criminal, clownish, stupid, menacing and immoral—except to keep him in his place, just as we are now doing? The ideal of equality may be all right in theory, the bigot concludes, but it was never meant to apply to criminals, imbeciles or black men.

The ultimate ally of anti-Negro prejudice is the sex rumor. Negroes are repeatedly represented as plotting to cross the color line and commit the sin of miscegenation. The stories invariably concern the relations between Negro men and white women, not the far more frequent liaisons of white man and Negro woman. There are stories of rape and attempted rape, and less lurid versions representing Negroes as approaching white women, following them on the streets, trying to hold their hands, and so on. One wartime story asserted that Negroes who were not drafted (the disloyalty theme) were saying to the white men who left for the war that they would "take care of" the white women back home. Though especially common in the South, Negro sex rumors are frequent also in the North. In a New England city, known for its relatively peaceful race relations, a local story circulated to "explain" why the washroom in a certain restaurant had been boarded up. The reason alleged—and wholly fictitious—was that two Negroes had taken a white woman into that particular washroom and raped her.

The motivational current here runs deep. In the American Puritan tradition, all matters pertaining to sex are likely to have a high emotional charge and, for this reason, to spill over easily into other regions of strong passion. Sex, as a proposition for topical interest, is a never failing target for rumor. Like the measurement of status, it is also a source of heavy guilt-feeling. To blame ourselves for our sexual sins, as for our sins against the American creed, is never agreeable; better, by far, blame someone else for his real or imagined lapses. The resemblance between the sex and the minority-group rumor is close—projection in the interest of guilt-evasion is common to both—and this resemblance facilitates fusion. Why not escape guilt by heaping the blame for our own sexual lapses upon the very same persons who threaten our social position?

Deep inside, many people feel insecure in their status, or in their economic future, or in their own sexual morality. All of these matters are intimate and central in their lives, and such intense and pivotal interests cannot well be kept separate: a threat to one is a threat to the others. Hence the Negro scapegoat is seen not only as socially arrogant but also as pressing upon us vocationally, and as sexually more potent and less inhibited than we. In him we perceive all the grabbing, climbing, lewd behavior we might indulge in if we let ourselves go. He is the sinner. Even if we are not blameless, his misdeeds—as recounted in rumor—are more overt and worse than ours. Why, then, should we feel guilt at our peccadillos?

While all this rationalizing is going on, we may, perversely enough, find the Negro's "animal" qualities darkly fascinating. If so, we must severely repress this satanic attraction and, through reaction formation—that is, by turning against the fascination that we disapprove of—fight the devil even harder.[4] We do so by adopting the most sacred of taboos: undeviating opposition to racial amalgamation. The very thought fills us with horror (or does it?). Were it violated, the way would be opened for a collapse of all our moral and economic standards. We would admit defeat at the hands of the black and evil stranger whom, in our unconscious, we regard in part as our own unhallowed alter ego.

Complicated as this analysis of anti-Negro rumors may be, it does not exaggerate the intricacy of the emotional and cognitive fusions that account for their appeal. It seems to be the rule that people *personify* the forces of evil and center them in some visibly different, near-lying *minority group*. The commonest, but by no means the only, "demons" today are "Communists," Jews and Negroes. Since the blame ascribed to them is certainly in excess of their just deserts, we technically call them *scapegoats*.

Case Studies in Rumor

Let us now examine in closer detail two samples of rumor-discourse. The fact that both samples seem out of date itself illustrates the ephemeral quality of rumor. "Propositions for belief" are likely to be short-lived, simply because the panorama of human interest changes rapidly. Much may be learned, however, from a study of standard examples drawn from different social atmospheres, even if they are dated.

The analysis of any given rumor can never be perfect, because the precise psychological and social conditions under which it is told are known only in part and often through inference alone. Further, no single story can be expected to illustrate all the principles of rumor; but the basic formula should be detectable in every case.

CASE ONE. Immediately following the San Francisco earthquake on April 18, 1906, the wildest rumors were afloat in the city. Four of these were recounted by Jo Chamberlain in the Baltimore *Sunday Sun* (March 31, 1946): (a) a tidal wave had engulfed New York at the same time as the San Francisco quake; (b) Chicago had slid into Lake Michigan; (c) the quake had loosed the animals in the zoo, and they were eating refugees in Golden Gate Park; and (d) men were found with women's fingers in their pockets, for they had not had time to take the rings off. In these last stories, the ghouls were always strung up to the nearest lamp post.

Comment: The suspicious reader may wonder whether these rumors, recounted forty years after their circulation, may not have suffered considerable additional sharpening and other distortion in the interim. An example, perhaps, is the word "always" in Rumor (d): it would certainly be difficult to prove that this ghoulish story *invariably* was accompanied by the denouement of summary justice. The rumors circulating after the catastrophe were, however, recorded at the time; and we may assume, for purposes of our analysis, that they did not differ greatly from those listed above. ·

1. One obvious principle illustrated in this series is the *fecundity of rumor*. Prodigious importance and vast ambiguity conspired in the manufacture of one wild story after another, many of which were merely slight variations of others. The chain of associations is simple: one big city has been destroyed, why not others? The fecundity makes for sharpening through a multiplication of catastrophes.

2. The disturbed population is trying to gauge the importance of the event as one phase of its *effort after meaning*. Metaphorically, people were saying "things just couldn't be more horrible." Having lost home and perhaps loved ones, they underlined their feelings of anxiety and desolation by adding the ravages of wild beasts or ghouls and the destruction of an additional metropolis or two. Through these embellishments, the sense of total disaster is metaphorically conveyed.

3. In their effort after meaning, people likewise drew many *inferences*—some plausible, some not. Among the more reasonable inferences is the possibility that the quake might have liberated

animals from the zoo. Whether there was a kernel of truth in this statement we do not now know; it is possible that the shattered cages permitted *some* animals to escape. But it is likely that, as the rumor spread, many qualifying phrases were leveled out, so that the extent of the stampede was sharpened. And it seems probable that *condensation* brought in the gruesome fate of the refugees. Imagination—in rumor as in dreams—often unifies discrete events, drawing simplicity out of multiplicity and a specious order out of confusion. In this case, animals were in Golden Gate Park, and refugees were in Golden Gate Park; the latter were condensed into the maws of the former.

4. The hanging of the ghouls represents a *moralized closure* and a fantasied revenge. The vast frustrations engendered by the catastrophe had no personal cause. The despoiler of the dead was the only accessible scapegoat in a cataclysm brought on by an act of God.

5. Panic-rumors such as these correspond to the final stage of *riot-rumors*. Nothing is too wild to be believed, provided it somehow explains or relieves the current excitement. But, unlike riot-rumors, the tales nourished by panic do not have preceding stages of build-up unless the panic itself developed gradually—a rather unusual situation.

6. There is no evidence here for *rumor-chains*. The catastrophe forged so complete a unity of interest that we can well imagine a survivor telling these stories to a complete stranger. We cannot, however, imagine a citizen of New York or Chicago believing the tales of destruction of his own city. Dwellers in each metropolis had their own secure standards of evidence, making such tales impossible. It is doubtful, too, that the press published any rumors that could be readily checked. Many *unverifiable* stories, however, were published on hearsay evidence alone and were believed widely throughout the country until the quake was no longer a subject of topical interest.

7. One can easily imagine *prestige* accruing to the teller of such horror stories. The whole nation was in a state of agitation and eager for news of any kind. As soon as the outlines of the catastrophe became known, details to fill in the picture were greedily grasped, and a neighbor who supplied latest bits of "news" was welcomed and eagerly listened to. Such a neighbor may oblige by adding lurid inventions.

CASE TWO. The following story circulated during the visit of Madame Chiang Kai-shek to America in 1943. The scene of the incident was usually said to be Baltimore. One day, the story goes, a gentleman entered a jewelry store and asked for a $500 watch.

The jeweler did not carry such expensive stock, but finally managed to find several high-grade timepieces for his customer to choose from. The purchaser selected, in all, $7000 worth of watches and jewelry. When asked by the proprietor how they were to be paid for, the customer replied that he was Madame Chiang's secretary and requested that his purchase be charged to Chinese lend-lease.

Comment: This was typical of the World War II *wedge-driving* rumors, intended to divide the United States from its allies. Such stories gave government officials grave concern. Of the same stamp were the tales that the Russians were using lend-lease butter to grease their guns, and that the British were using their aid funds to purchase nylon stockings and other scarce and luxurious articles, thus depriving our own citizens of the coveted goods.

1. Evidence shows that we can expect such stories to circulate only among a limited *rumor-public.* The Madame Chiang scandal would appeal to people with a pre-existing grudge against China or, more probably, against the Democratic administration in Washington.

2. Like hostility rumors generally, this one is a product of frustration, much of the resulting aggression being *displaced.* Wartime shortages were annoying and high taxes aggravating. If goods in short supply are going abroad and tax revenue is being squandered recklessly by a prodigal administration, why should we not feel annoyed? We are willing to make sacrifices for the war, but it is not the war we are complaining about; it is the scandalous inefficiency of that radical set of long-haired professors and "that man" in Washington. The rumor represents a subtle fusion of antipathies and frustrations, and serves to explain and justify our political animosities.

3. The motivation may also entail *guilt-evasion.* During the wartime boom, many people indulged in luxuries that they could not afford in peacetime and that were hardly compatible with the wartime emphasis upon self-sacrifice and the purchase of war bonds. But our petty extravagances could easily be forgotten and forgiven in the face of the blatant self-indulgence of Madame Chiang, one of the most prominent wartime personages, wantonly wasting *our* national funds in the purchase of fabulous luxuries.

4. There may be an element of *assimilation* to the widely current belief in the waste and corruption of high officials in China. But this factor, if present, is minor, since the victims of the animus are more apparently the American than the Chinese officials.

5. *Concreteness* is used to lend plausibility to the story; precise amounts—$500 and $7000—are mentioned. Part of the rationalizing process is to surround the item with the pseudo-authority of detail.

6. Although the locale of this story was not always given as Baltimore, we know that the *label* first conferred upon an incident tends to remain unchanged, especially if it introduces the story. First items in a series are well retained.

7. Had the story been told without introducing the name of Madame Chiang, its essential function would have been unchanged. But to specify a well-known individual is a common device for personalizing a rumor and for assimilating it to common and conventional subject matter of current interest.

Guide for the Analysis of Rumor

The reader is now invited to make his own analysis of additional cases—selected from the final section, Additional Cases for Analysis, or from his own daily intake of rumor. In undertaking his analyses, he may find the following questions helpful. Each is based on an established principle of rumor; but, needless to say, not all the questions are applicable to all samples of rumor.

1. Is the story a proposition for belief of topical reference?
2. Do teller and listener lack secure standards of evidence for its verification?
3. Are ambiguity and importance both present? Which factor is more prominent?
4. In what way does the rumor reflect an effort after meaning?
5. Does it offer an economical and simplified explanation of a confusing environmental or emotional situation?
6. Does it explain some inner tension?
7. Is the tension primarily emotional or nonemotional?
8. Is the tension anxiety, hostility, wish, guilt, curiosity or some other state of mind?
9. Does the story justify the existence in the teller of an otherwise unacceptable emotion?
10. What makes the story important to the teller?
11. In what sense does the telling of the rumor confer relief?
12. What elements of rationalization are present?
13. Does the rumor contain possibilities of projection?
14. Does it resemble a daydream?
15. May it serve the function of guilt-evasion?
16. Does it reflect displaced aggression?
17. In telling it, is the teller likely to acquire prestige?
18. Might it be told to please a friend or to confer a favor?

19. Might it serve in phatic communication? (That is, does it serve to avoid an awkward silence by giving "someone something to say"?)

20. Can one detect the kernel of truth from which it probably developed?

21. Is it a home-stretch rumor?

22. Might there have been errors in the initial perception?

23. What might have been the course of the creative embedding?

24. Is it likely that it contains elaboration? If so, of what type?

25. Does it probably suffer from a distortion of names, dates, numbers or time?

26. Does its label or locale persist?

27. Is there likely to have been a complete shift of theme?

28. Is there evidence of conventionalization? moralization?

29. What cultural assimilations does it seem to reflect?

30. Does it partake of the character of a legend?

31. Could it conceivably contain a reversal to truth?

32. Does it contain tendency-wit?

33. Do the conditions underlying its circulation illustrate the fecundity of rumor?

34. What may have become leveled out?

35. Have oddities or perseverative wording persisted in the telling?

36. Has there been sharpening through multiplication?

37. Have movement, size or familiar symbols played a part in sharpening?

38. Has there been concretization or personalization?

39. What closure tendencies may be illustrated?

40. Does it deal with current events?

41. Does it contemporize past events?

42. Does it reflect relatively more intellectual or more emotional, assimilative tendencies?

43. Are all details assimilated to the principal theme?

44. May condensation of items have occurred?

45. Is there evidence of good-continuation?

46. In what way is assimilation to expectancy shown?

47. Is there assimilation to linguistic habits?

48. Has there been assimilation to occupational, class, racial or other forms of self-interest?

49. Is there assimilation to prejudice?

50. Is it conceivable that any part rests on verbal misunderstanding?

51. What is the expressive (metaphorical) signification of the rumor?

52. Does it represent a fusion of passions or antipathies?

53. Does it probably travel in a rumor-chain? What is its public? Why?

54. Are people suggestible to this particular tale because their minds are "unstuck" or "overstuck"?

55. Could it be classified as a fear, hostility or wish rumor?

56. Could it be part of a whispering campaign?

57. What relation, if any, does it bear to news? to the press?

58. Is the story labeled rumor or fact? Is it ascribed to an authoritative source? With what effect?

59. Might it perhaps represent a stage in crisis (riot) rumor-spreading?

60. What might be the best way to refute it?

Additional Cases for Analysis

The reader may wish to try his hand at analyzing the following rumors:

CASE THREE. Twenty-four hours before a sizable contingent of navy men were to receive their honorable discharges from the service, a rumor spread among them that the commanding officer had announced they must wait two weeks longer for their discharges, until the ship they were working on had been decommissioned.

CASE FOUR. The Russians, it is said, "nationalize their women."

CASE FIVE. Every few years a story reappears to the effect that a sea serpent has been seen in Loch Ness, Scotland.

CASE SIX. In the early days of World War II, it was rumored that the Philippine Islands (in some versions, the Panama Canal as well) had been attacked by the Japanese a whole week before the Pearl Harbor assault, but that news of this attack had been withheld from the public.

CASE SEVEN. Before taking off on a combat mission, many squadrons were plagued with rumors to the effect that their equipment was in some way defective; that the target was almost inaccessible because of antiaircraft protection; and that the enemy had recently perfected a new and dreadful defense weapon, which would almost certainly be employed against the squadron.

CASE EIGHT. Workers in a New England manufacturing town during the darkest days of the depression in the 1930s believed that the rich were running over the children of the poor in their elegant cars and never caring; also, that the whole depression was some sort of plot by the upper classes to cut the wages of the workers.

REFERENCES

1. R. H. Knapp, "A psychology of rumor," *Publ. Opin. Quart.*, 1944, 8:22-37.
2. H. W. Odum, *Race and rumors of race: challenge to American crisis*, Chapel Hill: University of North Carolina Press, 1943.
3. G. Myrdal, *An American dilemma*, New York: Harper, 1944.
4. H. V. McLean, "Psychodynamic factors in racial relations," *Ann. Amer. Acad. Pol. Soc. Sci.*, 1946, 244:159-66.

Expectancy and war

Psychology tells us that what a child or an adult expects will determine in large part what he learns, thinks and does. Countless experiments have proved this fact in the nursery, classroom and laboratory.

This essay broadens the point. It argues that the scourge of war is also to a large extent a result of expectancies. If we wish to work for peace, we must direct much effort to altering the anticipations of individuals—both the leaders and the led. The task is one for the classroom no less than for mass media, for individual citizens as well as for world assemblies.

Certainly the causes of war are not wholly psychological. But political and economic solutions will not be effective unless they entail a radical change in the expectancies of mankind. It is encouraging to note that recent programs involving exchange of persons, good will tours and summit conferences recognize the validity of this argument.

The essay grew out of a Conference of the UNESCO "Tensions Project" held in Paris in July 1948. It first appeared in the volume *Tensions that cause wars* (1950) under the title "The role of expectancy."

The people of the world—the common people themselves— never make war. They are led into war; they fight wars; and they suffer the consequences—but they do not actually make war. Hence, when we say (as does the Preamble to the UNESCO Charter) that "wars begin in the minds of men," we can mean only that under certain circumstances, leaders can provoke and organize the people of a nation to fight. Left alone, people themselves could not make war.

Having said this, we must hasten to admit that circumstances prevailing today make it tragically easy to fabricate a warlike spirit in the minds of men and to instill in them obedience to war-minded leadership. The crux of the matter is the fact that, while most people deplore war, they none the less *expect* it to continue. *And what people expect determines their behavior.*

Expectations are themselves a complex matter, only partially conscious and only partially rational. To change warlike expectations to peaceful expectations requires, first of all, a careful analysis of the blend of personal and social factors that determines the anticipations of people in the world today.

Extreme Views of Aggressive Nationalism

Among the many attempts to explain national aggressiveness we find two that are fatally one-sided. One errs in attributing the aggressiveness wholly to the idiosyncrasies of the individual, the other in attributing it wholly to history and the economic imbalances of world society. We shall see that the concept *expectation of war* is a crystallization of both sets of factors.

Those who locate the sole cause of aggressive nationalism in human nature sometimes say that every person has an instinct of pugnacity. What is more natural than for him to rush to war whenever this biological instinct is provoked? Even if instincts are left out of the explanation, the frustrations of life are said to be so great that anger, hostility and resentment flow in every bosom, only to vent themselves ultimately through war. Personal aggression, we are told, becomes displaced upon an external enemy. The enemy becomes a scapegoat and attracts the wrath aroused by the frustrations we encounter in our occupation or in our unsatisfactory family life.

The fallacy of this purely personal explanation lies in the fact that, however pugnacious or frustrated an individual may be, he lacks the capacity to make organized warfare. He is capable of temper tantrums, chronic nagging, biting sarcasm and personal cruelty; but he alone cannot invade an alien land or drop bombs upon a distant enemy to give vent to his own emotions. Furthermore, whereas national aggressiveness is total—all citizens being involved in offensive and defensive efforts—relatively few citizens feel personally hostile toward the enemy. Studies of soldiers in combat show that hate and aggression are less commonly felt than fear, homesickness and boredom. Few citizens in an aggressive nation actually *feel* aggressive. Thus their warlike activity cannot be due solely to their personal motivations.

An interpretation exclusively in terms of personal life, therefore, will not work. How is it with the historical-economic approach (favored, for example, by Marxist thinkers)? Here too a fatal one-sidedness is evident. No social system has yet succeeded in abolishing war. Aggressive nationalism has flourished under communism as well as under capitalism, in both Christian and non-Christian countries, among illiterate and literate peoples, under authoritarian and democratic political structures. True, some nations, such as Switzerland, have been relatively successful in avoiding war. And some social systems may increase the *probability* of aggression; fascism, for example, by its very nature, engenders a war-minded leadership. But to hold that only one type of social system automatically excludes war, and that all others automatically engender war, is to violate the evidence of history up to the present time.

The Marxist theory of the causes of war overlooks the indispensable role of expectancy. It pivots on the alleged impossibility of achieving basic (and needed) reforms in production and ownership without violence, since the owners of the tools of production (stereotyped as "monopolistic capitalism") will presumably not relinquish their grasp without violence (stereotyped as "class warfare"). "Monopolistic capitalism," the argument runs, "will not destroy itself but must be destroyed." This simple and, I fear, war-engendering formula is itself a reflection of dogmatic expectancy.

Historic inevitability is not involved here. There are, rather, two sets of expectancy—one in the "have-nots," and one in the "haves." Both sets of expectancy have to be built up through psychological stimulation. Poor people, history shows, do not automatically resort to warfare to obtain a fairer share of the world's loot. They must first be led to perceive their interests as their leaders perceive them, and then must be exhorted and pushed into organized revolt.

Similarly history shows that the owners of the tools of production often yield peacefully to the expanding force of nationalization. In many progressive countries, mines, sugar refineries, banks, factories and transportation facilities are leaving private hands without violence. And it is by no means uncommon for peacefully minded owners in certain capitalistic countries to yield gracefully to an effective partnership with labor. On the other hand, the owners' apprehension may be crystallized into a horror of the "commies" and, with the aid of private and public propaganda, into a rigid expectancy that war alone will safeguard the owners' prerogatives.

Class warfare thus reduces largely to the anticipations of the contending parties. So, too, do the "imperialistic wars" decried by Communists—and by decent men everywhere. Wars of expansion, of exploitation or simply of distraction have not been limited to a capitalistic form of social organization. Belligerent sorties have occurred whenever or wherever greedy leaders have succeeded in inducing enough men (usually mercenaries) to carry out their inhuman raids. Highly collectivistic societies have been as guilty of such raiding parties as have the more individualistic societies.

In short, the indispensable condition of war is that people must *expect* war and must prepare for war before, under war-minded leadership, they make war. It is in this sense that "wars begin in the minds of men." Personal aggressiveness does not itself render war inevitable; it is simply a contributing cause when people *expect* to vent their emotions in warfare. Similarly the alleged economic causes of war are effective causes only when people think war is a solution to problems of poverty and economic rivalry. What men expect determines their behavior.

Personal Factors in the Expectancy of War

Expectancy, as I have said, is a complex state of mind. To imply that men anticipate war only in a simple, conscious way, as they anticipate the arrival of a commuter's train on schedule or a change in weather, would be an oversimplification. The deeper the emotions involved, the more unconscious and evasive are the determinants of our expectancies. Let us, therefore, look more closely at the personal conditions involved in hostile expectancies.

Some men have an apparently unbounded capacity for bitter hate, prolonged resentments and envy. Yet, paradoxically, men also have an unlimited capacity for love, friendship and affiliative behavior. No person ever seems able to love or be loved enough to satisfy him. The best psychological thinking, in my opinion, holds that hate and jealousy result from interference with affiliative relationships. Hate springs from interference with love. Aggressive nationalism, therefore, in so far as it entails elements of hate, represents in some devious way an interference with man's basic capacity for affiliative living and loyalty.

Such interference takes a complex course of development. The infant, we know, is at first in a friendly, symbiotic relationship with his mother. Anger is likely to surge up in him whenever this happy situation is interrupted, perhaps in connection with weaning or perhaps when younger brothers or sisters are born. A child who feels thus rejected is likely both to hate and to love the rejecting parent. Since hate and love conflict painfully, the hate may not be recognized. It may be repressed. Outwardly the child lives at peace with his parents, but his bottled up resentment may slip out in unusual ways against many "parent figures"—teachers, policemen, rulers, clergy.

According to this line of thinking, aggression may exist in a personal life and yet be almost unrecognized. The individual is ripe for a channelizing of his hatred upon substitute objects. Freud goes so far as to hold that the common feeling of bitterness and hate toward Jews is due to people's resentment toward God Himself for demanding so much of us. This hatred, repressed through fear of God, gets displaced upon the Jews, who taught us about God and are commonly accused of killing Christ, the son of God. In a deeper sense, the theory continues, we ourselves would like to kill Christ for expecting so much of us. Since we deplore this impulse in ourselves, we blame the Jews, who, legend tells us, have actually carried it out.

It is not necessary to accept Freud's somewhat involved theory of anti-Semitism to recognize that man's hostile impulses are subtle and are capable of much strange channeling. For our purpose, it is enough to note that channeling of hostility in the direction of war or racial and religious prejudice is an authentic possibility. Strange crystallizations take place around the myths available in our folklore. Originally, of course, these myths were created and maintained by like-minded individuals who felt a need to project their personal conflicts outward. In this way, Jews became the mythological cause of people's inner unrest; Communists—or capitalists—became a threat to their very existence. The legend adopted by the individual is available to him in his culture and is often forced on him by his parents, teachers or leaders.

The dark-skinned races, we hear, are ready to pollute our "blood." Symbolisms and displacements of this sort are legion. The conflicts within our bosoms are personified outward. In the myth we find the mirror image of our own disordered lives. When one can no longer tolerate one's own problems, one often seizes upon the institutional interpretation and legend. After a time, organized hostility comes to seem inevitable. In warfare one may act out symbolically the buried and unrecognized conflicts in one's own private life.

Such an analysis as this—appropriate to *some* people—shows how deeply buried the roots of expectancy of war may lie. But men differ exceedingly in the causes of aggression in their lives, in the amount and type of aggression they sustain and in the manner in which it is expressed. Many people are virtually aggressionless; frustrations, deprivations and slights to their pride affect them very little. They have serene and benevolent minds, even when they deal with individuals who are hotbeds of hatred. No doubt genetic factors of temperament that we know little about are involved in aggression. But whether for reasons of inheritance or of training, some men are clearly *extropunitive* and some *intropunitive*. The former will readily blame others when things go wrong; the latter tend to blame themselves and refuse to project their own guilt upon others.

Yet, for all this diversity, it is not difficult to marshal plenty of resentment against a "common enemy." Any society contains a large nucleus of extropunitive aggressors. All that is needed is to persuade these individuals that a particular enemy is responsible for the vague discomfort in their personal lives.

This line of reasoning must not lead us to the mistaken assumption that within every nation there is a fixed reservoir of hostility—hostility that *must* be released somehow, through local conflicts, class prejudices or external warfare. Oddly enough, one does not relieve aggression by expressing it in one channel rather than in another. A country with many internal explosions does *not* have fewer external explosions. Studies show the opposite: nations and tribes that are aggressive within the group are also aggressive outside, while peaceful social units tend to be peaceful in both their internal and their external relations. The Arapesh, though much undernourished, are a placid and peaceful folk at home and abroad. The Dobu are suspicious, vicious and hateful, both among themselves and among strangers. Hence, in speaking of the channeling of aggression, we must avoid the "steam-boiler-with-multiple-valves" fallacy.

The fact is that aggression breeds aggression. One comes to *expect* aggression as a response to problems. Conversely, peaceful relations breed expectancy of peaceful relations. Thus aggression is pretty much of a habit; the more you express it, the more you have of it. It is not enough, therefore, to find a "moral equivalent for war" (that is, a harmless outlet for aggression); it is equally important to change people's false expectancy that *any* outlet for aggression will automatically bring a solution. If wars were simply a relief from tension, they might conceivably have their justification. But experience shows that one war not only engenders another but also brings fierce domestic postwar strain and conflict into the nation itself.

It is true that, while a war is actually in progress, a nation often feels united and friendly within its own borders. This fact, among others, leads some theorists to argue that friendly social relations demand a "common enemy." We never feel so firmly cemented with our friends, they say, as when we are united with them in ridiculing, criticizing or fighting a common opponent. And if a common enemy is needed to guarantee affiliative relations with our allies, is not the vision of one world chimerical? If all nations were friendly, who would be the enemy to cement our internal loyalty?

Three answers come to mind: (1) Whether a common enemy is needed in a more advanced stage of human development is not yet known. (2) If such an enemy is needed, may we not point to the ravages of uncontrolled nature, disease and ignorance—all of which may, if necessary, be personified to satisfy our need for a tangible villain? (3) In the foreseeable future there will certainly be criminals—both domestic and international—as well as dissident outlawed groups against which globally minded citizens may unite in their wrath. The expectancy of peaceful relations with all men will be at best a gradual achievement.

Personal aggressiveness, then, exists in large amounts and in devious forms; it plays many unhappy tricks with our own essential longing for friendship, love and peace. Mental hygiene is profoundly concerned with these ravages of hate, anxiety and envy in the personal life. In complex ways, such individual states of mind intrude themselves into international relations. Sometimes the person with unresolved aggression regards war as a good means of evading a family difficulty and gladly follows a call to the colors. Sometimes he sees in the enemy, with or without some justification, a cause of his own misery. Sometimes he merely wishes to submit to a leader, as many Germans submitted to Hitler, in order to escape from the responsibilities of making the difficult decisions of maturity. "Let the leader be my conscience," says such a person. "If the leader himself is disordered in his inner life—a prey to mythical notions and unresolved hatreds—no matter. I shall follow wherever he calls, for I am too weary with my own conflicts to resist him. Decision is too much of a burden for me. Let the leader interpret the political and economic scene. I will follow."

Social Factors in the Expectancy of War

Left alone, the distress in each personal life would take so many forms and seek so many solutions that a concerted, national, warlike effort would not occur. But the members of a group are, after all, imbued with common values and sentiments. They "know" from their ancestors that their group is much sinned against, that the boundaries of their land are unjustly narrow. They "know" also that theirs is an inherently superior group and therefore most deserving.

One important reason why every national and cultural group feels superior is that, in fact, there existed for this group a golden age—a time when it was superior in culture, prosperity, science or power to all surrounding groups. This golden age may have been a hundred, a thousand or two thousand years ago; but at some time or other it had—as every cultural group has had—a high mark of artistic, material or intellectual distinction. Motivated by our personal pride, we find it easy to identify ourselves with the golden age of our people. What we deserve today we are inclined to estimate by this age of exaltation.

Such ethnocentricism is well-nigh universal among all peoples. Its roots are deep, as deep as our own boundless self-esteem. Expectancy of war grows in part from the latent resentments we hold against other groups who, perhaps centuries ago, violated the rights of our ancestors with whom we now identify ourselves. The fixity of these self-adulating sentiments may be estimated from the ethnocentric tone of much social science. Openly or implicitly, many a social scientist frames his theories and his observations so that his own culture emerges most glamorous and his own nation sinless. Until social science becomes truly transnational, we must heed the criticism that comes from the sociology of knowledge. We cannot expect too much of ordinary citizens, who often follow the myths manufactured by their intellectuals and build their own expectations upon them.

To some youths, war is definitely appealing. It arouses expectations of adventure, novelty and exalted comradeship. It removes the heavy burden of maturity, since in military service one has few important decisions to make. Economic insecurity, family troubles and overbearing or possessive parents are, for the time being, disposed of.

Can peace be made equally exciting? Can it possibly provide expectancies as satisfying as the prospect of war? This particular question has led to an experiment, now rapidly expanding, with what are commonly called "work service camps." In 1920 a small group of internationally minded volunteers, with the permission of local authorities, started to clear and reconstruct the land and buildings around Esnes-Verdun. In April 1921, however, the prefect of the district declared that "recent developments in Franco-German politics" had made it necessary to suppress the work. The first experiment thus ended under duress from aggressive nationalism.

But the efforts continued, particularly in times of local catastrophe. Groups of volunteers have been organized to assist in rebuilding regions affected by flood, fire or avalanche. In the summer of 1948, at least 130 voluntary service camps were flourishing in Europe, principally under the auspices of the *Service Civil Interna-*

tional. In the United States and in Mexico, under the auspices of the American Friends Service Committee, a score more were under way. Nearly all camps are international in composition; all are designed for collaborative work of mutual service without financial profit to the participants. The tasks have a positive social value, and the labor is not regarded by ordinary paid laborers as offering dangerous competition.

Slight though the impact of such work service camps is when viewed on a world scale, their appeal and their success indicate that youth may find constructive peacetime projects both exciting and satisfying. While conscription and military training affect the anticipation of youth in the direction of aggressive nationalism, work service camps affect their anticipations in the direction of internationalism, constructive activity and friendly human relationships. One important purpose of the *Service Civil International* is to persuade governments to accept voluntary service of this order as an alternative to compulsory military training. This goal has obviously not yet been reached, but the issue has been well drawn: *will nations permit youth to have alternative expectations concerning their public duties—expectations entailing international cooperation and constructive service rather than preparation for war?* The prospect seems utopian, but the question illustrates the type of decision that nations will be forced to make if they ever become sufficiently enlightened to consider the psychological importance of expectation on the attitudes of youth.

Like traditions and a sense of adventure, symbols are an important factor in expectancy. Germans think of themselves as belonging to the land of Beethoven and Goethe; Norwegians preserve the relics of the Vikings and in fantasy share in their fabulous exploits. Greeks do not forget Praxiteles and Demosthenes. Flags, martial music and noble ruins are profoundly significant to the citizen whose security and self-esteem are inseparable from the tradition of his people.

Most symbols are of an exclusively parochial order. They mark off my country, or my religion, or my caste, from yours. World symbols are virtually lacking: there are no world parks, gardens and universities; no world currency; no genuine world capital. A few fine words have been spoken—the Atlantic Charter, the United Nations Charter, the Preamble to the UNESCO Charter—but these documents are little known and still fail to rally appreciable loyalty. Yet, just as the diversified egos within a nation cannot be fused into one "we" except with the aid of tradition and symbol, so international loyalty cannot be achieved without the common focus of thought and the common uplift that come from symbols of transnational unity.

Our existing national symbols are not necessarily mischievous. A very considerable amount of national loyalty is compatible with world loyalty. But at times these symbols are deliberately employed for war-making purposes by leaders of government and of public opinion. Patriotic phrases repeated over and over in a warlike context will habituate people to the expectation of war. Nationalistic bureaus of "propaganda and enlightenment" deliberately frame the expectancies of men.

When people's minds have become habituated to accepting a designated enemy as a menace, the next step is to set the final expectation that will lead to war. Leaders usually do this with a formulation of national demands. An ultimatum is sent to the enemy. When it is rejected, people feel that no path other than war remains open.

An ultimatum is a momentous matter. Take the case of two individuals: when they meet to discuss their aims and their needs, they have a fair chance of finding a friendly, common solution; but when one confronts the other with an ultimatum, a fight ensues. If one party yields momentarily under duress, it is only for the purpose of building up his resources for later revenge. So it is with nations in disagreement: demands and prefabricated solutions usually increase tensions, simply because they deny the other fellow a right to participate in matters affecting his own destiny. The price he would pay in loss of pride is too great. He prefers to fight.

Pride of position is the immediate cause of every war. So decisive and final have been the demands made by each national spokesman that to yield ground would be felt humiliating and shameful. Expectancies have become frozen. It is "Fifty-four forty or fight." At this point, war is indeed inevitable.

Before this stage is reached, the art of resolving difficulties through the mutual discussion of desires and needs (in place of demands and ultimata) must be cultivated. The desires and needs of people are seldom incompatible; more often they are parallel and reciprocal, because one nation generally has something to spare that the others require. Since all men need and want freedom from destructive poverty, from irrational fear and from debilitating ignorance, it is plainly through joint action that the pathway to a common goal can best be discovered. The prerequisite of peace lies in developing the habit of discussing *needs* and *desires,* rather than (as now) stating arranged solutions.

Ignorance and Expectancy

One of the most important barriers to international understanding is ignorance of the other fellow's intentions and of his way of life. Ignorance may be of two kinds: *simple ignorance of the facts,* or *distortion of facts* to accord with one's own motives or with the motives of demagogic leaders who have much to gain from misrepresentation.

Simple ignorance is the easier of these two kinds to repair. Crusades against illiteracy, now under way from Mexico to India and from Nigeria to Siberia are exciting and gratifying in their results. Psychological studies have shown that an appreciable relationship does exist between a high level of general education and freedom from prejudice. The relationship, however, is far from perfect. Even scholars may be intense bigots. Salvation does not lie in schooling alone.

Ignorance due to distortion of facts is harder to remedy. Some distortions are simple and understandable, though often damaging, as when certain white children recoil from colored people because they look "dirty." One's personal history often creates the emotional ground for a distortion, as in the case of the youth who hated "the Irish" because his rather cruel father happened to be of Irish descent. The most mischievous capacity of the human mind is its impulsive tendency to categorize and endow all members of a particular group with one set of alleged attributes. My cruel father is Irish, therefore all Irish are cruel.

A hostile image, once formed, is peculiarly resistant to the onslaught of contrary evidence. An Oxford student is said to have remarked, "I despise all Americans—but I have never met one I didn't like." Thus do tabloid generalizations persist, even when every ounce of firsthand experience contradicts them. We know of no remedy for this mental-emotional tabloidism except the inculcation of habits of discriminating perception and critical thought. Systematic training is possible even in the lower schools.

The emotional economy of a group stereotype is easily seen in the image many Americans hold of the Soviet Union. When the Russians were our allies in World War II, they were readily perceived as courageous, cheerful, progressive and liberty-loving people.

In the postwar period, when circumstances had shifted, the image became one of a cruel, oppressed, atheistic and double-dealing folk. Thus perceived, Russia came to serve as a satisfactory scapegoat—a distant menace capable of explaining many of our frustrations. Communists became the symbolic cause of evil at home. Is my employment jeopardized? Blame the Communists! Am I inconvenienced by inflation? Blame the Communistic labor leaders! Are the colleges advocating dangerous internationalism? Oust the Communist professors! A study has shown that the dislocations in America after World War I were blamed on a diversity of scapegoats: Bolsheviks, hyphenated-Americans, monopolists, the IWW. After World War II the image had sharpened; the ubiquitous villain is simply the "Communist."

Now, in order for a villain to become common property, communication and propaganda are needed. Unless newspapers, politicians and special pleaders of all kinds join in painting the picture, people will not focus their diversity of negative emotions upon one clearly identified menace. Expectancy of a new war within twenty-five years increased in America from 40 per cent of the population in August 1945 to 65 per cent in July 1946. In the same interval, the enemy became clearly identified as Russia. The services of news agencies and public opinion molders were essential to this shift.

But is expectancy never rooted in fact? Are there no natural and inevitable wars, provoked by differences in ideology or by intransigence in one party to a dispute? Are expectancies only a product of designing propagandists or irresponsible leaders and publicists, busily watering the seeds of aggression in the individual life?

The answer, I believe, is as follows: While some serious and basic conflicts of interest may be unavoidable, warlike solutions spring always from warlike expectancies and preparation. The confirmed Marxist who sees class warfare—world-wide revolution preceded by imperialistic wars—as inevitable is merely *seeing* them as inevitable. If enough people on both sides of a dispute expect it to result in a war, then of course war *becomes* inevitable. (I shall have more to say shortly about defensive wars.)

Unfortunately, the images we have of other people are more often condescending or hostile than friendly. Textbooks, legends, traditions, leaders and mass media of communication conspire to keep them so. The reason, I presume, is that hostile images accord best with people's desires to hold firmly to provincial islands of security. That the world itself is our natural island of security is a conception too spacious for our fragmented egos to grasp. But, fortunately, even hostile images are susceptible to change. They change when films, radio, newspapers and textbooks change. They change when people travel observantly and sympathetically. They change when people engage as participants in shared projects of work or recreation. They change when people gain insight into the myth-making process of their own minds as it is manipulated by publicists.

Let me repeat that school knowledge is insufficient. As Sorokin points out, the twentieth century marks the highest educational level in all of human history. At the same time, it is immeasurably the bloodiest century, in terms of civil and international wars, persecution of minorities and criminal violence of all types. One reason is that schools are seldom international in their emphasis. More often, at all hours of the day, they din national glories into the children's minds.

Yet even a new, internationally minded curriculum would not be a magic cure. For intellectual knowledge is not emotional knowledge. Only the sound mind, free from cramping complexes, can turn book learning into international understanding. A scholar may be familiar with all ethical systems and may himself be the author of an altruistic doctrine of ethics; yet in his personal life he may be blatantly egoistic, chauvinistic and war-minded. A man may understand human frailties and the techniques of propaganda, as Goebbels did, and use them to destroy his fellow men.

The Personal Philosophy of Life

It is here that moral and religious leaders have a strong point to make. Only when knowledge is deeply rooted in acceptable values does it become socially effective. Moral inclination is still an essential part of the story of war and peace.

Recent empirical studies have shown an important relationship between one's philosophy of life and one's tendency to hostility. People who are afraid of life, who say that the world is a hazardous place and that men are basically evil and dangerous, are people with much race and religious prejudice. Usually they hate Catholics, Negroes and Jews; they are superpatriotic and find their security only in nationalistic strength and sovereignty. They are generally institution-minded, docile outwardly to parents and traditions. They like fraternities and sororities, and find binding security only in small in-group attachments. They are peculiarly rigid in their approach to practical problems, even to the solution of simple arithmetical tasks. This pattern of rigidity marks the aggressor-personality. It constitutes a belligerent philosophy of life. International and intercultural understanding requires a degree of relaxation and peace with oneself that such personalities lack.

A Jesuit priest, a student of mine, studied the amount of prejudice against Negroes within a Catholic parish. Without being told the purpose of the research, a devoted layman was asked to give the names of members whom he would regard as deeply Christian in their faith and in their lives, and to give names of other members whom he felt were merely "institutional" Catholics, conforming to the rules but not genuinely Christian in respect to their outlook. These two groups were then studied by means of a well-framed questionnaire designed to measure anti-Negro feeling. It turned out that the "institutional" Catholics were vastly more bigoted. To them, apparently, the church was an island of security in a hostile world. Outsiders were objects of distrust. The essential teachings of Christianity had not penetrated into their personalities. They were living their lives rigidly, holding fast to in-group security and hating outsiders. Although this particular study did not deal directly with nationalistic sentiments, it strongly suggests that war-mindedness is closely associated with a philosophy of life that is tense, in-groupish and dependent on small platforms of organized security, not daring to embrace the world as a whole within its view.

We thus have reason to believe that two types of personality formation are especially likely to be swept into the stream of national aggressiveness. One—the most obvious—is the unintegrated, many-minded person, easily controlled through suggestion and through momentary appeals by leaders and publicists. He will see demons where the morning paper puts them. Being unsure of his own values, he will yield to the demagogue and follow the prevailing fashion in blame.

The other type is the individual who has himself developed an authoritarian character structure. To him the world is a jungle. He needs a safety island in his group, his own nation; beyond the in-group he feels helpless. He suspects, rejects and hates the stranger. Such a person quickly perceives menace in a harmless minority group in his own land, or in any foreign power that is pointed out to him as a threat.

We need corresponding studies of the altruistic and world-minded citizen, the man who has no difficulty enlarging his circles of loyalty. Wendell Willkie was no less a good Hoosier or good American for embracing the cause of "One World." On the basis of available evidence, psychologists are inclined to believe that men are less likely to be swayed into irrational fears and national antagonisms if they have spent reasonably secure childhood years in an atmosphere where affection prevailed and where high ideals of altruism were not only taught but practiced. But childhood security is undoubtedly only one of the factors making for strong attitudes of trust and relaxation in dealing with one's fellows. We need to know the other factors involved.

The Role of Parent and Leader in Building Expectancies

The child's philosophy of life grows chiefly from seeds planted by his parents. Studies show that, in general, those who mirror the parents' views in respect to religion, politics and ethics are likely to be bigoted unless the parents' views were exceptionally altruistic. The mature and benevolent outlook on life is not likely to be found among those who cling blindly to parental patterns of security.

Yet, for better or for worse, parental attitudes are always in some degree adopted. Few parents realize that they are imparting attitudes unsuited to life in a world greatly altered since their childhood. To some degree, schools and colleges modify the parental influence, but the content of instruction in schools and colleges is more often parochial than international.

Political leaders and other figures of public importance also play a vital part. If feelings of insecurity prevail, their interpretations of these inward jitters may become decisive factors in our view of the world at large. If I am told by a person to whom I accord prestige that the Jew is threatening my job, or that the Negro endangers my sexual prerogatives, or that a certain foreign country threatens my preferred way of life, I am likely to accept the interpretation and prepare myself perhaps for violent action—or, at least, for a future suspicious separation.

Marxist thinkers and others insist that leaders are mere incidents in the stream of history. Leaders, they say, are not much more than puppets that reflect prevailing tensions and transmit to the individual the dominant ideology. In only a limited sense is this true. Leaders are, of course, subject to their own fears, just as are their followers. They are influenced by current myths, by their predecessors and by the prevailing nationalistic tradition. But aggressive nationalism cannot break out unless war-minded individuals are seated in positions of dominance. The leader is decisive in matters of war and peace, precisely because his followers are themselves ambivalent, or many-minded or charged with hostility. He can play upon the latent hostility or upon the affiliative impulses of his group. It is he who calls the tune.

An important distinction in respect to leadership is between what we may call "person-minded" leaders and "object-minded" leaders. The former are mindful of the human factor, of their responsibility to their constituents and of their constituents' interests. Object-minded leaders love power and pursue a goal forcibly and heedlessly. To them, human beings are mere *things* to be manipulated in the service of a cause. Object-minded leaders often set their eyes on aggressive nationalism and, in the course of their activity, raise people's expectancies to accord with their own desires. People are made to see no other way out but war.

Along with object-minded leaders we may, I think, include a great many incompetent leaders in the international field—men who stumble into war because their position puts demands on them that are too great for their skill in human relations. They quickly reach the point in international dealings where they can engage only in recrimination. Such bunglers drag the people along with them. Their own maladroitness is interpreted by them as villainy on the part of the enemy.

Person-minded leaders hate war because they habitually reckon the human consequences. They are indisposed to utilize propaganda and manipulative techniques, to create false images and over-simplified categories around which to rally their followers. It is harder to be consistently skillful in advancing the interests of persons than of an aggressive cause. But modern experiments in social psychology indicate that it might be possible to train person-minded leaders. Until now we have allowed leadership to rise in haphazard fashion. It was more or less chance whether the leader turned out to be person-minded or object-minded.

Whether the expectations of a population are directed toward war or toward peace, toward arbitration or open break, toward person-centeredness or object-centeredness, depends largely upon the deeds done and the symbols invoked by national leaders. The greatest menace to the world today are leaders in office who regard war as inevitable and thus condition their people for armed conflict. For if men regard war as inevitable, it is inevitable.

Social Structure and Expectancy of War

I have said that war has flourished under all known social systems. The differentiating factor between war and peace, therefore, is not a surface matter of social organization, but deeper human factors of expectancy and channelizing of attitude. Personality is so unstable a unit in nature that it can be swayed to national aggression or to international amity. War can be avoided as soon as we learn how to prevent the swaying of expectancies toward warfare. Or am I overstating the case?

What, for example, about defensive warfare? A peaceful people, invaded by a warlike neighbor, would normally seize weapons in self-defense. In this case, is not expectation irrelevant? No; in such a case, *unilateral* expectation was the cause of war. One side in the conflict regarded attack as inevitable. If war is to be avoided, *no* nation can be permitted to have warlike expectations, for one war-minded land endangers all others and keeps war-mindedness alive through fear.

What of the "economic causes" of war, so much under discussion today? I do not for a moment hold such causes to be unimportant. Prolonged hunger, especially in the face of plenty, will engender an understandable violence if no other solution is available. Raids and counter-raids on surrounding tribes are as old as human history. Often the motives have been hunger; but at times they have also been desire for revenge and for excitement, escape from boredom and personal frustration (channelized by the leader). Economic wars are not the only kinds of war. There are ideological wars, religious wars, wars of envy and wars of boredom.

And, as I have said, certain political systems make expectancy of war almost inevitable, while others render this mode of life relatively unpopular and unlikely. The tradition of a culture may exalt martial virtues, or it may condemn the outlay of funds and the exercise of military prowess. Political systems make for war or for peace, according to the expectancies they create.

The factor of expectancy is decisive. The wants of men, even acute hunger, do not lead to violence unless people *think* violence is the way to satisfy them. When those who "have" refuse to yield to those who "have not" they increase the expectancy of war by making it seem a reasonable mode of behavior to the "have-nots." To refuse to negotiate is a way of creating expectancy of violence. The proud and unbending kings of France brought on the Revolution by destroying every other alternative in the minds of their subjects.

Organization for war is a peculiarly low-grade form of social organization, even though in modern times it takes elaborate and ingenious forms. Young draftees are herded into camps, given routine tasks to perform, drilled in specialties and discouraged from thinking as integrated personalities. Essentially, only the young man's capacity for obedience is played upon, stimulated by patriotic symbols; and the process fulfills some momentary function in relieving personal frustration. The war machine is thus a primitive organization of human resources. As a form of social structure, it segmentalizes the individual; whole personalities are not involved. It is for this reason that the aftermath of war usually brings about demoralization, criminality and shattered personalities.

The way up from this primitive form of social organization is long and hard. We have always had wars because they have been seen as the simplest mode of solving conflicts between groups of people. If wars had not today become so disastrous, we might be tempted to let this easy "solution" of social conflict remain. But we have now no alternative except to change mankind's habit of expecting armed conflict to solve its disagreements.

Summary in Terms of World Organizations

Man's moral ideals, as expressed in the great creeds of the human race, are at a fairly high level. But his capacity to profess one thing and act the opposite seems almost unlimited. At the present time, he appears completely unable to bring his conduct in line with his expressed ideals.

We have seen three principal reasons why this fatal chasm exists:

1. Men's personalities are seldom well unified. There are anxieties and repressions, unsatisfied wants and unrequited love, shame, guilt and awe before the unknown. Pressed between two oblivions, man's life is to him mysterious and fearful, yet vaguely beautiful and intensely interesting. Seldom is he able to unite his basic desire for love and understanding of the world about him with an underlying feeling of trust for his fellow men. Relatively few personalities are integrated to such an adequate degree, or so free from fear.

2. This basic ambivalence in life, and its confusedness, make man a prey to slanderous conceptions of his fellow men. Security is found only within the in-groups—within the family, the church, the tribe, the nation. All else appears hazardous and unknown. Myths arise exalting the in-group, and legends depicting the menace or inferiority of the out-group. This view of the out-group often entails an expectancy of armed conflict. Images of the "enemy" seldom correspond to reality, because people are ignorant of the facts and because they tend to oversimplify the motives and characteristics of the out-group in order to justify their inimical sentiments.

3. *Such vaguely hostile expectancies are easily manipulated by war-minded leaders, or by the incompetent who slip willy-nilly into patterns of nationalism.*

For these reasons a state of cynicism results, and men despair of ever achieving their desire for peace. They expect war—and this expectancy itself brings war. Only by changing the expectation, in leaders and followers, in parents and children, shall we eliminate war.

Our perspective on this giant task of attitude change is still limited and the outlook still discouraging. Yet we find hope in the fact that, within the past few years, three significant quasi-global organizations have been formed. The function of each in its own area is to alter the mode of human anticipation from one of war to one of peace. The area of activity of these three organizations corresponds well to the three obstacles I have just enumerated.

World Health Organization. The aim of the World Health Organization, as stated in its constitution, is "the attainment by all peoples of the highest possible level of health." Health is defined as "a state of complete physical, mental and social well-being and not merely the absence of disease or infirmity." Since "mental and social well-being" is included, it is clear that this organization is dedicated to the development of integrated, peaceable personalities, capable of handling personal and interpersonal tensions without resort to violence. Mental hygiene—health on the level of personality—is of primary concern to this organization. With improvement in mental health, the number of relaxed, wholesome, internationally minded citizens will surely increase.

There are, of course, many other agencies whose aim is constructive action on this same level. Wise physicians, parents, teachers, psychiatrists and clergymen, individually and in their professional organizations, work ceaselessly for the same end.

Unesco. This organization is dedicated to erecting the "defenses of peace" in the minds of men. In terms of our analysis, the special function of UNESCO is to correct the distorted images that make for war and thus to diminish expectations of war and rationalizations of war. In its program of international education and cooperation, UNESCO tries to reduce strangeness and strain among the peoples of the world. It facilitates the contributions of schools, international voluntary work camps, artists, publicists and scholars to the process of altering belligerence into friendliness. UNESCO represents only one line of constructive effort in this direction, but its international character makes it particularly significant.

The United Nations. At the level of political and economic relations between nations, the United Nations is dedicated to the task of altering expectancies. It provides a means for seeking peaceful solutions of conflicts, and it brings the leaders of nations together. But public confidence in the efficacy of this activity is still weak. The success of the United Nations will be guaranteed as soon as the people and their leaders really *expect* it to succeed. The great majority of the people of the world have by now heard of the United Nations and know of its efforts. *Confidence* in the United Nations is itself a key to the prevention of war.

These three organizations, and other bodies with analogous functions, are hard at work. Their endeavor in all cases is to build expectancy of peace and to provide machinery for its achievement. That men are hopefully yearning for their success is the first step in acquiring a new expectancy. Yearning may gradually turn into confidence. And when men are fully confident that international organizations can eradicate war, they will, at last, succeed in doing so.

Guidelines for research in international cooperation

This essay argues that prompt and energetic research in the broad field of social science may play a significant role in the prevention of World War III. While it was first published shortly after the close of the last war—in the *Journal of Social Issues* (1947)—its content is no less relevant and urgent today.

The head of a philanthropic foundation, interviewing an applicant for a grant, once asked, "Do you regard your project as 'basic research,' or do you really have something in mind?" This paper shows that the needed social and psychological research can be both scientifically basic and intensely practical.

Confronted with the cheerless spectacle of the modern world, an increasing number of today's prophets are saying that our international troubles are wholly *moral*. Technical progress, they point out, brought in its wake a perilous secularization of life. Among its macabre consequences we reckon technological unemployment, technological warfare and now the black portent of atomic destruction. The present century, in spite of its unexampled inventiveness, has been the bloodiest century on record in terms of international, civil and criminal violence.

Secularization, these prophets insist, led mankind to forget the Commandments of Moses, the ethics of Confucius, the self-discipline of Krishna and the vision of Christian Brotherhood. It were better now, they say, for each man to look to his own salvation. Let religion revive. Let character be restored. Only then may we expect human relations to improve.

Can one doubt that these advocates of moral reformation are right in arguing that the great moral creeds of the world, *if taken in their purity*, would help control the ravages of technology? Were men to backtrack from the present gulf of secularization, were they to start practicing their creeds, peace on earth would be more readily achieved.

The manifest difficulty in accepting this apparently simple counsel lies not in the falseness or inapplicability of our creeds but in their sheer antiquity. Many, perhaps most, inhabitants of the earth would recognize "Love thy neighbor as thyself" as a worthy imperative. But

347

this commandment tells twentieth-century man very little about how he can translate his affectionate purposes into action. How, in an age of giant industries, bureaucracy, instant communication and atomic energy, shall one effectively love one's neighbor?

Suppose a factory owner, a man of good will, wishes to practice the Golden Rule. What does the Rule tell him about fair and just wages? Without research into living costs, the needs and aspirations of his employees and the standards for safety and health, he cannot intelligently be a Christian. The age of shepherds and Sadducees bequeathed him a sound moral orientation but none of the skills or knowledge needed to implement his ideals.

Suppose I am persuaded that I should love my neighbor as myself—or, at least, that I should live at peace with him. My neighbors, I know, are almost three billion in number. What concretely shall I do in my capacity as a world citizen? Shall I press for the Quota Force Control amendment to the United Nations Charter? Shall I work for birth control in India and for a gigantic loan for industrial up-building in that country? Shall I approve or disapprove Scheme X for the international control of crime? Only social research, focused upon overlapping problems of nations, will tell the answers.

Sound moral purpose is by no means lacking in the world. It still flows from the great creedal literature of past ages, even while it is being reinterpreted in the light of modern conditions. The present chasm between technology and morals has formed chiefly because physical engineering has outstripped social engineering, because physical science has been allowed to outdistance social science. The worship of technological efficiency for its own sake is an almost universally recognized evil, but its control through moral efficiency awaits knowledge and instrument.

Policy, Research and Operations

Perhaps the most heartening event of our times is the establishment of the Economic and Social Council of the United Nations and its dependent specialized agencies including UNESCO. The last of these, in the Preamble to its Charter, strikes the keynote of a new era: "Since wars begin in the minds of men it is in the minds of men that the defenses of peace must be constructed." The implications are crystal clear: man's moral sense condemns war; let us therefore study scientifically the sources of this evil in men's minds and scientifically remove them.

But here an initial misgiving arises. Can research into the causes of war be translated effectively into action? A certain pessimism has descended upon many of the world's most resourceful social scientists. Aiming to improve morale in wartime, industrial relations in peace-time and amity between races, they have pressed ahead with research and have proffered solutions. For the most part, their findings have been disregarded and their zeal correspondingly dampened. Political expediency, power politics and selfish national purposes have con-spired to overlook—to "place on file"—their counsel. Atomic scientists, likewise, were listened to respectfully in their capacity as technological producers; but when they spoke earnestly regarding the moral and economic implications of their discovery, a chorus of special interests tried to drown them out. Today amoral technology is in the saddle; the socially minded engineer is a pedestrian left far behind.

The situation can be remedied in three ways:

First: boldness in taking risks is called for. Everyone knows there are serious inherent limitations in social research. It is likely that social investigation can never attain an exactness equivalent to that of physical technology, whose ravages it aims to control. Unlike physical and chemical research, social studies are infrequently addi-tive, and their powers of generalization are limited. But we cannot know precisely the inherent limitations of social science until it is given an opportunity of adequate scope. The imperfections of social engineering is no excuse for failing either to encourage its growth or to employ its aid wherever practicable.

The United States alone spent two billion dollars on the inven-tion of the atomic bomb. Would it be absurd to spend an equivalent sum, if necessary, on the discovery of means for its control? And, as the Preamble to the UNESCO Charter states, it is undoubtedly in the minds of men that the defenses of peace must be sought. Success cannot be guaranteed; it is entirely possible that social engineering may fail to implement the moral sense of mankind and that mankind may go under. But we shall never know the potential value of social science unless we take the risk.

Second: policy makers (I include the Department of State as well as the highest policy authorities in the United Nations) *can and should open their minds continually to the documented advice of social scientists.* When it is good, they should follow it. Publicity given to relevant research, to the recommendations of social scientists and to the policies finally adopted will reveal the extent to which international practices are determined by selfishness and momentary expediency, and the extent to which they conform to the best social knowledge available.

Third: let social scientists continually strive to attain a standard in research that merits respect. Too often in the past, their findings have been trivial or incompetent. Equally often, they have failed to make even the soundest of their principles intelligible or their applicability clear. Psychologists, sociologists, anthropologists and economists have much to learn about practical orientation of their studies and about effective means for communicating their results to policy makers.[1]

If developments move in the direction of the three suggestions just offered, the integration between policy bodies and social scientists will be greatly improved. Much encouragement comes from the knowledge that, during recent years, some beneficial coordination has been achieved. In numerous instances during World War II, social science gave indispensable aid to the war effort. In spite of resistance and some hostility, social science scored triumphs, notably in the areas of psychological warfare, personnel selection, morale building and effective communication between the government and the public.[2] The scope of this success is sufficiently great to raise our hopes high for the potential results of teamwork between social scientists and administrators in the area of international cooperation.

While the natural scientist or the medical scientist, operating alone in his individual laboratory, may do significant research of importance to the entire world, it is safe to say that almost no social research of international significance can be successfully carried forward in this manner. Even if a whole nation should concentrate its energy upon social investigations, it is unlikely to accomplish much of *world* significance. A single nation's culture-bound outlook is restrictive. True, in the past, social scientists have occasionally traveled abroad in their quest for data, but their reports have seldom been broad-gauged enough and free enough from provincialism to serve as a guide to international policy of any type whatsoever.

At the present time, barriers of language, inadequate facilities (especially in smaller and poorer countries), meagerness of intercommunication and lack of incentive to focus upon common problems conspire to separate and segregate the social scientists of the world. As yet the resources of their knowledge and skill, as well as their eagerness to aid, have not been tapped in the interests of world peace. To obtain the concerted effort of the world's social scientists, even in regard to limited and special topics, we now need international stimulation, facilities and coordination. Thousands of highly skilled physical scientists worked in collaboration on a *national* scale for the production of the destructive atomic bomb. The control of its destructive potential and the realization of its latent benefits will require equally many, and equally able, minds cooperating on an *international* scale.

What Is Known and What Is Needed

International social research need not start at scratch. Already much initial work has been done. A sufficient number of general principles are known, and widely enough agreed upon, to set the guidelines for urgently needed investigations. More important, these principles might *immediately* be applied with immense profit to the conduct of international relations, if the proper officials were so disposed.

As we examine these principles and their usefulness as guides to concrete research and policy, two limitations should be held in mind. *First:* they are offered as illustrations, not as a final system. An adequate survey should have the benefit of wide discussion and concerted approval by a large number of social scientists assembled from many nations.[3] *Second:* the discussion is limited largely to psychological principles, with some borrowing from social anthropology and sociology. The potential contributions of economics, geography, political science and history are unquestionably large; but these disciplines fall outside the range of the present survey.

Trends toward collective security. Perhaps the first principle to which the social scientist would call attention is the unidirectional historical trend toward the formation of a world government. From the cave man to the twentieth century, human beings have formed larger and larger working and living groups. At some time in the dim past, families became clans. Clans turned into tribes and states. Federations followed; empires had their day; commonwealth and regional unions flourished. During the past century, nonpolitical international organizations have sprung up in bewildering numbers, especially among scientific, professional and recreational groups. The League of Nations, followed by Hitler's sinister and abortive New Order, were chapters in the same saga. The United Nations is the latest and best hope mankind has devised. Yet it is not necessarily the final effort; even now it is unclear whether one world is the next step in the series, or whether mankind is doomed first to live through a divided period, a pro- and anti-Russian world.

The social scientist also warns that, though it is bound to come about, the form of the future world government is as yet undetermined. A tyrannical global system is a distinct danger. Precisely for this reason, a maximum effort in study and research is needed to insure that future developments shall be such as to implement the moral sense of mankind. Unless social engineering hastens to the support of democratic ideals, a tyrannical form of world government or an additional period of divisiveness and war may be expected to occur. Almost as bad would be the creation of a benevolent bureaucracy from which individual initiative and participation were excluded. No social structure is solid unless the citizens themselves feel that they themselves have a part to play in shaping their mortal destinies.

Participation in one's own destiny. Various lines of research in recent years have demonstrated the inescapable importance of personal participation in matters affecting one's own welfare. People almost always want to solve their problems for themselves, or at least feel that they play an important part in the process of achieving a solution. International relief organizations have learned that charitable handouts seldom strengthen the recipient or win his gratitude. Apathy, bootlicking or resentment may accompany "benevolence" of any sort, whether it be alms or an imposed political system. On the other hand, personal efforts at upbuilding and rehabilitation are usually undertaken with joy by a person who feels that the product he achieves will be his own and will not suffer destruction or expropriation.

Thus human progress and human happiness seem to depend, not upon what one has in hand, but upon one's freedom to grow and to build. Shortly after World War II, the inhabitants of certain villages in Poland and in Czechoslovakia rebuilt their destroyed communities through cooperative efforts, declaring that they were supremely happy in the process. But in many localities of the world, freedom to build is denied; and the people who are denied such freedom become reactive, bitter, resentful and destructive.[4]

Though the guideline here is clear, and is fortified by much research in group dynamics and industrial relations, we still know far too little about the process of eliciting participation and encouraging cooperative enterprise. We know too little about the techniques of linking the basic motives of self-interest to the best of all means for attaining it—namely, mutual aid. There are also cultural differences to be taken into account, though all peoples seem potentially capable of cooperation. How best to engage this capability, and how best to extend the circle of cooperative endeavor until it reaches an international orbit—these are subjects demanding immediate research.

Economic and social insecurity. Persons who feel that their livelihood or safety is threatened generally make poor citizens—of a town, a nation or the world. They tend to be defensive, restless, suspicious. Since poverty is well-nigh universal and social insecurity widely prevalent, it becomes imperative to determine the types of provisions, guarantees and reassurances that are most needed to allay fear and unrest. What are the standards of security and well-being below which no people can fall without incurring social disaster? Up to now, these standards have been guessed at through intuition and in terms of expediency, but only the results of an objective investigation will serve as a reliable basis for action.

Certain minimum guarantees against starvation and disease may be a legitimate objective for all nations acting in concert at a governmental level. But human interests are best served when people themselves are consulted and permitted to play an active part in providing for their own security. The precise forms of self-help to be encouraged, and the ideal order of priority, are subjects for research, not speculation.

We know that criminality, especially among children, can often be traced directly to feelings of psychological insecurity. National unrest, likewise, is often derived from apprehensiveness. War springs in part from conditions of chronic suspicion and deprivation. All these social ills cry for sustained research into the conditions of, and remedies for, intolerable insecurity. Some available studies suggest that a certain amount of social and economic uncertainty is conducive to personal growth, but that privations which bring morbid anxiety lead to antisocial conduct.

One form of insecurity especially injurious to the cause of peace arises from the frequent inconsistency of national and international policy. An important factor in the downfall of democratic Germany and the rise of Hitler was the German people's dismay at the shifting policies of the Allies. To the Germans, Versailles meant one thing, the Dawes Plan another; reparations indicated one attitude, nonenforcement of reparations another. Punitive treatment was inconsistently mixed with friendship. By such an inconsistent administering of rewards and punishments in a laboratory, a rat can be made neurotic. Under similar circumstances, a child, an adult or a social group grows restless and embittered. It is necessary for each nation to know, at any given moment, precisely where she stands in the international family.

Psychological security on an international scale, therefore, requires a policy of clear commitment, frequently reiterated and carried forward with unvarying consistency. To arouse hopes and let them fall; to start one ill-considered policy and switch it in midstream; to invite cooperation and then reject it—all these are fatal errors. Research seems scarcely needed to prove this point, but the fact should be clearly recorded and prominently advertised in order to influence continually the operations of policy and deliberative bodies.

International conference procedure. At the root of much of the vagueness and inconsistency of international decisions lie the human failings that come to light in the work of committees and assemblies. Men, even trained statesmen, do not know how to deliberate efficiently. Up to now, in social science, only a bare beginning has been made in the study of the processes of discussion, group criticism and decision. We may expect much basic work to be done in the future even without international support. But so essential is it for international groups to learn how to employ the most effective conference procedures that money and time would be well invested in additional investigations.

The parliamentary problems of international bodies are unique, for when individuals come together from contrasting cultural backgrounds, employing different languages and reflecting diverse traditions, the ordinary difficulties of efficient mental coordination are exaggerated. How shall representatives of different nations learn most effectively to deliberate together unless international support and encouragement are given to this vital line of research?

Focusing on children. Social scientists know that within the next generation it is theoretically possible to have a world language, to build universal loyalty to a world state, and to eliminate most racial and national prejudices. They know equally well that the goal cannot be achieved in practice, for it is from their parents that children chiefly learn their social attitudes. The older generation unfortunately inclines to be firmly set in its bitterness and its blindness; and children, with their almost limitless plasticity, will acquire much of this burden. Yet children still constitute the best possible focus for our internationalizing efforts. They can readily identify with symbols of world unity, even while holding inviolate their loyalty to family, neighborhood and nation.

To overlook children is to be stupidly inefficient from the standpoint of social engineering. Twenty-five years is not too long to await results in the perspective of social evolution. Social scientists might reasonably advise that adults be largely disregarded in favor of children. The establishment of health centers, nutritional standards, curricular standards, welfare stations, model schools, a children's village, research in social attitudes, social training and appropriate symbols might well hold the center of the stage. The children of today are the custodians of the United Nations of tomorrow. The problems we cannot solve they will inherit, and their ability to cope with these problems will exceed ours only if their loyalties are stronger and their initial training sounder.

There is a simple psychological reason why international bodies tend to overlook children. Delegates assemble in an atmosphere of cameras, microphones and bald heads. Where are the children? While in an adult world, adults tend to forget them. Would it not be well to arrange the entrance to the General Assembly, the Security Council and the UNESCO headquarters so that it would lead the delegates through a nursery school play yard—just as a reminder?

To focus upon child welfare, education, health and juvenile research would have an extra advantage. What every parent wants (with few exceptions) the wide world over is a better opportunity for his child than he himself had. A United Nations devoted to providing such an opportunity would win the allegiance of adults far faster than through a direct appeal to their adult-centered interests.

One dare not minimize the political obstacles in the way. To take a single example, the task of teaching the children of the world scientific facts about race will turn out to be a vexatious problem. Sovereign rights will seem to be threatened. The senator from Mississippi will scarcely welcome scientific facts about race in Mississippi's public schools, especially if the curriculum is devised in consultation with Russian and Negro scholars. Children are plastic and willing; adults are the bigots. Yet even here, research and patience may discover not only a scientifically sound curriculum for international use, but also, in time, the effective means for introducing this curriculum into backward areas.

The common ground of human nature. To teach children the ways of peace requires, among other things, a factual knowledge of the peoples of the world. What, up to now, have anthropologists given us? And what have the schools been teaching? Broadly speaking, both have accented the *differences* that divide the families of mankind. There has been little malice in the practice; yet the results have often been harmful. The American child, for example, learns with horror about headhunters and infanticide; he learns to laugh at the Dutch, who clop in wooden shoes, and at the quaint observances of Easter among adherents to the Orthodox faith. The implication of inferiority is a usual by-product of our present method of teaching cultural and national differences. Less dramatic, but far sounder, would be the teaching of the common considerations of justice and morality that are identical over vast areas of the earth. Practices that may *seem* to differ dramatically often indicate common aspirations and common values. The prayer wheels of Tibet and the silent Quaker meeting have virtually identical functional significance; so, too, the initiation rites of the Pawnee and the American high school commencement.

Except for the work of some anthropologists—notably the Cross Cultural Survey developed under the direction of George P. Murdoch of Yale University—little effort has been spent in the search for the common ground of mankind. A vast project of investigation, absolutely basic to the interests of peace and to the success of the United Nations, is the preparation of an encyclopedia of the uniformities and similarities of the world's peoples in respect to their aspirations, beliefs and practices. The successful execution of this project would call for the cooperation of many kinds of social scientists in many countries. Such a set of volumes, sure to be epoch making, would serve as a reference guide for innumerable aspects of world policy for years to come.

One large aspect of this research will inevitably deal with the problem of national character. Here lies much virgin territory to be explored. The common ground for mankind cannot be fully understood or intelligently employed unless the national and ethnic variants are objectively known for what they are.

The desires and opinions of the common man. It is not only the enduring uniformities and equivalences in culture that need to be known, but also the *current* state of world needs and world opinion. Here, too, internationally sponsored social research is indispensable.

In the modern day it is unnecessary to remain in ignorance of the aspirations, hopes, wishes or judgment of the common man. Particularly when statesmen find themselves deadlocked through their incompatible demands for solutions to international problems, it would be salutary to know what the people of the world think. In many cases, a knowledge of public opinion would aid in redefining the issues and devising peaceful solutions.

One cannot deny that adults in every nation are frequently as belligerent and uncompromising as their statesmen in matters pertaining to boundaries and sovereignty. But a study of the view of the majority of the common people would probably reveal that more important to them than boundaries are matters of self-respect, pride, food, shelter, marriage, the welfare of their children and the opportunity to identify with some successful group—not necessarily with their own belligerent nation. A focus on matters of prior importance to the citizenry would often bring a redefinition of the issues and disclose unexpected solutions. For the root-desires of two people are seldom incompatible: when they confront each other with their basic *desires,* they can usually satisfy both sets of interests through cooperation. But when they confront each other with rigid *demands,* there is often no solution short of war. (Cf. Chapter 11.)

In brief, the time has come for a continuing international service in public opinion. Polling now exists in more than a dozen countries. Facilities and talent are available; they await international coordination and utilization.

Communication. A reciprocal research service is required in order to achieve effective communication to the public of all lands. How may radio, motion pictures, television, books, news services, periodicals and lecturers be best employed in order that people everywhere may be informed in affairs of international import? Purely local research, such as that done in America, is inadequate. It overlooks entirely the difficulties of polylingualism or varying habits, tastes and practices in other lands. The task of communicating effectively with a world audience requires internationally sponsored research.

A special phase of the communication problem deals with the strategies of propaganda. It is recognized today that propaganda has its uses in the service of good causes, but that it may be a device of doubtful ethical justification. To what extent propaganda techniques may legitimately be employed in the interests of international cooperation is a subject for searching discussion. But such discussion cannot profitably take place unless the essential features, the strategies and the tactics of propaganda are first scientifically analyzed.

Condescension and its perils. A principle upon which social scientists almost unanimously agree is that human relations founded upon an attitude of condescension are perilous. So far as is known, no group of people is content to think of itself as inferior to any other group, nor is any single individual normally willing to regard himself as of less worth or merit than another. In some periods of history, slavery or feudalism seemed to lead a temporarily peaceful existence; but it may be safely asserted that policies based on condescension will sooner or later lead to violence. In the world today the unrest of citizens formerly regarded as second-class is manifest. Dark-skinned people are moving ahead toward independence. The white-skinned third of the world's population cannot prevent the movement; the English-speaking tenth certainly cannot do so. Any attempt to preserve the older imperial and colonial systems is doomed to breed violence and war.

Perhaps the basic principle of the science of human relations is that, to deal effectively with any other mortal, it is necessary to find out how he feels. Xenophobia and condescension give way in the face of psychological knowledge. Mutual understanding grows. Projects of investigation in this area range from the analysis of the genesis and nature of race prejudice to the assembling of a world-wide collection of self-told narratives, graphically illustrated, to serve as material for broadening our appreciation of people who represent other colors, other creeds and other nationalities. Research in the fields of ethnic differences, ethnic similarities and interracial understanding is almost limitless in scope. We must rely upon social engineering derived from this type of research to offset the ravages of hostility and condescension that in the past have poisoned our ethnic attitudes.

Need of symbols. For most people the concept of a single, democratically oriented world is difficult to hold in mind. As a rule, personal loyalty can adhere to an abstraction only when the abstraction is richly symbolized. Christianity rivets attention upon the cross; nations, upon their flags. Greece has its Acropolis, America its Statue of Liberty. The Moslem faces Mecca. International mercy is represented by the Red Cross. On his lapel the serviceman bears insignia of his military history and his status.

The great majority of symbols are now nationalistic. Artists and musicians, architects and designers are to a large extent culture-bound; inevitably their productions favor single nations rather than the concert of nations. Does it not follow that an early and urgent task is to stimulate, by commission or competition, the devising of adequate world symbols? It should be done on an international scale; and to carry out this task successfully, research is indispensable.

With modern techniques, world opinion can be consulted. Proposed symbols can be pretested before adoption. Business uses market research to determine the effectiveness of trade marks; why should not the United Nations do the same? Tastes in music can be ascertained; so, too, inclinations respecting a common language. If schools were to teach the vernacular and, in addition, one universal tongue, what should the latter be?

It would be fanciful, of course, to assume that symbols can be arbitrarily or synthetically created. They grow out of a deep feeling and are accepted only on the basis of conviction. But millions of people already have the requisite feeling and conviction; in their search for symbols, they need stimulus and incentive, guidance and research. In time, more and better symbols will inevitably emerge, but they will have a fairer chance of success if deliberate attention is paid to the course of their development. It is in this connection that international parks and universities should be considered. Quite apart from their utilitarian significance, they have profound symbolic meaning as well.

Summary

My plea is for an accelerated development of social engineering based on social research, to the end that we may overtake and control the ravages of a rampant and amoral technology. I am convinced that the basic moral sense of mankind is sufficiently established in direction and motive power to employ with profit the principles and instruments which the nascent science of human relations has already developed—and which it will continue to develop at a rapid rate if adequate support is given.

The principles stated in this paper derive from psychology, sociology and social anthropology. In all probability they would be endorsed by most specialists in these disciplines. But a far more complete list of principles and a fuller account of applications would result if many social scientists were to work in concert upon these problems. Such concerted action should be instigated on an international scale.

Should any "hard-headed" statesman scorn the guidelines here offered as an expression of futile idealism, he himself would stand revealed as the most impractical of men. Scientific facts in the social field, as in any field, can be disregarded only with peril. The Einsteinian equation $e = mc^2$ was once dismissed as pedantry; yet the formula led to the release of atomic energy. The "pedantry" of social science might even now contribute enormously to the establishment of peace and international cooperation if its applications were understood and employed by policy makers.

Social science has as yet by no means realized its potential power as a welder of international relations, nor will it do so until adequate support is given on both a national and an international scale. Since the most urgent challenges pertain to world-wide problems, international support is most acutely needed. The cooperation of social scientists all over the world, though as yet meager, would not be difficult to achieve.

Some of the research required for international policy is of an *ad hoc* and momentary character, often statistical in nature. The pivotal investigations needed for long-range planning, however, fall for the most part in the areas this essay has surveyed. The research here recommended is, in all cases, intimately related to basic principles of social science. These principles, as far as they are now known—and as rapidly as new ones are formulated inductively with the aid of research—should be allowed to direct policy.

By way of summation, let me outline the essential areas of research mentioned above. The list is only a hint of the total research needed, but the topics included are all accessible and important. The list is intended to serve as a starting point for discussion among interested groups of social scientists and policy makers:

1. Prepare a historical survey of the trend toward larger and larger units of collective security.

2. Determine the conditions for democratic mass participation:
   A. The conditions required for a sense of freedom to build
   B. The conditions for linking self-interest to the techniques of mutual aid
   C. The conditions for widening the individual's circle of cooperative enterprise

3. Determine the effects of economic and psychological insecurity:
   A. Under what circumstances, and to what degree, does insecurity serve as an incentive?
   B. Under what circumstances, and beyond what point, does insecurity engender morbid and antisocial reactions?
   C. What is the relation between childhood insecurity and the formation of delinquent and hostile attitudes?
   D. What forms of insecurity lead to national unrest and warlike sentiments?

E. What international policies, if consistently maintained, would lead to an optimum sense of security?

4. Investigate international conference procedures:
    A. What are the requirements of effective deliberation and group decision in large assemblies? In committees?
    B. How are these requirements modified when participants are from different cultural and linguistic backgrounds?

5. Direct main efforts upon children:
    A. Determine how multiple loyalties can be created without mental conflict
    B. Explore the possibilities of a children's village for shaping favorable international attitudes.
    C. Prepare international standards for health and nutrition
    D. Investigate the conditions for the formation of attitudes
    E. Devise model curricula to eliminate ethnic prejudice and explain the interdependence of nations
    F. Determine on a world-wide scale parental aspirations for children
    G. Devise methods for keeping policy bodies aware of children and their needs
    H. Explore methods for the installation of child training projects in all countries

6. Determine objectively the common ground of mankind:
    A. Prepare an encyclopedia of the uniformities and similarities of cultures
    B. Interpret cultural difference in terms of functional equivalences
    C. Explore in detail the conception of national character

7. Ascertain current opinion:
    A. Establish a continuing operation for revealing the state of men's needs, aspirations and opinions. (Start in countries where machinery is already available)
    B. Center attention upon common needs rather than upon divisive demands
    C. Translate findings into implications for policy

8. Investigate channels of communication:
    A. Study the merits of all media in respect to their value for international cooperation
    B. Experiment with programs and determine their effectiveness

c. Determine the strategy and tactics of propaganda and devise methods for building immunity

D. Trace the dissemination of ideas through rumor, through both illicit and authoritative channels

E. Explore continually the problems of polylingualism and the conditions for a world language

9. Clarify the problem of race:

A. Solve the problem of identities and differences in racial abilities and temperament

B. Prepare authoritative ethnographic maps

c. Examine the psychological effects of policies of condescension

D. Estimate in advance the probable effects of proposed policies respecting bases and trusteeships

E. Determine the causes of xenophobia

F. Determine the conditions for mutual understanding among individuals of diverse backgrounds

10. Develop symbols of international cooperation:

A. Identify the symbols that appeal to diverse groups

B. Pre-test plans for world centers, music, parks, universities and other symbols of unity

c. Determine means for encouraging the development of effective world symbols

REFERENCES

1. Suggestions for bridging the chasm in communication and for improving the relevance of social research are made by A. H. Leighton, *The governing of men,* Princeton: Princeton University Press, 1945, especially pp. 390-97; and in Chapters 12 and 13 of the present volume.

2. Some indication of the variety and nature of the successful wartime applications of social science to administrative policy can be obtained from D. Cartwright, "American social psychology and the war," *J. Consult. Psychol.,* 1946, 10:67-72.

3. The list of principles here offered is not, however, quite as individual and arbitrary as may appear. Several of them are contained in "Human nature and the peace," a statement subscribed to by 2,058 American psychologists, all members of the American Psychological Association. The "Psychologists' statement" is published in full in the *Psycholog. Bull.,* 1945, 42:376-78; also in G. Murphy (ed.), *Human nature and enduring peace* (Yearbook of the Society for the Psychological Study of Social Issues, Boston: Houghton Mifflin, 1945).

4. See Chapter 12 of the present volume.

Bibliography

Gordon W. Allport

BOOKS, MONOGRAPHS AND TESTS

A-S reaction study (with F. H. Allport), Boston: Houghton Mifflin, 1928; rev. ed., Boston: Houghton Mifflin, 1949.

A study of values (with P. E. Vernon), Boston: Houghton Mifflin, 1931; rev. ed. (with G. Lindzey and P. E. Vernon), Boston: Houghton Mifflin, 1951; 3rd ed. (with G. Lindzey and P. E. Vernon), Boston: Houghton Mifflin, 1960.

Studies in expressive movement (with P. E. Vernon), New York: Macmillan, 1933; microfilm ed., Ann Arbor: University Microfilms, 1959.

The psychology of radio (with H. Cantril), New York: Harper, 1935. Reprinted in part as "Speaker versus loudspeaker" (with H. Cantril), in G. E. Swanson, T. M. Newcomb and E. L. Hartley (eds.), *Readings in social psychology* (rev. ed.), New York: Holt, 1952, Part I, A, pp. 96-103.

Trait-names: a psycho-lexical study (with H. S. Odbert), *Psychol. Monogr.*, 1936, 47:1-171 No. 211.

Personality: a psychological interpretation, New York: Holt, 1937. Also published as *Persönlichkeit: Struktur, Entwicklung, und Erfassung der menschlichen Eigenart* (trans. by H. von Bracken), Stuttgart: Klett Verlag, 1949; 2nd ed., Meisenheim/Glan: Verlag Anton Hain, K.G., 1959.

The use of personal documents in psychological science, New York: Social Science Research Council, 1942, Bull. 49.

The psychology of rumor (with L. Postman), New York: Holt, 1947. Also published in Japanese (trans. by T. Minami), Tokyo: Iwanami Gendai Sōsho, 1953; and in Spanish as *Psicologia del Rumor* (trans. by J. Clementi), Buenos Aires: Editorial Psique, 1953.

The individual and his religion, New York: Macmillan, 1950. Also published in Japanese (trans. by T. Haratani), Tokyo: Iwanami Gendai Sōsho, 1953; and in Greek (trans. by S. N. Papadaki), Athens: Christian Union of Christian Workers, 1960.

The nature of personality: selected papers, Cambridge: Addison-Wesley, 1950.

The nature of prejudice, Cambridge: Addison-Wesley, 1954; Boston: Beacon; abridged ed., Garden City: Doubleday Anchor, 1958. Chap. 1 reprinted in W. O. Sutherland and R. L. Montgomery (eds.), *The reader: a study of form and content*, Boston: Little, Brown, 1960.

Becoming: basic considerations for a psychology of personality, New Haven: Yale University Press, 1955. Also published in Danish as *Personlighedens Udformning* (trans. by A. Madsen), Copenhagen: Nyt Nordisk Forlag Arnold Busck, 1956; in Swedish as *Personlighetens Utveckling* (trans. by A. Asker), Stockholm: Alfa Boktryckeri, 1957; in German as *Werden der Persönlichkeit* (trans. by H. von Bracken), Bern: Verlag Hans Huber, 1958; in Japanese (trans. by H. Toyosawa), Tokyo: Risosha Ltd., 1959; and in Korean (trans. by Tong-He Choo), Seoul: Tong-Shin Co., 1960.

Personality and social encounter, Boston: Beacon, 1960.

Pattern and growth in personality, New York: Holt, Rinehart and Winston, 1961; also London: Holt, Rinehart and Winston, 1963.

ARTICLES AND REVIEWS

1921

"Personality traits: their classification and measurement" (with F. H. Allport), *J. Abnorm. Soc. Psychol.*, 1921, 16:6-40.

"Personality and character," *Psychol. Bull.*, 1921, 18:441-55.

Reviews:

W. H. Pyle, *The psychology of learning*, *J. Abnorm. Soc. Psychol.*, 1921-22, 16:414-15.

M. S. Pittman, *The value of school supervision*; W. S. Herzog, *State maintenance for teachers in training*; and A. G. Peaks, *Periodic variations in efficiency*, *J. Abnorm. Soc. Psychol.*, 1921-22, 16:415.

1922

Reviews:

L. Berman, *The glands regulating personality*, *J. Abnorm. Soc. Psychol.*, 1922, 17:220-22.

E. S. Bogardus, *Essentials of social psychology*, *J. Abnorm. Soc. Psychol.*, 1922, 17:104-06.

1923

"Germany's state of mind," *New Republic*, 1923, 34:63-65.

"The Leipzig congress of psychology," *Amer. J. Psychol.*, 1923, 34:612-15.

1924

"The study of the undivided personality," *J. Abnorm. Soc. Psychol.*, 1924, 19:132-41.

"Eidetic imagery," *Brit. J. Psychol.*, 1924, 15:99-120.

"Die theoretischen Hauptströmungen in der amerikanischen Psychologie der Gegenwart," *Zeitschrift f. Pädagog. Psychol.*, 1924, 4:129-37.

"The standpoint of Gestalt psychology," *Psyche*, 1924, 4:354-61.

Reviews:

M. P. Follett, *Creative experience*, *J. Abnorm. Soc. Psychol.*, 1924, 18:426-28.

W. W. Smith, *The measurement of emotion*; and H. Eng, *Experimentelle Untersuchungen über das Gefühlsleben des Kindes im Vergleich mit dem des Erwachsenen*, *J. Abnorm. Soc. Psychol.*, 1924, 18:414-16.

1925

Review:

W. B. Munro, *Personality in politics*, *J. Abnorm. Soc. Psychol.*, 1925, 20:209-11.

1926

Reviews:

K. Dunlap, *Social psychology*, *J. Abnorm. Soc. Psychol.*, 1926, 21:95-100.

O. Selz, *Über die Persönlichkeitstypen und die Methoden ihrer Bestimmung*, *Amer. J. Psychol.*, 1926, 37:618-19.

1927

"Concepts of trait and personality," *Psychol. Bull.*, 1927, 24:284-93.
Reviews:
A. A. Roback, *A bibliography of character and personality*, *Psychol. Bull.*, 1927, 24:309-10.
A. A. Roback, *Psychology of character*, *Psychol. Bull.*, 1927, 24:717-23.
W. S. Taylor (ed.), *Readings in abnormal psychology and mental hygiene*, *J. Abnorm. Soc. Psychol.*, 1927, 21:445-48.

1928

"The eidetic image and the after-image," *Amer. J. Psychol.*, 1928, 40:418-25.
"A test for ascendance-submission," *J. Abnorm. Soc. Psychol.*, 1928, 23:118-36.

1929

"The study of personality by the intuitive method: an experiment in teaching from *The locomotive god*," *J. Abnorm. Soc. Psychol.*, 1929, 24:14-27.
"The composition of political attitudes," *Amer. J. Sociol.*, 1929, 35:220-38.
Reviews:
E. T. Clark, *The psychology of religious awakening*, *Psychol. Bull.*, 1929, 26:710-11.
W. McDougall, *The group mind*, *J. Abnorm. Soc. Psychol.*, 1929, 24:123-26.
H. Meltzer and E. Bailor, *Developed lessons in psychology*, *Dartmouth Alumni Bull.*, 1929.
T. Munro, *Scientific method in aesthetics*, *Psychol. Bull.*, 1929, 26:711.
C. Murchison, *Social psychology*, *Psychol. Bull.*, 1929, 26:709-10.
M. Prince, *Clinical and experimental studies in personality*, *Psychol. Bull.*, 1929, 26:711-12.
L. T. Troland, *Fundamentals of human motivation*, *J. Abnorm. Soc. Psychol.*, 1929, 23:510-13.

1930

"Some guiding principles in understanding personality," *The Family*, June 1930, pp. 124-28.
"The neurotic personality and traits of self-expression," *J. Soc. Psychol.*, 1930, 1:524-27.
"The field of personality" (with P. E. Vernon), *Psychol. Bull.*, 1930, 27:677-730.
"Change and decay in the visual memory image," *Brit. J. Psychol.*, 1930, 21:133-48.
Reviews:
J. E. Downey, *Creative imagination*, *Psychol. Bull.*, 1930, 27:408-10.
K. Young, *Social psychology*, *Psychol. Bull.*, 1930, 27:731-33.

1931

"What is a trait of personality?" *J. Abnorm. Soc. Psychol.*, 1931, 25:368-72.
"A test for personal values" (with P. E. Vernon), *J. Abnorm. Soc. Psychol.*, 1931, 26:231-48.

1932

Reviews:

W. Boven, *La science du caractère*, Amer. J. Psychol., 1932, 44:838-39.

J. C. Flugel, *The psychology of clothes*, Psychol. Bull., 1932, 29:358-59.

D. Katz and F. H. Allport, *Students' attitudes*, Psychol. Bull., 1932, 29:356-58.

F. Künkel, *Vitale Dialektik*, Psychol. Bull., 1932, 29:371-73.

A. A. Roback, *Personality*, Psychol. Bull., 1932, 29:359-60.

J. J. Smith, *Social psychology*, Psychol. Bull., 1932, 29:360.

P. M. Symonds, *Diagnosing personality and conduct*, J. Soc. Psychol., 1932, 3:391-97.

1933

"The study of personality by the experimental method," *Char. & Pers.*, 1933, 1:259-64.

"The determination of personal interests by psychological and graphological methods" (with H. Cantril and H. A. Rand), *Char. & Pers.*, 1933, 2:134-51.

"Recent applications of the *study of values*" (with H. Cantril), *J. Abnorm. Soc. Psychol.*, 1933, 28:259-73.

Reviews:

C. Bühler, *Der menschliche Lebenslauf als psychologisches Problem*, Sociologus, 1933, 9:336-38.

N. D. M. Hirsch, *Genius and creative intelligence*, Psychol. Bull., 1933, 30:365-66.

L. Klages, *The science of character* (trans. by W. H. Johnston), Psychol. Bull., 1933, 30:370-71.

M. A. McLaughlin, *The genesis and constancy of ascendance and submission as personality traits*, Amer. J. Psychol., 1933, 45:779-80.

1934

"Judging personality from voice" (with H. Cantril), *J. Soc. Psychol.*, 1934, 5:37-55.

Reviews:

A. Goldenweiser, *History, psychology, and culture*, Psychol. Bull., 1934, 31:363-64.

A. A. Roback, *Self-consciousness and its treatment*, Psychol. Bull., 1934, 31:370.

1935

"Attitudes," in C. C. Murchison (ed.), *A handbook of social psychology*, Worcester: Clark University Press, 1935, Chap. 17.

"The radio as a stimulus situation," *Acta Psychol.*, 1935, 1:1-6.

"The nature of motivation," *Understanding the child*, Jan. 1935, pp. 3-6.

1936

"Are attitudes biological or cultural in origin?" (with R. L. Schanck), *Char. & Pers.*, 1936, 4:195-205.

Review:

G. K. Zipf, *The Psycho-biology of language*, Psychol. Bull., 1936, 33:219-22.

1937

"The functional autonomy of motives," *Amer. J. Psychol.*, 1937, 50:141-56. Also published in C. L. Stacey and M. F. DeMartino (eds.), *Understanding human motivation*, Cleveland: Howard Allen, 1958, pp. 69-81.

"The personalistic psychology of William Stern," *Char. & Pers.*, 1937, 5:231-46. Also published (abridged) in H. Brand (ed.), *The study of personality*, New York: Wiley, 1954, pp. 149-61.

1938

"The Journal of Abnormal and Social Psychology: an editorial," *J. Abnorm. Soc. Psychol.*, 1938, 33:3-13.

"William Stern: 1871-1938," *Amer. J. Psychol.*, 1938, 51:770-74.

"Personality: a problem for science or a problem for art?" *Revista de Psihologie*, 1938, 1:1-15.

Review:

L. B. Murphy, *Social behavior and child personality*, *J. Abnorm. Soc. Psychol.*, 1938, 33:538-43.

1939

"Dewey's individual and social psychology," in P. A. Schilpp (ed.), *The philosophy of John Dewey*, Evanston and Chicago: Northwestern University Press, 1939, Chap. 9.

"Recent applications of the A-S reaction study" (with R. Ruggles), *J. Abnorm. Soc. Psychol.*, 1939, 34:518-28.

"The education of a teacher," *The Harvard Progressive*, 1939, 4:7-9.

1940

"The psychologist's frame of reference," *Psychol. Bull.*, 1940, 37:1-28. Also published as El marco de referencia de los psicologos (trans. by A. Bernal del Riesgo), Havana: University of Havana, 1946.

"Fifty years of change in American psychology" (with J. S. Bruner), *Psychol. Bull.*, 1940, 37:757-76.

"The psychology of newspapers: five tentative laws" (with J. M. Faden), *Publ. Opin. Quart.*, 1940, 4:687-703.

"Motivation in personality: reply to Mr. Bertocci," *Psychol. Rev.*, 1940, 47:533-54. Also published in H. Brand, *The study of personality: a book of readings*, New York: Wiley, 1954, pp. 83-99; and in C. L. Stacey and M. F. DeMartino (eds.), *Understanding human motivation*, Cleveland: Howard Allen, 1958, pp. 105-20.

"Liberalism and the motives of men," *Frontiers of Democracy*, 1940, 6:136-37.

Foreword to H. Werner, *Comparative psychology of mental development* (trans. by E. B. Garside), New York: Harper, 1940; rev. ed., Chicago: Follett Pub. Co., 1948.

1941

"Liabilities and assets in civilian morale," *Ann. Amer. Acad. Pol. Soc. Sci.*, 1941, 216:88-94.

"Psychological service for civilian morale," *J. Consult. Psychol.*, 1941, 5;235-39.

"Personality under social catastrophe: ninety life-histories of the Nazi revolution" (with J. S. Bruner and E. M. Jandorf), *Char. & Pers.*, 1941, 10:1-22. Also published in C. Kluckhohn and H. A. Murray, *Personality in nature, society, and culture*, New York: Knopf, 1948, Chap. 25; and in C. Kluckhohn, H. A. Murray and D. M. Schneider, *Personality in nature, society and culture*, New York: Knopf, 1953, Chap. 27.

"Morale: American style." *Christian Science Monitor* (Weekly Magazine Section), Apr. 26, 1941, pp. 1-2, 13.

Review:

J. M. MacKaye, *The logic of language*. *J. Abnorm. Soc. Psychol.*, 1941, 36:296-97.

1942

"The nature of democratic morale," in G. Watson (ed.), *Civilian morale*, Boston: Houghton Mifflin, 1942, Chap. 1.

"Defense seminars for morale study and morale building," *J. Soc. Psychol.*, SPSSI Bull., 1942, 15:399-401.

"Report on the third front: at home," *Christian Science Monitor* (Weekly Magazine Section), Sept. 5, 1942, pp. 6, 14.

"Morale and its measurement," in *Public Policy*, Cambridge: Littauer School of Public Administration, 1942, 3:3-17.

Review:

F. C. Bartlett, *Political propaganda*, Sat. Rev. Lit., 1942, 25:18.

1943

"The productive paradoxes of William James," *Psychol. Rev.*, 1943, 50:95-120.

"Test tube for rumors," *Coronet*, 1943, 14:136-40.

"Psychological considerations in making the peace: editorial note," *J. Abnorm. Soc. Psychol.*, 1943, 38:131.

"This clinical supplement: editorial note," *J. Abnorm. Soc. Psychol.*, 38:3-5.

"Do rosy headlines sell newspapers?" (with E. C. Winship), *Publ. Opin. Quart.*, 1943, 7:205-10. Reprinted in D. Katz, D. Cartwright, S. Eldersveld and A. McG. Lee, *Public opinion and propaganda*, New York: Dryden Press, 1954:271-74.

"Social psychology and the civilian war effort" (with H. R. Veltfort), *J. Soc. Psychol.*, SPSSI Bull., 1943, 18:165-233.

"The ego in contemporary psychology," *Psychol. Rev.*, 1943, 50:451-78. Also published in C. L. Stacey and M. F. DeMartino (eds.), *Understanding human motivation*, Cleveland: Howard Allen, 1958, pp. 140-58.

"Morale research and its clearing" (with G. R. Schmeidler), *Psychol. Bull.*, 1943, 40:65-68.

"Restoring morale in occupied territory," *Publ. Opin. Quart.*, 1943, 7:606-17.

Reviews:

E. P. Aldrich (ed.), *As William James said*, J. Abnorm. Soc. Psychol., 1943, 38:119-120.

M. D. Allers, *The psychology of character*, Amer. Sociol. Rev., 1943, 8:735-36.

M. A. May, *A social psychology of war and peace*, Ann. Amer. Acad. Pol. Soc. Sci.*, 1943, 229:186-87.

A. A. Roback, *William James: his marginalia, personality and contribution*, *New England Quarterly*, 1943, 16:143-44.

C. Schrodes, J. van Gundy and R. W. Husband (eds.), *Psychology through literature*, *J. Abnorm. Soc. Psychol.*, 1943, 38:203 (No. 2, Clin. Suppl.).

E. C. Tolman, *Drives toward war*, *J. Abnorm. Soc. Psychol.*, 1943, 38:293-96.

1944

Prefaces to *Educational opportunities in greater Boston*, Cambridge: Prospect Union Educational Exchange, 1944 and annually thereafter.

"The quest of Nellie Wise Allport," privately printed, 1944.

"The roots of religion," *Advent Paper*, No. 1, Boston: Church of the Advent, 1944. Reprinted as "La radici della religione" (trans. by Sac. Prof. G. Zunini), *Orientamenti Pedagogici*, 1958, 4:158-74.

"ABC's of scapegoating" (ed. and author of Foreword), Chicago: Central YWCA College, 1944; rev. ed., *Freedom Pamphlet Series*, New York: Anti-Defamation League of B'nai B'rith, 1948; revised, 1959. Also reprinted as *Treibjagd auf Sündenböcke* (trans. by K. C. Knudsen), Berlin: Im Christian-Verlag, 1953.

"This clinical number: editorial," *J. Abnorm. Soc. Psychol.*, 1944, 39:147-49.

"Social psychology and the civilian war effort" (with G. R. Schmeidler), *J. Soc. Psychol.*, SPSSI Bull., 1944, 20:145-80.

"The bigot in our midst," *Commonweal*, 1944, 25:582-86. Also published in *The Catholic Digest*, 1944, 9:93-96; and in *Common Sense* (Johannesburg, South Africa), 1945, 6:154-56. Rev. ed., New York: Community Relations Service, 1950.

1945

"The psychology of participation," *Psychol. Rev.*, 1945, 52:117-32. Also published in *Occup. Psychol.* (London), 1946, 20:54-62; in S. D. Hoslett (ed.), *Human factors in management*, Parkville, Mo.: Park College Press, 1946; and in D. F. Sullivan (ed.), *Readings in group work*, New York: Association Press, 1952, pp. 239-58, Chap. 19.

"Human nature and the peace," *Psychol. Bull.*, 1945, 42:376-78.

"Is intergroup education possible?" *Harv. Educ. Rev.*, 1945, 15:83-86.

"Catharsis and the reduction of prejudice," *J. Soc. Issues*, 1945, 1:1-8.

"The basic psychology of rumor" (with L. Postman), *Trans N.Y. Acad. Sci.*, Section of Psychology, 1945, 8:61-81. Also published in G. E. Swanson, T. M. Newcomb and E. L. Hartley (eds.), *Readings in Social psychology* (rev. ed.), New York: Holt, 1952, Part II, b, pp. 160-71; in E. E. Maccoby, T. M. Newcomb and E. L. Hartley, *Readings in social psychology* (3rd ed.), New York: Holt, 1958, pp. 54-65; in D. Katz, D. Cartwright, S. Eldersveld and A. McG. Lee, *Public opinion and propaganda*, New York: Dryden Press, 1954, 394-404; and in W. Schramm (ed.), *The process and effects of mass communication*, Urbana, Ill.: University of Illinois Press, 1954, pp. 141-55.

Review:
G. Gallup, *A guide to public opinion*, *J. Abnorm. Soc. Psychol.*, 1945, 40:113-14.

1946

"Personalistic psychology as science: a reply," *Psychol. Rev.*, 1946, 53:132-35.
"Controlling group prejudice" (ed. and author of Foreword), *Ann. Amer. Acad. Pol. Soc. Sci.*, 1946, vol. 244.
"Psychology and social relations at Harvard University" (with E. G. Boring), *Amer. Psychol.*, 1946, 1:119-22.
"Some roots of prejudice" (with B. M. Kramer), published as a separate and in *J. Psychol.*, 1946, 22:9-39; rev. ed., *Roots of prejudice*, New York: American Jewish Congress, Pamphlet Series *Jewish Affairs*, 1946, 1:13.
"Geneticism *versus* ego-structure in theories of personality," *Brit. J. Educ. Psychol.*, 1946, 16:57-68.
"Effect: a secondary principle of learning," *Psychol. Rev.*, 1946, 53:335-47.
Preface to E. Simmel (ed.), *Anti-Semitism: a social disease*, New York: International Universities Press, 1946.
"The priest and the psychologist," *Bull. of General Theological Seminary*, Sept. 1946.
"An analysis of rumor" (with L. Postman), *Publ. Opin. Quart.*, 1946-47, 10:501-17. Also published in *Science Digest*, 1947, 22:58-61.
Introduction to Swami Akhilananda, *Hindu psychology*, New York: Harper, 1946.

Review:

A. H. Leighton, *The governing of men*, *J. Abnorm. Soc. Psychol.*, 1946, 41:89-92.

1947

"Guide lines for research in international cooperation," *J. Soc. Issues*, 1947, 3:21-37. Also published in T. H. Pear (ed.), *Psychological factors of peace and war*, London: Hutchinson & Co., 1950, Chap. 7.
Introduction to M. I. Rasey, *Toward maturity, the psychology of child development*," New York: Hinds, Hayden and Eldredge, 1947.
"The genius of Kurt Lewin," *J. Pers.*, 1947, 16:1-10. Also published in *J. Soc. Issues*, 1948, 4:14-21, Suppl. series 1.
"Scientific models and human morals," *Psychol. Rev.*, 1947, 54:182-92. Also published as "Modelos cientificos y moral humana," *Rev. Psicol. Gen. Apl.* (Madrid), 1948, 3:425-47; and "Modelos cientificos y moral humana," *Actas del Primer Congreso Argentino de Psicologia*, 1 (Universidad Nacional de Tucuman, Ministerio de Educacion de la Nacion), 1955.

1948

Foreword to K. Lewin (G. W. Lewin, ed.), *Resolving social conflicts*, New York: Harper, 1948.
"Psychology," in *College reading and religion*, New Haven: Yale University Press, 1948, Chap. 3.
"The religion of the post-war college student" (with J. M. Gillespie and J. Young), published as a separate and in *J. Psychol.*, 1948, 25:3-33. Also published in J. Seidman (ed.), *The adolescent: a book of readings*, New York: Dryden Press, 1953.

Reviews:

D. Jacobson, *The affairs of dame rumor*, Boston Sunday Post, Oct. 24, 1948.

E. Mayo, *Some notes on the psychology of Pierre Janet, Survey Graphic,*
1948, 37:5, 267.

A. Schweitzer, *The psychiatric study of Jesus, Christian Register,* Apr.
1948.

1949

"Psychology and the fourth R," *New Republic,* Oct. 17, 1949, pp. 23-26.

Editorial note, *J. Abnorm. Soc. Psychol.,* 1949, 44:439-42.

1950

Foreword to M. G. Ross, *Religious beliefs of youth,* New York: Association
Press, 1950.

"How shall we evaluate teaching?" in B. B. Cronkhite (ed.), *A handbook for
college teachers,* Cambridge: Harvard University Press, 1950, Chap. 3.

"The role of expectancy," in H. Cantril (ed.), *Tensions that cause wars,*
Urbana, Ill.: University of Illinois Press, 1950.

"A psychological approach to the study of love and hate," in P. A. Sorokin
(ed.), *Explorations in altruistic love and behavior,* Boston: Beacon Press,
1950, Chap. 5.

"Prejudice: a problem in psychological and social causation" (Kurt Lewin
Memorial Lecture), *J. Soc. Issues,* 1950, Suppl. Series. Also published
in T. Parsons and E. A. Shils (eds.), *Toward a general theory of action,*
Cambridge: Harvard University Press, 1951, Part 4, Chap. 1.

Reviews:

S. A. Stouffer *et al., The American soldier* (2 vols.), *J. Abnorm. Soc.
Psychol.,* 1950, 45:168-73.

"A five-volume shelf about a sickness of both individuals and society:
prejudice" [M. Horkheimer and S. H. Flowerman, eds., *Studies in
prejudice* (5 vols.), New York: Harper, 1950], *Sci. Amer.,* 1950,
182:56-58.

1951

"The situation we face: a psychological analysis," in A. W. Loos (ed.),
Religious faith and world culture, New York: Prentice-Hall, 1951, pp.
35-48. Also published in *New Outlook* (Santa Monica, Calif.), 1955,
8:82-87.

"Basic principles in improving human relations," in K. W. Bigelow (ed.),
Cultural groups and human relations, New York: Teachers College-
Columbia University, 1951, Chap. 2.

Foreword to M. H. Wormser and C. Selltiz, *How to conduct a community
self-survey of civil rights,* New York: Association Press, 1951.

Foreword to H. E. Kagan, *Changing the attitude of Christian toward Jew,*
New York: Columbia University Press, 1951.

Foreword to E. Powers and H. Witmer, *An experiment in the prevention of
delinquency,* New York: Columbia University Press, 1951.

Review:

J. La Farge, S.J., *No postponement, Thought,* 1951, 26:471-472, No. 102.

1952

"An evaluation of AFSC volunteer work service camps in Germany," in
H. W. Riecken, *The volunteer work camp: a psychological evaluation,*
Cambridge: Addison-Wesley, 1952, Appendix A, pp. 185-220.

"Resolving intergroup tensions, an appraisal of methods," in L. A. Cook (ed.), *Toward better human relations,* Detroit: Wayne University Press, 1952, Chap. 3.

"The individual and his religion," *The Andover Newton Bulletin,* 1952, 44:3-10.

"The resolution of intergroup tensions," an *Intergroup Education Pamphlet,* New York: National Conference of Christians and Jews, 1952.

"The mature personality," *Pastoral Psychol.,* 1952, 2:19-24.

"What is on the student's mind?" proceedings of the Thirtieth Annual Meeting of the *American College Health Association, Bulletin* No. 32, Stanford: Stanford University Press, 1952.

"Why do people join?" interview in *Adult Leadership,* 1952, 1:10-12.

"Reading the nature of prejudice," *Claremont College Reading Conference, Seventeenth Yearbook* (Claremont, Calif.), 1952, pp. 51-64.

1953

"The trend in motivational theory," *Amer. J. Orthopsychiat.,* 1953, 25:107-19. Also published as "Bemerkungen zu dem gegenwärtigen Stand der Theorie der Motivation in den USA" (trans. by H. von Bracken and Leo Canders), *Psychol. Beit.,* 1953, 1:10-28; and in C. E. Moustakas (ed.), *The self: explorations in personal growth,* New York: Harper, 1956; in E. L. and R. E. Hartley, *Outside readings in psychology,* 2nd ed., New York: Crowell, 1957, Chap. 22; and in C. L. Stacey and M. F. DeMartino (eds.), *Understanding human motivation,* Cleveland: Howard Allen, 1958, pp. 54-65.

"The teaching-learning situation," *Publ. Hlth. Rep.,* 1953, 68:875-79.

"The psychological nature of personality," *The Personalist,* 1953, 34:347-57.

Review:

H. G. Trager and M. R. Yarrow, *They learn what they live, The Child,* 1953, 18:30.

1954

"Techniques for reducing group prejudice," in P. A. Sorokin (ed.), *Forms and techniques of altruistic and spiritual growth,* Boston: Beacon, 1954, Chap. 24.

"The historical background of modern social psychology," in G. Lindzey (ed.), *Handbook of social psychology,* Cambridge: Addison-Wesley, 1954, Vol. I., Chap. 1.

Introduction to J. Evans, *Three men,* New York: Knopf, 1954.

"A psychologist views the Supreme Court ruling on segregation," *Nieman Reports,* 1954, 8:12-13.

Comments on: J. L. Moreno, Transference, countertransference and tele: their relation to group research and group psychotherapy. *Group Psychother.,* 1954, 7:307-08.

1955

Youth's outlook on the future (with J. M. Gillespie), New York: Doubleday, Doubleday Papers in Psychology, 1955 (distributed by Random House).

"The limits of social service," in J. E. Russell (ed.), *National policies for education, health and social services* (Columbia University Bicentennial Conference Series), New York: Doubleday, 1955, pp. 194-213.

Reviews:
  R. B. Perry, *Realms of value: a critique of human civilization*, J. Abnorm. Soc. Psychol., 1955, 50:154-56.
  S. A. Stouffer, *Communism, conformity, and civil liberties*, Saturday Rev. Lit., 1955, 28:14-15.

1956

"Prejudice in modern perspective," *The Hoernlé memorial lecture 1956*, Durban, South Africa: The South African Institute of Race Relations, 1956.

"The participant citizen," *The sixth annual George Denny lecture*, September 4, 1956, Durban, South Africa: Natal Technical College.

Review:
  M. Freedman, *A minority in Britain: social studies of the Anglo-Jewish community*, Amer. Anthrop., 1956, 58:401-02.

1957

"European and American theories of personality," in H. P. David and H. von Bracken (eds.), *Perspectives in personality theory*, New York: Basic Books, 1957, Chap. 1.

"Cultural influence on the perception of movement: the trapezoidal illusion among Zulus" (with T. F. Pettigrew), *J. Abnorm. Soc. Psychol.*, 1957, 55:104-13.

Review:
  P. A. Bertocci, *Free will, responsibility, and grace*, Religion in Life, 1957, 26:612-13.

1958

"What units shall we employ?" in G. Lindzey (ed.), *Assessment of human motives*, New York: Rinehart, 1958, Chap. 9. Reprinted as a paperback, New York: Grove Press, 1960.

Foreword to G. V. Coelho, *Changing images of America: a study of Indian students' perceptions*, Glencoe, Ill.: The Free Press, 1958.

Foreword to E. Mira y Lopez (L. Bellak *et al.*, eds.) *M. K. P. Myokinetic Psychodiagnosis* (trans.), New York: Logos Press, 1958.

"Perception and public health," *Health Education Monographs*, Oakland, Calif.: Society of Health Educators, 1958, No. 2, pp. 2-15.

"Binocular resolution and perception of race in South Africa" (with T. F. Pettigrew and E. O. Barnett), *Brit. J. Psychol.*, 1958, 49:265-78, Part 4.

"Personality: normal and abnormal," *The Sociological Review*, 1958, 6:167-80.

Review:
  P. Lafitte, *The person in psychology: reality or abstraction?* Contemp. Psychol., 1958, 3:105.

1959

"Normative compatibility in the light of social science," in A. H. Maslow (ed.), *New knowledge in human values*, New York: Harper, 1959, pp. 137-50. Also published in *Relig. Educ.*, 1958, 53:62-68.

Preface to V. E. Frankl, *From death-camp to existentialism*. Boston: Beacon, 1959 (trans.).

"Religion and prejudice," *The Crane Review*, 1959, 2:1-10.

1960

"Uniqueness in students," in W. D. Weatherford, Jr. (ed.), *The goals of higher education*, Cambridge: Harvard University Press, 1960, pp. 57-75.

"Psychology and religion," in J. Clark (ed.), *The student seeks an answer*, Chap. 2. Ingraham Lectures in Philosophy and Religion, Waterville: Colby College Press, 1960, pp. 35-49.

"The open system in personality theory," *J. Abnorm. Soc. Psychol.*, 1960, 61: 301-310. Also published in E. P. Hollander and R. G. Hunt (eds.), *Current perspectives in social psychology*, New York: Oxford University Press, 1963, pp. 151-162; and as "Il sistema aperto nella teoria della personalità" (trans. by P. G. Grasso), *Orientamenti Pedagogici*, 1960, 7: 664-682.

"Wahrnehmung und öffentliche Gesundheitspflege" (trans. by L. Canders), of "Perception and public health" (see 1958), *Psychol. Beit.*, 1960, Heft 3-4/IV:384-404.

1961

Introduction to W. James, *Psychology: the briefer course*, New York: Harper Torchbooks, 1961.

Foreword to C. E. Lincoln, *The black Muslims in America*, Boston: Beacon Press, 1961.

Comment, in R. May (ed.), *Existential psychology*, Chap. 6, New York: Random House, 1961.

William Douglas (The man of the month), *Pastoral Psychology*, 1961, 12:6 and 66.

"Approach to mental health," reprint of portions of *The individual and his religion* (1950), *Sci. of Mind*, 1961, 34:6-11; 37-42.

"Values and our youth," *Teachers Coll. Rec.*, 1961, 63:211-219. Also published in *Image of man* (Proceed. 1961 Summer Conf.), Bellingham, Wash.: Western Washington State College *Bull.*, 1961, 3; and in R. E. Grinder (ed.), *Studies in adolescence*, New York: Macmillan, 1963, pp. 17-27.

"The psychologist's image of man," *Image of man* (Proceed. 1961 Summer Conf.), Bellingham, Wash.: Western Washington State College *Bull.*, 1961, 3.

"Prejudice in perspective" (Lucile P. Morrison Lecture), La Jolla, Calif.: Western Behavioral Sciences Institute, *Report No. 1*, 1961.

"The trend in motivational theory," reprinted (see 1953) in T. K. Menon (ed.), *Recent trends in psychology*, Calcutta: Orient Longmans Ltd., 1961; and in Martha T. and S. A. Mednick (eds.), *Research in personality*, New York: Holt, Rinehart and Winston, 1963, pp. 63-74; and in B. C. Birney and R. C. Teevan (eds.), *Measuring human motivation*, Princeton: Van Nostrand Insight Book, 1962, pp. 164-181.

1962

"The general and the unique in psychological science," *J. Person.*, 1962, 30: 405-422. Also published in *Image of man* (Proceed. 1961 Summer Conf.), Bellingham, Wash.: Western Washington State College *Bull.*, 1961, 3.

"Das Allgemeine und das Eigenartige in der psychologischen Praxis," *Psychol.*

Beit., 1962, 6:630-650. Also published as "Il generale e l'unico nella scienza psicologica" (trans.), *Bollettino di Psychol. Applicata*, 1963, 57-58:3-16.

"Cultural influence on the perception of movement" (with T. F. Pettigrew), reprinted (see 1957) in J. A. Dyal (ed.), *Readings in psychology: understanding human behavior*, New York: McGraw-Hill, 1962, Selection 27; also published in *Reprint Series in the Social Sciences*, Indianapolis: Bobbs-Merrill, P-5.

Desenvolvimento da personalidade (trans. of *Becoming*, 1955, see books, monographs and tests section), Sao Paulo, Brazil: Editora Herder, 1962.

Review:

G. C. Zahn, *German Catholics and Hitler's wars*, *Unitarian-Universalist Register-Leader*, 1962, 143:21.

1963

"Behavioral science, religion, and mental health," *J. Relig. & Health*, 1963, 2:187-197. Also published in *The Northeast*, Diocese of Maine, 1963, 90:13-22.

Foreword to N. L. Farberow (ed.), *Taboo topics*, New York: Atherton Press, 1963.

"The emphasis on molar problems," in M. H. Marx (ed.), *Theories in contemporary psychology*, New York: Macmillan, 1963, pp. 258-271, reprinted from "Scientific models and human morals" (see 1947).

Index of Names

Ackerman, N. W., 256
Addams, J., 272
Adler, A., 28, 52
Adorno, T. W., 216, 235
Aldington, R., 15
Allport, F. H., 37, 47, 54, 117, 126, 129, 191-92, 198, 300, 309
Allport, G. W.: Bibliography, 363-74
Ambrose, Saint, 259, 262
Amen, E. W., 90
Amiel, H. F., 6
Anderson, J. E., 83
Angell, R. C., 176, 180
Angyal, A., 159, 185, 188, 197-98
Apple, D., 297, 309
Augustine, Saint, 259
Axelrad, S., 292
Axline, V. M., 249, 256

Bainton, R. H., 262, 266-67
Bair, J. H., 185, 197
Baldwin, A. L., 124, 126, 129
Baldwin, M. V., 108
Bales, R. F., 235
Barbellion, 13
Barrabee, E. L., 293
Barron, F., 161, 166, 168, 303, 310
Bartlett, F. C., 46, 80, 92
Bayton, J. A., 93
Beethoven, van, L., 335
Bellis, E., 310
Belmont, L., 109
Bentley, M., 132
Berg, I. A., 292
Bergson, H., 95
Bernard, L. L., 112-13, 128
Bertalanffy, von, L., 42, 53
Bertocci, P., 29, 35, 38, 67-68, 150
Beth, M., 90
Bettelheim, G., 150, 216, 250, 256
Bie, de, P., 175, 180
Bills, A. G., 197
Birch, H. G., 109
Bismarck, von, O., 45, 272
Bisno, H., 276, 293

Blake, R. W., 310
Blake, W., 253
Blenkner, M., 292
Bohnengel, C., 197
Bohr, N., 52
Boring, E. G., 67
Boswell, J., 12
Bowlby, J., 159, 285
Brentano, F., 60, 73
Bridgman, P. W., 42, 49, 53
Brightman, E. S., 17-18, 25, 35-38
Bronner, A. F., 293
Brown, E., 115
Brozek, J., 108
Bruner, J. S., 37, 303
Brunner, E. de S., 235
Buber, M., 47
Buchler, J., 301, 310
Buck, R. C., 49, 54
Burma, J. H., 256
Burrow, T., 224
Burt, C., 137, 142-51
Byington, S. T., 90

Cabot, R. C., 272-73, 276, 278, 285, 292-93
Calkins, M. W., 18, 36, 72
Calvin, J., 260
Campbell, E. Q., 257, 266
Cannell, C. F., 292
Cannon, W. B., 43, 53, 60, 67
Cantril, H., 46, 77, 91-92, 224
Carlson, A. J., 67
Cartwright, D., 37, 362
Casanova, G., 13
Cassel, J., 310
Cassirer, E., 64, 68
Castellio, S., 262, 265
Cattell, R. B., 120, 122-23, 129
Chamberlain, J., 320
Chang, H. T., 54
Chase, S., 224, 235, 256
Chein, I., 108, 256
Chesterton, G. K., 9
Citron, A. F., 256

377

Coffey, H. S., 292
Coghill, G. E., 132
Collins, M. E., 228, 235
Combs, A. W., 38, 46
Comte, A., 284
Conant, J. B., 107
Confucius, 347
Cook, L. A., 242, 255
Cook, S. W., 228, 235, 255
Coutu, W., 37, 115, 129
Cranston, R., 108
Cromwell, O., 263
Crosby, B., 250, 312
Cusa, Cardinal, 262
Cushing, H., 46

Darwin, C., 95, 112
Delgado, H., 90
Demosthenes, 335
Derryberry, M., 309
Descartes, R., 219
Deutsch, M., 228, 235, 255
Deutscher, M., 256
Dewey, J., 37, 179, 181-82, 185,
    191-93, 197-98
Dickens, C., 10
Dickson, W. J., 87, 93, 216, 235
Dollard, J., 150
Dryden, J., 12
Durkheim, E., 184

Edwards, A. L., 80-81, 92
Einstein, A., 42
Elizabeth I, Queen, 260
Elkin, F., 49, 54
Emerson, H., 272
Emerson, R. W., 271-72
Empedocles, 111, 203
Ericksen, C. W., 303, 310
Erikson, E. H., 46, 159
Escalona, S. K., 216
Eysenck, H. J., 235, 292

Federn, P., 90
Feigl, H., 50, 53
Field, D. D., 263
Finesinger, J. E., 293
Flaubert, G., 6
Fliess, W., 160
Flugel, J. C., 176, 180
Follett, M. P., 172, 179, 190, 198
Forster, E. M., 210, 214

Fox, R., 309
Francis of Assisi, Saint, 265
Frank, J. D., 97, 93
Frankl, V., 45, 54, 166
Franklin, L. M., 237
Freedman, M., 266, 292
French, D. G., 274
French, R. M., 75, 91-92, 103
Frenkel-Brunswik, E., 42, 53, 80, 92,
    216, 235, 303, 310
Freud, A., 103
Freud, S., 26, 28-29, 44, 52, 59-60,
    75, 77, 89, 91, 95f., 103-4, 106,
    112, 118, 120, 137-39, 144, 160-
    1, 163, 199, 204-5, 207, 209,
    224, 285-86, 331
Friedrich, C. J., 198
Frings, J., 292
Fromm, E., 38, 103, 166
Fromm-Reichmann, F., 38

Galen, 111
Gandhi, M. K., 51, 178, 222, 246,
    257, 265
Gates, A. I., 184, 197
Gelasius I, Pope, 262, 265
Getzels, J. W., 98, 105, 108
Gillespie, J. M., 267
Glueck, E. T., 272, 292-93
Glueck, S., 272, 292-93
Goethe, von, J. W., 230, 335
Goldstein, K., 42, 46, 68, 76, 91,
    107, 109, 166, 188, 198, 303,
    310
Gooddy, W., 46, 54
Goodell, H., 310
Gosse, E., 12
Gregory of Nyssa, Saint, 259
Griffiths, W., 301, 310
Grinker, R. R., 107-8, 150
Guetzkow, H., 108
Guilford, J. P., 120, 122, 129
Guttman, L. P., 39

Haggard, E. A., 184, 197
Haggard, H. W., 235
Hall, C. S., 168
Halmos, P., 158-61, 165, 168
Harding, J., 256
Harley, J. D., 310
Hartley, E. L., 54
Hartmann, G. W., 81, 92

Hartmann, H., 75, 91, 103, 138, 150
Hartshorne, H., 91
Harvey, W., 111
Hastings, P. K., 303, 310
Hastorf, A. H., 43, 53
Hay, M., 266
Healy, W., 285, 293
Heath, C. W., 129
Hebb, D. O., 47, 54, 112, 128, 310
Hendrick, I., 75, 91
Henry, P., 317
Herbart, J. F., 183
Hertzman, M., 129
Herzog, E., 292
Hilgard, E. R., 38, 57, 67
Hill, O., 272
Hippocrates, 111
Hobbes, T., 40, 203-4, 211
Hoch, P., 293
Hoernlé, R. F. A., 219-20, 222, 234
Hollingshead, A. B., 310
Holt, E. B., 57, 172, 179, 182
Hoppe, F., 84, 86-87, 92
Horney, K., 38, 103, 113
Horowitz, E. L., 38, 90
Hoslett, S. D., 179
Hovland, C. I., 256
Huddleston, T., 265
Hull, C. L., 52, 61, 68, 114
Hume, D., 204
Hunt, J. McV., 275, 293
Huntley, C. W., 85, 92
Huxley, A., 266
Huxley, J., 59, 67

Inkeles, A., 235
Innocent VIII, Pope, 260
Israeli, N., 84, 92-93

Jaco, G. E., 310
Jahoda, M., 255-56
James, W., 22, 27, 37, 71-73, 75, 91, 115, 125, 129, 182-83, 242
Jandorf, E. M., 37
Janowitz, M., 216, 250, 256
Jarrett, M., 285
Jellinek, E. M., 235
Jenkin, N., 309
Jensen, G., 91
John Chrysostom, Saint, 259, 266
Johnson, D. M., 91

Jordan, W. K., 267
Jung, C. G., 46, 96, 159, 166

Kagan, H. E., 244-45, 256
Kardiner, A., 102-3, 108
Kant, I., 60, 179
Kelly, G. A., 121, 125-26, 129
Kendler, T. S., 256
King, M. L., 265
Kinsey, A. C., 156
Klapper, J. T., 256
Klein, D. B., 186, 197
Klein, G. S., 53, 78, 92, 121, 303, 310
Klein, M., 286
Klineberg, O., 142, 150, 255
Kluckhohn, C. M., 227, 235
Knapp, R. H., 326
Knutson, A., 303
Koffka, K., 75-77, 88, 90-91, 138, 150
Kogan, L. S., 275, 293
Köhler, W., 26, 138, 197
Korzybski, A., 224
Kraepelin, E., 122
Kramer, B. M., 216, 255
Kramer, H., 266
Krech, D., 53
Kretschmer, E., 122
Kris, E., 103, 108
Kroeber, A. L., 235
Kropotkin, P., 204
Kubie, L. S., 293
Kurtz, R. H., 293
Kutner, B., 306, 310

La Guardia, F., 312
Lamb, C., 298, 309
Langfeld, H. S., 182
La Rochefoucauld, de, F., 203
Latourette, K. S., 267
Leary, T., 292
Le Bon, G., 184
Lecky, P., 38, 62, 68
Le Dantec, F., 74, 76-77, 90, 203
Lederer, H. D., 309
Lee, P. R., 272
Leibnitz, F. W., 52
Leighton, A. H., 68, 189, 198, 262
Leonard, W. E., 13
Levin, H., 310
Levine, J. M., 81, 92

Levine, R., 108
Levinson, D. J., 216, 235
Lewin, K., 25, 37, 47, 76, 86, 88,
     91, 118, 132, 138, 186, 189,
     197-98, 216, 246, 256
Lewis, H. B., 129, 198
Likert, R., 179
Lindzey, G., 101, 121, 168, 235
Lippitt, R., 256
Lippman, W., 224
Lipps, T., 183
Locke, J., 52, 263
Lowenstein, R. M., 256
Lully, R., 262
Lundholm, H., 90

Maccoby, E. E., 54, 310
MacCorquodale, K., 114, 129
MacCrone, I. D., 230, 235
Machiavelli, N., 203
Machover, K., 129
MacKinnon, D. W., 91
Madison, J., 263
Malherbe, E. G., 228, 235
McCarthy, J., 280
McCary, J. L., 129
McClelland, D. C., 118, 129
McCormick, M. T., 293
McDougall, W., 25, 30, 39, 46, 67-
     68, 75, 91, 95-96, 112, 141-42,
     147, 149-50, 199
McGranahan, D. V., 109
McGregor, D., 188, 198
McLean, H. V., 326
Margineanu, N., 3
Marks, E., 79, 92
Marquis, D. G., 57, 67, 123, 129
Marshall, J., 312
Maslow, A. H., 46, 159, 161-62,
     166, 168-69, 177-78, 256
May, M., 91
Mead, M., 82
Meehl, P. E., 114, 129
Meissner, P., 129
Merton, R. K., 54
Meyer, A., 285
Meyers, G., 266-67
Miles, H. W., 293
Mill, J. S., 39
Miller, J. G., 49, 54
Milner, P., 54
Milton, J., 263

Montaigne, de, M. E., 262
Moore, J. S., 90
Moreno, J. L., 224
Morgan, L., 132
Morris, C., 64-65, 68
Mowrer, O. H., 43, 53
Murdoch, G. P., 356
Murphy, G., 19, 37, 47, 54, 72, 78,
     81, 90-92, 108, 262
Murray, H. A., 32, 38, 41, 88, 91,
     93, 96, 118, 129, 300, 309
Myrdal, G., 241, 243, 317, 326

Newbigin, L., 259, 266
Newcomb, T. M., 54
Newman, J. H., 266
Nietzsche, F. W., 160, 203
Nyswander, D. B., 295

Odum, H. W., 326
Olds, J., 54
Ossorio, A., 292
Ovesey, L., 102-3, 108

Pareto, V., 184
Parsons, Talcott, 23-24, 37-38, 47,
     54, 309-10
Parsons, Theophilus, 199
Pasteur, L., 51
Paul, B., 299, 309-10
Paul, Saint, 258, 291
Pear, T. H., 180
Pearl, R., 289
Pearson, K., 276
Perl, R. E., 293
Perry, R. B., 125-26, 129, 172, 179
Petrullo, L., 129
Pettigrew, T. F., 257, 266
Piaget, J., 74, 174-75, 177, 179-80,
     265
Plato, 179, 297
Plog, S., 40
Polansky, N., 151
Postman, L., 301, 303, 310-11
Powers, E., 216, 273, 282, 292, 294
Praxiteles, 335
Preston, M. G., 93
Prince, M., 72, 132
Proust, M., 6
Pumpian-Mindlin, E., 42, 53-54

Rabelais, F., 276
Ramsey, G., 310
Rank, O., 285-86
Rapaport, D., 104, 109
Rashkis, H. A., 293
Redlich, F. C., 310
Rich, G. J., 293
Richmond, M., 272, 276, 283, 293
Riesman, D., 24, 37
Roberts, B. J., 306, 310
Robinson, V. P., 294
Roby, T. B., 54
Roethlisberger, F. J., 87, 93, 179, 216, 235
Rogers, C. R., 29, 38, 88, 93, 160, 185, 197
Romanes, J. G., 33
Roosevelt, E., 250, 316
Roosevelt, F. D., 56, 62, 312
Rorschach, 96-98, 100, 116, 120
Rose, A. M., 256
Rose, R. J., 184, 197
Rosenzweig, S., 84, 92, 98, 108
Rousseau, J. J., 13
Roy, R. L., 267
Royce, J., 182, 197, 220, 222
Rupp, I. D., 235

Sanford, R. N., 108, 216, 235
Sapir, E., 40
Scheerer, M., 310
Schilpp, P. A., 197
Schoenfeld, N., 78, 92
Schopenhauer, A., 60, 95, 203
Scriven, M., 54
Schweitzer, A., 265
Schwenkfeld, K., 262, 265
Sears, R. R., 310
Sells, S. B., 81, 92, 293
Selltiz, C., 256
Servetus, M., 260
Shaftel, G., 256
Shaftel, R. F., 256
Shaskan, D. A., 293
Sheldon, W. H., 120
Sherif, M., 76-77, 82, 91
Sherrington, C., 128, 132
Shils, E. A., 37-38, 310
Shoben, E. J., 157, 165, 168
Simmel, E., 216, 256
Simmons, O. G., 310
Simon, A. J., 293

Simons, M., 223, 235, 258, 266
Sixtus IV, Pope, 260
Smith, A., 204
Smith, H., 54
Smith, K., 250
Snygg, D., 38, 46
Socrates, 262
Sorokin, P. A., 169, 177-78, 180, 199, 237, 339
Southard, E., 285
Spencer, H., 289
Spiegel, J. P., 107-8, 150
Spinoza, B., 179, 219-20
Spitz, R. A., 310
Spoerl, H. D., 38, 198
Spranger, E., 121, 183, 197
Springer, J., 266
Stagner, R., 43, 53, 97, 108
Stein, G., 72
Stern, W., 18, 26, 35-38, 132, 183
Stirner, M., 74, 76-77, 90
Stouffer, S. A., 172, 179, 202, 215-16, 235
Summers, M., 266
Suttie, I., 59, 67, 199, 203, 205, 207, 215-16
Symonds, P. M., 38, 91

Taft, R., 249
Tagiuri, R., 129
Tannenbaum, A. S., 117, 129
Tarde, G., 184
Taylor, J. G., 54
Terman, L. M., 83, 92
Tertullian, 262, 267
Teuber, H. L., 197, 282, 294
Thackeray, W. M., 9
Theis, S., 272, 292
Theophrastus, 6, 8
Thomas Aquinas, Saint, 112, 221
Thoreau, H., 271-72
Thorndike, E. L., 64, 68
Thouless, R., 224
Thurstone, L. L., 39, 120, 122, 132
Titchener, E. B., 27
Toch, H. H., 43, 53
Tolman, E. C., 57-59, 67, 301, 310
Torquemada, de, T., 260
Towley, L. H., 294
Toynbee, A., 272
Troland, L., 132

Trow, W. C., 91
Tyler, R. W., 291, 294

Urban II, Pope, 260

Vernon, P. E., 101, 109, 121, 123, 129

Wale, F. G., 292
Walkley, R. P., 228, 235
Wapner, S., 129
Washburn, M. F., 182
Watson, G., 87
Watson, J. B., 24, 39, 57
Watson, R. I., 293
Watson, W. S., 81, 92
Webb, S., 278, 293
Weider, A., 119
Weil, A., 180
Wells, H. G., 13
Wertheimer, M., 9, 60
White, R., 46
Whitehead, A. N., 200
Whitehorn, J. C., 102, 108
Whorf, B. L., 40
Wilkie, W., 79, 340

Williams, R., 263, 265
Williams, R. M., 255
Wilner, D. M., 228, 235
Witmer, H., 216, 273, 292
Withey, S. B., 292
Witkin, H. A., 121, 129, 302-3, 310
Wittgenstein, L., 224
Witty, P., 150
Wolff, C., 112
Wolff, H. G., 310
Wolff, W., 85, 159, 168
Woodworth, R. S., 46, 53, 119, 121, 123, 129, 132, 142, 297, 309
Wormser, M. H., 256
Wundt, W., 27, 40, 90, 184
Wyatt, F., 197

Yerkes, R. M., 64, 68
Young, J., 267

Zborowski, M., 305, 310
Zilboorg, G., 52
Zillig, M., 81, 92
Zimmerman, W. S., 122, 129
Zweig, S., 6

Index of Subjects

Abnormality, 155-68
Action emphasis, 181-98
Action research, 237-55, 273
Act-psychology, 60, 183
Adjustment, 156
Affiliation, 63, 162, 171, 199-215, 330
Aggression, 204, 317, 328-30, 332
Altruism, 210, 255, 271, 341
Ambiguity and rumor, 312
American character, 24, 182-84
American Friends Service Committee, 265, 335
Anabaptist, 223, 258
Anglo-Boer war, 232
Animal model, 57-68
Anomie, 156
Anthropology, 5, 11, 165, 231-32, 350, 359
Anticipatory goal response, 61
Anti-Semitism, 212, 221, 231, 245, 251, 253, 261, 263, 265, 331
Anxiety, 229, 250
Apathy, 195, 288-89
Apperception, 300
Arapesh, 332
Art *versus* science, 3-15, 148-49
Asceticism, 170
Aspiration level, 85-87, 116
Assessment of motives, 95-108, 111, 129
Attitudes, 111, 113, 120-21, 131, 183, 238, 250, 290, 300-301
Authoritarian, 170, 192, 206, 213-14, 229, 339
Axiology, 32, 276; see also Value

Bantu, 173, 227, 229
Becoming, 44
Behavior primacy, 46, 53
Behavioral science, 44
Behaviorism, 3, 39, 56, 64, 182
Belief-value matrix, 301
Bigotry. See Prejudice
Biography, 11-14, 101-2, 125

Biology, 4, 44, 285
Biophysical, 21
Biosocial, 21
Body-mind problem, 20, 35-36, 40
Brainwashing, 307
Brotherhood, 257, 261, 347
Buddhism, 47

Cambridge-Somerville Youth Study, 273-74, 284
Catharsis, 252-55
Cathexis, 58-59, 119
Catholic Interracial Councils, 265
Character writing, 7-9
Charity organization, 277
Child training, 230, 263-64, 286, 308, 339, 341, 354-55
Church history, 257-66
Citizen Sam, 187
Civil rights, 240
Civil War, 232
Client-centered, 29, 138, 185
Coding, 44
Cognitive style, 48, 113, 177-78, 213, 302-4
Collective security, 351-52
Collective structure, 118
Common enemy, 332-33
Communism, 80-81, 212, 224, 228, 319, 329, 331, 338
Community Chest, 278-79
Compensation, 83
Competence, 46
Complementarity, 52
Completion test, 98-99
Concentration camp, 45
Condescension, 357-58
Conference procedure, 354, 361
Conflict, 169-80
Confrontation, 164
Conscience, 45, 75, 276
Conscientious objectors, 97-98
Conscious report, 100-9
Contact, equal status, 225, 228, 232, 241, 246-47

Continuity-discontinuity, 163
Coward, 7
Creativity, 160
Cross-cultural studies, 305-7
Cultural influence, 76-77, 82, 165
Cultural relativity, 62, 350
Cultural universals, 227, 355-56, 361
Culture and personality, 5, 48
Cumulation, principle of, 241
Curiosity rumors, 313-14

Decentering, 174-77
Definitions, of personality, v, 21, 27, 36, 145-46
Delinquency, 272-74, 353
Democracy, 167, 181-98, 213, 277, 288-89
Desire:
  and demand, 171-72, 356-57
  for affiliation, 199-215
  for meaning, 306, 313, 320
Direct methods, 95-109
Discrimination, 172-80
Distortion, in rumor, 314-26
Dobu, 332
Drives. *See* Motivation

Educational programs, 242-49
Elements of personality, 111-29, 131-35
Ego (*see also* Self):
  autonomy, 104
  bodily, 307
  concept of, 71-93
  defense, 163, 224, 244
  dominance, 74
  extension, 162
  fighter for ends, 75
  functions, 196
  involvement, 77-93, 145, 187-91
  knower, 72, 90
  level, 86
  localization, 73, 90
  object of knowledge, 73
  psychology, 29, 75, 95, 138
  reactive, 188-96
  recognition, 171
  strength, 139, 162
  structure, 107, 137-51
  system, 76

Egocentricity, 74, 174-75, 210
Egoism, 63, 203, 211
Emergence, 30, 35
Empathy, 183
Empty organism, 24-26
Equimindedness, 178, 222, 257, 263
Essential characteristics, 124-25
Ethics, 155, 169-82, 224, 277, 291; *see also* Value
Ethnic judgments, 79, 305-6
Ethnocentricism, 174, 334; *see also* Prejudice
Ethology, 39
Evaluation. *See* Research
Evolution, social, 289
Exclusionist style, 210, 212-13, 215, 264
Exhortation, 251
Existentialism, 39, 45, 160, 291
Expectancy, 57-59, 327-46
Expressive traits, 105-6, 121
Extrinsic religion, 257, 264-66

Fabians, 272
Factor analysis 19, 30, 122-23, 126, 146, 148
Faculty psychology, 111-13
Fashions in phychology, 39, 53, 55, 71-72, 95, 285
Fear rumors, 316, 320
Field-dependence, 121, 302-4
First Amendment, 263
Flight from tenderness, 199-200
Four Freedoms, 62
Frame of reference, 81-82
Friendship theory, 282-83, 287
Functional autonomy, 28-29, 51, 117, 140-47, 164, 211
Functionalism, 40, 54, 182
Future, importance of, 61, 84, 89, 101

General systems theory, 49-50
Geneticism, 61, 96, 104, 137-51
Gestalt, 3, 25-26, 42, 58, 76, 138
Goals of social work, 275-77
Group:
  differences, 226-28, 243
  libel, 240-42
  retraining, 247-49
  tensions. *See* Prejudice

Growth of personality, 159, 165-66, 275-77
Guilt, 229-30, 318, 322

Habits, 24, 39, 114, 131-32, 145
Harry Holzer, 49
Hate, 199-215, 316, 321-22, 330
Health, public, 295-309
Healthy personality, 155-68
Hedonism, 170, 181
Hindu psychology, 45
Homeostasis, 43, 46, 53, 160, 196
Hospitalism, 307
Hostility, 199-215, 225, 337
Hugenots, 260
Humanism, 276
Humoral phychology, 111
Hypothetical construct, 114

Iconic, 65
Identification, 28, 86, 104
Identity, search for, 46
Ideomotor theory, 183
Idiographic method, 52, 125, 146-47, 149
Incident control, 248
Inclusion of interests, 169-80, 210
Indirect methods, 95-109
Industrial psychology, 87, 187-90
Industrial relations, 201-203, 224-25, 352
Infant model, 57-68, 141
Informational approach, 242-43
Inquisition, 260, 262
Instincts, 112-13, 137-51, 207-9
Institute of Race Relations, 219, 234
Integration, 99, 105, 108, 158, 192, 196, 301
Intelligence, 83-84, 88, 120, 186
Intention, 50, 58-60, 183
Intercultural education, 242-49
Interest, 82-83, 121, 169-80
International relations, 175-77, 190, 280-81, 327-62
Interpersonal behavior, 113
Interstructurance, 117
Intervening variable, 24, 114
Interviewer bias, 80
Intrinsic religion, 257, 264-66
Intuition, 30
Irenicism, 262

J-curve, 227
Japanese relocation, 189-90
Job-satisfaction, 87, 201-2

Know-Nothings, 261

Leadership, 341-42
Learning, 82-84, 184, 208-9, 230-31
Legislation, 240-42
Leveling in rumor, 314-15, 320-25
Leviathan, 40
Literary characterology, 3-15
Little Rock, 257
Logotherapy, 46, 166
Love, psychology of, 199-215
Loyalty, 220

Marxism, 328-29, 338, 341
Mass media, 249-50, 327, 338-39, 357
Matching method, 11
Maturity of personality, 105, 211
Mechanical models, 56-68
Medical sciences, 295-309
Metaphors, 55-68
Methods, 11, 95-109, 119
Minnesota Multiphasic Inventory, 119, 121, 161
Models, 39, 54-68
Moral science, 56, 63
Moral sense, 55, 134, 344, 347-48
Morale, 65, 139, 171, 349
Motivation (see also Functional autonomy):
  affiliative, 199-215
  assessment, 111-29
  dependable, 142
  dominance, 74
  drives, 51, 58, 83-86, 91, 112, 132, 142
  ego-involved, 85-86, 145, 187-91
  existential, 45
  growth versus deficiency, 46
  hunger, 97-98, 103, 106
  interest, 82-83, 121, 169-80
  love and hate, 199-215
  passive, 75
  rumor, 313-26
  sexuality, 59, 63, 156, 199, 204, 230, 313, 318-19
  social service, 281-82

theory, 26-30, 95-109
traits as, 132, 137-51
unconscious, 120
unhealthy, 106
values, 107
will, 60
Motor mimicry, 183
Motor psychology, 181-86
Movement in case work, 275
Multivariate scales, 119-20

National character, 24, 186, 356
Nationalism, 174-75, 328-30, 341, 345
Natural science, 42, 196
Naturalism, v, 157-60, 169
Needs, 58, 120
Negro, 173, 206, 208, 211, 228-29, 232, 239, 241, 243-44, 246-47, 253-54, 261, 263, 265, 316-19, 340, 355
Neo-Freudianism, 29
Neurosis, 62, 99, 119, 163, 173, 285
New Deal, 80-81, 272, 316
Nomothetic, 20, 26-27, 52, 147-48
Non-directive therapy, 29, 138, 184
Norm, 155-56, 158
Normal distribution, 156, 163
Normality, 105, 123, 145, 155-68, 275

Office of War Information, 311-12
Olympic games, 177
Operationism, 24
Oral aggression, 205

Pain, 305
Parataxic dyad, 282
Participation, 181-98
Peace, 63, 334, 342, 362
Pearl Harbor, 311
Pelagians, 259
Perception, 39, 114-15, 162, 295-309
Person-centered, 17-19, 26, 272
Person perception, 39, 114-15
Personal cluster analysis, 126
Personal constructs, 121, 125
Personal Security Scale, 303
Personalism, 17-38
Personality:
    and culture, 5, 21-22, 48

basic, 22
consistency of, 8-12, 52, 78
criteria for theory, 20-38
definitions, v, 21, 27, 36, 145-46
democratic, 195
growth in, 159, 165-66, 275-77, 284, 352
health, 155-168
idiographic approach, 12, 30, 125, 146-47, 149
integumented, 20-24, 47
levels, 50
literary approach, 3-15
mature, 155-68, 211
modal, 22
normal vs. abnormal, 105, 123, 145, 155-68, 275
structure, 108, 111-29
system, 24, 39-54
tests, 30
theory, 17, 26, 28-30, 45
trait theory, 31-33, 111-29, 131-35
uniqueness, 31, 145
units of, 32-33, 111-29
Phenomenology, 46, 60, 228-29
Philanthropy, 271-92
Philosophy, 5, 17-38, 162-67, 169-81, 203-5, 219-20, 272, 277
Philosophy of life, 162, 339
Phylogenetic model, 57-68, 142
Physical science, 3, 10, 42, 55-56, 147
Police, 253
Positivism, 24-25, 43, 72
Praise, 83
Preferred patterns, 107
Prejudice, 173-78, 188, 202, 206-15, 219-34, 237-55, 257-66, 274, 331, 358
Proaction, 41, 44, 46, 50, 52
Proception, 79-82, 295, 301-9
Professionalism, 274, 281-84
Projection, 282, 314
Projective methods, 95-109, 116-17
Propaganda, 249-50, 336, 338, 357, 362
Propriate, 51
Psychoanalysis, 13, 27-29, 44, 46, 60, 72-73, 75, 102-3, 106, 251-52, 285-86
Psychic surface, 96

Psychodiagnostic methods, 95-109
Psychodrama, 247
Psychodynamics, 101-2, 229
Psycholinguistics, 40-41, 64-65
Public health, 295-309
Public service, 55-56, 90; see also Social policy
Public vs. private, 277-81, 290

Quaker, 262, 356

Race differences, 225-27, 243-44, 362
Race relations. See Prejudice
Radix, 9
Reactive, 41, 44, 188-96
Recentering, 238
Reciprocity, 175, 265
Reinforcement, 50-51, 58, 84, 201
Religion, 45, 47, 104, 140, 194, 202, 204-5, 219, 222-24, 251, 257-66, 276, 347
REP Test, 126
Research:
  basic, 347, 360
  design, 239
  evaluative, 237-55, 272-77
  in affiliation, 178-79
  international, 347-62
  on race, 226
Resolution of conflict, 169-80
Revelation, 258-59
Reward. See Reinforcement
Rights and duties, 280
Rival, 177, 212, 215, 247
Role, 22, 47-48, 116, 247-49
Role Construct Repertory (REP) Test, 126
Rorschach Test, 97, 100, 116, 120
Rumor, 311-26

St. Bartholomew's Eve, 260
Scapegoating, 188, 193, 262, 319, 331; see also Witchcraft
Schemata, 121
Secularism, 347
Security, 264, 303, 344, 353, 360
Segregation, 172, 225, 229, 231, 241, 246, 265
Self (see also Ego):
  actualization, 46, 91, 166

confrontation, 9
control, 158
definition, 35
esteem, 34, 74-75, 145, 171, 199, 202, 211, 215
factotum, 33
hierarchy, 26
image, 29, 34, 62, 160-1
in illness, 298
insight, 34-35, 164, 252
interest, 224, 264, 360
judgment, 80, 85
Jung, 46
love, 207
objectification, 162
phenomenology of, 34
psychology, 183
regard, 46, 87
Selves, multiple, 115-16
Sensory deprivation, 307
Sexuality, 59, 63, 156, 199, 204, 230, 313, 318-19
Sharpening in rumor, 314-15, 320-25
Signs, 64
Situationism, 114-17, 134
Sleeper effect, 240, 250
Social:
  diagnosis, 283-84
  engineering, 349, 352, 358-59
  Ethics Department (Harvard), 271
  policy, 169-80, 181-98, 214, 226-34, 237-55, 271-92, 347-62
  service, 271-92
  structure, 23, 48, 191-92, 289, 342-45
Socius, 82
Soul, 71-80, 90, 196
Soundness of personality, 155-68
South Africa, Union of, 173, 219-20, 228, 233, 258, 305
Specialism, 282-83
Stereotype, 221, 224, 253, 337-38
Structure of personality, 107, 111-29
Study of Values Test, 101, 121
Survival norm, 159-60, 177
Symbiosis, 204-5
Symbols, 64-65, 335, 354, 358-59, 362
Syndrome, 123
System theory, 39-54
Systematic relevance, 9

Task-involvement, 187-91
Technology, 57, 155, 195, 347-49
Temperament, 111, 120
Tension reduction, 44, 61, 96, 107, 160
Thematic Apperception Test, 100
Themes, college, 10-11
Theocracy, 223, 259, 263
Theology, 200, 258-60
Theories of personality, 17, 26, 28-30, 40, 45, 52, 59, 95-96
Thomism, 221, 277
Thumbsucking, 61-62
Tinsit, 115
Traces, 26, 80, 114
Traits:
    common, 135, 148-49
    concept of, 8, 13, 131-35
    dynamic, 132
    expressive, 121
    general *vs.* specific, 78, 132
    independence of, 133
    individual, 108, 135, 148-49
    measures of, 116, 133
    motives, 132, 137-51
    primary, 123
    source, 122
    stylistic, 121
    surface, 122
    theory of, 31-33, 111-29
    variability, 115-17

Transactionalism, 47-49
Transistasis, 160
Trends, 111, 117, 126

Unconscious, 95-109, 120, 165
UNESCO, 327, 335, 345-46, 348
Uniqueness, 31, 111, 123-28, 131-35, 145-49
Unitarian Service Committee, 265
United Nations, 175, 233-34, 346, 348-49, 351, 355, 359
Units of personality, 111-29, 131-35
Utopias, 170

V–J Day, 311
Values, 32-33, 107, 155, 181, 222-24
Vicarious approach, 245-47
Voting, 190-91

Walden, 271
War, 226, 329-46
Whorfian hypothesis, 40
Witchcraft, 221, 229, 306
Woodworth Personal Data, 119, 121
Work Service camps, 334
World Health Organization, 345
Würzburg School, 183

Xenophobia, 358, 362

Zululand, 305-6

$$25.25$$
$$1.18$$
$$2\overline{)2.36}$$

$$26.43$$
$$33.61$$